CARDIOVASCULAR MRI AND MRA

CARDIOVASCULAR MRI AND MRA

CHARLES B. HIGGINS, MD

Professor
Department of Radiology
University of California San Francisco
San Francisco, California

ALBERT DE ROOS, MD

Professor and Vice Chairman
Department of Radiology
Leiden University Medical Center
Leiden, The Netherlands

With Contributions by 51 Authors

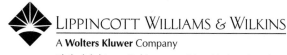

LIPPINCOTT WILLIAMS & WILKINS
A **Wolters Kluwer** Company
Philadelphia • Baltimore • New York • London
Buenos Aires • Hong Kong • Sydney • Tokyo

Acquisitions Editor: Joyce-Rachel John
Developmental Editor: Delois Patterson
Manufacturing Manager: Colin Warnock
Production Editor: Timothy Prairie
Cover Designer: Christine Jenny
Compositor: Maryland Composition
Printer: Maple Press

Printed in the United States of America
9 8 7 6 5 4 3 2 1

Library of Congress Cataloging-in-Publication Data

Cardiovascular MRI and MRA / [edited by] Charles B. Higgins, Albert de Roos.
    p. ; cm.
  Includes bibliographical references and index.
  ISBN 0-7817-3482-7 (hardcover : alk. paper)
    1. Cardiovascular system—Magnetic resonance imaging. 2. Cardiovascular
system—Diseases—Diagnosis. I. Higgins, Charles B. II. Roos, Albert de, 1953–
    [DNLM: 1. Heart Diseases—diagnosis. 2. Magnetic Resonance Angiography. 3.
  Magnetic Resonance Imaging. 4. Vascular Diseases—diagnosis. WG 210 C2685 2002]
  RC670.5.M33 C375 2002
  616.1′07548—dc21

                                                                    2002072995

*To our residents and fellows
whose work has contributed to
progress in cardiovascular
MRI and MRA*

CONTENTS

CONTRIBUTING AUTHORS

Haydar Akbari, MD   Research Fellow, Department of Radiology, University of California San Francisco, San Francisco, California

Charles M. Anderson, MD, PhD   Associate Professor, Department of Radiology, University of California San Francisco; Chief of MRI, Department of Radiology, San Francisco VA Medical Center, San Francisco, California

Philip A. Araoz, MD   Clinical Instructor, Department of Radiology, University of California San Francisco, San Francisco, California

Frank M. Baer, MD, PhD   Associate Professor, Klinik III für Innere Medizin, Universität zu Köln, Köln, Germany

W. L. F. Bedaux, MD   Research Fellow, Department of Cardiology, Vrije Universiteit Medical Center, Amsterdam, The Netherlands

René M. Botnar, PhD   Visiting Scientist, Cardiovascular Division, Harvard Medical School; Senior Scientist, Cardiovascular Division, Beth Israel Deaconess Medical Center, Boston, Massachusetts

Lawrence M. Boxt, MD   Professor of Clinical Radiology, Department of Radiology, Albert Einstein College of Medicine; Chief of Cardiovascular Imaging, Department of Radiology, Beth Israel Medical Center, New York, New York

Arno Bücker, MD   Associate Professor, Department of Diagnostic Radiology, University Clinic Aachen, Aachen, Germany

Shalini G. Chabra, MD   Research Fellow, Department of Radiology, Weill Medical College of Cornell University; Resident, Department of Internal Medicine, Metropolitan Hospital, New York, New York

Graham R. Cherryman, FRCR   Professor, Department of Radiology, University of Leicester; Honorary Consultant and Clinical Director, Department of Radiology, University Hospitals of Leicester, Leicester, United Kingdom

Kelly M. Choi, MD   Cardiology Fellow, Department of Medicine/Cardiology, Duke University; Cardiology Fellow, Duke Cardiovascular Magnetic Resonance Center, Duke University Medical Center, Durham, North Carolina

Jozo Crnac, MD   Abteilung für Kardiologie, Sankt Katharinen Hospital Frechen, Frechen, Germany

Jörg F. Debatin, MD, MBA   Professor and Chairman, Department of Diagnostic and Interventional Radiology, University Hospital Essen, Essen, Germany

Albert de Roos, MD   Professor and Vice Chairman, Department of Radiology, Leiden University Medical Center, Leiden, The Netherlands

Martijn S. Dirksen, MD   PhD Research Student, Department of Radiology, Leiden University Medical Center, Leiden, The Netherlands

Qian Dong, MD   Researcher, Department of Radiology, University of Michigan, Ann Arbor, Michigan

Joost Doornbos, PhD   Scientist, Department of Radiology, Leiden University Medical Center, Leiden, The Netherlands

Rossella Fattori, MD   Assistant Professor and Chief, Cardiovascular Unit, Department of Radiology, S. Orsola University Hospital, Bologna, Italy

Zahi A. Fayad, PhD   Associate Professor, Departments of Radiology and Medicine (Cardiology), Mount Sinai School of Medicine; Director, Cardiovascular Imaging Research, The Zena and Michael A Weiner Cardiovascular Institute, Mount Sinai Medical Center, New York, New York

Mathias Goyen, MD   Assistant Professor, Department of Diagnostic and Interventional Radiology, University Hospital Essen, Essen, Germany

Willem A. Helbing, MD, PhD   Professor and Head, Division of Pediatric Cardiology, Department of Pediatrics, Erasmus MC-Sophia Children's Hospital, Rotterdam, The Netherlands

Charles B. Higgins, MD   Professor, Department of Radiology, University of California San Francisco, San Francisco, California

Robert M. Judd, PhD   Associate Professor, Department of Medicine, Duke University Medical Center, Durham, North Carolina

J. Wouter Jukema, MD, PhD, FESC, FACC   Associate Professor of Cardiology, Head, Interventional Cardiology, Department of Cardiology, Leiden University Medical Center, Leiden, The Netherlands

Philip J. Kilner, MD, PhD   Consultant, Cardiovascular Magnetic Resonance Unit, Royal Brompton Hospital, London, United Kingdom

Raymond J. Kim, MD   Associate Professor, Department of Medicine (Cardiology), Duke University; Clinical Director, Duke Cardiovascular Magnetic Resonance Center, Duke University Medical Center, Durham, North Carolina

Kraig V. Kissinger, BS, RT (R) (MR)   Senior Cardiac MR Technologist, Cardiac MR Center, Beth Israel Deaconess Medical Center, Boston, Massachusetts

Gabriele A. Krombach, MD   Department of Radiology, University of Technology (RWTH-Aachen), Aachen, Germany

Hildo J. Lamb, PhD   Senior Scientist, Department of Radiology, Leiden University Medical Center, Leiden, The Netherlands

Warren J. Manning, MD   Associate Professor of Medicine and Radiology, Harvard Medical School; Section Chief, Non-invasive Cardiac Imaging, Cardiovascular Division, Beth Israel Deaconess Medical Center, Boston, Massachusetts

Eike Nagel, MD   Director of Cardiovascular Magnetic Resonance, Department of Cardiology, German Heart Institute, Berlin, Germany

Johannes C. Post, MD, PhD   Resident, Department of Cardiology, Vrije Universiteit Medical Center, Amsterdam, The Netherlands

Martin R. Prince, MD, PhD   Professor of Radiology, Department of Radiology, Weill Medical College of Cornell University; Chief of MRI, Department of Radiology, New York Presbyterian Hospital, New York, New York

Frank Rademakers, MD   Professor, Department of Cardiology, Catholic University Leuven; Department of Cardiology/Non-invasive Imaging, University Hospital Gasthuisberg, Leuven, Belgium

Gautham P. Reddy, MD, MPH   Assistant Professor of Radiology, Associate Director of Residency Program, Department of Radiology, University of California San Francisco, San Francisco, California

Johan H. C. Reiber, PhD   Professor of Medical Imaging, Department of Radiology, Division of Image Processing, Leiden University Medical Center, Leiden, The Netherlands

Arno A. W. Roest, PhD   Research Fellow, Department of Pediatric Cardiology, Leiden University Medical Center, Leiden, The Netherlands

Anna Rozenshtein, MD   Assistant Professor of Clinical Radiology, Department of Radiology, College of Physicians and Surgeons of Columbia University; Attending Radiologist, Department of Radiology, St. Luke's-Roosevelt Hospital Center, New York, New York

Stefan G. Ruehm, MD   Associate Professor, Department of Diagnostic and Interventional Radiology, University Hospital Essen, Essen, Germany

Maythem Saeed, DVM, PhD   Professor, Department of Radiology, University of California San Francisco, San Francisco, California

Hajime Sakuma, MD   Associate Professor, Department of Radiology, Mie University Hospital, Tsu, Mie, Japan

David Saloner, PhD   Professor, Department of Radiology, University of California San Francisco; Director, Vascular Imaging Research Center, San Francisco VA Medical Center, San Francisco, California

Matthias Schmidt, MD   Oberarzt, Klinik und Poliklinik für Nuklearmedizin, Universität zu Köln, Köln, Germany

Penelope R. Sensky, MRCP   Specialist Registrar, Department of Cardiology, Glenfield Hospital, Leicester, United Kingdom

Lars Søndergaard   Department of Cardiology, Rigshospitalet, Copenhagen, Denmark

Freddy Ståhlberg   Professor, Department of Radiation Physics, The Jubileum Institute, Lund University Hospital, Lund, Sweden

Matthias Stuber, PhD   Visiting Scientist, Cardiovascular Division/Cardiac MRI, Harvard Medical School, Boston, Massachusetts

Carsten Thomsen   Department of Radiology, Rigshospitalet, Copenhagen, Denmark

Rob J. van der Geest, MSc   Assistant Professor, Department of Radiology, Division of Image Processing, Leiden University Medical Center, Leiden, The Netherlands

Ernst E. van der Wall, MD   Department of Cardiology, Leiden University Medical Center, Leiden, The Netherlands

Albert C. van Rossum, MD, PhD   Professor and Head of Outpatient Clinic, Department of Cardiology, Vrije Universiteit Medical Center, Amsterdam, The Netherlands

Martin N. Wasser, MD   Radiologist, Department of Radiology, Leiden University Medical Center, Leiden, The Netherlands

Norbert Watzinger, MD   Assistant Professor, Department of Medicine, University of Graz, Graz, Austria

PREFACE

Magnetic resonance imaging (MRI) is a mature imaging modality for nearly all regions of the body. Cardiovascular MRI remained, however, immature and unfamiliar even after two decades of evolution. The first MR images of the human heart were produced around 1982. Now, twenty years later, many diagnosticians of cardiac and vascular diseases still are not fully cognizant of the extensive capabilities of this modality. Developments during the past five years, including improved MR gradient systems and new imaging sequences, have provided new and more practical MR techniques for the evaluation and precise quantification of cardiovascular morphology and physiology.

Our goal in writing this book was to provide updated information on the use of MRI and MRA for the evaluation of both cardiac and vascular diseases. Recognizing that the technology involved in cardiovascular MRI continues to change, we embarked upon a schedule for writing this book that spanned less than a year from conception to completion of the manuscript.

The book consists of five parts. The first part contains information about the technology and scientific basis for clinical applications. The second, third, and fourth parts describe the applications in specific cardiac diseases. Appropriately, the nine chapters that make up Part III focus on the multifaceted role of MRI in ischemic heart disease. The fifth part addresses the numerous uses of MRA for the assessment of vascular diseases.

The authors include basic scientists, cardiologists, and radiologists from around the world. These experts have had a long involvement in fostering the development of cardiovascular MRI and MRA.

Charles B. Higgins, MD
Albert de Roos, MD

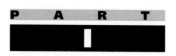

BASIC PRINCIPLES

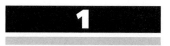

CLINICAL APPROACH TO CARDIOVASCULAR MRI TECHNIQUES

HILDO J. LAMB
JOOST DOORNBOS

The techniques used in cardiovascular MRI continue to change rapidly, and cardiovascular MRI is currently in an exciting and crucial phase of its final clinical acceptance. The main technical limitations have now been overcome by the development of improved scanner hardware, software, and image-processing tools. In this chapter, basic and advanced techniques of cardiovascular MRI are discussed in the context of their clinical application. The discussion is based on a virtual patient examination, with a focus on techniques used in the functional evaluation of heart disease. MRI techniques for perfusion imaging, visualization of delayed enhancement, coronary artery MRA, and vessel wall imaging are discussed in greater detail in other chapters and are only briefly mentioned here.

COILS

Clinical cardiac examinations can be performed with the standard body coil, although image quality is suboptimal. The main problem is the limited in-plane spatial resolution, which is about 3 mm^2. A high degree of spatial resolution is

especially important for an accurate assessment of abnormalities of wall motion caused by, for example, myocardial infarction. In the past, reliable images were obtained with the body coil in the assessment of global and regional myocardial wall motion (Fig. 1.1). For an imaging center that is particularly interested in cardiovascular MRI, a surface coil is a worthwhile investment, such as a single circular coil with a diameter of approximately 14 cm; with this type of coil, image quality and spatial resolution are improved substantially. The best alternative is a dedicated cardiac phased-array coil constructed of multiple elements. This type of coil is now commercially available from most manufacturers of scanners (Fig. 1.1). The main advantages are that it further improves image quality and spatial resolution and provides a larger field of view. An additional advantage is that phased-array coils make it possible to apply the sensitivity encoding (SENSE) imaging technique (1). SENSE, which is based on parallel imaging with use of all the coil elements, represents a revolutionizing technology in cardiovascular MRI. Each coil has a different sensitivity profile; this feature can be exploited to reduce the density of the acquired k-space data and thereby accelerate scan time. With the use of SENSE, a twofold increase in imaging speed can currently be obtained, but in an experimental setting, up to fourfold increases were achieved. In general, SENSE is believed to

H. J. Lamb and J. Doornbos: Department of Radiology, Leiden University Medical Center, Leiden, The Netherlands.

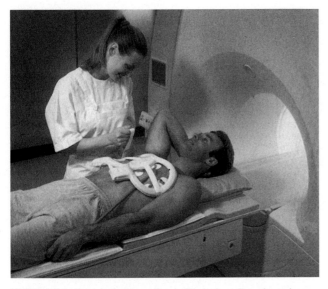

FIGURE 1.1. Practical setup of a dedicated cardiac phased-array coil and vector electrocardiogram. The standard body coil is integrated with the magnet bore. (Courtesy of Philips Medical Systems, Best, The Netherlands.)

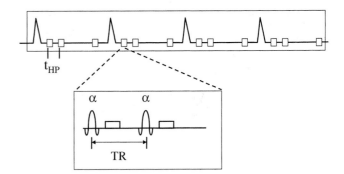

FIGURE 1.3. Schematic diagram of the basic principle of a turbofield echo (TFE) MRI sequence in relation to timing within the cardiac cycle. After each radiofrequency (rf) excitation pulse (α), one line in k-space is acquired, which is repeated two times in this case (turbo factor 2), so that a total of 2 k-lines are acquired per heart phase image segment per cardiac cycle *(enlarged detail)*. In total, four heart beats are shown, resulting in an image of 8 k-lines. If an image of 120 k-lines is required, the procedure must be repeated 15 times, for a total of 60 heart beats. At a heart rate of 60 beats/min, the acquisition can be completed during continuous breathing within 60 seconds. *White squares* indicate heart phase image segments; t_{HP}, time between each heart phase (temporal resolution); TR, repetition time between rf excitations.

have contributed significantly to the clinical acceptance of cardiovascular MRI because it reduces MRI scan time, making it comparable with that of ultrasonographic or computed tomographic examination.

CARDIAC MOTION COMPENSATION

Cardiac motion compensation is accomplished by synchronizing image acquisition with the electrocardiographic (ECG) signal. Image formation in MRI is based on filling "k-space" during data acquisition (see the appendix at the end of this chapter); this concept is not explained further here because many thorough and comprehensive articles on the topic have been published (2–6). ECG triggering is aimed at filling k-space in multiple steps, based on timing within the cardiac cycle (Figs. 1.2 to 1.6). For example, to construct a movie of a cardiac slice, approximately 20 cardiac phases (time frames) are needed to obtain sufficient temporal resolution. In general, a temporal resolution of less than 40 milliseconds per cardiac phase image is needed to enable selection of the end-systolic time frame and calculate,

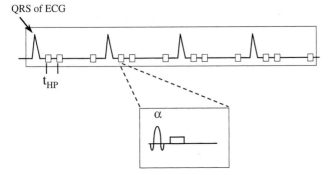

FIGURE 1.2. Schematic diagram of the basic principle of a gradient-echo, or fast-field echo (FFE), MRI sequence in relation to timing within the cardiac cycle. After each radiofrequency (rf) excitation pulse (α), one line in k-space is acquired *(enlarged detail)*. In total, four heart beats are shown, resulting in an image of 4 k-lines. If an image of 120 k-lines is required, the procedure must be repeated 30 times, for a total of 120 heart beats. At a heart rate of 60 beats/min, the acquisition can be completed during continuous breathing within 2 minutes. *White squares* indicate heart phase image segments; t_{HP}, time between each heart phase (temporal resolution).

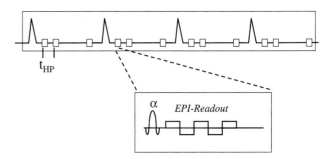

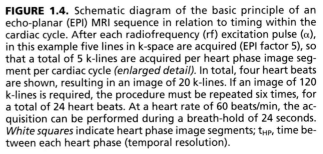

FIGURE 1.4. Schematic diagram of the basic principle of an echo-planar (EPI) MRI sequence in relation to timing within the cardiac cycle. After each radiofrequency (rf) excitation pulse (α), in this example five lines in k-space are acquired (EPI factor 5), so that a total of 5 k-lines are acquired per heart phase image segment per cardiac cycle *(enlarged detail)*. In total, four heart beats are shown, resulting in an image of 20 k-lines. If an image of 120 k-lines is required, the procedure must be repeated six times, for a total of 24 heart beats. At a heart rate of 60 beats/min, the acquisition can be performed during a breath-hold of 24 seconds. *White squares* indicate heart phase image segments; t_{HP}, time between each heart phase (temporal resolution).

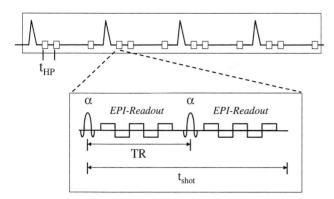

FIGURE 1.5. Schematic diagram of the basic principle of a turbo-field echo-planar (TFEPI) MRI sequence in relation to timing within the cardiac cycle. After each radiofrequency (rf) excitation pulse (α), in this case five lines in k-space are acquired (EPI factor 5), which is repeated two times per shot (turbo factor 2), so that a total of 10 k-lines are acquired per heart phase image segment per cardiac cycle *(enlarged detail)*. In total, four heart beats are shown, resulting in an image of 40 k-lines. If an image of 120 k-lines is required, the procedure must be repeated three times, for a total of 12 heart beats. At a heart rate of 60 beats/min, the acquisition can be performed during a breath-hold of 12 seconds. *White squares* indicate heart phase image segments; t_{HP}, time between each heart phase (temporal resolution); TR, repetition time; t_{shot}, shot duration.

for example, the end-systolic volume or ejection fraction. These 20 cardiac images per slice cannot be obtained at once. Therefore, ECG triggering was developed to synchronize partial k-space filling with the cardiac cycle. Suppose we need 128 k-lines for the first cardiac phase image but can acquire only 12 k-lines for the image per heart beat, so that

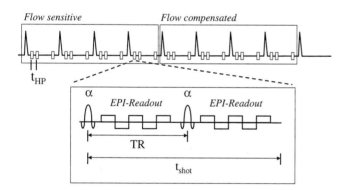

FIGURE 1.6. Schematic diagram of the basic principle of a turbo-field echo-planar (TFEPI) MRI flow sequence in relation to timing within the cardiac cycle. After each radiofrequency (rf) excitation pulse (α), in this case five lines in k-space are acquired (EPI factor 5), which is repeated two times per shot (turbo factor 2), so that a total of 10 k-lines are acquired per heart phase image segment per cardiac cycle *(enlarged detail)*. In total, four heart beats are shown for the flow-sensitive image, in addition to four heart beats for the flow-compensated image, resulting in images of 40 k-lines for each image type. If 120 k-lines are required for images with a sufficiently high degree of spatial resolution, the procedure must be repeated three times, for a total of 24 heart beats. At a heart rate of 60 beats/min, the acquisition can be performed during a breath-hold of 24 seconds. *White squares* indicate heart phase image segments; t_{HP}, time between each heart phase (temporal resolution); TR, repetition time; t_{shot}, shot duration.

11 heart beats are needed to complete k-space filling for the image. A breath-hold of approximately 11 seconds would be required at a heart rate of 60 beats/min. Of course, all 20 cardiac phases are acquired at once, so that within 11 seconds, a full movie of a cardiac slice can be obtained.

Currently, two ECG triggering methods are available. The first is prospective triggering, in which image acquisition starts immediately after the QRS complex of the ECG and stops after about 80% of the cardiac cycle has elapsed; consequently, the 20 cardiac phases are distributed over this 80% of the cycle, and the last 20% of the cardiac cycle is not imaged. This technique is suitable for imaging systolic heart function. When one is interested in the last part of the cardiac cycle for an evaluation of diastolic heart function, a different method can be applied. In retrospective ECG gating, image data are acquired irrespective of the ECG, and the ECG is recorded in parallel. Once the MRI acquisition is finished, the computer retrospectively calculates the appropriate cardiac phases based on the stored ECG and k-space data. In this way, the last part of the cardiac cycle can also be imaged. This technique has been applied clinically, mostly in conjunction with MR flow mapping (see below), because it allows an estimation of, for example, the diastolic filling pattern or regurgitation volume in a patient with mitral valve insufficiency. Recently, retrospective gating became available in combination with faster scan techniques, such as echo-planar imaging and fast balanced gradient-echo acquisitions (see below), so the standard nowadays is retrospective ECG triggering for most cardiovascular MRI purposes.

A major problem in the clinical application of cardiovascular MRI is the practical worry of obtaining a reliable ECG signal from a patient inside an MRI scanner. In about 2% to 5% of clinical cases, no reliable ECG signal can be obtained. The electric ECG signal is distorted by the interaction of the magnetic field and the pulsating blood flow through the aortic arch (magnetohemodynamic effect). Recently, a new approach was launched to correct for this problem. The vector ECG is based on the three-dimensional orientation of the QRS complex and T wave of the ECG and the distorting component (7). Thus, the MRI acquisition is triggered by the QRS complex only, and not mistakenly by the T wave or ECG distortions or by signal induced by gradient switching. The vector ECG, in conjunction with the dedicated cardiac synergy surface coil and SENSE, has revolutionized the clinical application of cardiovascular MRI. Today, the only practical limitations to cardiovascular MRI are the conventional MRI exclusion criteria, such as the presence of implanted metal objects or pregnancy.

RESPIRATORY MOTION COMPENSATION

A second source of image distortion is respiratory motion. A decade ago, MRI acquisitions were so time-consuming that it was impossible to perform breath-hold imaging. At that time, an inventive technique was introduced that was called *respiratory-ordered phase encoding* (ROPE) (8) or *phase-encoding artifact reduction* (PEAR). It was based on a special k-line reordering technique combined with a respiratory tracking device placed around the patient's abdomen. When k-lines acquired during breathing were positioned in the periphery of k-space (this part of k-space is less sensitive to motion), breathing artifacts were decreased. With this type of artifact reduction, image quality was improved, but not yet optimal.

After the development of faster MRI techniques, such as echo-planar imaging and turbo-field echo imaging, it became possible to acquire image data during a short breath-hold of about 15 seconds. The general disadvantage of breath-hold acquisitions is that the reproducibility of the breath-hold level is quite low. In a multislice, multiple breath-hold acquisition, errors may be introduced, for example, into the summed end-diastolic volumes of different slices acquired during different breath-holds. If the patient is not properly instructed, the measurements may be highly variable, or, even worse, the clinical data may be inaccurate. Therefore, when breath-hold acquisitions are being obtained, it is necessary to instruct patients carefully to hold their breath in expiration; doing so minimizes the problem of breath-hold level reproducibility.

With some high-resolution MRI acquisitions, longer acquisition times are required than can be obtained during a breath-hold. For example, coronary artery MRA can be performed during a short breath-hold, but optimal quality can be achieved only by using the respiratory navigator technique (9,10). Respiratory navigation is based on a one-dimensional image positioned at the interface between lung and liver, so that the motion of the diaphragm can be tracked. Usually,

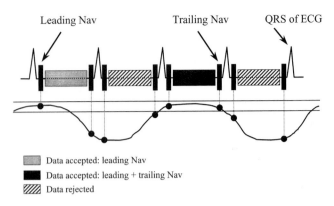

FIGURE 1.8. The MRI acquisition is gated to a predefined acceptance window *(two solid horizontal lines)* based on the traced respiratory signal *(curved solid line)* around end-expiration. The k-space data are acquired continuously, but only data are stored that fulfill the requirement that (a) before data acquisition, the navigator was within the acceptance window (leading navigator); or (b) before and after data acquisition, the navigator was within the acceptance window (leading and trailing navigator). Other acquired image data are deleted. This is the principle of a real-time prospective respiratory navigator.

the navigator beam is positioned on the right hemidiaphragm (Fig. 1.7) and its 1D image is acquired before and after every MRI data acquisition block (Fig. 1.8), with an acquisition duration of only 30 milliseconds. The acquisition is then gated to the automatically traced breathing signal derived from the respiratory navigator. A window around the end-expiration position of the diaphragm is defined by determining the positions in which MRI data are accepted. For example, a 3-mm acceptance window means that in end-expiration, a variation of less than 3 mm in diaphragm position is accepted. Respiratory navigators can also be used for slice

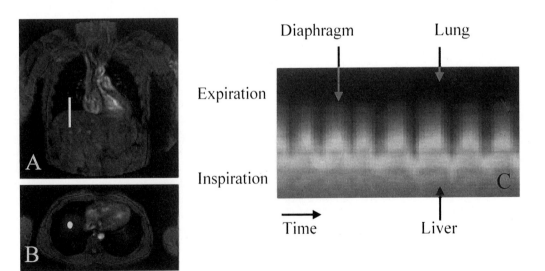

FIGURE 1.7. The respiratory navigator pencil beam (A, *white line*; B, *white dot*) is positioned on the right hemidiaphragm at the interface between lung and liver, based on a survey image in the coronal **(A)** and sagittal **(B)** planes. The one-dimensional navigator image is acquired repeatedly over time to construct an image of diaphragmatic motion **(C)**. The edge between lung and liver is traced automatically to yield a breathing curve similar to that represented in the diagram of Figure 1.8.

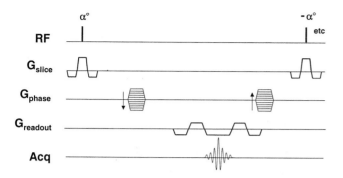

FIGURE 1.9. Balanced fast-field echo (FFE) pulse sequences belong to the group of steady-state free-precession techniques. Time-balanced gradients are applied for all gradient directions: slice selection, phase encoding, and frequency readout. In combination with the alternating phase of the excitation pulse, this enables acquisition of both free induction decay and echo signals. The sequence produces a high degree of image intensity for tissues with a high T2-to-T1 ratio independently of the repetition time (TR). Balanced FFE images are obtained after field shimming because field homogeneity is very important.

lowing an evaluation only of changes in ventricular volume and some rough estimation of wall motion abnormalities. In the future, a combination of ultrafast acquisition schemes with SENSE may allow higher-resolution imaging.

Another promising development is real-time imaging of the heart. Real-time cardiac imaging was introduced in the early days of MRI (12). More recently, data have been presented showing full ventricular coverage in real time without the need for ECG triggering or breath holding (13,14). Ventricular function has been accurately quantified in these preliminary studies. In combination with future real-time image analysis, this technique may revolutionize the applications of cardiac MRI.

SURVEY

The first step in a cardiovascular MRI examination is the acquisition of a localizer to determine the general anatomy, which forms the basis for further acquisitions. The purpose of the first scan is to image the cardiac region in the three basic orientations—the coronal, transverse, and sagittal planes. Fifteen 10-mm slices are obtained for each orientation. A decade ago, such "scout" images were obtained by using a multislice spin-echo technique, sometimes in combination with turbo spin echo. This technique can still be used if your local MR scanner does not support faster imaging techniques. A faster method for acquiring survey images is, for example, a turbo-field echo or turbo-field echo-planar MRI sequence.

Recently, balanced gradient-echo [balanced fast-field echo (FFE), true fast imaging with steady precession (FISP)] techniques have become available, yielding images that provide a high degree of contrast between blood and myocardium (Figs. 1.9 and 1.10). Survey images can be acquired during continuous breathing, with use of the respiratory navigator, or during a breath-hold. Currently, excellent images can be obtained by using balanced FFE with continuous breathing; the acquisition time is only 15 seconds.

tracking, in which the slice position is adjusted according to breathing changes detected by the navigator. In this way, the acquisition is not gated to a certain predefined acceptance window; rather, all scanned data are acquired. The combination of these two techniques currently appears to be the best solution. Within an acceptance window of, say, 3 mm, the remaining respiratory motion is compensated for by using the tracking technique. Good results of coronary MRA have been obtained with this technique (11).

Very recent technical advances have made it possible to acquire a stack of 12 slices, each comprising about 25 cardiac phases, in a single breath-hold of up to 20 seconds. These ultrafast techniques combine turbo-field echo, echo-planar, and spiral k-space acquisition. Their primary application is in the assessment of cardiac function; the single breath-hold eliminates the previously mentioned problem of slice level reproducibility in multiple breath-hold approaches. However, the spatial resolution of this technique is still quite low, al-

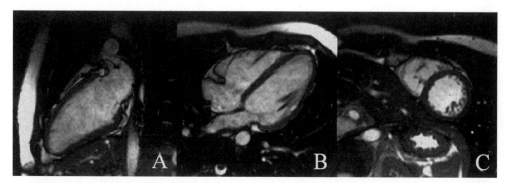

FIGURE 1.10. Example of balanced fast-field echo (FFE) images acquired in the two-chamber view **(A)**, four-chamber view **(B)**, and short-axis view **(C)**. Each image consists of 25 cardiac time frames, which were acquired during a breath-hold of 12 seconds for each view. Images are shown in the end-diastolic time frame. Note the excellent contrast between blood and myocardium, in comparison with the echo-planar images in the other figures of this chapter.

PLANSCAN

Based on the survey images, further MRI scans can be planned. Planning can be performed manually with the planning tools available in the standard scanner software. Since the beginning of the new millennium, it has been possible to carry out planning in real time, even in combination with balanced FFE. With a real-time planning tool, changes made manually in the imaging plane are immediately executed by the free-running MRI acquisition. In this way, the optimal imaging plane can be found within seconds. Once the desired imaging plane has been reached, the geometry settings can be stored for later use during the cardiovascular examination. The time efficiency is increased substantially with use of the real-time planning tool, allowing routine application of cardiovascular MRI.

Another approach is to use survey images as input for an algorithm that plans the desired imaging planes automatically (15). The software finds the position of the heart in the survey images automatically and uses this information to plan other acquisitions. This operator-independent automatic planscan method reliably quantifies, for example, end-diastolic volume or ejection fraction and reduces inter-examination variability substantially. Therefore, this method is eminently suitable in patient follow-up to evaluate the therapeutic effects of, say, antihypertensive or lipid-lowering drugs. However, the automatic planscan procedure is currently available only off-line as a research tool, and the time efficiency of the real-time planning alternative appears to be greater.

ANATOMY

Today, the most frequent indication for a clinical referral to undergo MRI is congenital heart disease. The primary interest of the referring physician is usually the global cardiovascular anatomy. The purpose of these MRI scans is to image the heart in three dimensions, so that complex con-

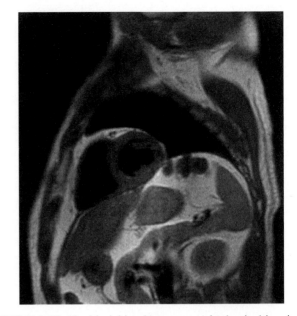

FIGURE 1.12. The black blood image was obtained with a dual-inversion fast spin-echo technique in combination with SENSE (SENSitivity Encoding) (factor 2). Echo spacing, 4.3 milliseconds; field of view, 350 x 350 mm; matrix, 192 × 146; slice thickness, 8 mm. Scan time was 6 seconds. (Courtesy of Philips Medical Systems, Best, The Netherlands.)

genital cardiac deformations can be diagnosed and followed over time to plan surgical correction of the anomalies. In the past, the time-consuming (turbo) spin echo was the technique of choice. Its major disadvantage was that the presence of major breathing artifacts hampered reliable evaluation of the cardiac anatomy.

Nowadays, several alternatives are available. The latest is a multiple breath-hold dual-inversion black blood turbo spin-echo technique (Figs. 1.11 and 1.12), which yields images of excellent quality (16). A disadvantage of this approach is that each slice must be imaged during a separate breath-hold, with again the risk for low breath-hold level reproducibility. The expectation is that in the future this technique will be further optimized, perhaps by combining it

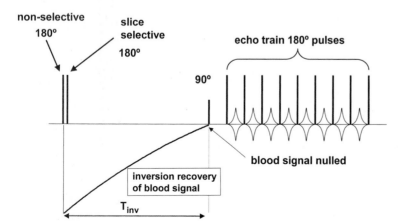

FIGURE 1.11. Schematic diagram of a black blood pulse sequence. A nonselective 180-degree pulse inverts all signals. Subsequently, a slice-selective 180-degree pulse resets the signal of the studied slice. Blood with an inverted signal flows into the slice plane. After a delay (T_{inv}, inversion time), the blood signal is nulled, and data acquisition is performed with a fast spin-echo pulse train. The image is obtained in a breath-hold. Note that the inversion time depends on the heart rate.

with SENSE, so that single breath-hold or respiratory navigator-gated acquisitions will be possible.

FUNCTION

The second step in a cardiovascular MRI examination is an evaluation of cardiac function. The second most frequent indication for cardiac MRI is an evaluation of myocardial wall motion abnormalities in patients with suspected myocardial ischemia. Nowadays, most of these patients have previously undergone echocardiography and have proved hard to image with ultrasonography. They are usually obese or have pulmonary emphysema. The expectation is that because of the experience that cardiologists are obtaining with MRI in this group of patients, the demand for MRI analysis of cardiac function will increase in the future.

As in echocardiography, the short-axis view of the left ventricle (LV) is the "work horse" view in cardiac MRI. Before the short-axis view can be acquired, two long-axis views must be acquired, which in themselves yield diagnostic information, especially concerning the apical wall motion pattern of both ventricles. First, the vertical long-axis, or two-chamber, view is acquired (Fig. 1.13). Based on a transverse survey image at the level of the mitral valve, the center of the slice is positioned approximately in the middle of the mitral valve and angulated in such a way that the slice cuts through the LV apex on a lower transverse survey image. For selection of the end-systolic cardiac time frame, the two-chamber view must be acquired with a dynamic gradient-echo technique. This can be accomplished by us-

ing a conventional gradient-echo technique during continuous breathing, but better results are obtained when an ultrafast breath-hold technique, such as echo-planar imaging, is used (17). Currently, the best option is a balanced FFE sequence because it provides excellent contrast between blood and myocardium.

Next, the horizontal long-axis, or four-chamber, view must be acquired (Fig. 1.14). Planning of the four-chamber view is based on the diastolic and systolic images of the two-chamber view. First, the center of the slice must be positioned at the lower third of the mitral valve on the end-systolic two-chamber image; then the slice must be angulated through the apex. After this, the position of the slice on the diastolic two-chamber image is checked to ensure that the atrium is imaged properly. The four-chamber image also must be acquired with a dynamic imaging technique, preferably balanced FFE. The two- and four-chamber views yield some important clinical information, mainly concerning ventricular anatomy and dimensions, presence of hypertrophy, valve insufficiencies, and the like.

The final step in the evaluation of ventricular function is planning the short-axis view itself (Fig. 1.15). A stack of 10 to 12 slices, each 8 to 10 mm thick, is positioned perpendicular to the long axis of the LV, defined as extending from the midmitral point to the LV apex based on the systolic and diastolic images of the four-chamber view and the systolic two-chamber view. The entire ventricle in end-diastole, which can be checked on the end-diastolic images, must be included. This is important for calculation of the end-diastolic volume, stroke volume, ejection fraction, and derived functional parameters.

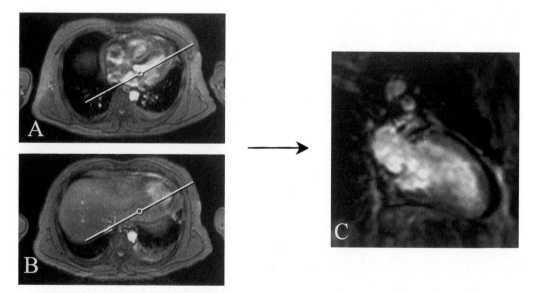

FIGURE 1.13. The vertical long-axis, or two-chamber, view is planned in the following way: Based on a transverse survey image at the level of the mitral valve **(A)**, the center of the slice is positioned approximately in the middle of the mitral valve and angulated in such a way that the slice intersects with the left ventricular apex on a lower transverse survey image **(B)**. An end-diastolic two-chamber image is shown here, acquired during a 12-second breath-hold in expiration with echo-planar MRI **(C)**.

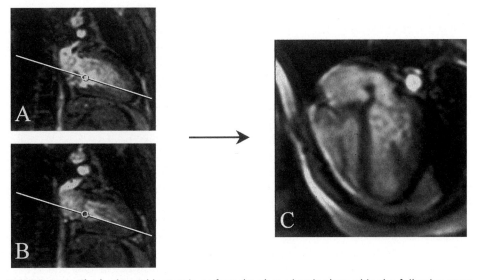

FIGURE 1.14. The horizontal long-axis, or four-chamber, view is planned in the following way: The center of the slice must be positioned at the lower third of the mitral valve on the end-systolic two-chamber image **(B)**; then, the slice must be angulated through the apex (A,B). Next, the position of the slice is checked on the diastolic two-chamber image **(A)** to ensure that the atrium is imaged properly. An end-diastolic four-chamber image is shown here, acquired during a 12-second breath-hold in expiration with echo-planar MRI **(C)**.

The short-axis scan, with 10 to 12 slices covering the ventricles in their entirety, can be acquired in a conventional gradient-echo sequence during continuous breathing, which is very time-consuming. A better alternative is a breath-hold acquisition with echo-planar imaging, but again, the best technique available today is the balanced FFE MRI sequence (Fig. 1.10). Nowadays, these scans are performed using multiple breath-holds in expiration, with the associated problems previously mentioned. In the near future, it is expected that the entire short-axis stack of slices will be acquired within a single breath-hold of up to 15 seconds with the use of balanced FFE-SENSE, perhaps in com-

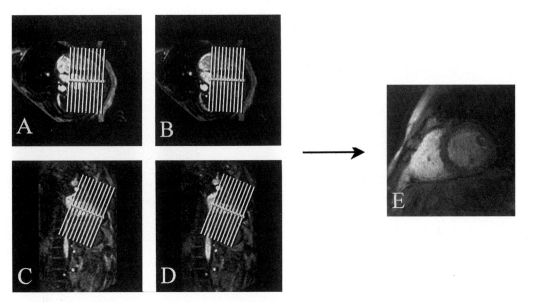

FIGURE 1.15. The short-axis view is planned in the following way: A stack of slices is positioned perpendicular to the long axis of the left ventricle (LV), defined as extending from the midmitral point to the LV apex based on the diastolic **(A)** and systolic **(B)** images of the four-chamber view and the diastolic **(C)** and systolic **(D)** two-chamber view. The entire ventricle must be included in end-diastole; this can be checked on the end-diastolic images (A,C). An end-diastolic short-axis image is shown here, acquired during a 12-second breath-hold in expiration with echo-planar MRI **(E)**.

bination with spiral k-space acquisition. One step further into the future may lead to real-time imaging of the short-axis stack, although this poses several problems during off-line image processing. Real-time imaging of the short-axis view currently seems perfectly suitable for cardiac stress imaging during continuous increasing dosing with dobutamine.

PERFUSION

Myocardial perfusion of the ischemic heart can be studied with MRI (18). Most approaches to perfusion analysis make use of intravenously injected gadolinium-based contrast agents. This type of contrast media temporarily changes the T1 relaxation time and therefore the MR signal intensity of well-perfused tissues. After contrast injection, ischemic myocardial regions show up as areas with no or little signal intensity change in comparison with well-perfused myocardium. To visualize the passage of a bolus of injected material, fast T1-weighted MR techniques should be used. The first reports on visualization of perfusion defects in human patients described the acquisition of a single slice level (19). Currently, perfusion studies apply fast gradient-echo pulse sequences (magnetization-prepared turbo-field echo/echo-planar/fast low-angle shot), which enable the repetitive registration of three or more anatomic levels at every heart beat, or alternatively six levels with a temporal resolution of every other heart beat (20). A recent development is the "interleaved notched saturation" method, which enables rapid coverage of seven levels (19).

Quantitative image analysis yields parameters to characterize passage of the bolus immediately after administration of the contrast agent. Some parameters obtained from the image series describing this first pass are rate and level of enhancement, time to peak, and mean transit time. These characteristic parameters may be obtained for each image pixel and can be graphically displayed in so-called parametric images that visualize the anatomic location of abnormalities (21).

DELAYED ENHANCEMENT

After a low-molecular-weight contrast agent is injected, its plasma concentration reaches a maximum value and then rapidly decreases through diffusion to the interstitial space and renal washout. Contrast agent that diffuses to the interstitial space is resorbed into the capillary bed and undergoes renal excretion. However, when tissue is damaged, as in infarction, the resorption rate of the contrast agent is diminished. At 15 to 30 minutes after contrast injection, washout is complete in normal myocardium, but not in infarcted or edematous tissue. This phenomenon is the basis of "delayed enhancement imaging." Various authors (22,23) have de-

scribed the relation between myocardial viability and size of the area displaying delayed enhancement. In MR images, the contrast agent can be detected as a bright area on images acquired with T1-weighted MR pulse sequences ranging from basic spin-echo methods to more sophisticated gradient-echo sequences in which an inversion or saturation prepulse is used. Currently, the principle "bright is dead," indicating that bright areas on a delayed MR image after contrast injection correspond to nonviable myocardium, is subject to lively debate (24–26).

FLOW

One of the advantages of MRI in cardiovascular diagnosis is its ability to measure flow velocity (in centimeters per second) and flow volume (in milliliters per second). MR flow measurement is based on the principle of "spin phase" (27). Usually, MR images use only the absolute value of the MR signal arising from the slice under investigation. However, the acquired data also contain information regarding a property called *spin phase*. MR data acquisition and postprocessing can be set up in such a way that two images of each slice are produced: an image with gray values representing spatial localization of the tissues, and an image with gray values representing the velocity of the tissue present in each image element. The latter image is called the *velocity map* (Fig. 1.16). In a velocity map, pixels of static tissue are displayed with an intensity of zero, whereas pixels of, for example, moving blood have a positive or negative value, depending on the direction of flow. The use of additional magnetic field gradients in the imaging pulse sequence is the basis of velocity mapping. These field gradients may be applied "in plane" or "through plane," thus encoding different components of the flow direction. In most instances, the imaging slice is positioned to measure through-plane flow, but it is also feasible to quantify flow in all three dimensions by adding additional data acquisitions.

To obtain useful data on blood flow, it is necessary to measure flow in a vessel or valve of interest at many instances during the cardiac cycle. For example, flow velocity can be measured in a region of interest at many time frames to produce a flow velocity-versus-time curve (see below), which provides information on changes in flow velocity during the cardiac cycle. In such a flow velocity curve, the area under the curve is computed to obtain the stroke volume—that is, the amount of blood passing through the region of interest during a cardiac cycle. Other valuable hemodynamic parameters related to cardiac contraction and relaxation may also be gleaned from the flow velocity curve (28).

Flow-encoding MR scans are based on gradient-echo pulse sequences in combination with prospective ECG triggering or retrospective ECG gating. For an evaluation of diastolic ventricular function, retrospective ECG gating

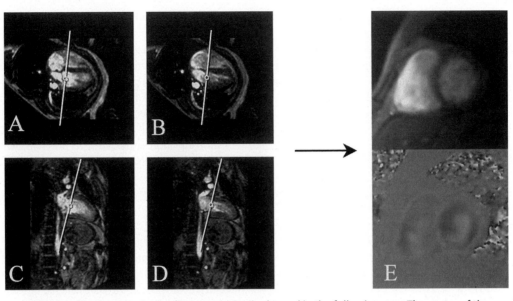

FIGURE 1.16. The mitral valve flow acquisition is planned in the following way: The center of the slice is positioned in the middle of the mitral valve on the end-systolic two-chamber **(D)** and four-chamber **(B)** images and angulated parallel to the mitral valve, also on the end-diastolic two-chamber **(C)** and four-chamber **(A)** images. An end-diastolic image of the mitral valve is shown here **(E)**. The upper image is the normal, or modulus, image; the lower image is the velocity-encoded image (velocity map).

is required because prospective ECG triggering images only the first 80% of the cardiac cycle, and the atrial contribution to ventricular filling occurs in the last 10% to 20% of the cardiac cycle. Currently, a flow measurement has a duration of 2 to 3 minutes, and the result represents the average flow during the acquisition period. Recent developments in scanner hardware and software have enabled real-time flow measurement (29) in a clinical setting (30), so that phenomena with fast changes in flow can be investigated with MR.

The clinically most relevant cardiac flow acquisitions are through the mitral valve, tricuspid valve, ascending aorta, and pulmonary artery:

The mitral valve flow acquisition is planned on the two- and four-chamber views in end-systole (Fig. 1.16). The center of the slice is positioned in the middle of the mitral valve on the end-systolic two- and four-chamber images and angulated parallel to the mitral valve. A typical mitral valve flow curve is shown in Figure 1.17.

The tricuspid valve flow acquisition is based on an extra survey image—the right ventricular (RV) two-chamber view (Fig. 1.18). This view is planned on the end-systolic four-chamber view. The center of the slice is positioned in the middle of the tricuspid valve and angulated through the apex of the RV. The tricuspid valve flow acquisition is first planned on the end-systolic four-chamber view (Fig. 1.19). The center of the slice is positioned on the center of the tricuspid valve and angulated parallel to the tricuspid valve. Thereafter, the slice is angulated on the RV two-chamber view parallel to the tricuspid valve. A typical tricuspid valve flow curve is shown in Figure 1.20.

The acquisition to measure blood flow velocities and volume through the ascending aorta is planned on the original survey images in the coronal and sagittal views (Fig. 1.21). An unangulated slice is positioned perpendicular to the ascending aorta on a coronal image, usually at the level of the bifurcation of the pulmonary artery. On a

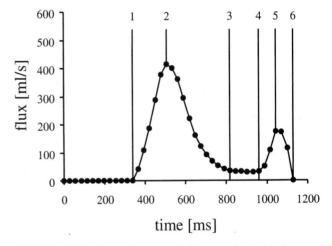

FIGURE 1.17. Typical mitral valve flow curve obtained after tracing the orifice of the valve in all cardiac time frames on the velocity-encoded images. The integration of velocity data over time for all pixels enclosed in the traced area results in a volume–flow (flux) curve. The early peak filling rate *(2)* is a result of the pressure difference between the left atrium and left ventricle and is a passive process. The atrial peak filling rate *(5)* is a result of left atrial contraction and is an active process. Another functional parameter that can be derived from the curve is the fastest change in flux between, for example, *2* and *3*, the so-called early deceleration peak. Note the diastase between *3* and *4*.

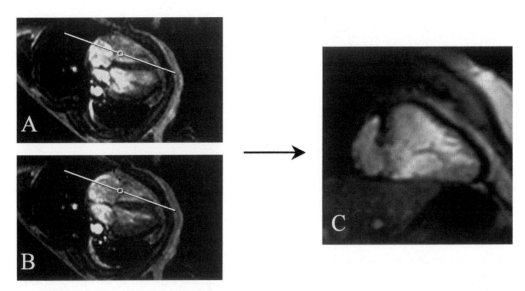

FIGURE 1.18. The tricuspid valve flow is based on an additional survey image—the right ventricular (RV) two-chamber view. The RV two-chamber view is planned on the end-systolic four-chamber view **(B)**. The center of the slice is positioned in the middle of the tricuspid valve and angulated through the apex of the RV based on the end-diastolic **(A)** and end-systolic images (B). An end-diastolic RV two-chamber image is shown here, acquired during a 12-second breath-hold in expiration with echo-planar MRI **(C)**.

sagittal image of the original survey, the angulation can be adjusted if necessary, but this is usually not the case. A typical flow curve through the ascending aorta is shown in Figure 1.22.

The acquisition to measure blood flow through the pulmonary artery is planned on original survey images in the coronal and transverse views (Fig. 1.23). First, another survey image must be acquired of one to three slices in the center of and parallel to the pulmonary artery based on an original sagittal image. Then, the pulmonary artery flow acquisition can be planned perpendicular to the pulmonary artery based on the angulated survey image, as pre-

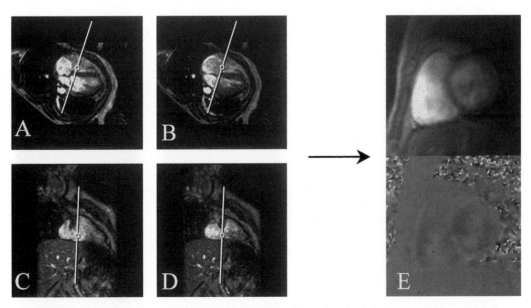

FIGURE 1.19. The tricuspid valve flow acquisition is planned in the following way: The center of the slice is positioned on the center of the tricuspid valve on the end-systolic four-chamber view **(B)** and angulated parallel to the tricuspid valve based on the end-diastolic four-chamber view **(A)**. Thereafter, the slice is angulated on the end-diastolic **(C)** and end-systolic **(D)** right ventricular two-chamber view parallel to the tricuspid valve. An end-diastolic image of the tricuspid valve is shown here **(E)**. The upper image is the normal, or modulus, image; the lower image is the velocity-encoded image.

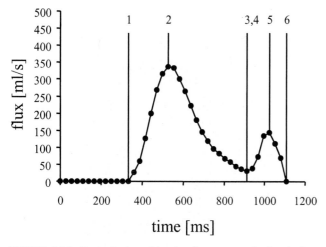

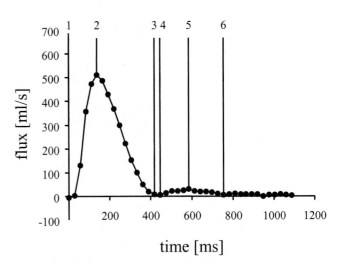

FIGURE 1.20. Typical tricuspid valve flow curve obtained after the orifice of the valve has been traced in all cardiac time frames on the velocity-encoded images. The early peak filling rate *(2)* is a result of the pressure difference between the right atrium and right ventricle and is a passive process. The atrial peak filling rate *(5)* is a result of left atrial contraction and is an active process. Another possible functional parameter that can be derived from the curve is the fastest change in flux between, for example, *1* and *2,* the so-called early acceleration peak.

FIGURE 1.22. Typical flow curve through the ascending aorta obtained after the contour of the ascending aorta has been traced in all cardiac time frames on the velocity-encoded images. The peak ejection rate *(2)* is a result of left ventricular (LV) contraction. The area under the curve between *1* and *3* is the LV stroke volume. Another interesting functional parameter that can be derived from the curve is the fastest change in flux between, for example, *1* and *2,* the so-called aortic acceleration peak.

viously described, and on the original sagittal survey image (Fig. 1.23). In addition, the slice position in the caudocranial direction must be positioned just before the bifurcation of the pulmonary artery on a transverse image of the original survey. A typical flow curve through the pulmonary artery is shown in Figure 1.24.

CORONARY MRA

Coronary MRA is not discussed in great detail in this chapter; the reader is referred to later chapters for an indepth explanation of techniques and procedures. For now, it suffices to mention three major points of concern in

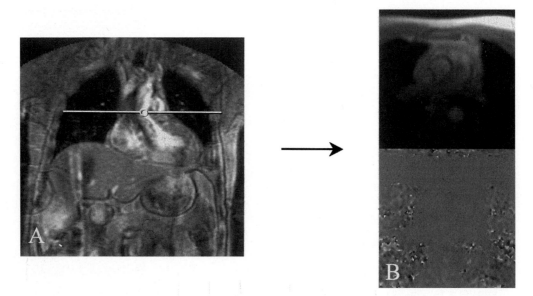

FIGURE 1.21. The flow acquisition through the ascending aorta is planned in the following way: An unangulated slice is positioned perpendicular to the ascending aorta on a coronal survey image **(A)**; usually, this is at the level of the bifurcation of the pulmonary artery. On a sagittal image of the original survey, the angulation can be adjusted if necessary, although this is usually not the case (not shown). An end-diastolic image of the ascending aorta is shown here **(B)**. The upper image is the normal, or modulus, image; the lower image is the velocity-encoded image.

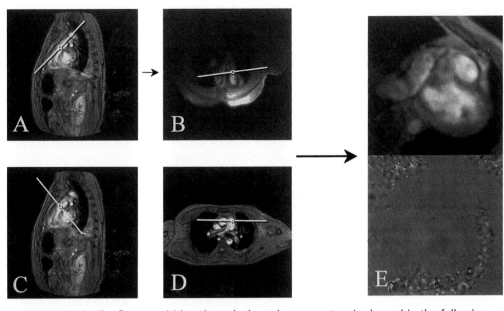

FIGURE 1.23. The flow acquisition through the pulmonary artery is planned in the following way: First, another survey image must be acquired of one to three slices in the center of and parallel to the pulmonary artery based on an original sagittal survey image **(A)**. Then, the pulmonary artery flow acquisition can be planned perpendicular to the pulmonary artery based on the angulated survey image **(B)** and on the original sagittal survey image **(C)**. In addition, the slice position in the caudocranial direction must be positioned just before the bifurcation of the pulmonary artery on a transverse image of the original survey **(D)**. An end-diastolic image of the pulmonary artery is shown here **(E)**. The upper image is the normal, or modulus, image; the lower image is the velocity-encoded image.

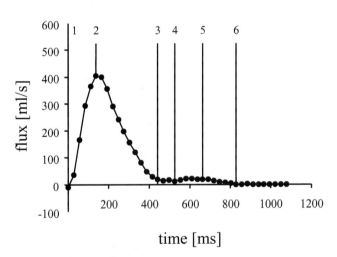

FIGURE 1.24. Typical flow curve through the pulmonary artery obtained after the contour of the pulmonary artery has been traced in all cardiac time frames on the velocity-encoded images. The peak ejection rate *(2)* is a result of right ventricular (RV) contraction. The area under the curve between *1* and *3* is the RV stroke volume. Another interesting functional parameter that can be derived from the curve is the fastest change in flux between, for example, *2* and *3,* the so-called pulmonary deceleration peak.

coronary MRA. The first is cardiac motion itself, which limits the shot length of image acquisition to less than 100 milliseconds. The second is respiratory motion, which can be corrected for by using respiratory navigators with residual respiratory motion of up to 3 mm. Currently, the in-plane image resolution is limited to 0.7 mm because of the 100-millisecond shot duration; within this period of time, some cardiac motion still occurs and causes image blurring. In theory, an in-plane resolution of about 0.3 mm can be reached, but this is currently hampered by the long shot duration of about 100 milliseconds. With further improvements in scanner hardware and software, it is expected that isotropic resolution of 250 μm will be reached in the near future, possibly by performing coronary MRA at 3 tesla (T) instead of the standard clinical field strength of 1.5 T. All major MRI machine manufacturers now offer 3-T MRI scanners.

The third point of concern is the way image contrast between a coronary vessel and surrounding tissue is optimized. Basically, two alternatives are available: (a) the T2 preparation technique and (b) the use of a contrast agent in combination with spiral k-space filling, which is discussed in detail in a later chapter. It is important to realize that it is perhaps more important to suppress signal from surrounding tissue perfectly than to enhance the signal inside the coronary arteries.

VESSEL WALL IMAGING

In this chapter, vessel wall imaging is not discussed in detail; the reader is referred to later chapters for an in-depth explanation of techniques and procedures. In general, vessel wall imaging is an important feature of cardiovascular MRI that currently cannot be accomplished noninvasively with other imaging modalities. Therefore, much effort is currently being expended to develop MRI techniques capable of imaging, for example, coronary vessel walls (31). Again, a switch to a fieldstrength of 3 T may improve earlier results in this area. One of the future applications of vessel wall imaging will be to determine the composition and stability of atherosclerotic plaque. In the far future, vessel wall imaging may be combined with interventional cardiovascular MRI and interventional MRI procedures, such as dottering and stenting under MRI guidance.

CARDIOVASCULAR MR IMAGE PROCESSING

One of the main, if not the main, obstructions to the routine clinical application of cardiovascular MRI is the relatively underdeveloped state of cardiac image analysis. Currently, the only option for obtaining reliable measurements is to perform image analysis manually. Drawing endocardial and epicardial contours is a very time-consuming part of the cardiac examination. Several software packages are available to assist in this tedious task, such as MASS and FLOW software (MEDIS, Medical Imaging Systems, Leiden, The Netherlands) (32,33). Recently, a new technique was developed to detect myocardial borders fully automatically, without any user interaction. This approach uses the "active appearance model" algorithm, which is based on a statistical description of the possible shape of myocardial contours in four dimensions (34). The method showed excellent first results; therefore, it may for the first time allow an accurate,

fully automated evaluation of cardiac function. It may be possible to apply this technique in the future to analyze perfusion and delayed enhancement images.

Future developments in image processing are aimed at designing a single software package to evaluate function, perfusion, delayed enhancement, and coronary MRA images. Analogous to the development of a single comprehensive cardiac acquisition scheme, "one-stop-shop" cardiac image processing is now within reach. A further step will be the ability to analyze cardiovascular MR images in real time; performing a clinical evaluation based on quantification while the patient is still in the MRI scanner will allow online quality control of the previous acquisitions. In the ideal world, real-time cardiovascular MR image acquisition and real-time image analysis are combined, the latter being not completely unrealistic on the time scale of a decennium.

APPENDIX: CALCULATIONS ON K-SPACE

Image formation in MRI is based on filling "k-space" during data acquisition. The concept is not explained further in this context because many thorough and comprehensive articles on this topic are available (2–6). Aspects of k-space relevant to a practical understanding of MRI are the calculation of the number of k-lines to be acquired and a determination of the spatial resolution of cardiac images.

The number of k-lines in the phase-encoding (Y) direction can be calculated by applying the following formula:

$$\begin{aligned}\text{Number of k-lines} = \ &\text{Acquisition Matrix}\\ &\times \text{Rectangular Field of View}\\ &\times \text{Symmetric Reduction}\\ &\times \text{Asymmetric Reduction}\end{aligned}$$

where symmetric reduction factor equals scan percent and asymmetric reduction factor equals halfscan (Figs. 1.25 and 1.26). For example, with an acquisition matrix of 256, a

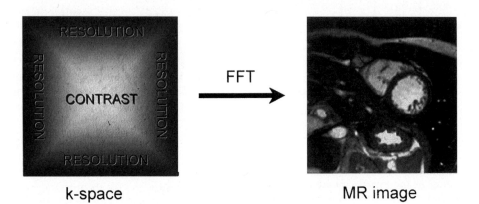

FIGURE 1.25. Schematic diagram of the relation between k-space and the MR image. The center of k-space contains relatively more information on contrast, whereas the periphery contains more information on resolution. Note that each point in k-space is related to all points in the MR image. The image shown was acquired by using balanced fast-field echo during a breath-hold of 15 seconds. *CONTRAST,* gray values in larger areas; *RESOLUTION,* visibility of small structures; *FFT,* fast Fourier transform.

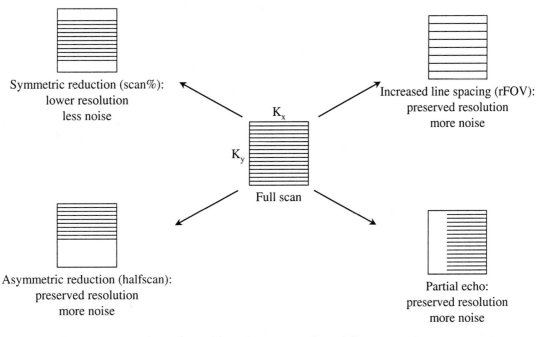

Symmetric reduction (scan%):
lower resolution
less noise

K_x

K_y

Full scan

Increased line spacing (rFOV):
preserved resolution
more noise

Asymmetric reduction (halfscan):
preserved resolution
more noise

Partial echo:
preserved resolution
more noise

FIGURE 1.26. MRI can be performed faster by acquiring fewer k-lines per MR image. Symmetric reduction and increased line spacing are the most frequently used techniques to reduce the number of k-lines. Symmetric reduction means that on both the extreme edges of k-space in the Y-resolution (phase-encoding direction), the part that determines image resolution (Fig. 1.25), k-lines are not acquired. As a result, an image with fewer k-lines is acquired, but the tradeoff is a reduction in planar spatial resolution. Increased line spacing decreases the density of k-lines in k-space, whereas the entire k-space is still traversed. In this way, the image resolution remains the same, the image noise increases, and the field of view is rectangular. Another way of reducing the number of k-lines is to acquire only, for example, a five-eighth portion of k-space with the same k-line density; this asymmetric reduction results in more image noise. Another way to speed up the MRI acquisition is not to reduce the number of k-lines, but to reduce the part of the generated echo that is sampled; this procedure increases image noise because fewer image data are acquired.

rectangular field-of-view factor of 0.6, a symmetric reduction factor of 0.8, and an asymmetric reduction factor of 1 (meaning no halfscan), the number of k-lines equals 256 × 0.6 × 0.8 × 1, or 122.

The image pixel resolution can be calculated according to the following formulas:

X-resolution (Echo Readout Direction)
= Field of View/Acquisition Matrix

Y-resolution (Phase-Encoding Direction)
= Field of View/(Acquisition Matrix × Symmetric Reduction)

For example, with a field of view of 300 mm, an acquisition matrix of 256, and a symmetric reduction factor of 0.8, X-resolution will be 300/256, or 1.2 mm, and Y-resolution will be 300/(256 × 0.8) = 1.5 mm. Reconstructing to a 256 × 256 matrix, meaning that the Y-resolution is interpolated to the X-resolution (in this case 1.2 mm), results in an apparent in-plane image resolution of 1.2 mm × 1.2 mm, and with a slice thickness of 8 mm, yielding a final resolution of $1.2 \times 1.2 \times 8$ mm^3, at a field of view of 300 × 180 (= 300 × 0.6) mm^2.

REFERENCES

1. Pruessmann KP, Weiger M, Scheidegger MB, et al. SENSE: sensitivity encoding for fast MRI. *Magn Reson Med* 1999;42:952–962.
2. Boxerman JL, Mosher TJ, McVeigh ER, et al. Advanced MR imaging techniques for evaluation of the heart and great vessels. *Radiographics* 1998;18:543–564.
3. Boxt LM. Primer on cardiac magnetic resonance imaging: how to perform the examination. *Top Magn Reson Imaging* 2000;11:331–347.
4. Duerk JL. Principles of MR image formation and reconstruction. *Magn Reson Imaging Clin N Am* 1999;7:629–659.
5. Reeder SB, Faranesh AZ. Ultrafast pulse sequence techniques for cardiac magnetic resonance imaging. *Top Magn Reson Imaging* 2000;11:312–330.
6. Sakuma H, Takeda K, Higgins CB. Fast magnetic resonance imaging of the heart. *Eur J Radiol* 1999;29:101–113.
7. Chia JM, Fischer SE, Wickline SA, et al. Performance of QRS detection for cardiac magnetic resonance imaging with a novel vectorcardiographic triggering method. *J Magn Reson Imaging* 2000;12:678–688.
8. Bailes DR, Gilderdale DJ, Bydder GM, et al. Respiratory ordered phase encoding (ROPE): a method for reducing respiratory motion artefacts in MR imaging. *J Comput Assist Tomogr* 1985;9:835–838.
9. Wang Y, Rossman PJ, Grimm RC, et al. Navigator-echo-based real-time respiratory gating and triggering for reduction of respi-

ration effects in three-dimensional coronary MR angiography. *Radiology* 1996;198:55–60.

10. Danias PG, McConnell MV, Khasgiwala VC, et al. Prospective navigator correction of image position for coronary MR angiography. *Radiology* 1997;203:733–736.

11. Stuber M, Botnar RM, Danias PG, et al. Submillimeter three-dimensional coronary MR angiography with real-time navigator correction: comparison of navigator locations. *Radiology* 1999; 212:579–587.

12. Chapman B, Turner R, Ordidge RJ, et al. Real-time movie imaging from a single cardiac cycle by NMR. *Magn Reson Med* 1987;5: 246–254.

13. Weber OM, Eggers H, Spiegel MA, et al. Real-time interactive magnetic resonance imaging with multiple coils for the assessment of left ventricular function. *J Magn Reson Imaging* 1999;10: 826–832.

14. Yang PC, Kerr AB, Liu AC, et al. New real-time interactive cardiac magnetic resonance imaging system complements echocardiography. *J Am Coll Cardiol* 1998;32:2049–2056.

15. Lelieveldt BPF, van der Geest RJ, Lamb HJ, et al. Automated observer-independent acquisition of cardiac short-axis MR images: a pilot study. *Radiology* 2001;221:537–542.

16. Simonetti OP, Finn JP, White RD, et al. "Black blood" T2-weighted inversion-recovery MR imaging of the heart. *Radiology* 1996;199:49–57.

17. Lamb HJ, Doornbos J, van der Velde EA, et al. Echo planar MRI of the heart on a standard system: validation of measurements of left ventricular function and mass. *J Comput Assist Tomogr* 1996; 20:942–949.

18. Wilke N, Jerosch-Herold M, Stillman AE, et al. Concepts of myocardial perfusion imaging in magnetic resonance imaging. *Magn Reson Q* 1994;10:249–286.

19. Cullen JH, Horsfield MA, Reek CR, et al. A myocardial perfusion reserve index in humans using first-pass contrast-enhanced magnetic resonance imaging. *J Am Coll Cardiol* 1999;33:1386–1394.

20. Lauerma K, Virtanen KS, Sipila LM, et al. Multislice MRI in assessment of myocardial perfusion in patients with single-vessel proximal left anterior descending coronary artery disease before and after revascularization. *Circulation* 1997;96:2859–2867.

21. Dromigny-Badin A, Zhu YM, Magnin I, et al. Fusion of cine magnetic resonance and contrast-enhanced first-pass magnetic resonance data in patients with coronary artery disease: a feasibility study. *Invest Radiol* 1998;33:12–21.

22. Gerber KH, Higgins CB. Quantitation of size of myocardial infarctions by computerized transmission tomography. Comparison with hot-spot and cold-spot radionuclide scans. *Invest Radiol* 1983;18:238–244.

23. de Roos A, Doornbos J, van der Wall EE, et al. MR imaging of acute myocardial infarction: value of Gd-DTPA. *AJR Am J Roentgenol* 1988;150:531–534.

24. Kim RJ, Fieno DS, Parrish TB, et al. Relationship of MRI delayed contrast enhancement to irreversible injury, infarct age, and contractile function. *Circulation* 1999;100:1992–2002.

25. Kim RJ, Wu E, Rafael A, et al. The use of contrast-enhanced magnetic resonance imaging to identify reversible myocardial dysfunction. *N Engl J Med* 2000;343:1445–1453.

26. Gerber BL, Rochitte CE, Melin JA, et al. Microvascular obstruction and left ventricular remodeling early after acute myocardial infarction. *Circulation* 2000;101:2734–2741.

27. van Dijk P. Direct cardiac NMR imaging of heart wall and blood flow velocity. *J Comput Assist Tomogr* 1984;8:429–436.

28. Lamb HJ, Beyerbacht HP, van der LA, et al. Diastolic dysfunction in hypertensive heart disease is associated with altered myocardial metabolism. *Circulation* 1999;99:2261–2267.

29. Guilfoyle DN, Gibbs P, Ordidge RJ, et al. Real-time flow measurements using echo-planar imaging. *Magn Reson Med* 1991;18: 1–8.

30. Klein C, Schalla S, Schnackenburg B, et al. Magnetic resonance flow measurements in real time: comparison with a standard gradient-echo technique. *J Magn Reson Imaging* 2001;14:306–310.

31. Botnar RM, Stuber M, Kissinger KV, et al. Noninvasive coronary vessel wall and plaque imaging with magnetic resonance imaging. *Circulation* 2000;102:2582–2587.

32. van der Geest RJ, Buller VG, Jansen E, et al. Comparison between manual and semiautomated analysis of left ventricular volume parameters from short-axis MR images. *J Comput Assist Tomogr* 1997; 21:756–765.

33. van der Geest RJ, Niezen RA, van der Wall EE, et al. Automated measurement of volume flow in the ascending aorta using MR velocity maps: evaluation of inter- and intraobserver variability in healthy volunteers. *J Comput Assist Tomogr* 1998;22:904–911.

34. Mitchell SC, Lelieveldt BP, van der Geest RJ, et al. Multistage hybrid active appearance model matching: segmentation of left and right ventricles in cardiac MR images. *IEEE Trans Med Imaging* 2001;20:415–423.

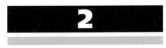

2

MRA TECHNIQUES

DAVID SALONER

A number of features of MRI make it well suited for the evaluation of vascular disease. The principal advantage of MRI is that it can cover an extended vascular territory and provide information at all points in three-dimensional (3D) space, yet the modality is noninvasive or, in the case of venously injected contrast-enhanced imaging, only minimally invasive. The 3D data sets obtained make it possible to display vessels of interest in a variety of formats; contiguous slices can be oriented in any obliquity, or a projection format can be used. MRA has been used primarily to obtain images of the vascular lumen, although interest is growing in the use of MRA to delineate disease processes by imaging vessel walls.

Like other MRI methods, MRA is least successful when substantial gross motion occurs during data acquisition. Gross motion can be caused by poor patient compliance or may represent physiologic motion, such as cardiac motion during imaging of the coronary arteries or breathing during imaging of the visceral vessels. Also, blood flow itself can degrade the quality of images of the vascular lumen when the flow is either extremely low, extremely high, or disordered.

Techniques for obtaining high-quality MR angiograms have evolved along with improvements in MR instrumentation. Indeed, the performance requirements for high-quality MRA have been the driving force behind a number of advances in MR instrumentation. As new performance capabilities become available, new techniques become feasible, and this trend can be expected to continue. In this chapter, a number of different methods of obtaining MR angiograms are discussed. Methods for displaying data are also presented.

FLOW DYNAMICS

The signal intensity measured in MRA studies of flowing blood depends on the distribution of blood flow rates and directions, and variations in these values (e.g., resulting from cardiac pulsatility) during the time that data are acquired. The design and implementation of imaging strategies and the choice of imaging parameters, therefore, require careful consideration of the anticipated hemodynamics in the vessels of interest, both in the normal and diseased conditions. Setting aside the problem of gross motion for the moment, MRA methods provide accurate images of the lumen when the image resolution is sufficiently high to provide several pixels across the diameter of the lumen; when the rate of flow is sufficiently high that blood traveling through the imaging volume receives only a small number of radiofrequency (RF) excitations; and when flow patterns remain regular and reproducible throughout the cardiac cycle. Deviations from these flow conditions can occur in both healthy and diseased vessels (1–3).

D. Saloner: Department of Radiology, University of California San Francisco, San Francisco, California.

Variations in flow conditions can result from large differences in systolic and diastolic flow. These can be particularly pronounced; for example, in the arteries of the lower extremities, a pronounced interval of rapid antegrade flow is followed by a short, smaller retrograde component, which is in turn followed by an extended diastolic interval during which flow velocities are extremely low. *In vivo,* flow patterns are also profoundly affected by variations in geometry. Even in healthy persons, blood vessels are curved, with numerous branches and bifurcations. Such geometric variations can substantially affect the velocity fields, so that flattened profiles may be seen across the vascular lumen at the entrance to branch vessels, or helical flow patterns in curved vessels such as the aortic arch. However, in the absence of disease, flow is generally laminar and reproducible from cycle to cycle. In regions of atherosclerosis, the vascular wall can be very irregular, with a residual lumen that is highly asymmetric and markedly variable in diameter. These geometric variations can create regions of disturbed flow, such as velocity jets that emanate from a tight stenosis accompanied by the shedding of flow vortices; these represent turbulent flow that varies from one cycle to the next.

PRIMARY MRA METHODS

All MRA techniques aim to create a high level of contrast between spins that are moving and spins that are stationary (4–9). MRI methods are capable of measuring both the magnitude of the transverse magnetization and the orientation of that magnetization in space (the phase). Methods have therefore been devised that are designed to create large differences in either the magnitude or phase of the magnetization between spins that are stationary and spins that are moving (5,7). MR sequences that rely on blood flow to transport fully magnetized blood into the imaging volume and thereby create a substantial difference between the magnetization of flowing and stationary spins are generally referred to as *time-of-flight (TOF) methods,* and they display the magnitude of the transverse magnetization (4). MR sequences that rely on contrast agents injected into the blood stream to enhance the vascular signal are referred to as *contrast-enhanced methods,* and these also create images that display the magnitude of the transverse magnetization (10). Images that display the phase of the magnetization are referred to as *phase-contrast images* (11). These methods rely on the motion of spins with respect to the imaging gradients for vessel-to-stationary tissue contrast.

FLOW COMPENSATION

Accurate spatial localization, providing images with a high signal-to-noise ratio, is accomplished by ensuring that in the center of the readout interval, an echo is formed in which the orientation of the transverse magnetization of all excited material is the same (rephased). In general, when imaging gradients are applied, spins accumulate a phase shift. Conventional imaging gradients, which are designed to generate a signal echo from stationary material, do not account for the motion of flowing spins, and at the center of the echo, moving spins accumulate a phase that depends on their motion between RF excitation and the time the echo is collected. In a voxel containing blood spins moving with a spread of velocities, a variety of phases will be present. The mean magnetization in the voxel is the sum of all the individual vectors, and because of the spread of phases, a drop in signal strength will occur that is referred to as *intravoxel phase dispersion.* With many MRA sequences, it is important that gradient waveforms be implemented to correct for blood motion such that the magnetization of moving spins is also rephased at the center of the echo (12,13). These are referred to as *motion compensation gradients* (14). Whereas conventional gradient-echo sequences use gradient waveforms consisting of two lobes of gradient field strength applied with opposite polarity, flow compensation gradients require additional lobes of applied gradients. In principle, flow compensation can be pursued to include all orders of motion (15). In practice, however, the added gradient lobes needed for higher-order motion compensation require additional time to play out, so that the echo time (TE) is lengthened. If motion compensation is used, the most effective method for improving signal retention from moving spins, even in disturbed flow, which contains high-order motion terms, is to rephase constant velocity terms only (16–19).

Most MRA sequences incorporate velocity compensation gradients along the directions of the slice selection and frequency-encoding gradients. The phase-encoding direction is not compensated; the short duration of the phase-encoding gradients minimizes the effects of motion during the application of those gradients.

TIME-OF-FLIGHT METHODS

The contrast obtained in an MRA study is closely related to the strength of the longitudinal magnetization in flowing blood relative to that in stationary tissue (6,20,21). In a gradient-echo sequence (flip angle <90 degrees), the strength of the longitudinal magnetization of spins subjected to a series of RF pulses decreases with each excitation. The longitudinal magnetization of spins continues to decrease as the number of RF excitations received increases, a process referred to as *saturation,* until it reaches a steady-state value that is determined by the flip angle, the repetition time, and the Tl relaxation time for that tissue. Stationary material remains in the imaging volume throughout data acquisition, and therefore the magnetization strength of stationary spins decreases to the steady-state value. In blood vessels, the longitudinal magnetization of spins at any given location depends on how many RF excitations those spins have received between entering the imaging volume and reaching that location. Fast-moving blood may receive only a few RF pulses and so retain substantial magnetization strength. Slowly moving spins may receive a large number of pulses, and the longitudinal magnetization of those spins, like that of stationary spins, may drop to the steady-state value. In magnitude images, spins that have received many RF pulses and are strongly saturated appear dark, whereas spins that retain substantial magnetization strength appear bright.

TWO-DIMENSIONAL TIME-OF-FLIGHT METHODS

The technique of engendering strong contrast between the longitudinal magnetization of flowing and stationary spins and then using flow-compensated gradients to encode the transverse magnetization correctly has been used to good effect in thin-slice strategies, also called *sequential 2D TOF* (22,23). In the thin-slice strategy, a single slice perpendicular to the blood vessel is acquired in a flow-compensated gradient sequence (Fig. 2.1). Making the slice very thin ensures that the slice will be replenished with relaxed blood and that it will not become saturated, even if moderately large flip angles are applied. Each single-slice acquisition

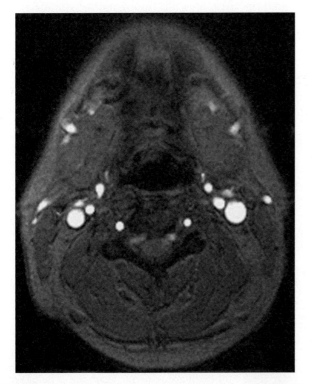

FIGURE 2.1. A two-dimensional gradient-echo sequence slice through the neck. Arteries and veins are shown with high contrast relative to stationary tissue. Repetition time/echo time/flip angle = 35/9/30 degrees.

requires a time on the order of 8 seconds. The sequence can be repeated multiple times, with the position of the slice shifted each time to permit acquisition of a large set of consecutive slices in a reasonable imaging time. In standard multislice imaging, the images are collected simultaneously; here, however, the images are collected sequentially so that blood is not saturated by one slice before entering another. A high level of signal contrast is attained between blood vessels and the stationary surround. This procedure provides a full 3D data set, and the single slices can then be reformatted by stacking them and calculating the desired plane of projection.

Shortcomings of Two-Dimensional Time-of-Flight Methods

Sequential 2D TOF techniques provide strong inflow enhancement when the slices are perpendicular to the vessels of interest. When the vessels are in the same plane as the slice, or reenter the slice, the blood becomes saturated and contrast is progressively lost. This effect is more pronounced when the slices are thick. In addition, in examinations such as an axial carotid artery study, a superior presaturation slab is applied that is close to and moves along with the current slice. This maneuver removes venous structures. Vascular loops are sometimes found, especially in the cervical vertebral arteries of older patients. If the loop is large enough, inferiorly moving arterial blood may also be presaturated and yield no signal. For this reason, the method is most effective when the course of the vessel of interest is straight.

When slices are collected perpendicular to the vessel of interest, projected images are obtained in which the plane of viewing (i.e., along the length of the vessel) corresponds to the axis with poorest resolution. Resolution is improved if very thin slices are acquired, but this may not be practical because the total imaging time depends on the number of slices collected. In addition, thinner slices have a lower signal-to-noise ratio and require longer TEs.

In many cases, particularly in the abdomen, reduced resolution in the projection view can be successfully addressed by acquiring slices in the same plane as the desired projection. In-plane saturation of the inferior vena cava during the acquisition of coronal slices may be reduced by using small flip angles at the expense of contrast.

THREE-DIMENSIONAL TIME-OF-FLIGHT METHODS

The major shortcoming of the thin-slice strategy is the limited resolution that can currently be achieved in the direction of slice selection. In 2D techniques that use flow-compensation gradients, the slice thickness chosen is typically 2 mm or greater. The use of 3D techniques permits the acquisition of a full 3D data set with isotropic voxels of less than 1 mm (3,4,7,24). High-resolution voxels are critical for the visualization of small branch vessels, which may otherwise be obscured by partial voluming. They also provide a clear depiction of tortuous vessels with equal fidelity in each spatial dimension.

The use of 3D methods further permits the acquisition of data sets with TEs shorter than those achieved with 2D methods. In acquiring data from a 3D volume, the excitation volume in the "slice select" direction is chosen to be a slab with a thickness of approximately 40 mm. In comparison with 2D methods, an additional cycle of phase encoding is imposed to allow the data to be reduced to a set of partitions. With 3D acquisitions, substantially longer acquisition times are required than with 2D methods, but 3D acquisitions provide the advantage of an increased signal-to-noise ratio. Blood flowing through the excitation volume receives many more excitation pulses in 3D acquisition than in 2D imaging. To avoid excessive saturation effects, the flip angle must be reduced (<30 degrees).

PRESATURATION

In many cases, it is confusing to evaluate an arterial structure when it is obscured by an overlying vein, and vice versa. To eliminate the signal from these vessels, a presaturation band with a flip angle of 90 degrees can be placed adjacent to the imaging slice or volume so that blood is saturated before it enters the slice (25,26) (Fig. 2.2). For example, to remove an inferior vena cava signal from a

study of the origin of the renal artery, one can place a transverse presaturation band across the abdomen inferior to the kidneys. Despite their utility, the application of presaturation pulses requires careful attention because their existence in a given acquisition is often not directly noted in the resultant images if they are placed outside the imaging volume. Care must be taken to ensure that the vessel of interest is not similarly presaturated.

PARAMETER CHOICES

In generating an MR angiogram, parameter choices are often made that optimize one feature of the angiogram at the expense of others. In choosing optimal pulse sequence parameters, one has to take into account the expected flow velocity, the thickness of the imaging volume that must be traversed, and the acceptable level of contrast between flowing and stationary material.

Repetition Time

The selection of the most suitable repetition time (TR) is a compromise. The shorter the TR, the more saturated the signal from stationary material. However, if the TR is shortened, blood receives more RF excitations in traversing the same distance than it would with a longer TR. This problem is illustrated in Fig. 2.3, which is a transverse 3D acquisition through the circle of Willis from a normal volunteer. The most suitable TR depends on the rate at which blood

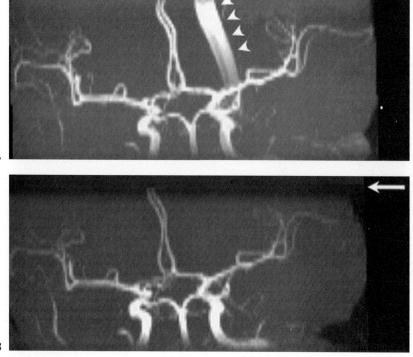

A

B

FIGURE 2.2. A maximum intensity projection on the coronal plane of a three-dimensional time-of-flight acquisition through the circle of Willis. **A:** With no presaturation, the sagittal sinus is clearly depicted *(arrowheads)* and overlies the arterial signal. **B:** A superior axial saturation band *(arrow)* eliminates signal from venous blood.

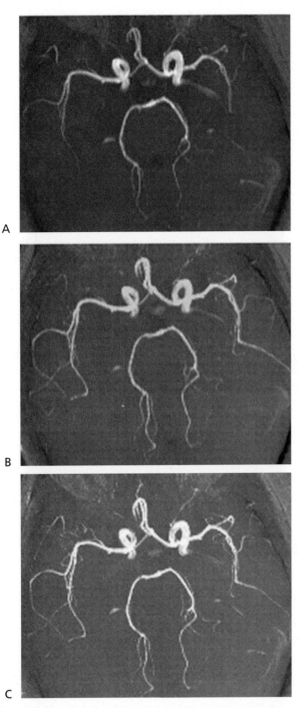

FIGURE 2.3. Time-of-flight acquisitions through the circle of Willis with variation of the repetition time. As the repetition time increases, less saturation of the stationary tissue and retention of the more distal arterial signal occur. Repetition time/echo time/flip angle values were 25/7/10 degrees **(A)**, 35/7/25 degrees **(B)**, and 45/7/40 degrees **(C)**.

Flip Angle

The choice of flip angle (α) is similarly a compromise. An increased value of α more heavily suppresses stationary signal but more rapidly saturates signal from blood that receives multiple excitations (Fig. 2.4). Again, the choice of this variable depends on flow dynamics. With a steady flow, the distribution of magnetization strength across the excited region reflects the flip angle, and the variation is larger with a larger flip angle. However, this variation is temporally constant, and each phase-encoding step samples the same dis-

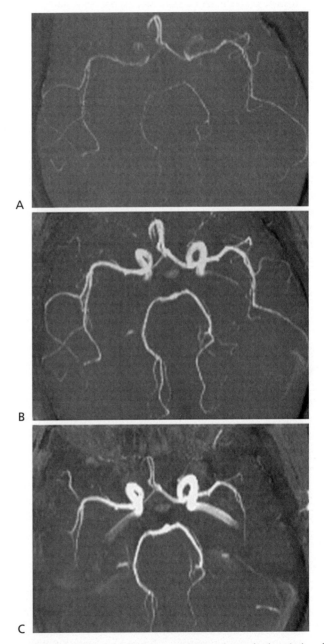

FIGURE 2.4. Time-of-flight acquisitions through the circle of Willis with variation of the flip angle. As the flip angle increases, increasing saturation of the stationary tissue and reduction of the more distal arterial signal occur. Repetition time/echo time/flip angle values were 35/7/10 degrees **(A)**, 35/7/25 degrees **(B)**, and 35/7/40 degrees **(C)**.

transits a slice; therefore, it varies from vessel to vessel and, for a given vessel, is somewhat patient-dependent. One should also note that a longer TR dictates a longer total study time and hence an increased possibility of motion on the part of the patient, which can substantially degrade image quality.

tribution of magnetization. With a pulsatile flow, the distribution of magnetization varies from cycle to cycle. The resulting pulsatile ghosting artifacts can be reduced by reducing the flip angle.

DISORDERED BLOOD FLOW

Laminar flow becomes unstable at high flow velocities and breaks down into turbulent flow. In regions where true turbulence exists, such as immediately distal to a critical stenosis, the flow patterns are complicated by the fact that flow is laminar in some regions and turbulent in others; furthermore, in some intermittent regions, flow randomly fluctuates between these two conditions. In that case, the different phase-encoding steps required to build up the MRA image are collected with different signal distributions. The fluctuations result in inconsistent data and image degradation (27,28). In addition, disturbed flow implies that between RF excitation and signal readout, protons will move through complicated trajectories described not only by constant velocity terms but also by high-order motion terms that are not rephased by constant velocity compensation. At the time of readout, some voxels will contain protons with a range of motion histories and a corresponding range of accumulated phases. Such voxels will have a reduced net transverse magnetization strength and will appear in the MR image with reduced signal intensity. The artifactual loss of signal associated with disturbed flow can mimic the appearance of vessel stenosis in vessels of normal caliber and can lead to an overestimation of the degree and extent of stenosis in diseased vessels.

ALTERNATIVE MRA METHODS

Although significant progress has been made with conventional TOF methods, a series of innovative strategies have been pursued to improve MRA further. Specialized sequences have been proposed to reduce the well-known loss of signal noted at sites of disturbed flow. Other approaches have been pursued to enhance the contrast between flowing spins and stationary spins, either by more effectively suppressing the signal from stationary spins or by retaining flow signal in the more distal portions of the vessels of interest.

Short-Echo Sequences

In general, the effects of disturbed flow, which result in intravoxel phase dispersion, can be reduced by shortening the duration of the encoding gradients (17,19,29–32). The extent to which this can be done is limited by the rate at which the magnetic field gradients can be altered (the slew rate) and the maximum achievable gradient strength. Furthermore, acquiring data with a strong frequency-encoding gradient results in a reduced signal-to-noise ratio. Nevertheless, significant improvement in MRA quality has been achieved with the development of better-performing gradients.

In selecting the TE of TOF MRA sequences, it is important to consider the dependence of the background signal on the TE. In voxels with significant contributions from protons attached to fat and protons attached to water, the signal strength depends on the phase relationship between those two components. The phase relationship is determined by the slight difference in precessional frequencies of protons in the two different environments. At 1.5 tesla (T), for example, the fat and water signals are out of phase at odd multiples of 2.3 milliseconds and in phase at even multiples of 2.3 milliseconds. Therefore, background suppression is more effective in images acquired with a TE of 7 milliseconds than in images acquired with a TE of 5 milliseconds (33) (Fig. 2.5). Nevertheless, the benefits of short-TE MRA are still apparent in regions with little fat contribution, such as the brain.

Sequences with a reduced TE can also be achieved by relaxing the requirement that the full echo be placed symmetrically in the data acquisition window. Conventional MRA sequences sacrifice a fraction of the echo and place the echo closer to the excitation pulse to reduce the TE. The slight loss in resolution that results from dropping the high-order frequency components is compensated for by the reduced sensitivity to flow disturbance (34,35). This strategy can be further pursued with the use of partial Fourier techniques, in which highly asymmetric echoes are acquired. In this case, the loss in resolution is unacceptable, and additional postprocessing steps must be taken by using the inherent symmetry of the Fourier data to reconstruct the missing information.

Ramped Radiofrequency Excitation

TOF sequences depend on the contrast between unsaturated flowing spins and partially saturated stationary spins to identify blood flow. As vessels pass through a volume of excitation, blood in the more distal portions becomes increasingly saturated. This tendency can be counteracted by designing an RF excitation pulse tailored to reduce such saturation (36). These pulses are designed to reduce saturation for spins entering from one side of the volume of interest. The RF pulse is asymmetric and provides a relatively small excitation angle for spins on the proximal side of the slab. This excitation angle becomes progressively larger across the slab. In this way, spins entering the slab retain their signal strength until, at the distal side of the slab, they are fairly heavily pulsed to sample the remaining magnetization most effectively without consideration of yet more distal portions of the vessel. The resulting magnetization response along the length of the vessel is then flatter when compared to what one obtains with a constant flip angle excitation (37,38) (Fig. 2.6). These pulses have been termed *tilted optimized nonsaturating excitation* (TONE).

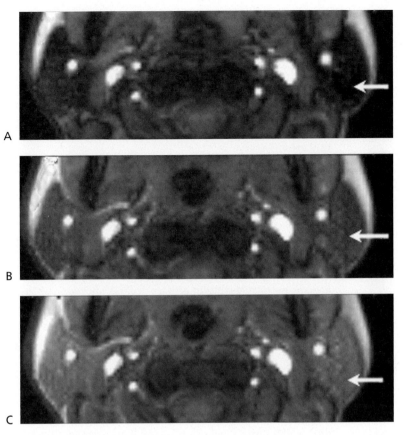

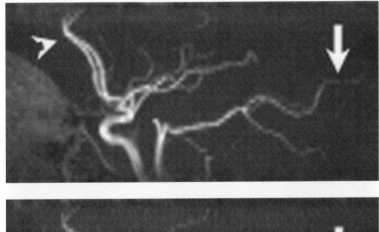

FIGURE 2.5. Single-slice partitions from three-dimensional acquisitions through the neck. Signal cancellation of lipids and free water within the same voxel is greatest at multiples of 2.3 milliseconds. This is clearly noted in the neck muscles *(arrows)*. Repetition time/echo time/flip angle values were 35/7/25 degrees **(A)**, 35/6/25 degrees **(B)**, and 35/5/25 degrees **(C)**.

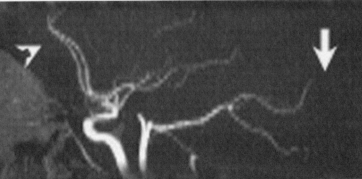

FIGURE 2.6. Time-of-flight acquisitions through the circle of Willis. Use of a ramped radiofrequency (RF) excitation profile is compared with use of a constant RF excitation profile. The ramped profile retains signal more distally in the anterior *(arrowhead)* and posterior *(arrow)* cerebral arteries. **A:** Ramped RF excitation, repetition time/echo time = 35/7; flip angle increasing linearly from 15 degrees at the proximal edge of the slab to 35 degrees at the distal edge of the slab. **B:** Single-slab repetition time/echo time = 35/7; constant flip angle = 25 degrees.

Sequential Three-Dimensional Methods

The distal saturation of blood flow that occurs in 3D TOF sequences can also be reduced by reducing the thickness of the excitation slab and by using multiple 3D volumes to cover the region of interest. This method has been termed *multiple overlapping thin-slab acquisition* (MOTSA) (39). In this approach, the 3D slabs are placed orthogonal to the principal direction of flow (e.g., axial slabs for studies of the extracranial carotids). To avoid bands of signal loss where the RF profiles trail off at the slab edges, substantial overlap of consecutive slabs is provided. This comes with a penalty of increased total acquisition time. Patient motion between acquisition of consecutive slabs is seen (as in sequential 2D studies) as a sharp discontinuity of the luminal edge. The reduced slab thickness limits the length of time that spins remain in the excited volume and results in a better retention of signal in the distal vessels (Fig. 2.7). This method provides the high-resolution capabilities of 3D sequences (40).

Spiral Scan

An artifact that was recognized in early clinical studies is the so-called misregistration artifact (41,42). Signal from spins that move obliquely with respect to the phase- and frequency-encoding axes appear at a spatial location in the image other than the lumen of the vessel. This can be noted as a bright vessel running diagonally and parallel to a dark lumen. The artifact occurs because in conventional 2D Fourier encoding, phase encoding occurs at an earlier time than does frequency encoding. Consequently, the location

of flowing spins in the image is mismapped. One approach to correcting the problem is to replace the phase-encoding gradient lobe with a bipolar lobe designed to encode spins moving with constant velocity with the phase appropriate to their location when the center of the frequency-encoding axis occurs (43). Although helpful, this approach again corrects only for spins moving with a constant velocity, and displacement artifacts for spins moving with higher-order motion are still seen.

A more fundamental approach to correcting displacement artifact is to use pulse sequences such as spiral scan, in which spatial information along both axes is acquired simultaneously. Spiral scan methods build up k-space by designing gradient trajectories that start in the center of k-space and spiral out to the edge (44,45). In the case of flow, spiral scan methods have the attraction that the two dimensions of spatial encoding take place simultaneously in time. Therefore, little or no misregistration artifact occurs. They are also attractive because they greatly reduce TEs, particularly for the low spatial frequency information in the center of k-space, thereby increasing insensitivity to disturbed flow.

Cardiac Synchronized MRA

Arterial flow is characterized by pulsatile variations. These differ in different parts of the body and change in vascular disease. Pulsatile flow can produce flow patterns that are markedly different in systole and diastole. In particular, the blood in many vessels is virtually stationary during diastole, which can be the major fraction of the cardiac cycle. In other vessels, particularly in regions distal to a stenosis, systolic

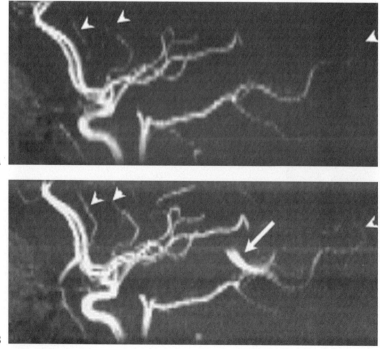

A

B

FIGURE 2.7. A comparison of a single-slab excitation through the circle of Willis with a two-slab multiple overlapping thin-slab acquisition (MOTSA) acquisition. The MOTSA acquisition retains signal in the distal small arteries *(arrowheads)* and also shows signal in the lower slab, representing the venous signal *(arrow)* entering from above (no presaturation). **A:** Single-slab repetition time/echo time = 35/7. **B:** Two-slab MOTSA, repetition time/echo time/flip angle = 35/7/25 degrees.

flow can be turbulent while diastolic flow is relatively ordered. It is then advantageous to capture signal in the desirable portion of the cardiac cycle and skip the interval with undesirable flow characteristics.

One method of accomplishing this is to use a gating approach, in which the cardiac signal is monitored and a selected gate window is chosen to cover the desired interval (46–48). This technique is very effective in studies of the lower extremities, where slow flow in diastole leads to a significant saturation of flow signal in conventional MRA studies. Placing a 200-millisecond-wide data acceptance window over peak systole ensures that data are acquired during strong inflow enhancement. On the other hand, in studies of stenotic lesions of the carotid bifurcation, gating the data acquisition to diastole makes it possible to avoid systole, in which flow is disordered.

Black Blood

Bright blood MR angiograms are limited in their ability to define the luminal edge clearly at locations of disturbed flow. At a site distal to a tight stenosis or at an acutely angled bifurcation, flow eddies may be generated. Sequences designed to refocus spins moving with constant velocity may fail to rephase the signal from the regions of disturbed flow, and a signal loss is the result. This can lead to an overestimation of the degree and particularly the extent of a stenosis. Black blood angiography is used in an attempt to avoid such overestimation (49–53).

The earliest manifestation of blood flow in clinical studies was noted in single-slice spin-echo sequences, in which flowing blood appeared as a signal void. Spin-echo sequences can

be further modified to obliterate signal from moving spins more fully while signal from stationary spins is retained. This is accomplished by adding presaturation pulses to saturate spins selectively before they enter the vessel segment of interest. Furthermore, flow compensation is removed, and the gradient lobes can be designed to accentuate intravoxel phase dispersion. Increased TEs also increase the likelihood that flowing spins will leave the selected slice during the interval between the 90-degree and 180-degree pulses, so that echo formation for those spins is prevented.

Although these techniques may be effective in reducing flow signal, it is important that signal from the stationary spins be fully captured, which is difficult to do if regions of low signal intensity, such as air or bone, are close to the vessel of interest. This situation can occur at sites such as the carotid siphon. These sequences are also unreliable in depicting a vessel lumen in which calcified plaque is present, and the appearance of a patent lumen results in an underestimation of the degree of stenosis (Fig. 2.8). The other potential problem is that slow or recirculating blood may not appear black.

Once a series of black blood slices have been acquired, the problem becomes one of display. The maximum intensity projection (MIP) algorithm, which displays structures with high signal intensity, must be modified to retain regions of minimum signal. The algorithm must also not incorporate regions of low signal intensity that are not of interest, such as bone and air.

Despite the technical limitations noted above, black blood techniques remain interesting because they are insensitive to two of the major limitations of conventional MRA methods: (a) intravoxel phase dispersion secondary to flow disturbance and (b) signal saturation, which results from the

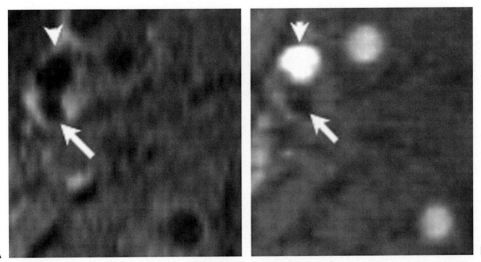

A

B

FIGURE 2.8. A comparison of a black blood image with a time-of-flight image at the same level through the neck of a patient with calcified plaque in the internal carotid artery. **A:** A T1-weighted spin-echo sequence shows a black, patent lumen *(arrowhead)* and a region of calcification *(arrow)* that has the appearance of an ulceration into the plaque. **B:** A single partition from a three-dimensional time-of-flight study at the same level shows the patent lumen as bright *(arrowhead)* and the calcification as black *(arrow)*.

repetitive pulsing of spins in transit through the excitation volume.

Radiofrequency Excitation Pulses

Much of the progress in the development of MRA has been based on improved methods of manipulating the magnetic field gradients. Additionally, the pulse programmer can use tailored RF pulses to modify signal characteristics. Although the TONE pulses referred to above are designed to retain signal from flowing blood more effectively, alternative pulses have been proposed that can selectively reduce the signal from stationary tissue while leaving the signal from flowing spins unaffected.

One such RF pulse is the fat saturation pulse, which is designed for the selective excitation of protons attached to lipids (54,55). This method makes use of the property that protons attached to lipids see a slightly different chemical environment than do protons attached to free water. Protons in fat and protons in water experience slightly different local magnetic fields and so have precessional frequencies that differ by about 220 Hz at 1.5 T. A saturating pulse (90 degrees) can therefore be delivered at the resonant frequency of fat protons to leave the magnetization of flowing blood unchanged but effectively eliminate the fat signal from the MR image. The efficiency with which this technique can be performed depends on the homogeneity of the magnetic field over the volume of excitation. In regions of the body such as the lower extremities, it can be very useful in suppressing the signal from subcutaneous fat and the signal from bone marrow, which is otherwise high (Fig. 2.9).

A mediating mechanism can also be used that exploits the different relaxation properties of protons attached to free water versus those of protons bound to membranes and other macromolecules. Bound protons have a very short T2 relaxation time and a broad spectrum of precessional frequencies. They can therefore be excited with pulses that are far from the resonance of mobile protons to saturate their magnetization strength. This in turn reduces the signal strength of mobile protons in the tissue parenchyma, which undergo a rapid exchange with the bound protons. Moving spins do not participate in this mechanism, and the magnetization of flowing blood is largely unaffected by these off-resonance excitation pulses (Fig. 2.10). This approach is termed *magnetization transfer saturation* (56–58). Both magnetization transfer saturation pulses and fat saturation pulses impose additional time requirements on pulse sequences and lengthen the minimum possible TR.

PHASE-DIFFERENCE METHODS

The contrast provided by the *longitudinal* amplitude methods described above depends on the difference in longitudinal magnetization strength between material that has received few prior excitation pulses and stationary material that has received numerous excitations during application of the RF acquisition pulse. A different approach to angiographic contrast is to modulate the phase of the *transverse* magnetization between the time of RF excitation and the time of signal acquisition (11,59).

In this approach, the phase of moving spins is purposely altered by appropriate gradient waveforms. An additional phase-modulating gradient is added to a sequence that is otherwise flow-compensated. This gradient produces a phase accumulation for a moving spin that is proportional to the ve-

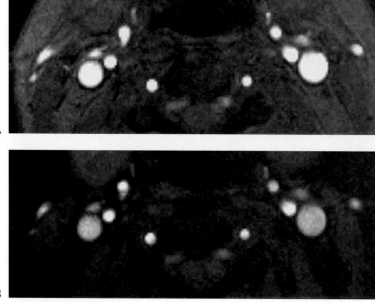

A

B

FIGURE 2.9. Comparison of images acquired with and without fat saturation. **A:** Two-dimensional single slice through the carotid bifurcation without fat saturation. **B:** Two-dimensional single slice through the carotid bifurcation with fat saturation showing strong suppression of signal and improved delineation of the blood vessels.

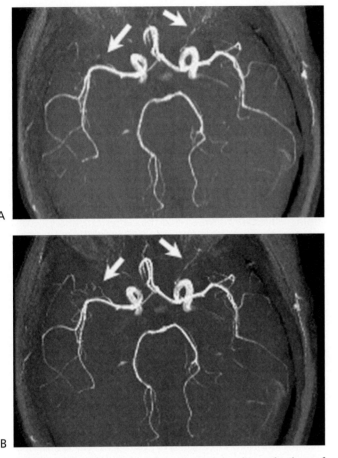

A

B

FIGURE 2.10. Comparison of maximum intensity projections of three-dimensional time-of-flight images acquired through the circle of Willis with and without magnetization transfer saturation. **A:** Without magnetization transfer saturation, small vessels *(arrows)* are hard to see because of the low level of contrast with respect to stationary tissue. **B:** With magnetization transfer saturation, increased signal saturation of the parenchyma and improved delineation of the smaller vessels are noted *(arrows).*

locity of the spin. A second image is acquired with the sense of the phase-modulation gradient reversed. In this case, the magnitude of the transverse magnetization is identical for both images, but the phase of the transverse magnetization is proportional to the flow velocity and to the duration and magnitude of the phase-modulation gradients. Provided the gradients are not too great, an image can be constructed from the raw data of the two images by subtracting their magnetization vectors. Stationary tissue magnitude and phase are identical in both data sets, and therefore the stationary tissue has no signal in the subtraction image.

The gradient strength should be selected in proportion to the velocity of flow in the vessel under investigation. With strong gradients, the method can be tailored to provide a high degree of sensitivity to slow blood flow, such as that in veins. The signal-to-noise ratio in a phase-contrast image increases as the phase difference of the magnetization of flowing spins, which is what is represented in the subtracted images, increases. However, if the combination of blood

velocity and gradient strength is too high, a phase-aliasing artifact will occur that causes signal dropout in areas of the vasculature where flow velocities are high.

Like TOF studies, phase-contrast angiograms can be obtained of 2D or 3D volumes. However, in phase contrast, because of the excellent suppression of stationary tissue signal, 2D slabs can be acquired with a thickness of several centimeters while projection views of the vasculature with good contrast properties are retained. Two-dimensional cine phase-contrast studies are capable of generating informative displays of flow dynamics as it varies over the cardiac cycle.

Because the signal intensity is proportional to the velocity of flow, the phase-contrast method can be used to determine flow velocities. Flow components can lie along any of three orthogonal directions, and it is necessary to repeat the measurements for all three spatial directions to acquire a total flow map. The total time can be reduced by acquiring one reference image and three encoded images, although the total acquisition time is still long relative to that required for the TOF method, and the phase-contrast method is susceptible to machine imperfections, such as eddy currents. Nevertheless, because of the relative insensitivity of this method to flow saturation effects and the strong suppression of signal from stationary tissue, it remains an attractive technique for slow-flow situations.

CONTRAST-ENHANCED MRA

Signal contrast in MRA is determined predominantly by blood flow patterns, whereas in conventional MRI, T1 and T2 values are of critical importance. Contrast agents have been used to advantage in MRA studies exploiting their short T1 properties (60,61). When contrast agents are used, much the same type of analysis is required as in other angiographic methods, such as spiral computed tomographic angiography, in which the initiation and duration of the contrast bolus injection relative to the interval of data acquisition must be carefully timed.

T1 Shortening

At the dosages applied in MRA studies, contrast agents act to reduce the T1 relaxation time of intraluminal blood. The T1 relaxation time of blood is of the order of 1.2 seconds at a field strength of 1.5 T, the field strength of a high-field magnet. When gadolinium contrast agents are used at sufficiently high concentrations, the T1 relaxation time of blood is reduced to less than 150 milliseconds, well below the T1 relaxation time of all tissue material. As a consequence, contrast-enhanced blood rapidly recovers magnetization and has a high degree of signal strength, even for short values of the TR.

When an MR angiogram is acquired with the use of a contrast agent, a different approach is required than in standard MRA. After a bolus injection of the contrast agent has been administered, the agent is in the arterial phase for a short interval (62,63). It is important to time the MR data acquisition so that it coincides with the period of peak arterial signal. After the arterial signal reaches a peak, its strength decreases, and the venous signal starts to increase. In conventional MRA studies of arteries, presaturation pulses are applied superior or inferior to the volume of interest to eliminate signal from the veins. In contrast-enhanced MRA, the application of presaturation pulses is not a viable strategy for eliminating venous signal. Most contrast-enhanced studies rely on the use of parameters providing the shortest possible data acquisition time, and the addition of a presaturation pulse substantially increases that time. In any event, presaturation is of limited utility because the reduced T1 values of the blood rapidly restore saturated magnetization strength.

In certain applications, it is important to be able to acquire a 3D study in a short time. For example, when extracranial carotid arteries are imaged, a short interval occurs during which the first pass of the bolus provides maximal intraarterial signal while venous enhancement, which begins shortly after the arterial phase because of the effect of the blood–brain barrier, has not yet begun. Similarly, short acquisition times are desirable in imaging vessels of the abdomen, so that studies can be obtained within a breath-hold. The use of current high-performance gradient systems permits the TE to be reduced to less than 2 milliseconds and the TR to be of the order of 5 milliseconds. This very short TR value permits the acquisition of 3D studies within 10 to 20 seconds. Conventional TOF MRA methods rely on spins with full magnetization strength flowing into the imaging volume between one excitation pulse and the next. With extremely short TR values, inflow enhancement is minimal. The signal strength in contrast-enhanced studies therefore depends heavily on the T1 relaxation time of the material in the volume.

Phase-Encoding Considerations

To achieve a rapid acquisition time, it is desirable to choose a small number of phase-encoding lines. However, one is limited by the need to achieve adequate resolution, which is the pixel size varying as field of view (FOV) divided by the number of phase-encoding lines. The FOV along the phase-encoding axis must also be large enough to accommodate the anatomy along that axis. Failure to choose a sufficiently large FOV results in misinterpretation of signal and the appearance of "wrap-around" artifact. When the vessels of interest are in the center of the anatomy, this edge artifact can be tolerated.

The overall contrast in an MR image is largely dictated by the signal measured at the center of k-space, whereas much of the high-resolution detail is determined by the periphery of k-space. Because of the time course of intravascular magnetization strength following contrast injection, the use of linear phase encoding can result either in large portions of k-space being measured before the magnetization

enhancement occurs or in the center of k-space being sampled well after the peak enhancement is over.

A wide range of alternative methods can be used to sample the k-space data points needed to create an image. Of particular relevance to contrast-enhanced MRA methods are techniques that permit the center of k-space to be measured during peak magnetization strength. One such method is centric phase encoding. For 2D, this consists first of collecting the echo with zero y-phase encoding strength, then moving out from the center of k-space to the periphery, collecting echoes with alternately positive and negative values of phase-encoding strength. The method can be extended to 3D, in which both the z-phase encoding and y-phase encoding values are varied so that the center of k-space is collected at the beginning of the data acquisition and the edges of k-space are collected later. This process has been referred to as *elliptical centric phase-encoding view order* (63).

Acquisition Timing

As in other angiographic techniques in which a contrast agent is used, the timing of image acquisition relative to passage of the contrast agent is of key importance in contrast-enhanced MRA. In some applications, multiple injections of contrast material can be administered. However, to reduce the effects of venous enhancement and exploit fully the high level of magnetization strength that prevails immediately following injection of the contrast agent, the timing of data acquisition remains important. Appropriate timing depends on the specifics of the acquisition strategy (discussed below) but can be achieved with several different approaches.

Acquisition Timing: Test Bolus

A straightforward approach to timing a sequence is the use of a test bolus (62,64). A small amount of contrast agent (e.g., 2 mL of gadolinium) is injected and followed immediately with a saline solution flush to ensure that the contrast agent does not remain in the injection tubing. A rapid imaging sequence is applied covering the anatomy of interest, and images are collected at 1-second intervals for about 50 seconds. If the image acquisition is correctly prescribed (e.g., use of a thick slab in the plane of the vessel of interest or of saturation slabs), no temporally varying inflow enhancement effects will occur, and the arrival of contrast agent at the target area will be readily apparent. This method provides a determination of the time interval between injection and peak magnetization enhancement in the region of interest.

The full study is then performed based on the previously determined time delay between injection and peak magnetization strength. The volume of gadolinium appropriate for the target vessels in question is injected, again followed by a saline solution flush, and after a delay time, the contrast-enhanced MRA sequence is initiated. Generally, the delay time in a contrast-enhanced MRA sequence is chosen such that the center of k-space is collected when the magnetization strength reaches a peak. Because the center of k-space determines the overall contrast properties of the image, this strategy ensures maximum contrast between blood and stationary material. With this approach, the high spatial frequency data are collected when magnetization strength is lower, although this compromise, which results in edge blurring, is not readily apparent in contrast-enhanced MRA images.

Acquisition Timing: Signal-Initiated Acquisition

An alternative approach to the test bolus technique is an automated method (63,65,66). A pulse sequence is initiated that samples the magnetization strength in the vessel of interest, or in a parent vessel. The sampling sequence is chosen to be a low-resolution 2D study with a rapid image acquisition time and with immediate reconstruction and display of images—a method referred to as *MR fluoroscopy*; alternatively, a line scan study is used in which signal can be sampled as often as every 20 milliseconds. After contrast injection, the sampling study is terminated as soon as signal enhancement exceeds a preset threshold, and the contrast-enhanced MRA study is begun. This technique accounts for variations in transit time that may occur when a test bolus is injected rather than a full dose. Because the contrast agent has already begun its rapid enhancement phase when the leading edge is detected, it is important to use an imaging sequence that is constructed to acquire the central portion of k-space early in the data acquisition period. For this purpose, the centric or elliptic phase-encoding strategy can be used.

Acquisition Timing: Dynamic Subtraction Contrast-Enhanced MRA

The ideal solution to the problem of determining injection timing would simply be to collect 3D image sets continuously, beginning before the injection and ending well after the agent has passed into the venous phase. If that were possible, it would no longer be necessary to synchronize data collection with the injection. Magnetization enhancement following a bolus injection occurs relatively rapidly (in 5 to 10 seconds), and to capture the phase of strong magnetization enhancement and differentiate the arterial from the venous phase, it is desirable to collect k-space data for the full 3D volume in an interval of, say, 5 seconds. Currently, 3D data sets require acquisition times that are generally of the order of 10 seconds.

This limitation can be addressed by constructing image data sets that are close in time and share k-space data (67,68). In this method, a desired temporal resolution is specified. Three-dimensional data sets can then be created within any desired temporal window by using the k-space data that are actually acquired in that window and k-space

data that are created by interpolation of the measurements made before and after the desired time window that are closest in time to the specified interval. Many specific implementations of this strategy are possible, and a typical approach is to sample the blocks of k-space that cover the middle of k-space more frequently than the blocks that cover the periphery of k-space. This method increases the likelihood that the important regions of k-space determining the overall contrast-to-noise ratio are captured during the phase when intravascular magnetization strength is high.

Zero-Filled Interpolation

Because of contrast passage considerations, contrast-enhanced MRA acquisitions are designed to collect the necessary data in as short a time as possible. Apart from the saving of time provided by the reduction in TR, scan time is often shortened by reducing the number of phase-encoding steps used, particularly along the slab select direction. The slab volume often cannot be commensurately reduced because vessel coverage would otherwise be compromised, with a loss in spatial resolution. Image presentation then suffers, particularly when the data are viewed on a plane containing the reduced resolution dimension. Image appearance can be made more visually appealing by applying an interpolation algorithm. Zero-filled interpolation operates on the basic feature of MRI that MR data are acquired with a discrete matrix (69).

When an MR image is acquired, data are collected from the true underlying magnetization distribution of the object. This magnetization distribution is continuous. In the process of image acquisition, a finite matrix of data is collected for a given FOV, which defines the image resolution. This process is the equivalent of convolving or "blurring" the continuous magnetization distribution with a point spread function that has a width equal to the acquisition resolution. The blurred image is the closest that one can get to the underlying "true" magnetization distribution. However, it is standard for MR images to present the continuous data in a lower display format; for example, for a 256-mm FOV and a 256-data matrix, the image is formed by sampling the blurred signal intensity distribution at 1-mm spatial intervals and linearly interpolating the intensities between these points. The "raw" data (i.e., magnetization magnitude and phase) are collected in any event and contain all the information necessary to construct the variations in intensity of the "blurred" image correctly at arbitrarily small spatial intervals. This process of reconstructing the image at smaller spatial steps than those of the acquired resolution is termed *zero-filled interpolation.*

In practice, the process of zero-filled interpolation doubles the data file size with every successive order of interpolation, and it is unusual for zero-filled interpolation to be performed with other than a factor of two increases in image matrix size. It is important to realize that even with infinitely small image reconstruction steps, the final reconstructed image will only approach the "blurred" image, and the image acquisition resolution simply remains the value obtained by dividing the FOV by the matrix. Another way of saying this is that zero-filled interpolation does not improve the inherent resolution of the acquired data, but it restores some of the resolution that conventional MR image reconstruction loses through linear interpolation.

Imaging Parameters

The MR technologist is able to select several imaging parameters that affect the quality of a contrast-enhanced MR angiogram. These include the flip angle and timing parameters, such as TR and TE. Other parameters, such as the phase-encoding ordering schemes, are determined by the pulse sequence programmer. In conventional MRA, evaluating the specific impact of parameter variations on image appearance is straightforward. However, it is more difficult in contrast-enhanced MRA because the initial contrast bolus affects the image appearance of all subsequent injections. Parameters have been chosen based on theoretic considerations, phantom studies, and limited human studies.

The choice of TR is dictated by the desirability of very short acquisition times that permit breath-hold studies and capture the phase as the contrast material reaches peak concentration in the arteries. The minimum value of TR that can be prescribed depends on the structure of the pulse sequence. This again is related to the need to apply gradients of magnetic field to encode the spatial location of the magnetization, and particularly to form and measure the "echo." Increasing the strength of the applied gradient used while the echo is measured decreases the time needed to measure the signal. However, it also decreases the signal-to-noise ratio. The minimum TR is therefore a compromise between signal-to-noise ratio and acquisition time.

In conventional TOF MRA, the flip angle is a sensitive determinant of the overall quality of the image. In particular, because the T1 of blood is longer than that of most tissue, a flip angle greater than 30 degrees in a 3D study typically results in saturation of signal in the distal territories of the vessels of interest. In contrast-enhanced MRA, the T1 of blood is significantly shorter than that of the surrounding tissue; these studies are more forgiving with respect to the specific flip angle chosen, and flip angles between 30 and 60 degrees are found to be satisfactory. The optimal flip angle depends somewhat on the TR chosen, and some saturation will occur for larger flip angles with very short TR values.

Advantages of Contrast-Enhanced MRA

The use of contrast agents in MRA offers three main advantages. First, the total time required to collect data for a 3D study is quite short, of the order of 10 to 20 seconds. This means that gross patient motion can be substantially re-duced. Studies of the visceral arteries can be performed in a single breath-hold (70–72). With TOF methods, studies of the extracranial carotid arteries take up to 10 minutes to acquire, and patient activities such as swallowing, snoring, and neck movements can substantially degrade image quality. Short-duration contrast-enhanced MRA largely avoids these problems (Fig. 2.11). The second major advantage is increased coverage. Because TOF methods rely on inflow enhancement, signal strength in distal vessels is diminished, and the only way to ensure a uniformly high vascular signal through a large volume is to use multiple overlapping subvolumes to cover the region of interest. This results in long acquisition times, inefficient data because of overlap requirements, and the increased possibility of patient motion. Provided contrast material fills the vessels of interest, contrast-enhanced MRA can be used to cover a very large volume with excellent contrast-to-noise properties (Fig. 2.12). The third major benefit of contrast-enhanced MRA is that because of the signal strength, sequences can be applied with a high bandwidth to allow very short TEs yet an adequate signal-to-noise ratio. All MRA sequences benefit from reduced echo times because they restrict the signal loss associated with disordered flow.

Limitations of Contrast-Enhanced MRA

Contrast-enhanced MRA also entails several disadvantages. A principal disadvantage is the need to inject a contrast agent, despite the low-risk profile of side effects of the agents in use (73). Although the actual data acquisition time is reduced, preparation time is increased because of the need to place an intravenous line before the patient enters the scanner. The administration of an injection requires the presence of additional personnel, which, together with the cost of the contrast agent, adds to the cost of the study. As noted above, a major concern is the presence of venous signal that increases with time following the injection. This has proved to be a major obstacle in studies of the intracranial circulation, particularly in the circle of Willis, where venous signal in the cavernous sinus obscures a delineation of the arterial lumen, and in the lower extremities, where veins and arteries abut each other. An additional limitation of contrast-enhanced MRA is the time constraint imposed by the need to capture the high-intensity signal during the short arterial phase. Even with the extremely short TRs used, 3D studies can be acquired only by compromising in terms of coverage or resolution.

The very strong suppression of signal from stationary material is advantageous for the visualization of vascular contours. Conventional MRA sequences also strongly suppress stationary material signal but retain considerably more signal than do contrast-enhanced MRA sequences. Stationary material signal can add valuable information to a study of vascular pathology. At regions of stenosis, conventional MRA sequences often show features of the

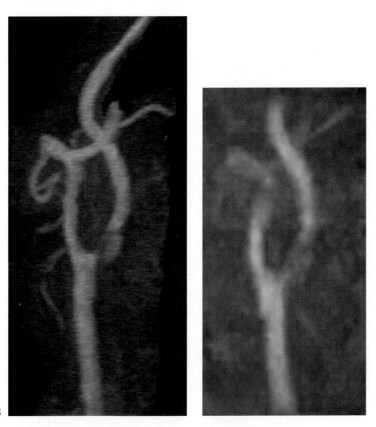

A,B

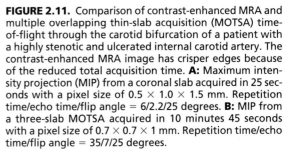

FIGURE 2.11. Comparison of contrast-enhanced MRA and multiple overlapping thin-slab acquisition (MOTSA) time-of-flight through the carotid bifurcation of a patient with a highly stenotic and ulcerated internal carotid artery. The contrast-enhanced MRA image has crisper edges because of the reduced total acquisition time. **A:** Maximum intensity projection (MIP) from a coronal slab acquired in 25 seconds with a pixel size of 0.5 × 1.0 × 1.5 mm. Repetition time/echo time/flip angle = 6/2.2/25 degrees. **B:** MIP from a three-slab MOTSA acquired in 10 minutes 45 seconds with a pixel size of 0.7 × 0.7 × 1 mm. Repetition time/echo time/flip angle = 35/7/25 degrees.

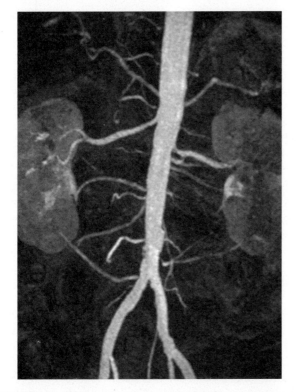

FIGURE 2.12. Maximum intensity projection from a contrast-enhanced MRA study of the aorta and renal arteries showing excellent signal retention through the aorta into the distal renal arteries and iliac arteries. Repetition time/echo time/flip angle = 4.6/1.8/25 degrees. Total acquisition time = 21 seconds.

atheromatous plaque that cannot be seen with contrast-enhanced MRA. The extent of atheroma can be assessed, and features such as high-signal hematomas are easily noted on TOF studies.

POSTPROCESSING AND DISPLAY

MRA studies cover a 3D volume either by acquiring multiple 2D slices or by providing an explicit 3D study of the volume of interest that produces a series of 2D partition images. Very rarely, a substantial portion of the vessel of interest lies within a single partition. More commonly, each slice contains a small segment of the vessel of interest. Overall interpretation of the relationship of one vessel segment to another is difficult. The analysis of complex vascular anatomy, in particular the tortuous 3D paths of most vessels, is greatly facilitated by postprocessing algorithms that provide a general overview of the anatomy. Several algorithms have been investigated that provide projection capability. The one most commonly used is the MIP technique (74).

Maximum Intensity Projection Algorithm

The MIP algorithm exploits the property of MRA sequences that signal from moving spins is high whereas that from stationary spins is low. It should be emphasized that the MIP is a postprocessing algorithm—it can be implemented any time after the data have been collected. Processing of the data can be performed without additional acquisitions or increased scan time.

The algorithm first specifies the desired viewing plane. Once the viewing plane has been specified, an imaginary ray is projected perpendicular to a given pixel in that viewing plane through the 3D data set. The algorithm then searches through all voxels in the acquired 3D data set that lie along the specified ray and determines the signal strength of the voxel with the highest signal intensity. That intensity value is then assigned to the image pixel in the viewing plane that is being generated. This process is repeated for every pixel in the viewing plane to create a projection image. This approach should be compared with the image created in x-ray projection. In that case, the projection image represents a summation of all attenuation effects along the path traversed by the x-ray. In MRA, stationary material typically has signal strength, albeit substantially less than that of the flow signal. If one were to perform a summation projection of an MR data set, the flow signal would be buried in the signal from the stationary background.

The MIP algorithm is attractive because it is not computationally intensive. It is easy to prescribe and extremely helpful in providing access to the projection views. The MIP provides a roadmap to overall vessel anatomy and can indicate sites of probable disease. Decisions can then be made, based on the appearance of the MIP, regarding whether to run an additional sequence focused on the suspect area and what volume the MRA sequence should cover.

Limitations of Maximum Intensity Projection

Although the MIP algorithm is quick and easy to use, it is known to generate significant artifacts (75,76). A common problem is that the strength of a low intravascular signal in the base images can appear to be less than that of stationary material (e.g., fat or hemorrhage, or after contrast agents have been administered). In that case, the stationary signal will be mapped to the projection image and information will be lost. This can result in images with the appearance of clinically significant disease, such as stenosis or occlusion. It is important to keep in mind that the MIP is only a convenience, and that the base images contain additional information that can be pivotal in correctly interpreting a study.

Because artifacts of the kind referred to above are a function of the volume of data being processed (the probability of including high-signal stationary material increases as the volume increases), it is important to limit postprocessing to as small a volume as possible to include the vessel of interest fully but exclude unwanted stationary signal. The probability of including a voxel from stationary material with a higher signal strength than that of the flowing material in-

creases as the thickness of the stationary material included in the data set increases. The contrast in the MIP can therefore be improved by restricting the MIP to a volume that includes only the immediate vicinity of the vessels of interest. This can be performed iteratively by using MIP images on three orthogonal planes as a guide in defining the volume to be included for postprocessing. This process is fairly user-intensive, although the algorithms are sufficiently fast that the data sets can be manipulated in a few minutes with the use of high-performance array processors. In addition, the technique can be used to eliminate overlapping vessels.

Reformatting

It is often extremely useful to view vascular contours in planes other from that of the native acquisition. A change in luminal cross-section, for example, is often more readily identified on longitudinal views of the vessel than on slices transverse to the vessel (77). Because no overlapping background signal is present that might obscure the vessel, this technique provides the strongest achievable contrast. Both 2D and 3D data sets covering a volume of interest can be reformatted to generate views with arbitrary orientations to the original data set. The presentation is particularly appealing for 3D data sets that have been acquired with isotropic voxels (i.e., voxels that have the same length along all three axes). In this case, reformatted images can be created with comparable resolution in any obliquity. The disadvantage of this approach is that it is labor-intensive. The appropriate planes must be interactively specified by the user and cannot be automated. Further, the resultant image provides a depiction of the data through only one plane. It is sometimes advantageous to create an MIP image of a small number of reformatted images to retain good contrast and acquire an overview of the vessels and a desirable viewing plane.

Further processing can be invoked that makes use of depth information. Volume-rendering techniques provide information on spatial relationships between vessels and soft-tissue structures (78,79). Surface rendering can also be used with virtual light sources to obtain images with intensity proportional to the surface gradients; these provide information on the texture of vessels.

SUMMARY

MR methods provide a wide range of approaches that can be used to obtain images of blood vessels with high contrast and good resolution. The ability to determine the course of a vessel through 3D space and the relation of the vasculature to surrounding soft tissue is of great value. MRA methods are extremely useful in the routine clinical evaluation of vascular disease. They are also valuable to the researcher interested in the onset and progression of vascular disease and in developing methods for treating these disorders.

ACKNOWLEDGMENTS

Support from a Veterans Administration MERIT Review Grant and National Institutes of Health grants HL56307 and HL61806 is acknowledged.

REFERENCES

1. Milnor WR. *Hemodynamics*. Baltimore: Williams & Wilkins, 1989:xii, 419.
2. Strandness DE, Sumner DS. *Hemodynamics for surgeons. Modern surgical monographs*. New York: Grune & Stratton, 1975:xi, 698.
3. Stroud JS, Berger SA, Saloner D. Influence of stenosis morphology on flow through severely stenotic vessels: implications for plaque rupture. *J Biomechanics* 2000;33:443–455.
4. Dumoulin CL, Cline HE, Souza SP, et al. Three-dimensional time-of-flight magnetic resonance angiography using spin saturation. *Magn Reson Med* 1989;11:35–46.
5. Dumoulin CL, Souza SP, Walker MF, et al. Three-dimensional phase contrast angiography. *Magn Reson Med* 1989;9:139–149.
6. Haacke EM, Masaryk TJ. The salient features of MR angiography. *Radiology* 1989;173:611–612.
7. Laub GA, Kaiser WA. MR angiography with gradient motion refocusing. *J Comput Assist Tomogr* 1988;12:377–382.
8. Lenz GW, Haacke EM, Masaryk TJ, et al. In-plane vascular imaging: pulse sequence design and strategy. *Radiology* 1988;166: 875–882.
9. Masaryk TJ, Tkach J, Glicklich M. Flow, radiofrequency pulse sequences, and gradient magnetic fields: basic interactions and adaptations to angiographic imaging. *Top Magn Reson Imaging* 1991;3:1–11.
10. Prince MR. Contrast-enhanced MR angiography: theory and optimization. *Magn Reson Imaging Clin N Am* 1998;6:257–267.
11. Moran PR. A flow velocity zeugmatographic interlace for NMR imaging in humans. *Magn Reson Imaging* 1982;1:197–203.
12. Constantinesco A, Mallet JJ, Bonmartin A, et al. Spatial or flow velocity phase encoding gradients in NMR imaging. *Magn Reson Imaging* 1984;2:335–340.
13. Pattany PM, Phillips JJ, Chiu LC, et al. Motion artifact suppression technique (MAST) for MR imaging. *J Comput Assist Tomogr* 1987;11:369–377.
14. Saloner D. Flow and motion. *Magn Reson Imaging Clin N Am* 1999;7:699–715.
15. Xiang QS, Nalcioglu O. Differential flow imaging by NMR. *Magn Reson Med* 1989;12:14–24.
16. Lee JN, Riederer SJ, Pelc NJ. Flow-compensated limited flip angle MR angiography. *Magn Reson Med* 1989;12:1–13.
17. Tkach JA, Lin W, Duda JJ Jr, et al. Optimizing three-dimensional time-of-flight MR angiography with variable repetition time. *Radiology* 1994;191:805–811.
18. Tkach JA, Ruggieri PM, Ross JS, et al. Pulse sequence strategies for vascular contrast in time-of-flight carotid MR angiography. *J Magn Reson Imaging* 1993;3:811–820.
19. Urchuk SN, Plewes DB. Mechanisms of flow-induced signal loss in MR angiography. *J Magn Reson Imaging* 1992;2:453–462.
20. Gao JH, Holland SK, Gore JC. Nuclear magnetic resonance signal from flowing nuclei in rapid imaging using gradient echoes. *Med Phys* 1988;15:809–814.
21. Saloner D. Determinants of image appearance in contrast-enhanced magnetic resonance angiography. A review. *Invest Radiol* 1998;33:488–495.
22. Gullberg GT, Wehrli FW, Shimakawa A, et al. MR vascular imaging with a fast gradient refocusing pulse sequence and reformatted images from transaxial sections. *Radiology* 1987;165:241–246.
23. Keller PJ, Drayer BP, Fram EK, et al. MR angiography with two-dimensional acquisition and three-dimensional display. Work in progress. *Radiology* 1989;173:527–532.
24. Ruggieri PM, Laub GA, Masaryk TJ, et al. Intracranial circulation: pulse-sequence considerations in three-dimensional (volume) MR angiography. *Radiology* 1989;171:785–791.
25. Edelman RR, Atkinson DJ, Silver MS, et al. FRODO pulse sequences: a new means of eliminating motion, flow, and wraparound artifacts. *Radiology* 1988;166:231–236.
26. Felmlee JP, Ehman RL. Spatial presaturation: a method for suppressing flow artifacts and improving depiction of vascular anatomy in MR imaging. *Radiology* 1987;164:559–564.
27. Gao JH, Holland SK, Gore JC. Effects of gradient timing and spatial resolution on the NMR signal from flowing blood. *Phys Med Biol* 1992;37:1581–1588.
28. Oshinski JN, Ku DN, Pettigrew RI. Turbulent fluctuation velocity: the most significant determinant of signal loss in stenotic vessels. *Magn Reson Med* 1995;33:193–199.
29. Duerk JL, Simonetti OP, Hurst GC, et al. Experimental confirmation of phase encoding of instantaneous derivatives of position. *Magn Reson Med* 1994;32:77–87.
30. Ehman RL, Felmlee JP. Flow artifact reduction in MRI: a review of the roles of gradient moment nulling and spatial presaturation. *Magn Reson Med* 1990;14:293–307.
31. Nishimura DG, Macovski A, Jackson JI, et al. Magnetic resonance angiography by selective inversion recovery using a compact gradient echo sequence. *Magn Reson Med* 1988;8:96–103.
32. Schmalbrock P, Yuan C, Chakeres DW, et al. Volume MR angiography: methods to achieve very short echo times. *Radiology* 1990;175:861–865.
33. Wehrli FW, Perkins TG, Shimakawa A, et al. Chemical shift-induced amplitude modulations in images obtained with gradient refocusing. *Magn Reson Imaging* 1987;5:157–158.
34. Gatenby JC, McCauley TR, Gore JC. Mechanisms of signal loss in magnetic resonance imaging of stenoses. *Med Phys* 1993;20:1049–1057.
35. Evans AJ, Richardson DB, Tien R, et al. Poststenotic signal loss in MR angiography: effects of echo time, flow compensation, and fractional echo. *AJNR Am J Neuroradiol* 1993;14:721–729.
36. Atkinson D, Brant-Zawadzki M, Gillan G, et al. Improved MR angiography: magnetization transfer suppression with variable flip angle excitation and increased resolution. *Radiology* 1994;190:890–894.
37. Roditi GH, Smith FW, Redpath TW. Evaluation of tilted, optimized, non-saturating excitation pulses in 3D magnetic resonance angiography of the abdominal aorta and major branches in volunteers. *Br J Radiol* 1994;67:11–13.
38. Nägele T, Klose U, Grodd W, et al. The effects of linearly increasing flip angles on 3D inflow MR angiography. *Magn Reson Med* 1994;31:561–566.
39. Parker DL, Yuan C, Blatter DD. MR angiography by multiple thin slab 3D acquisition. *Magn Reson Med* 1991;17:434–451.
40. Davis WL, Blatter DD, Harnsberger HR, et al. Intracranial MR angiography: comparison of single-volume three-dimensional time-of-flight and multiple overlapping thin slab acquisition techniques. *AJR Am J Roentgenol* 1994;163:915–920.
41. Nishimura DG, Jackson JI, Pauly JM. On the nature and reduction of the displacement artifact in flow images. *Magn Reson Med* 1991;22:481–492.
42. von Schulthess GK, Higgins CB. Blood flow imaging with MR: spin-phase phenomena. *Radiology* 1985;157:687–695.
43. Frank LR, Buxton RB, Kerber CW. Pulsatile flow artifacts in 3D magnetic resonance imaging. *Magn Reson Med* 1993;30:296–304.

44. Meyer CH, Hu BS, Nishimura DG, et al. Fast spiral coronary artery imaging. *Magn Reson Med* 1992;28:202–213.

45. Nishimura DG, Irarrazabal P, Meyer CH. A velocity k-space analysis of flow effects in echo-planar and spiral imaging. *Magn Reson Med* 1995;33:549–556.

46. de Graaf RG, Groen JP. MR angiography with pulsatile flow. *Magn Reson Imaging* 1992;10:25–34.

47. Saloner D, Selby K, Anderson CM. MRA studies of arterial stenosis: improvements by diastolic acquisition. *Magn Reson Med* 1994;31:196–203.

48. Selby K, Saloner D, Anderson CM, et al. MR angiography with a cardiac-phase–specific acquisition window. *J Magn Reson Imaging* 1992;2:637–643.

49. Finn JP, Edelman RR. Black-blood and segmented k-space magnetic resonance angiography. *Magn Reson Imaging Clin N Am* 1993;1:349–357.

50. Chien D, Goldmann A, Edelman RR. High-speed black blood imaging of vessel stenosis in the presence of pulsatile flow. *J Magn Reson Imaging* 1992;2:437–441.

51. Edelman RR, Chien D, Kim D. Fast selective black blood MR imaging. *Radiology* 1991;181:655–660.

52. Jara H, Barish MA. Black-blood MR angiography. Techniques and clinical applications. *Magn Reson Imaging Clin N Am* 1999;7:303–317.

53. Melhem ER, Jara H, Yucel EK. Black blood MR angiography using multislab three-dimensional TI-weighted turbo spin-echo technique: imaging of intracranial circulation. *AJR Am J Roentgenol* 1997;169:1418–1420.

54. Li D, Haacke EM, Mugler JP 3rd, et al. Three-dimensional time-of-flight MR angiography using selective inversion recovery RAGE with fat saturation and ECG-triggering: application to renal arteries. *Magn Reson Med* 1994;31:414–422.

55. Robison RO, Blatter DD, Parker DL, et al. Fat suppression in combination with multiple overlapping thin-slab 3-D acquisition MR angiography: proposed technique for improved vessel visualization. *AJNR Am J Neuroradiol* 1992;13:1429–1434.

56. Lin W, Tkach JA, Haacke EM, et al. Intracranial MR angiography: application of magnetization transfer contrast and fat saturation to short gradient-echo, velocity-compensated sequences. *Radiology* 1993;186:753–761.

57. Mathews VP, Ulmer JL, White ML, et al. Depiction of intracranial vessels with MRA: utility of magnetization transfer saturation and gadolinium. *J Comput Assist Tomogr* 1999;23:597–602.

58. Pike GB, Hu BS, Glover GH, et al. Magnetization transfer time-of-flight magnetic resonance angiography. *Magn Reson Med* 1992;25:372–379.

59. Bryant DJ, Payne JA, Firmin DN, et al. Measurement of flow with NMR imaging using a gradient pulse and phase difference technique. *J Comput Assist Tomogr* 1984;8:588–593.

60. Marchal G, Michiels J, Bosmans H, et al. Contrast-enhanced MRA of the brain. *J Comput Assist Tomogr* 1992;16:25–29.

61. Prince MR, Yucel EK, Kaufman JA, et al. Dynamic gadolinium-enhanced three-dimensional abdominal MR arteriography. *J Magn Reson Imaging* 1993;3:877–881.

62. Kim JK, Farb RI, Wright GA. Test bolus examination in the carotid artery at dynamic gadolinium-enhanced MR angiography [see Comments]. *Radiology* 1998;206:283–289.

63. Wilman AH, Riederer SJ, King BF, et al. Fluoroscopically triggered contrast-enhanced three-dimensional MR angiography with elliptical centric view order: application to the renal arteries. *Radiology* 1997;205:137–146.

64. Earls JP, Rofsky NM, DeCorato DR, et al. Hepatic arterial-phase dynamic gadolinium-enhanced MR imaging: optimization with a test examination and a power injector. *Radiology* 1997;202:268–273.

65. Foo TK, Saranathan M, Prince MR, et al. Automated detection of bolus arrival and initiation of data acquisition in fast, three-dimensional, gadolinium-enhanced MR angiography. *Radiology* 1997;203:275–280.

66. Ho VB, Choyke PL, Foo TK, et al. Automated bolus chase peripheral MR angiography: initial practical experiences and future directions of this work-in-progress. *J Magn Reson Imaging* 1999;10:376–388.

67. Korosec FR, Frayne R, Grist TM, et al. Time-resolved contrast-enhanced 3D MR angiography. *Magn Reson Med* 1996;36:345–351.

68. Mistretta CA, Grist TM, Korosec FR, et al. 3D time-resolved contrast-enhanced MR DSA: advantages and tradeoffs. *Magn Reson Med* 1998;40:571–581.

69. Du YP, Parker DL, Davis WL, et al. Reduction of partial-volume artifacts with zero-filled interpolation in three-dimensional MR angiography. *J Magn Reson Imaging* 1994;4:733–741.

70. Leung DA, Hany TF, Debatin JF. Three-dimensional contrast-enhanced magnetic resonance angiography of the abdominal arterial system. *Cardiovasc Intervent Radiol* 1998;21:1–10.

71. Leung DA, McKinnon GC, Davis CP, et al. Breath-hold, contrast-enhanced, three-dimensional MR angiography. *Radiology* 1996;200:569–571.

72. Prince MR, Narasimham DL, Stanley JC, et al. Breath-hold gadolinium-enhanced MR angiography of the abdominal aorta and its major branches. *Radiology* 1995;197:785–792.

73. Niendorf HP, Dinger JC, Haustein J, et al. Tolerance data of Gd-DTPA: a review. *Eur J Radiol* 1991;13:15–20.

74. Laub G. Displays for MR angiography. *Magn Reson Med* 1990;14:222–229.

75. Tsuruda J, Saloner D, Norman D. Artifacts associated with MR neuroangiography. *AJNR Am J Neuroradiol* 1992;13:1411–1422.

76. Anderson CM, Saloner D, Tsuruda JS, et al. Artifacts in maximum-intensity-projection display of MR angiograms. *AJR Am J Roentgenol* 1990;154:623–629.

77. Anderson CM, Lee RE, Levin DL, et al. Measurement of internal carotid artery stenosis from source MR angiograms. *Radiology* 1994;193:219–226.

78. Hu X, Alperin N, Levin DN, et al. Visualization of MR angiographic data with segmentation and volume-rendering techniques. *J Magn Reson Imaging* 1991;1:539–546.

79. Shapiro LB, Tien RD, Golding SJ, et al. Preliminary results of a modified surface rendering technique in the display of magnetic resonance angiography images. *Magn Reson Imaging* 1994;12:461–468.

CARDIAC PHYSIOLOGY: IMAGING ASPECTS

FRANK RADEMAKERS

The technical capabilities of cardiovascular MR (CMR), and consequently the clinical situations in which it can contribute to better patient management, continue to expand. However, to be able to translate technical improvements into improved patient care requires a good understanding of cardiovascular physiology and pathophysiology. The purpose of this chapter is therefore to (re)introduce some of the general concepts of cardiovascular physiology that can be of use in the interpretation of CMR still images, flow curves, and cine loops.

From the early days of Galen (about 200 A.D.) and through the times of Servetus (1511), Vesalius (1514), Harvey (1578), Frank (1895), Starling (1918), and many others, the anatomy and function of the heart have fascinated scientists all over the world (Fig. 3.1). Even today, not all the anatomic and functional aspects of the heart are fully understood. The fiber organization in bundles, laminae, and sheets remains a topic of discussion, and the famous Frank-Starling law cannot be fully explained by present knowledge. Although experimental techniques based on molecular technology are rapidly adding to our understanding of some of the basic mechanisms, a noninvasive method like CMR, with the ability to provide a comprehensive evaluation of anatomy, regional and global function, and flow and perfusion, can shed new light on the function and performance of the human heart *in vivo*. Cardiovascular disease remains the most important killer in the Western world, so

that a technique that provides comprehensive information noninvasively and repetitively in an aging population is of great value. Because of the need for a combination of advanced technical skills and a good knowledge of anatomy, physiology, pathophysiology, and patient management, a close cooperation between all disciplines involved will be required for the successful application of this technology.

In this chapter, the text in which the specific capabilities of CMR are discussed is italicized.

FUNCTIONAL ANATOMY

General Anatomy

The heart, as a muscle and pump, consists of two serial systems, joined in one organ enveloped by the pericardium. It weighs between 250 and 350 g and is located in the mediastinum. It extends obliquely from the second rib to the fifth intercostal space and spans about 13 cm.

The heart rests on the superior surface of the diaphragm and is flanked and partially covered by the lungs. Its broad base is directed toward the right shoulder, and the apex points inferiorly toward the left hip. It has four chambers, two inferiorly located ventricles and two superiorly located atria. The heart is divided longitudinally by the fibrous interatrial and the muscular interventricular septum. The right ventricle (RV) is the most anterior part of the heart, and the pulmonary trunk is the most anterior vessel. The left ventricle (LV) forms the inferoposterior part of the heart and the apex.

F. Rademakers: Department of Cardiology, Catholic University Leuven, Leuven, Belgium.

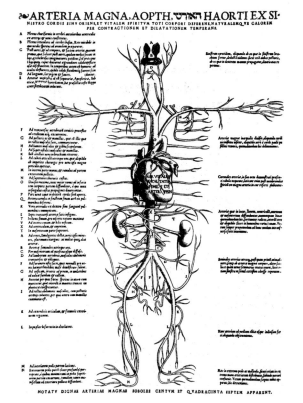

FIGURE 3.1. Andreas Vesalius (1514–1564) *Tabulae Anatomicae:* schematic of the circulation.

Several grooves (usually filled with epicardial fat) are visible on the surface of the heart, delineating the different cavities and carrying the blood vessels supplying the myocardium. The atrioventricular groove, or coronary sulcus, encircles the junction between the atria and ventricles and contains the right coronary artery, circumflex coronary artery, and coronary sinus. The anterior interventricular groove lies at the anterior junction of the RV and LV and contains the anterior descending coronary artery and the great cardiac vein. The posterior interventricular sulcus marks the same junction on the inferoposterior surface of the heart and contains the posterior descending artery, which can originate from the circumflex or right coronary artery, and the middle cardiac vein. The small cardiac vein runs along the right inferior margin of the heart and empties into the coronary sinus, just before the latter ends in the right atrium (RA).

Defining Regions and Surfaces

Defining the several surfaces and regions of the heart differs depending on the imaging technique, so that a great deal of confusion can arise when results of echocardiographic, nuclear, angiographic and CMR studies are compared. Part of the confusion derives from the reference point used and part from the changing position of the heart in the thoracic cavity that is associated mainly with aging but also with disease.

At a younger age, the heart is more vertically positioned, with a smaller "diaphragmatic" part and a larger "posterior" part.

With aging and in pulmonary disease, the heart assumes a more horizontal position, and the apex is more laterally located; as a result, the contact area with the diaphragm is larger, and the "posterior" face of the heart is more "inferior." It is clear that the confusion in nomenclature stems from definitions, which are based on either external references, body anatomy, or cardiac anatomy. A good example is a comparison of *echo* with *angio. Echo* adapts the acoustic window to obtain a standard view of the heart and from there defines the different regions; *angio* uses a standard external positioning of the x-ray tubes and defines regions from the projection boundaries thus obtained. *CMR provides an unlimited choice of image planes; one can therefore choose standardized two-dimensional slices of the heart (e.g., two-chamber, four-chamber, short-axis slices) and use intrinsic cardiac anatomy (insertion of RV, papillary muscles) as the reference for naming the different regions. On the other hand, because of its large field of view, it is extremely well suited to depict the relationship of the heart to the surrounding structures and to identify masses (i.e., tumors) extending from the surrounding area into the heart or vice versa. When standard transverse, sagittal, or frontal views are used, the same problems encountered with* angio *arise, and one has to be aware of the impact of different positions of the heart in the thorax on naming surfaces and regions.*

Circulation

The right side of the heart accepts desaturated blood from the body through the inferior and superior venae cavae and from the heart itself through the coronary sinus and pumps it through the pulmonary circulation. The left side of the heart receives oxygenated blood from the four pulmonary veins and pumps it into the aorta, from which it is distributed through the systemic circulation to the entire body.

Atria

Blood is continuously received in the thin-walled, muscular atria. During systole, when the atrioventricular valves are closed, the atria have a reservoir function, and during filling, they function as conduits. Only during atrial contraction do they have an active, boosting function, optimizing ventricular filling. Because no valves are present at the entrance of the veins into the atria, some retrograde blood flow occurs at the time of atrial contraction. Only the inflow regions of the atria are smooth; the auriculae and the anterior wall are muscular and even have muscle bundles, called the *pectinate muscles.*

Several other structures can be recognized, mainly in the RA. The origin of the inferior vena cava is delineated by the eustachian valve, which is intended to direct blood from the inferior vena cava toward the interatrial septum, where it crosses the foramen ovale in the prenatal circulation. After birth (and normally the closure of the foramen ovale, which remains as a depression on the interatrial septum), this flow deviation persists, often with some acceleration and turbulence. Higher in the atrium, but continuous with the eustachian valve, the Chiari network spans the atrium with small chords that can be mistaken for thrombi or vegetations. On the posterior surface of the atrium, the crista terminalis delineates the smooth inlet portion of the RA from the highly trabecular auricula and can sometimes be very prominent.

The left atrium (LA) receives the four pulmonary veins and has an appendage with a much smaller orifice than that in the RA. The LA appendage may contain thrombi, certainly in cases of atrial fibrillation, and can be the origin of thrombotic cerebral or peripheral disease.

CMR can accurately identify the veins emptying in the atria and abnormal (mostly) right venous return to the RA or superior vena cava. Flow in the pulmonary veins, used to analyze LV diastolic function, can be easily obtained, but optimal temporal resolution is required. Abnormal structures or masses seen on echocardiography can be identified as normal, anatomic variants or as true thrombi or tumors.

Valves

During diastole, blood flows from the atria into the ventricles through the mitral and tricuspid valves. The mitral valve, resembling a bishop's miter, has a larger anterior and a smaller posterior leaflet. Each leaflet is a flexible, thin sheath of connective tissue that is attached firmly to the mitral valve annulus. The annulus has the shape of a horseshoe, is flexible, does not lie in one plane, and changes shape during the filling phase. On the right side, the tricuspid valve has three leaflets (anterior, posterior, and septal) that differ in size and shape; therefore, this valve is very difficult to evaluate morphologically because it can never be captured in one plane. The mitral and tricuspid valves are suspended in the ventricles by the chordae tendineae. These are thin, tendinous structures connecting the free edges but also some neighboring parts of the valves to the papillary muscles, which are elongated protrusions of the muscular wall of the ventricles. Contraction of the papillary muscles during systole prevents the atrioventricular valves from prolapsing into the atria as pressure rises in the ventricles.

During systole, blood is expelled from the ventricles through the aortic valve and the pulmonary semilunar valve into the aorta and pulmonary artery, respectively. Both the aortic valve and the pulmonary valve are tricuspid, consisting of three pocket-like cusps that are freely suspended in the valve ring.

It is difficult with regular CMR to image fast-moving valve structures, but newer techniques (i.e., valve tracking) provide an accurate visualization of valve leaflets and openings and permit the direct quantification of a stenotic valve area. However, structures with fast, irregular movements, such as endocarditis lesions, can be missed.

Ventricles

The major difference between the left and right sides of the heart is the difference in load level. The pulmonary circulation is a short, low-pressure system that works at a peak pressure of 25 mm Hg, whereas the left side of the heart operates at pressures up to 125 mm Hg and drives a much longer circuit. This difference has major structural consequences; the wall of the right side of the heart is much thinner than that of the left side (2 to 3 mm vs. 9 mm). The purpose of this difference is to normalize wall tension and the tension on myocardial fibers in the wall (Fig. 3.2).

Tension is very difficult to measure or calculate, but it is roughly directly proportional to the pressure in the cavity and the diameter of the cavity and inversely proportional to the thickness of the wall. Other factors, such as the shape and curvature of the ventricle, also play a role. The more curved the surface, the lower the tension; the flatter the surface, the higher the tension.

A major consequence of the structural difference between the ventricles is the way in which they eject blood. The left ventricle must overcome a much larger afterload, and pressure in the cavity must increase to aortic pressure before ejection can start; the former is accomplished mainly by the contraction of fibers running circumferentially (in the midportion of the wall) and the latter by the contraction of more obliquely oriented fibers, which leads to thickening and longitudinal shortening, an inward motion of the endocardium, and ejection. On the right side, the pressure that must be overcome is much lower; therefore, ejection starts earlier (the pulmonary valve opens before the aortic valve) and is accomplished mainly by segmental shortening (mostly in the long axis) of the crescent-shaped ventricle rather than by wall thickening. Because the resistance to ejection is lower, the contraction continues for a longer time, and the pulmonary valve closes after the aortic valve.

CMR can image both ventricles in great detail, and the newer sequences [e.g., fast imaging with steady-state precession (FISP)] can show the marked intraventricular trabeculation. Because the entire ventricle can be imaged with a stack of short-

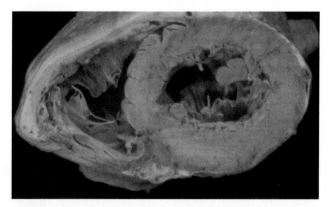

FIGURE 3.2. Transverse section through the left and right ventricles.

axis slices, the entire wall is encompassed, and the LV mass can be quantified with great accuracy and reproducibility. At the same time, intraventricular volumes are obtained, and when both end-diastolic and end-systolic frames are acquired, LV volumes, stroke volume, and ejection fraction can be calculated. True wall thickness, with tapering of the wall taken into account, can be determined by three-dimensional (3D) imaging combining short- and long-axis information.

Myofiber Structure

As alluded to, the myofiber structure in the walls of the ventricles is very intricate. Although some layers can be recognized in the RV, they are most prominent in the LV. The middle layer is mostly circumferential (circular in short-axis views), whereas the more epicardial and endocardial layers are obliquely oriented but in an opposite sense; when the ventricle is viewed with the base at the top, the epicardial fibers run from base left to apex right, the endocardial fibers run in just the opposite direction, and at the cavity edge several bundles run completely along the long axis of the ventricle (Fig. 3.3).

The consequence of this changing fiber orientation is that fibers at the epicardium and endocardium are nearly at a right angle to each other and show interaction or tethering; also, when the oblique fibers contract, the ventricle exhibits a twisting motion or torsion, which contributes to the efficiency of ejection. A physical effect of LV torsion is elevation and motion of the apex toward the chest wall, which can be felt as the apical impulse or apex beat; finally, long-axis shortening during systole, caused by oblique and longitudinal fibers, causes the base to move toward the apex, which is nearly stationary because the pericardium is fixed to the diaphragm (this fixation is partially lost after the pericardium has been opened, such as after cardiac surgery). As a result, when a short-axis slice of the LV is imaged near the base, different parts of the myocardium are visualized at end-diastole and end-systole, so that erroneous calculations of segmental shortening and thickening of the wall are possible.

Although diffusion imaging can identify local fiber orientation, this is very difficult to do in vivo, and on normal MR images, the wall appears as a solid structure. The consequences of the fiber structure—the various components of wall deformation (circumferential and longitudinal shortening, thickening, and shearing or twisting)—can be quantified, although for regional information, a marking or tagging technique must be used.

Collagen Matrix

The myocardium also has a "scaffold" structure, the fibrous skeleton, consisting of a network of collagen and elastin fibers. The fibrous skeleton supports the myofibers and transmits force throughout the myocardium. It is thicker in some regions, such as at the valvular rings and where the myocardium attaches to the great vessels. Because the fibrous skeleton is not electrically excitable, the ring plane joining the atrioventricular valves provides a barrier to the conduction of electricity between the atria and ventricles, which can be passed only at the atrioventricular node.

Because of its specific MR characteristics, the collagen skeleton at the valve plane can be easily identified.

Pericardium

The pericardium is a thin, fibrous structure that surrounds the entire heart except at the entry and exit of the great vessels. It consists of two layers, one adhering to the outer surface of the heart, and another in contact with the lungs and other surrounding tissues. The former, the visceral serous layer, is an integral part of the heart wall. The latter consists of a fibrous part and the parietal serous layer. The fibrous part is made of tough, dense connective tissue and anchors the heart to surrounding structures (the diaphragm and great vessels). Although the pericardium is somewhat stretchable, it resists large, sudden increases in cardiac volume.

The parietal serous layer lines the internal surface of the fibrous pericardium and is continuous with the visceral layer

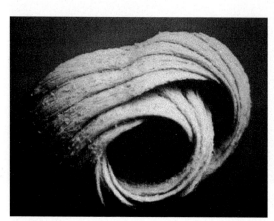
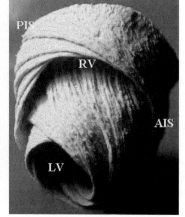

FIGURE 3.3. Dissection of myofiber layers (Torrent-Guasp).

as it folds over at points of attachment to the great vessels. The two serous layers are separated by a small amount of lubricating fluid, which accommodates the twisting and shortening movements of the heart during contraction and relaxation. Epicardial and pericardial fat is present in various amounts according to an individual's constitution. It is found mostly in the atrioventricular and interventricular grooves containing the epicardial vessels.

Increased amounts of epicardial fat are often mistaken for a pericardial effusion on echocardiography, which is readily recognized on CMR. Pericardial thickening, a cause of constrictive pericarditis (which is often difficult to diagnose), can be measured at various regions.

Interventricular Dependence

Because of the presence of the constraining pericardium and the fact that they share the interventricular and interatrial septum, the right and left sides of the heart show a great deal of interdependence, certainly in pathologic circumstances but also in cases of (sudden) ventricular enlargement and even in normal persons. The lower pressure and thinner wall of the right side of the heart make it more vulnerable to compressive forces, but the interdependence between the ventricles works both ways. When filling increases on the right side, as during inspiration, less filling occurs on the left side; in addition, pooling of blood in the pulmonary circulation decreases filling pressures in the left side of the heart. The reverse occurs during expiration, and an increase in intrathoracic pressure augments the LV afterload. Interdependence is increased when ventricular volumes are increased (dilated cardiomyopathies) or when the pericardium is relatively resistant to stretch (stiffer pericardium of constrictive pericarditis or increased intrapericardial pressure of pericardial effusion and tamponade). Pressures in the cavity should always be referred to the pressure in the pericardium, which in normal circumstances is about the same as the pleural pressure (0 to 2 mm Hg) and becomes negative during inspiration. In pathologic conditions, however, intracavitary pressure can be significantly increased by elevated intrapericardial pressure or effective pericardial resistance. Because this extra pressure is "felt" inside the heart but not in the supplying veins, a resistance to filling occurs; also, during some phases of the cardiac cycle, when the pressure in the atria and also in the (right) ventricle drops, pericardial pressure can become higher than the intracavitary pressure, so that collapse of the cavity ensues. Another example of the major impact of the pericardium on interventricular dependence is the change in regional motion that occurs after cardiac surgery in which the pericardium has been opened. The motion of the interventricular septum can be changed for months afterward, although thickening and intrinsic contractility are unhampered; this is a consequence of the changed interaction between left and right after removal of the constraints of an otherwise normal pericardium whereby the LV shows a more eccentric contraction and the interventricular septum is nearly immobile in an external reference system. If one were to reposition the images to fix the center of the LV on the screen, contraction would look much more normal, but the RV would tend to move outward.

The abnormal motion of the interventricular septum can easily be discerned on cine imaging. Causes of increased interdependence, such as a thickened pericardium, accumulation of pericardial fluid, and thrombi or blood present after cardiac surgery, can be differentiated.

Endocardium

The endocardium covers the entire inner surface of the heart and valves and has a very large surface area secondary to extensive trabeculation in both ventricles. Only the subaortic septal region is completely smooth. The function of the endocardium is still under investigation, but alterations, mainly to the relaxation phase, have been shown. The endocardium is continuous with the endothelial lining of the blood vessels as they enter or leave the heart.

Conduction System

The conduction system of the heart consists of specialized, spontaneously active cells and a conduction circuit. The trigger cells are concentrated in several areas (sinoatrial node and atrioventricular node), but impulses can originate all along the conduction system; however, the intrinsic frequency of the cells decreases from the sinoatrial node to the atrioventricular node to the bundle of His and further in the subendocardial Purkinje system. In normal circumstances, the sinoatrial node is the driving pacemaker of the heart, the average pace being 60 to 70 beats/min. Cardiac frequency is the result of a balance between parasympathetic and orthosympathetic tone, which at rest is shifted toward parasympathetic tone (the intrinsic rate of the sinoatrial node is about 100 beats/min).

The sinoatrial node is located in the posterior wall of the RA just inferior to the entrance of the superior vena cava. From the sinoatrial node, impulses spread through the gap junctions over both atria, activating atrial muscle and initiating atrial contraction. The impulse then reaches the atrioventricular node in the inferior part of the interatrial septum, where it slows for optimal timing and coordination between atrial and ventricular contraction (atrioventricular time delay is about 150 milliseconds). From there, the impulse runs through the His bundle and is conducted to the LV and RV over the bundle branches and finally the Purkinje fibers. Because the course of latter is subendocardial, the impulse must spread through the thick LV wall; it does so preferentially along the fiber bundles, which have an inward trajectory or imbrication angle and ultimately reach the epicardial and myocardial layers. The time between the onset of activation at the sinoatrial node and activation of the last ventricular myocyte is about 220 milliseconds in the normal heart. The cells that are activated last have the shortest action potential and therefore are inactivated first. The activation front therefore runs from endocardium to epicardium and the inactivation front from epicardium to endocardium, so that a T wave has the same orientation as the QRS complex on the surface electrocardiogram (ECG). Contraction starts at the endocardium and moves to the epicardium, but the epicardium relaxes first. In addition to this local inhomogeneity of activation and inactivation, the spread of the impulse over the ventricle, reaching the septum first, traveling toward the apex and free wall, and arriving at the basal parts last, causes an inhomogeneity in contraction and relaxation in respect to both timing and extent. Furthermore, regional inhomogeneity of contraction is caused by differences in local loading secondary to variations in wall thickness and curvature.

A fairly high degree of temporal and spatial resolution is required to appreciate this inhomogeneity fully, but it should not be mistaken for abnormalities of conduction (bundle branch block) or contraction (caused by ischemia, hypertrophy, or loading).

Knowledge of the microscopic and macroscopic anatomy of the heart is important in understanding the mechanics of the heart. A technique like CMR can contribute to a better characterization of cardiac anatomy by providing images with a very high level of spatial resolution and nearly "pathologic" characteristics. Imaging of the cavity and wall provides detailed information on volumes, mass, and global and regional deformation; it also provides quantitative information on shape and curvature, which make possible a better evaluation of local loading conditions. Knowledge of loading is needed, however, to derive intrinsic contractility or true systolic function from deformation.

CONTRACTION AND RELAXATION

Like skeletal muscle, cardiac muscle is striated, and the sliding myofilaments generate force and shortening. In contrast to the long, multinucleate fibers of skeletal muscle, the cardiac cells are short, wide, branched, and interconnected, with one or two nuclei. A loose connective tissue or endomysium surrounding the cells connects them to one other and to the fibrous skeleton of the heart. Whereas skeletal muscle fibers are structurally and functionally independent, cardiac cells are interlocked by intercalated disks containing desmosomes and gap junctions; in this way, the cells are firmly attached to one another, and electrical impulses can be easily transmitted from one cell to adjacent cells. Once stimulated, the heart contracts as a unit, although in sequence, as the electric impulse is spread through the conduction system and along the myocytes. The entire myocardium thus behaves as a large functional syncytium, structured in bundles and sheets and wrapped around the ventricles in a figure-of-eight arrangement; a bundle originating at the mitral valve ring can be followed at the epicardium as it runs obliquely over the heart and penetrates the wall to turn on itself at the apical dimple; it returns as an endocardial bundle, running again obliquely but at an angle of about 90 degrees to the epicardial part of its trajectory, and finally inserts again at the valve ring. Some investigators even believe that the entire heart, including the LV and RV, can be unwrapped in a single continuous bundle that is single-coiled for the RV and double-coiled for the LV.

Myocytes

Large mitochondria are abundantly present in the myocardial cells because these cells can operate nearly exclusively aerobically. On the other hand, cardiac myocytes can switch readily from metabolizing carbohydrates to metabolizing fats and even lactic acid; lack of oxygen, not lack of nutrients, is therefore the main cause of problems.

The myofilaments are typically organized in sarcomeres. They consist of thin actin filaments and thick myosin filaments. The head region of the myosin filament can attach to the actin to shorten the sarcomere (Fig. 3.4). Calcium is needed for this contraction.

Calcium homeostasis is governed by sarcolemmal and sarcoplasmic reticular transport (Fig. 3.5). Because of the long absolute refractory period, which is nearly as long as the contraction itself, cardiac myocytes cannot be tetanized.

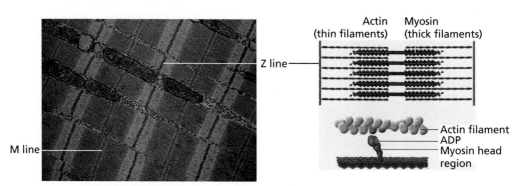

FIGURE 3.4. Sarcomeres and their actin and myosin components.

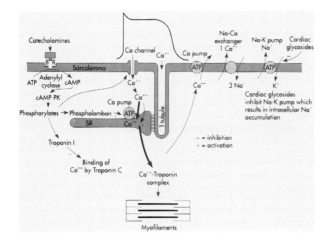

FIGURE 3.5. Calcium homeostasis.

Cardiac Cycle

As a result of the cyclic increase and decrease in intracellular calcium, the myocytes and myocardial syncytium exhibit a cycle of contraction and relaxation. The cardiac cycle can be described in terms of changes in blood volume and pressure and is divided into phases related to the opening and closing of the valves (Fig. 3.6).

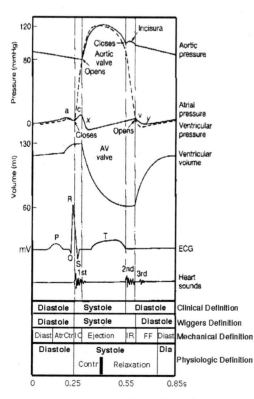

FIGURE 3.6. The cardiac cycle, divided into phases, according to different definitions.

With the onset of ventricular contraction, pressure increases in the cavity, and the atrioventricular valves are forced to close. Because the impulse through the Purkinje system is transmitted to the papillary muscles before the wall, the papillary muscles contract first and prevent the atrioventricular valves from bulging during the rising ventricular pressure. During the subsequent isovolumic contraction phase, in which both the atrioventricular and the ventriculoarterial valves are closed, pressure in the ventricular cavities rises to equal that in the aorta and pulmonary artery. Parts of the ventricles contract and shorten during this phase, thereby changing the shape of the ventricle and displacing blood in the cavity, mainly from the apical region toward the outflow tract, in preparation for the subsequent ejection. As soon as the pressure in the cavity is higher than in the connecting artery, the ventriculoarterial valve opens and blood is ejected. Although the ventricles start to relax after about 100 milliseconds (i.e., after one-third to one-half of the ejection phase has elapsed), flow is maintained because of inertia and compliance of the aorta (Windkessel effect). Relaxation of the ventricle is accompanied by a decrease in ventricular pressure to below aortic pressure. As soon as the pressure drops further and flow stops, the ventriculoarterial valve closes and the isovolumic relaxation phase starts. Again, this phase is characterized not only by a decrease in pressure but also by specific mechanical events. Untwisting of the LV occurs during most of this phase together with some longitudinal lengthening. As a consequence, the mitral ring starts to move upward, engulfing blood of the LA. The mitral valve, which was flattened toward the atrium during the high-pressure phase, returns to a more pointed configuration, and blood is shifted from the inflow region toward the apex. All these phenomena prepare the ventricle for an efficient subsequent filling. As soon as pressure in the ventricle, through active relaxation and the release of restoring forces, drops below the atrial pressure, the atrioventricular valves open, and fast, active filling follows. The "active" character of early filling is proven by the fact that ventricular pressure continues to drop, even while the ventricle starts to fill, which is incompatible with a passive filling phenomenon. After relaxation is completed, filling continues, but ventricular pressure now concomitantly rises. Flow is dependent on inertia only during this passive diastasis period. Once the atria are activated, they contract and further optimize ventricular filling by adding a final volume of blood.

In normal resting conditions at a heart rate of 60 beats/min, the cardiac cycle takes 1,000 milliseconds. Isovolumic contraction takes about 30 milliseconds, ejection 260 milliseconds, isovolumic relaxation 60 milliseconds, and filling the remaining 650 milliseconds. When the heart rate and contractility increase, it is mainly the filling period that is shortened; therefore, in normal circumstances, the diastolic or filling function is much more stressed during dynamic exercise than the systolic function.

Heart Sounds

Closure of the atrioventricular and ventriculoarterial valves is audible through the chest wall on auscultation. The first heart sound is caused by the nearly simultaneous closure of the atrioventricular valves. The second heart sound represents closure of the ventriculoarterial valves, with aortic valve closure preceding pulmonary valve closure. Respiration and ventricular interdependence cause an audible difference in the separation between the aortic and pulmonary components of the second heart sound; during inspiration, increased filling in the right side of the heart, prolonged ejection, and later pulmonary closure result in a wider splitting of the second heart sound.

LOADING AND CONTRACTILITY AS DETERMINANTS OF SYSTOLIC AND DIASTOLIC FUNCTION

All imaging techniques attempt to characterize motion and deformation of the heart optimally, but clinicians are really interested in cardiac performance. To go from motion to function or performance, several factors must be taken into account.

Intrinsic Deformation

Whole body motion of the myocardium (i.e., swinging or rotation) in the thoracic cavity must be "subtracted" to obtain intrinsic motion or deformation. This is the same as saying that myocardial deformation must be measured in a cardiac coordinate system (Fig. 3.7). When motion and deformation are referenced to the heart itself (i.e., when markers or references are used that are part of the cardiac structure), whole body motions are excluded. Similarly, when deformation of the myocardial wall must be quantified, a local cardiac coordinate system must be adopted; usually, a perpendicular coordinate system is used, in which one axis points outward

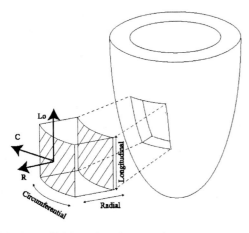

FIGURE 3.7. Definition of cardiac coordinate system.

perpendicular to the surface of the heart (radial axis, *R*), one is aligned to the short axis or circumference (circumferential axis, *C*), and one is perpendicular to the two other axes and is aligned to the long axis of the ventricle (longitudinal axis, *Lo*). At each site of the LV, such a coordinate system would have other orientations when viewed from the outside; for example, it would point a little downward near the apex to account for the tapering of the wall in this region.

Radial deformation, then, will everywhere quantify true 3D thickening and can be compared from region to region. Calculation of thickening from a simple short axis would give falsely high values near the apex because of the oblique cut through the wall. Although in most instances simple calculations of deformation will suffice for a given clinical indication, the limitations of not using true, oblique cuts and real 3D calculations of deformation must be remembered. Only by using a marker system (i.e., myocardial tagging) can all deformation components (normal and shear strains) be quantified in such a local cardiac coordinate system. One of these shear strains is the torsion motion of the ventricle, which has an important function in equalizing fiber load and optimizing LV performance (i.e., transforming 18% of fiber shortening into an ejection fraction of 70%). This can be accomplished only with an amplification mechanism in which the different layers of the LV myocardium work together and influence each other to enhance thickening in the endocardial part of the wall (endocardial thickening can exceed 70%, whereas epicardial thickening is only 20%).

No imaging technique except CMR is currently capable of true 3D imaging of the heart. With a combination of short- and long-axis information, the entire LV can be reconstructed and visualized in 3D. Although most clinical indications do not require such a reconstruction, improvements in automated contouring and segmentation may bring this into the clinical realm and provide useful information in regional cardiac pathology, such as ischemic heart disease.

Loading

Still, only deformation is quantified in this way, and whatever the level of sophistication of the technique used, deformation is only half of the contractility equation. The other part is load. The higher the load, the lower the deformation for a given degree of contractility. Conversely, a small deformation (small ejection fraction or little thickening) can be caused by decreased contractility, high loading conditions, or both. In most cases, we are interested in intrinsic contractility to make decisions on therapy and revascularization procedures. It is therefore important to be able at least to judge and qualitatively evaluate loading conditions because quantifying them has proved very difficult (Fig. 3.8).

Load is usually divided into preload and afterload, although the muscle feels only one load at each instant. Load has several components that depend on the size and shape of the ventricle. Although muscle load is what we are really interested in,

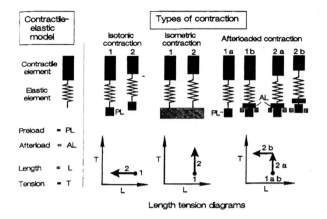

FIGURE 3.8. Definition of preload and afterload contractions.

crease in cavity size (endurance athletes) is compensated for by adequate hypertrophy, which consists of myofiber hypertrophy. This is in contrast with pathologic enlargement, in which hypertrophy is inadequate and consists of both myofiber hypertrophy (to a smaller extent) and hypertrophy of the collagen matrix with fibrosis. Fewer muscle fibers must carry an increased load, which leads to a vicious cycle of further dilation and ultimately cardiac failure.

CMR is uniquely appropriate to measure the different components of loading: cavity size, wall thickness, shape, and wall curvature. Although no absolute wall tension can be calculated, CMR thus far provides the best approximation that can be obtained.

tension at the myofiber level is extremely difficult to determine. We therefore try to infer tension in the wall from a simplification of Laplace's law: tension in the wall increases with a larger cavity size and a thinner wall for a given pressure.

During filling, the load is determined by pressure in the atrium, but resistance to flow by the mitral valve (including the subvalvular apparatus and mitral ring) and resistance to filling by the LV also determine the ultimate filling dynamics. The resistance to filling by the LV depends on the rate of myocardial relaxation and on the stiffness of the myocardium. The less compliant the myocardium, the more difficult it is to fill the ventricle, the higher the filling pressures, and the lower the filling volume.

Load during ejection depends mainly on the level of blood pressure. Aortic stenotic disease is an obvious cause of increased systolic load. Another is dilation without adequate compensatory hypertrophy or wall thinning, as in nontransmural myocardial infarction. Changes in the shape of the ventricle can also increase wall tension; a rounder ventricle, in comparison with a more ellipsoid normal ventricle, will have a higher load at the same pressure. In physiologic circumstances (intermittent volume or pressure load), an in-

Filling dynamics can be addressed by measuring the duration of isovolumic relaxation, the mitral inflow pattern, the pulmonary vein flow, and the dimensions of atrium and ventricle. In normal young persons, LV compliance is high and relaxation is fast, so that a large early filling volume and velocity and a smaller volume and velocity on atrial contraction are seen (Fig. 3.9, left). With aging, filling pressures may drop

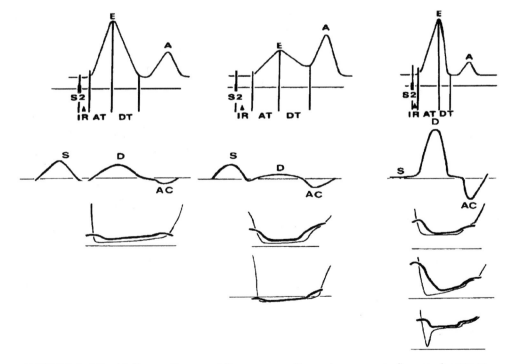

FIGURE 3.9. Mitral inflow patterns and the corresponding pulmonary vein flows and pressure tracings.

and relaxation may slow, so that isovolumic relaxation is prolonged and early filling volume and velocity are lower; in compensation, atrial filling increases, which is possible because the compliance of the ventricle is still normal (Fig. 3.9, middle). With hypertrophy caused by systolic overload (hypertension, aortic valve disease), a similar pattern develops, but mainly it results from prolonged ejection with a subsequent slowed relaxation. When the changes in the myocardium lead to a decreased compliance (fibrosis), filling pressures increase, thereby shortening the isovolumic relaxation time and increasing early filling velocity; because resistance to filling is greater at higher volumes (at atrial contraction after early filling), the volume/velocity on atrial contraction drops, and the pattern resembles normal values. This is called *pseudonormalization* (Fig. 3.9, right). In the early stages of disease, this pattern can be reversed to a "slowed relaxation, aging" pattern by decreasing the filling pressure, such as during a Valsalva maneuver. In the final stage of restrictive disease, such an intervention will no longer change the filling pattern; this stage is designated as "irreversible," and treatment will have little effect.

Such a restrictive syndrome can be the final stage of various cardiac abnormalities, such as ischemic heart disease, dilated cardiomyopathy, and hypertrophic heart disease (hypertension). It is also present in primary restrictive cardiomyopathies, which often are associated with some sort of infiltrative abnormality (amyloidosis, metabolic abnormalities). The same pattern, finally, can be found in constrictive pericarditis, in which the stiff pericardium does not allow any filling during the last phase of diastole (atrial contraction).

Differentiating constrictive pericarditis from restrictive cardiomyopathy can be very difficult; CMR can help by demonstrating a thickened pericardium, but the most important diagnostic tool (i.e., the influence of respiration on filling parameters) will have to await real-time velocity measurements (used in echo Doppler).

Contractility

Intrinsic contractility is governed by intrinsic and extrinsic factors. Intrinsic regulation is described by the Frank-Starling law of length-dependent activation; within certain limits, the more the muscle fibers are stretched, the more tension they can develop (Fig. 3.10).

At the organ level, this can be translated as follows: when the ventricle is filled more, the subsequent ejection is more forceful, stroke volume is increased, and end-diastolic volume returns to previous values. This positive length–tension relation of cardiac myocytes is made possible by the fact that under normal conditions, the length of cardiac myocytes is less than optimal. Any increase in stretch therefore increases the strength of contraction. An example of a physiologic factor that causes an increase in venous return and end-diastolic volume is dynamic exercise. Conversely, a very high

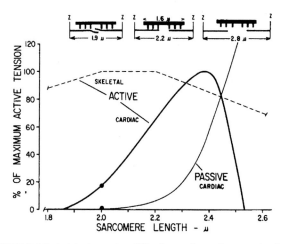

FIGURE 3.10. Intrinsic contractility depends on the stretch of the sarcomeres.

heart rate or bleeding with decreased filling can cause a decrease in intrinsic contractility. A second determinant of intrinsic contractility is heart rate per se; the contractile force of normal myocardium increases with the frequency of stimulation—the staircase phenomenon. This is not true for failing myocardium, which exhibits a negative staircase phenomenon (i.e., contractility decreases with increases in heart rate).

Extrinsic contractility is any change in contractile force independent of muscle stretch (i.e., independent of an increase in cellular calcium exchange). It can be caused by an increase in sympathetic stimulation, through nerve stimulation or circulating catecholamines. Thyroxine, glucagon, digitalis, and some other drugs also increase extrinsic contractility (positive inotropy), whereas acidosis, hyperkaliemia, hypocalcemia, and drugs such as calcium antagonists and beta blockers have a negative inotropic effect.

Parallel to the changes in systolic or ejection function, positive and negative lusitropic or filling effects can be described. In most instances, inotropic and lusitropic effects go hand in hand; when contraction force is increased, relaxation rate and filling velocities are also augmented.

EVALUATION OF CARDIAC FUNCTION: THE CARDIOVASCULAR MR PROTOCOL

Because the function of the heart is to deliver oxygen and nutrients to the cells and remove carbon dioxide and waste, the performance of the circulation can be described in terms of maintaining an appropriate cardiac output and blood pressure while keeping filling pressures at acceptable levels. Although these are referred to as *systolic function* and *diastolic function* and are viewed as independent tasks of the heart, they cannot really be separated. An abnormal systolic function causes a decreased stroke volume and subsequently an increased end-diastolic volume and pressure; conversely, a decreased filling volume, for whatever reason, immediately causes a diminished stroke volume. Symptoms of systolic or forward failure (decreased cardiac output, low blood pressure, fatigue, exercise intolerance) go hand in hand with symptoms of diastolic or backward failure (pulmonary congestion, dyspnea, peripheral edema). In a patient at a certain moment during the clinical evaluation, one or the other may be more prominent, but in essence they are inseparable.

Dimensions

The regulation and parameters of systolic and diastolic function, therefore, must be dealt with as a whole. To understand and describe cardiac function, it is essential first to observe ventricular and atrial dimensions. End-diastolic volume is the major determinant of intrinsic contractility, but on the other hand, the Frank-Starling relationship has its limits, and dilation without adequate compensatory hypertrophy increases load and decreases performance. Enlargement of the LV is the final common pathway in many disorders; it leads, through increases in load, to decreases in cardiac output and activation of the neurohumoral systems, which drive a negative vicious cycle. In a first phase, cardiac output at rest can be normal, even with a decreased ejection fraction, but an appropriate increase in cardiac output cannot be provided during exercise, and through further elimination of overloaded cardiomyocytes (apoptosis), a downward path is inevitable unless preventive measures are taken. Increases in atrial dimensions point to valvular abnormalities, increases in filling pressures, or both.

Deformation

Next, motion and deformation of the ventricles, with attention to circumferential and longitudinal shortening and thickening, must be addressed. This can be done by cine imaging in both true short- and long-axis orientations. Transverse images can also provide information but are often more difficult to interpret. Sometimes, SPAMM (spatial modulation of magnetization) tagging can be very helpful to clarify whether a certain region of myocardium is being pulled and moved by surrounding tissue or is undergoing true contraction and deformation.

When the entire ventricle is covered in cine mode by short-axis slices, the end-diastolic and end-systolic volumes, stroke volume, and ejection fraction can be obtained (Fig. 3.11). In the future, the combination of short- and long-axis information will make this technique even more reliable (partial volume effect at the apical slices, through-plane motion at the base with atrial volume in the most basal slice in systole).

Flow

Subsequently, flow can be obtained at the inflow and outflow regions. This determination provides a control value of

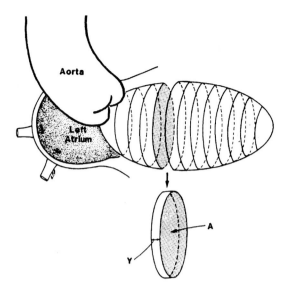

FIGURE 3.11. Multislice coverage of the ventricle allows accurate measurement of volumes.

stroke volume, information about the presence or absence of intracardiac shunts (comparing aortic with pulmonary flow volumes), and insight regarding diastolic performance, with a consideration of mitral and pulmonary vein flows.

Depending on the indication for the study, additional specifically directed information can then be acquired.

PERIPHERAL CIRCULATION

Blood is conducted through the systemic and pulmonary circulation via arteries, capillaries, and veins (Fig. 3.12). The exchange of oxygen, carbon dioxide, nutrients, and waste takes place in the capillaries, and the system tries to keep flow and pressure in this part of the circulation as stable as possible. Flow, however, depends on the existence of a pressure gradient, generated by the cyclic cardiac muscular pump. Pulsatile flow in the aorta must therefore be con-

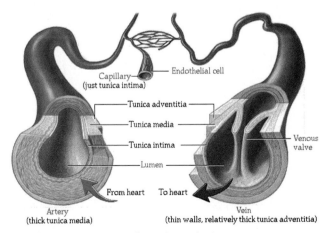

FIGURE 3.12. Structure of arteries and veins.

verted to continuous, laminar flow through the capillaries. The Windkessel effect in the aorta is a very important adaptive process whereby potential energy from the LV ejection is stored in the aortic wall and converted to kinetic energy (flow) during the subsequent diastole. Through the ever-increasing total surface area of the branching arterial tree, flow becomes more and more continuous (although the size of each vessel after branching is smaller than that of the original one, the total area after branching is larger than that of the one before).

The decreasing size of each single vessel and the presence of precapillary sphincters make this side of the circulation the resistance part; the greatest resistance to flow and the point of reflection (returning waves) are situated in the small arterial vessels or arterioles (Fig. 3.13).

On the other side of the capillary bed, the veins are capacitance vessels; they contain 63% of the blood volume in the circulation (arteries, 13%; arterioles and capillaries, 7%; heart, 7%; pulmonary circulation, 10%). Depending on gravity, muscle exercise, and the integrity of the venous valves, the capacitance of the veins can change and influence venous return and cardiac output.

Although the blood travels through the lumina of vessels at relatively low speed (in the aorta at 50 cm/s), the pulse wave travels through the arterial wall at high speed (1,000 cm/s) and is reflected in the small arterioles to return during the same cardiac cycle, so that it is superimposed on the forward-traveling pulse. The pressure measured at one point in the vasculature therefore represents both the forward and returning waves. In young healthy persons, the pulse wave velocity is slower and the returning wave in the aorta is superimposed after aortic valve closure, augmenting early

diastolic pressure and increasing the perfusion pressure of the coronaries. With aging and prematurely with hypertension, the arterial wall becomes stiffer, and the wave travels faster and is superimposed before aortic valve closure, during ejection. It therefore contributes to the ejection load, and the perfusion pressure of the coronaries is less optimal. This situation is less favorable for the myocardium; more energy must be spent to overcome the increased load and less efficient perfusion is available.

CMR can quantitatively measure flow and flow profiles in the large arteries. Although this type of study has not been pursued very intensively, a better insight into aortic flow could be important in deciding on specific therapy for a patient with arterial hypertension to decrease compensatory LV hypertrophy, an independent risk factor for cardiovascular events. LV mass as such can also be accurately measured, so that it is possible to assess the efficacy of therapy in an individual patient.

CORONARY BLOOD FLOW AND MYOCARDIAL PERFUSION

The coronary circulation provides the myocardium with the critically important oxygen supply, needed for the nearly exclusively aerobic metabolism of the myocytes. Although stenoses in the epicardial and large intramyocardial conductance vessels are obvious causes of perfusion abnormalities, deficiencies in the smaller resistance arterioles and capillaries (microcirculation) can also have a major impact on oxygen delivery to the myocardium.

Coronary atherosclerosis is a very long process that starts early in life, probably soon after childhood in the Western world. In the first phase, fatty streaks form; these develop into fatty lesions and expand outward, increasing the total vessel diameter without decreasing the lumen size. Such vessel remodeling is therefore invisible with "projection" techniques (i.e., coronary angiography, which visualizes only the coronary lumen). *Intravascular ultrasonography or CMR is required to observe the wall and the major changes that occur there early in the development of the disease.* Subsequently, the atherosclerotic lesion continues to grow and encroaches on the lumen, decreasing the diameter. Depending on the thickness and stability of the cap covering the lesion, it can rupture, causing a local thrombus and arterial occlusion, with a myocardial infarction as the consequence. Exercise or stress-induced complaints of angina, on the other hand, are caused most often by progressive narrowing of the lumen (possibly in steps by nonocclusive thrombi on ruptured plaques). A stenosis of more than 75% is usually needed to compromise flow.

Myocardial perfusion is phasic and occurs mainly during diastole because intramyocardial pressure is increased during systolic contraction. In normal conditions, flow and perfusion are governed by the driving pressure across the coronary bed (diastolic aortic pressure minus RA pressure) and

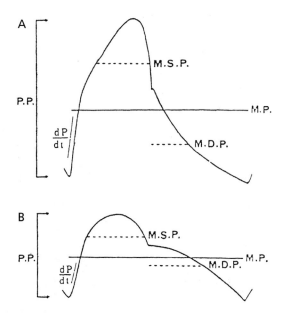

FIGURE 3.13. Returning wave superimposing in systole **(A)** and diastole **(B)**.

the resistance to flow in the small arterioles. Increases in diastolic volume and pressure (dilated cardiomyopathies) can therefore decrease perfusion pressure in the absence of any significant stenosis of the epicardial coronaries. Changes in the arteriolar resistance (hypertrophic disease) can have a similar effect.

Coronary flow and perfusion are maintained constant, irrespective of the coronary perfusion pressure, for a certain range of pressures (50 to 200 mm Hg); when pressure drops below this critical value, a steep decrease in flow is observed (coronary autoregulation). Conversely, during exercise, flow can be doubled or tripled by the increased mean perfusion pressure and the increased pulse pressure. In the presence of significant narrowing of an epicardial vessel, a pressure drop occurs across this lesion, and perfusion pressure in the poststenotic segment is decreased. When flow must increase during exercise, pressure in this segment can fall below the autoregulatory range, and a flow deficit ensues. Collateral flow can sometimes compensate for decreased antegrade flow but usually is unable to provide adequate perfusion during periods of greater demand (exercise).

The endocardial layers of the myocardium are subjected to greater stress and consume more oxygen, which could explain their greater vulnerability to ischemia. Similarly, after total coronary occlusion, infarcts expand in a wave front from the endocardium to the epicardium, with a greater expanse seen in the subendocardium.

CMR, with the use of first-pass techniques after contrast injection, can visualize myocardial perfusion (and regional perfusion deficits) and provide very good qualitative and semiquantitative analyses. Optimally, however, quantitative flow in milliliters per gram of tissue is desirable.

VENTRICULOARTERIAL COUPLING

The blood that is ejected by the LV must be "accepted" by the aorta. Although the resistance to flow in the aorta is the afterload for the ventricle, the stroke volume is the input function for the vasculature. If a system is to be efficient, input and output must be optimally matched (i.e., ventriculoarterial coupling must be fine-tuned, and an equilibrium situation must be reached). If not, performance of the system will be less than optimal, and more energy will be spent to obtain the same result (a specific combination of flow and pressure, i.e. cardiac output or stroke volume and blood pressure). Although these concepts are not widely used clinically, they can clarify ventricular dysfunction in some cases and also help to direct therapy (Fig. 3.14).

It is easiest is to consider equilibrium as the point where two performance lines (of ventricle and aorta) cross on a diagram of pressure and stroke volume. For the ventricle, the relation is inverse; the higher the pressure (afterload), the lower the stroke volume. For the arterial system, the relation is direct; the more blood entering the vessel, the greater the

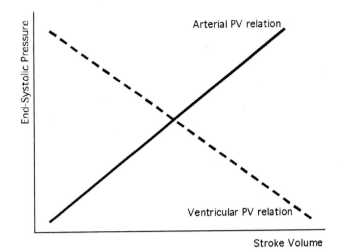

FIGURE 3.14. Ventriculoarterial coupling.

rise in pressure. Depending on ventricular performance and arterial compliance, the lines can be more or less steep, but equilibrium is where they cross. Here is where the transmission of energy is most efficient.

VALVULAR FUNCTION

The function of the valves is to direct blood flow through the circulation. They can be found in the heart and veins, and dysfunction is a major cause of symptoms and disease. In the heart, the atrioventricular and semilunar valves are quite different in structure, but they both must resist a high-pressure gradient in closed position while allowing opening and high-volume flow in low-gradient conditions. Problems can be caused by an increased resistance to flow (stenosis) or leakage (insufficiency). Quantification of these disorders is quite difficult but very important when decisions must be made regarding prognosis, therapy, and timing of intervention.

Stenosis

An evaluation of the severity of stenosis can be based on the stenotic area, gradient across the valve, or resistance to flow. A stenotic area can be measured directly with an imaging technique capable of choosing an image plane perpendicular to the valve and tracking valvular through-plane motion. *CMR has such capabilities.* The stenotic area can also be derived from gradient measurement and the continuity equation. In echo-Doppler, this technique is commonly used. The velocity at one site is measured together with the area at that site; the velocity at the stenotic site is also measured. Because the velocity integral times area equals flow volume and the flow at two sites of a continuous circuit must be the same, the one unknown, which is the stenotic area, can be computed. In echo-Doppler, the peak stenotic velocity is measured with continuous-wave Doppler, which captures the highest velocities along the trajectory, wherever they occur. This point, also called the *vena contracta,* is usually situated a little beyond the physically smallest opening because the flow lines of a stenotic lesion continue to converge after this smallest area has been passed.

With CMR, velocity can be measured in plane and through plane, but choosing the location where the highest velocity can be obtained is not always easy. Use of the void created by dephasing on cine imaging effectively detects the presence of a stenotic lesion but cannot quantify it.

Insufficiency

If quantifying stenosis is difficult, quantifying insufficiency is still more so. Many techniques have been used in echo-Doppler to quantify insufficiency, but all have significant disadvantages. Regurgitant orifice, fraction, and volume in addition to semiquantitative grading on color mapping have all been used.

CMR velocity mapping, especially when combined with valve tracking, effectively measures antegrade and retrograde flow over the valve, from which the regurgitant fraction can be readily calculated. To find the regurgitant orifice, the maximal gradient velocity must be measured, and this measurement entails the same difficulties as measurement of a stenotic valve.

SUMMARY

A good understanding of the functional anatomy and physiology of the heart and circulation is essential in interpreting CMR images. After basic morphologic and functional data have been acquired, the clinical problem and the results of this baseline study can direct further imaging. The detection of underlying mechanisms and diseases can indicate the diagnosis and suggest an optimal management strategy.

BIBLIOGRAPHY

Berne RM, Levy MN. *Cardiovascular physiology*, 8th ed. St. Louis: Mosby, 2001.
Bers DM. *Excitation–contraction coupling and cardiac contractile force.* Boston: Kluwer Academic Publishers, 2001.
Braunwald EM, Zipes DP. *Heart diseases*, 2nd ed. Philadelphia: Current Medicine, 2001.
McManus BM, ed. *Atlas of cardiovascular pathology.* Philadelphia: Current Science, 2001.
Page E, Fozzard HA, Solaro RJ, eds. *The heart.* New York: Oxford University Press, 2002.

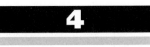

BLOOD FLOW MEASUREMENTS

HAYDAR AKBARI
GAUTHAM P. REDDY
CHARLES B. HIGGINS

The need for a precise, flexible, and noninvasive technique to quantify blood flow has motivated the application of MRI to the measurement of blood flow *in vivo*. One of the major advantages of using MRI to measure blood flow is that the flow itself is not affected by the measurement process. Moreover, unlike many of the alternative methods, MRI is noninvasive. These advantages make MRI the method of choice in both clinical diagnosis and physiologic investigation. MRI velocity mapping techniques, which can provide detailed, multidimensional information on flow, have been used to assess vessel morphology and blood flow patterns *in vivo* (1).

The use of MRI methods to measure blood flow began in the mid-1950s, and efforts to extend and improve flow measurements have continued since then (2,3). Early work on MRI blood flow techniques was reported in 1982 by Moran (4), who interlaced a velocity-encoding phase-modulation field gradient into a conventional MR sequence and thereby obtained quantitative images of flow. Van Dijk (5) reported the potential use of phase changes as a method for evaluating ventricular function in 1983. In 1984, Bryant et al. (6) reported the first clinical applications of MRI to flow measurements; they used a gradient-recalled echo sequence and a phase-difference technique. Flow was measured in the femoral and carotid arteries in healthy volunteers, and the measurements were validated *in vitro* with a continuous-flow-of-water phantom and *in vivo* with Doppler ultrasonography. Singer and Crooks (7) applied a time-of-flight (TOF) technique *in vivo* to measure the flow in internal jugular veins in humans. Subsequently, TOF techniques were used for blood flow measurements in other vessels (8,9).

Nayler et al. (10) described a specially designed gradient-echo technique for measuring blood flow that combined even-echo rephasing with a short-field echo time (TE) to avoid signal loss from flowing blood. Fast repetition of this sequence made it possible to acquire flow measurements at multiple points in the cardiac cycle. This method has been validated *in vivo* by comparing the aortic flow calculated from velocity maps with that measured by left ventricular (LV) stroke volume (11). In 1987, Underwood et al. (12) reported the initial clinical application of velocity-encoded cine (VEC) MRI in 13 patients with cardiovascular disease.

The development of velocity mapping as an extension of MRI can be compared with Doppler techniques in relation to echocardiography, except that MRI in many respects has capabilities beyond those of Doppler. MR velocity mapping can accurately measure velocities in pixels throughout the plane of acquisition. It can acquire data in any orientation, unrestricted by windows of access, and it allows a choice of the direction in which velocities are measured with respect to the imaging plane. The other major advantage of MR velocity mapping is that volume flow can be calculated with a high degree of accuracy because the mean velocity and area of the vessel are acquired simultaneously. Doppler echocardiography is accurate for measuring velocity, but not as good for assessing volume flow, especially when the flow pattern is complex (13). In addition, MR velocity mapping allows a comprehensive assessment of flow (three spatial dimensions, three velocity components, and time) and is well suited for studying both spatial and temporal patterns of flow. This is important because flow can be complex in cardiac chambers and in vessels that are curved or branching, with components of velocity in various directions. When compared with cardiac catheterization, MRI has both limitations and advantages. Like Doppler echocardiography, MRI is unable to measure pressure directly, but it has the advantage of noninvasiveness, the ability to measure flow and map velocities through obstructive lesions, and the ability to obtain tomographic views of complex three-dimensional anatomy (13).

H. Akbari, G. P. Reddy, and C. B. Higgins: Department of Radiology, University of California San Francisco, San Francisco, California.

TECHNIQUES

Flow-Sensitive Imaging

Several flow-sensitive MRI methods permit the measurement of blood flow in terms of either velocity or volume per time unit. Currently, the most popular flow-sensitive MRI technique, referred to as *phase-contrast, phase-shift,* or *VEC MRI,* is based on the principle that the phase of flowing spins relative to stationary spins along a magnetic gradient changes in direct proportion to flow velocity (14). This technique allows quantification of blood velocity profiles at different times during the cardiac cycle (15,16). VEC MRI is based on the acquisition of two sets of images, one with and one without velocity encoding; these are usually acquired simultaneously. The subtraction of the two sets of phase images allows the calculation of a phase shift that is proportional to flow velocity in the direction of the flow compensation gradient. The phase shift is displayed as variations in pixel signal intensity on the phase image. Stationary tissue appears gray on this image, flow in an antegrade direction along the flow-encoding axis appears bright, and flow in a retrograde direction appears dark. As a result, it is possible to differentiate antegrade from retrograde flow (17). Furthermore, as with Doppler ultrasonography, the phase map image can be color-coded to reinforce the differentiation between antegrade and retrograde flow. Velocity can be encoded in planes that are perpendicular to the direction of flow by using section-selective direction (through-plane velocity measurement), in planes that are parallel to the direction of flow by using phase-encoded or frequency-encoded directions (in-plane velocity measurement), or in three dimensions.

VEC MRI has certain limitations and potential sources of error (18). Because of the cyclic nature of the phase, aliasing may occur if more than one cycle of phase shift occurs. To avoid aliasing, which occurs when the velocity range is lower than the maximum velocity, the velocity threshold must be correctly selected before acquisition to maintain a phase shift of less than 180 degrees. Flow-related signal loss can be secondary to loss of coherence within a voxel, resulting in the inability to detect the phase of the flow signal above that of noise; to inappropriate selection of the velocity range, which in turn leads to poor detection of small vessels with slow flow; or to turbulence, which occurs in valvular stenosis and regurgitation. The latter can be overcome by using short-TE sequences. Partial volume averaging can occur in cases involving small vessels, improper vessel alignment, or a narrow inflow stream, particularly with in-plane velocity measurements and thick sections ($\geq$10 mm) (13).

VEC MRI can be used to calculate absolute velocity at any given time during the cardiac cycle at specified locations in the plane of data acquisition. Velocity can be measured for each pixel within a region-of-interest (ROI) encircling all or part of the cross-sectional vessel area or across a valve annulus. The instantaneous flow volume for each time frame during a cardiac cycle is calculated as the product of cross-sectional area (determined from the magnitude image) and spatial mean velocity (the average velocity for all pixels in the cross-sectional area on the phase image). Integration of all instantaneous flow volumes throughout the cardiac cycle yields the flow volume per heart beat (17–19). This technique has been evaluated both *in vitro* and *in vivo* by several investigators and shown to provide an accurate measurement of aortic and pulmonary arterial flow, which represent the stroke volumes of the left ventricle (LV) and right ventricle (RV), respectively (17–19). It has also been used to calculate the ratio of pulmonary to systemic flow, thereby allowing the noninvasive quantification of left-to-right shunts (20), and to measure differential blood flow in the right and left pulmonary arteries. Moreover, these measurements can be used in the evaluation and quantitative assessment of valvular regurgitation and stenosis.

Flow Measurement

A variety of MRI techniques of flow measurement have been investigated. MRI flow measurements can be classified into two major categories, one that makes use of longitudinal magnetization (TOF techniques) and one that uses transverse magnetization (phase techniques) (18,21–24). Techniques employing longitudinal magnetization detect the amplitude of MR signals. On the other hand, techniques using transverse magnetization detect spin phase changes resulting from flow in magnetic field gradient.

The two principal kinds of flow effects in MRI are TOF effects and phase shifts. TOF effects are caused by the persistence of local alterations in magnetization (e.g., those caused by selective excitation) for times comparable with the times between consecutive radiofrequency excitations; motion of the blood carries the altered magnetization with it, thus affecting the resulting signal at the next excitation. Phase shifts can result when excited spins in the blood move along magnetic field gradients such as those used in MRI; the change in signal phase relative to stationary material can be adjusted to be proportional to the component of the velocity along the gradient by suitably modifying the imaging pulse sequence (21,23,24).

Time-of-Flight Techniques

To quantify blood flow on the basis of the TOF principle, bolus tracking techniques have been used. The concept behind bolus tracking is to label blood at one point within the vessel and then determine the distance that the labeled blood has moved in a given amount of time. Usually, labeling is done by placing a dark line across the vessel with a saturation band. The distance that the saturation band moves is measured and compared with the delay time to compute the flow velocity as follows: $V = D/t$, where D is displacement and t is time. The method is sensitive to both forward and reverse flow, and the total acquisition (Σ15 seconds) can be performed within a breath-hold (22).

The major advantages of bolus tracking are its conceptual simplicity, rapidity, and lack of susceptibility to extraneous phase shifts. The fundamental limitation of this method is the necessity for careful slice positioning and the difficulty in computing flow volumes; only the peak velocity at the center of the vessel can be measured. Two-dimensional velocity profiles in a vessel cannot be determined. Therefore, a correct determination of the velocity at every point in a vascular cross-section is difficult with TOF methods. Furthermore, TOF techniques have proved difficult to use for quantifying flow because they rely on signal amplitude measurements, which depend not only on flow velocity but also on proton density, longitudinal relaxation time (T1), transverse relaxation time (T2), and particularly type of flow (10). This method has not been used in MR blood flow quantification as often as phase-shift techniques.

Phase-Contrast or Velocity-Encoded Cine Techniques

Flow-encoding phase shifts result from the application of bipolar magnetic field gradients, which are composed of two lobes with opposite signs. When the first lobe is applied, the spins of the stationary and moving tissues begin to accumulate phase. Immediately after the first lobe, the second lobe is applied, and the stationary protons lose their phase and accumulate a net phase of zero. Blood that moves during the time between these two gradients experiences unequal positive and negative gradients and therefore accumulates a net phase shift (10,23). The phase difference between the two sequences is proportional to flow in the velocity-encoded directions according to the following formula: δ phase = g $\times$ velocity $\times$ T $\times$ A_{g}, where g is the gyromagnetic ratio, T is the duration of the gradient pulse, and A_{g} is the area of each lobe of the gradient pulse. Velocity can be encoded in a single direction (e.g., in the flow direction) or in all three dimensions. Gradients can be varied in amplitude or duration to sensitize the experiment to fast or slow flow. The phase shift, which is proportional to the velocity, is displayed as variations in pixel intensity on the phase map image. Motion in the positive direction along the flow-encoding axis appears as bright (or dark) pixels; flow in the opposite direction appears as dark (or bright) pixels, and stationary tissue appears gray (22).

When cardiac gating, which is mandatory for pulsatile flow assessment, is performed, two (positive and negative) flow-encoded acquisitions are acquired as interleaved pairs at each point of the cardiac cycle. To suppress the background noise, the phase-encoded pixel intensities may be multiplied by the magnitude image, which is a by-product of the interleaved phase-difference technique. The resulting images are called *magnitude-weighted* or *flow images*.

To determine the profile of flow or the flow volume across the vessel lumen, usually, the magnitude-weighted images may be used to define the ROI. The ROI is superimposed in subsequent images throughout the cardiac cycle and can be adapted if any change in size and location occurs. The average velocity in the ROI measured on the phase images is then multiplied by the cross-sectional area to generate flow volume measurement (mean blood flow = spatial mean velocity $\times$ cross-sectional area of vessel). Pressure gradients are calculated by the modified Bernoulli equation: $\Delta P = 4v^2$, where ΔP is the pressure gradient in millimeters of mercury and v is the peak flow velocity in meters per second. VEC MRI permits the quantification of blood flow, flow velocity, and pressure gradients in central vessels or surgical conduits (23,24). VEC MRI flow measurements can be plotted on a graph, and the area under the curve can be integrated to derive the flow volume in one cardiac cycle (Fig. 4.1). These flow and pressure measurements can be used in a variety of clinical applications, including the measurement of shunt volumes, valvular regurgitation, pressure gradients across stenotic lesions, and differential flow in the pulmonary arteries (23–25). The development of automated computer programs has facilitated the use of VEC MRI. Further advances in automation should make this technique more accessible.

VEC MRI has several limitations. If the vessel of interest is not scanned in a plane perpendicular to the direction of flow or if partial volume averaging of the vessel occurs, velocity and flow may be underestimated. Aliasing is possible if the maximum velocity value is lower than the actual ve-

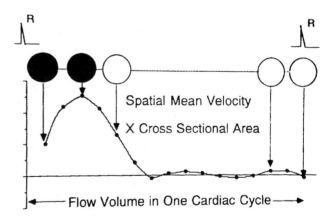

FIGURE 4.1. Velocity-encoded cine (VEC) MRI flow measurements. The diagram, of a flow-versus-time curve for blood flow in the aorta or pulmonary artery, demonstrates the outline of the cross-sectional area of the blood vessel *(arrow)* at each phase during the cardiac cycle, extending from one R wave to the next R wave. Each point on the curve represents the mean blood flow within the artery at a phase of the cardiac cycle. Each value is derived from a separate VEC MR image. The blood flow is a product of the spatial mean velocity and the cross-sectional area of the vessel. (From Higgins CB. Congenital heart disease. In: Higgins CB, Hricak H, Helms CA, eds. *Magnetic resonance imaging of the body*, 3rd ed. Philadelphia: Lippincott–Raven Publishers, 1997: 461–518, with permission.)

locity. In addition, very small vessels are poorly evaluated by VEC MRI. Pressure gradient measurement has additional pitfalls that can lead to an underestimation of the gradient; peak velocity may be at a site distal to the most severe stenosis and the vessel may not be scanned at the site of peak velocity (26), and velocities are averaged over the length of the acquisition because images are generally not acquired in real time (27).

Potential Sources of Error

The accuracy and limitations of blood flow quantification with MRI have been described by several groups (28,29). The major potential pitfalls and sources of error are the following: Flow-related signal loss may be induced by several factors, incorrect selection of the encoded velocity range can lead to poor visualization of small vessels or vessels with slow flow, and loss of phase coherence within a voxel results in an inability to detect the phase of flow signal above that of noise. Intravoxel dephasing and saturation of slow in-plane flow can be reduced by decreasing the voxel size and by increasing the repetition time (TR). A long TE may influence the accuracy of measurement of the velocities of jet flows. Signal loss caused by the turbulence associated with jet flows can be overcome by using a short TE (<4 milliseconds). Eddy currents, which may occur in regions of low signal intensity (outside the vessel), can cause undesired phase shifts. These phase errors add a bias to the measured velocity, which varies slowly across the image. Even though this velocity offset is generally a small fraction of the dynamic range of velocity, it can cause significant errors in estimates of flow volume. To minimize eddy currents, the use of shielded gradient coils or eddy compensation techniques has proved successful.

Misalignment is described as the interrelation between the true and measured flows. It is determined by the following equation: $F_{meas} = F_{true} (\cos \phi)$, where ϕ is the angle of misalignment, F_{meas} is the measured flow, and F_{true} is the true flow. This cosine relationship results in small errors; a misalignment of 20 degrees produces only a 6% error (30). Inaccuracy resulting from a perpendicular misalignment is minimized because measurement of the cross-sectional diameter varies with the obliquity of the section and proportionally offsets any error in measured velocity. Misalignment can be overcome by three-dimensional phase encoding.

Aliasing, or phase-wrap, occurs when velocity exceeds the anticipated range, resulting in phase displacement greater than 180 degrees. Higher-velocity spins will be displayed incorrectly and cannot be differentiated from flow in the opposite direction. Velocity aliasing can be reduced with algorithms that use spatial continuity to resolve ambiguity (31).

Partial volume averaging or averaging of flow phase data through the slice may be caused by large slice thickness, vessel obliquity, or small vessel size. The extent of error will be determined by the signal intensity of the surrounding tissue, which depends on tissue parameters (Tl, T2) and MR sequence parameters (TR, TE, flip angle). TOF techniques are unaffected by partial volume averaging and may be used in studies of complex tortuous vascular regions.

Signal misregistration is caused by motion occurring between the time of pulse excitation and the time of signal detection. The consequences are that flow signal cannot be compared directly with features on the magnitude images because of malpositioning of blood signal with respect to any stationary tissue, and that signal from flowing and stationary material is averaged if misregistration causes the flow signal to overlie any background signal. Signal misintegration is reduced by imaging in a plane perpendicular to the direction of flow.

Analysis and Display

Both temporal and spatial resolution are important to consider in an analysis of flow imaging. Because the blood vessel of interest may span relatively few pixels on an image, it may be difficult to avoid partial volume averaging near the vessel walls. In measurements of pulsatile flow, inadequate temporal resolution will distort the flow velocity as a function of the phase of the cardiac cycle. In any case, to find net flow through a vessel, it is usually necessary to integrate over both the vessel lumen and the cardiac cycle. The ROI for analysis may have to be modified in size and position at different phases in the cardiac cycle.

Display of the additional data provided by blood flow MRI can be a challenge. A single velocity component or a scalar speed can be displayed as a gray scale or color overlay on the image. The variation over time can be seen with a movie loop display or can be displayed as a graph of the values within an ROI as a function of time. However, multiple velocity components and multiplanar images are more difficult to display; fields of arrows or calculated particle paths can help visualize flow patterns (21).

Quantification of Stenosis by Velocity-Encoded Cine MRI

Velocity mapping of jets through a stenosis can be optimized by using a very short TE to avert severe signal loss in the jet. Kilner and colleagues (30) used a TE of less than 3.6 milliseconds with a 0.5-tesla (T) MRI system. Another report, in which a constant-flow phantom was used, demonstrated that jet velocities of up to 700 cm/s could be measured accurately ($r = .99$) when a TE of 6 to 7 milliseconds was used with a 1.5-T system (32).

With the use of phase maps, it has been shown that individual pixels in the vascular lumen or cardiac chamber from a large ROI can be interrogated to display an ensemble of velocities in the jet during peak systole (33). Peak jet velocities can then be estimated from the average of a number of pixels in the central region of the jet core.

As with Doppler ultrasonography, the modified Bernoulli equation can be used to estimate the gradient across a stenotic valve by measuring the peak velocity across the site of the stenosis: $\Delta P = 4v^2$, where ΔP is the peak pressure drop (millimeters of mercury) and v is the peak velocity (meters per second) across the stenosis. Studies comparing VEC MRI, Doppler ultrasonography, and cardiac catheterization have shown excellent correlation in patients with aortic and mitral valve stenosis (33,34). Kilner et al. (33) validated VEC MRI in 25 patients with cardiac valve stenosis and stressed some advantages of this technique over Doppler ultrasonography, especially at locations where acoustic access is limited. VEC MRI also has been applied to assess the severity of aortic stenosis by quantifying the valve area and cardiac output (34). Measurements of the valve area and cardiac output obtained with VEC MRI corresponded well with comparative measurements obtained with cardiac catheterization, Doppler ultrasonography, and indicator-dilution techniques. Heidenreich et al. (35) used VEC MRI to measure transmitral velocity in 16 patients with mitral valve stenosis. Significant correlation was shown between VEC MRI and Doppler measurements of peak (10-mm slice thickness, $r = .89$; 5-mm slice thickness, $r = .82$) and mean mitral valve gradients (10-mm slice thickness, $r = .84$ vs. 5-mm slice thickness, $r = .95$). Additionally, VEC MRI may provide more detailed information than Doppler ultrasonography in the hemodynamic assessment of asymmetric stenosis or complex flow patterns.

Global Ventricular Function

Systolic Performance

Parameters of LV function, such as stroke volume, ejection fraction, and cardiac output, are important diagnostic and prognostic indices of cardiac function in patients with heart disease. LV stroke volume has been quantified with VEC MRI measurements of aortic flow, and RV stroke volume with VEC MRI measurements of pulmonary flow (23). Stroke volume is calculated as the product of vascular cross-sectional area and flow velocity for all frames throughout the cardiac cycle. Kondo et al. (36) showed a high accuracy of VEC MRI measurements of aortic ($r = .80$) and pulmonary ($r = .91$) flow velocities in control subjects in comparison with measurements made by Doppler ultrasonography. RV and LV stroke volumes measured by VEC MRI were nearly identical and correlated closely ($r = .95$); they were similar to LV stroke volume determined by MRI volumetric analysis ($r = .98$) (37).

Diastolic Performance

Mitral inflow and pulmonary venous flow have been used as indices in the evaluation of LV diastolic function and mitral valve disease (38). Mohiaddin et al. (39) used VEC MRI to describe the flow patterns and flow velocities of mitral inflow and pulmonary veins in normal persons and patients with mitral valve stenosis. The mitral inflow in normal subjects was characterized by two positive peaks (early ventricular diastole and atrial contraction). In patients with mitral valve stenosis, the initial mitral inflow velocity persisted through diastole. Peak flow velocities in patients with mitral valve stenosis and in normal subjects have correlated well with values obtained with Doppler echocardiography (30,39). Pulmonary venous flow in normal persons showed two positive peaks (ventricular systole, ventricular diastole) and one negative peak (small backflow during atrial contraction).

VEC MRI has been used to measure the volume of blood flow across the mitral valve. In 10 normal volunteers studied by Hartiala et al. (40), the volume of blood flow across the mitral valve measured by VEC MRI ($5,610 \pm 620$ mL/min) was equivalent to the cardiac output measured by VEC MRI in the ascending aorta ($5,670 \pm 590$ mL/min) and by LV volumetrics derived from cine MRI ($5,440 \pm 614$ mL/min). In another study, VEC MRI was used to measure flow across the mitral valve to compare the contribution of atrial systole to LV filling in healthy subjects and in patients with LV hypertrophy (41). The VEC MRI-derived mitral inflow velocity pattern (E/A ratio) and left atrial contribution to LV filling (AC%) showed significant hyperbolic and linear correlation, respectively, with LV mass indices ($r = .95$ and $r = .86$).

Diastolic function of the RV has also been assessed with VEC MRI. The filling dynamics of the RV may be impaired in patients with right-sided valve lesions, pericardial disease, and several forms of cardiomyopathy (42,43). Mostbeck et al. (44) applied VEC MRI to measure flow velocities across the tricuspid valve and in the superior vena cava in 10 healthy volunteers to define normal RV relaxation. Values for peak early (E) and late (A) diastolic filling obtained with VEC MRI and the E/A ratio derived from VEC MRI and ultrasonography correlated closely ($r = .89$), but VEC MRI tended to overestimate the peak E and A velocities in comparison with Doppler ultrasonography. In another study, VEC MRI was used to quantify tricuspid inflow and superior vena cava flow in patients with arrhythmogenic RV dysplasia (ARVD) (45). The tricuspid flow curves in patients with ARVD differed distinctly from the curves in normal subjects, demonstrating A-wave predominance, and the right atrial contribution to diastolic inflow was significantly higher in the patients with ARVD than in normal persons ($37\% \pm 14\%$ versus $23\% \pm 2\%$).

CONGENITAL HEART DISEASE

MRI has been recognized as a method complementary to echocardiography in the evaluation of congenital heart disease (CHD) (46,47). MRI can depict both morphology and cardiac function and provide a quantitative assessment of the hemodynamics of CHD. This capability is particularly valuable when the usefulness of echocardiography is limited, as in the evaluation of the thoracic great vessels (48), the diagnosis of complex congenital anomalies, and follow-up after surgery (49). With advances in the surgical management of CHD, more and more patients require serial follow-up examinations postoperatively, and MRI may be an ideal modality for detecting residual defects and complications.

MRI has been used effectively in precisely demonstrating the morphology of CHD (46). However, evaluating function is of special importance in patients with cardiac disease, including those with congenital disease. As techniques have advanced in recent years, it has become apparent that MRI is useful for both qualitative and quantitative functional assessment of the heart and great vessels (46,50). Important capabilities of MRI in the quantitative evaluation of cardiac dimensions and function in CHD include measurement of the following: collateral blood flow and pressure gradients in coarctation of the aorta, intracardiac shunts and valvular regurgitation, differential blood flow in the right and left pulmonary arteries, and postoperative conduit blood flow and pressure gradients (25).

Coarctation of the Aorta

Coarctation of the aorta is a congenital stenosis. It is commonly located in the region of the ductus arteriosus at the junction of the aortic arch and descending aorta (aortic isthmus) just distal to the left subclavian artery. MRI can demonstrate the degree and the length of stenosis, associated aortic tubular hypoplasia, collateral pathways (internal mammary and posterior mediastinal arteries), post-stenotic dilation and relationship to the left subclavian artery, and degree of LV hypertrophy (51,52).

With the use of spin-echo MRI, the morphologic characteristics and enlarged collaterals of aortic coarctation can be demonstrated (Fig. 4.2). The physiologic severity of the coarctation can be measured with VEC MRI (53,54) (Fig. 4.2). These sequences are optimally obtained in an oblique sagittal orientation through the plane of the aortic arch. Each acquisition should be performed in a plane perpendicular to the direction of aortic blood flow. To calculate the quantity of collateral blood flow, the flow is estimated at two different locations, one at the proximal aorta 1 cm distal to the coarctation site and the other at the level of the diaphragm (54). In normal persons, flow is slightly greater in the proximal descending aorta than in the distal thoracic aorta. However, patients with coarctation may have greater blood flow distally, reflecting retrograde collateral blood flow into the aorta via the intercostal arteries and other branches of the thoracic aorta. To quantify the collateral circulation, the flow just distal to the coarctation site is subtracted from the flow at diaphragmatic level. Surgical management may depend on the degree of collateral flow. The

pressure gradient across the stenosis is the other hemodynamically important parameter in decision making. The peak flow velocity can be estimated with the use of VEC MRI through the most narrowed segment of coarctation (53), and the pressure gradient can be calculated with the modified Bernoulli equation: $\Delta P = 4v^2$, where ΔP is the pressure gradient in millimeters of mercury and v is the peak flow velocity in meters per second.

Balloon angioplasty and surgical flap repair are techniques commonly used to repair congenital aortic coarctation. In addition to perioperative complications, long-term changes may develop. Consequently, regular follow-up examinations and criteria for assessing clinical outcome are needed (55).

Noninvasive Detection and Quantification of Shunts

MRI is an effective means of demonstrating different portions of the atrial and ventricular septum and quantifying shunt lesions (46,56). Studies have confirmed the accuracy of VEC MRI in quantifying the pulmonary-to-systemic flow ratio (Q_p/Q_s) noninvasively, and correlation with catheterization and echocardiographic data has been good (20,23). VEC MRI is also a valuable method for monitoring shunt volume in CHD over time (23).

VEC MRI can be used to ascertain effective stroke volume and thereby quantify a shunt (Fig. 4.3). Blood flow is measured simultaneously in the ascending aorta and main pulmonary artery (20). In the absence of a shunt, blood flow is approximately equal in these two vessels. If a patient has a left-to-right shunt with an atrial septal defect, partial anomalous pulmonary venous connection, or ventricular septal defect, blood flow in the pulmonary artery will exceed flow in the aorta by the quantity of the shunt. In a patient with a patent ductus arteriosus, aortic blood flow is greater than pulmonary flow, and shunt volume is computed by subtracting pulmonary flow from aortic flow. The opposite relationship is true for right-to-left shunts. The pulmonary-to-systemic flow ratio as estimated by oximetry has been shown to correspond to the ratio obtained by VEC MRI (20).

Pulmonary Arteries

Because it does not rely on an imaging window, VEC MRI has the unique ability to measure blood flow in the pulmonary arteries (49). VEC MRI has been used to measure blood flow and velocity in the main and individually in the right and left pulmonary arteries. Because VEC MRI can measure blood flow separately in the right and left pulmonary arteries, it can provide important information in some patients who have complex CHD with a disparity in blood flow between the right and left pulmonary arteries (Fig. 4.4).

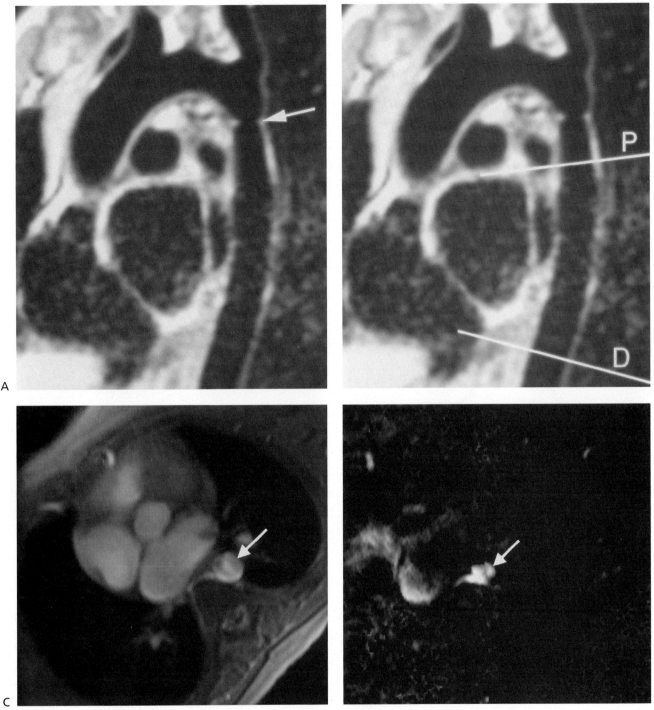

FIGURE 4.2. Coarctation of the aorta. **A:** Oblique sagittal electrocardiogram-gated spin-echo T1-weighted image demonstrates a discrete juxtaductal coarctation *(arrow)*. **B:** This image was used to prescribe velocity-encoded cine (VEC) MRI in planes through the proximal descending aorta *(line labeled P)* and distal descending aorta *(line labeled D)*. VEC MRI magnitude image **(C)** and phase image **(D)** through the proximal descending aorta *(arrow)*. *(continued)*

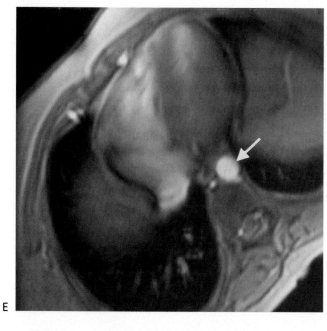

E

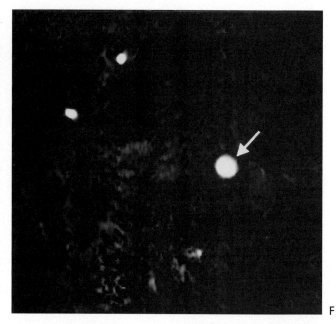

F

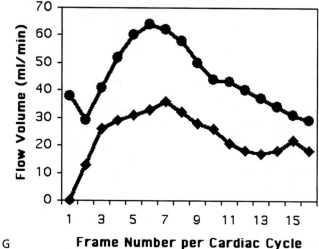

G

FIGURE 4.2. *(continued)* VEC MRI magnitude image **(E)** and phase image **(F)** through the distal aorta *(arrow)*. **G:** Flow curves derived from VEC MRI demonstrate a marked increase in flow in the distal aorta *(line joined by circles)* in comparison with the proximal aorta *(line joined by diamonds)*. The difference between the curves represents collateral circulation.

Caputo et al. (57) quantified right and left pulmonary artery flow volumes in normal subjects and in patients with CHD associated with disparate pulmonary flow. They acquired VEC MRI in planes perpendicular to the flow in each pulmonary artery in nine healthy subjects and demonstrated that the total blood flow within the left and right pulmonary arteries was nearly equal to the blood flow in the main pulmonary artery. The values for right and left pulmonary artery flow were 54% ± 5% and 46% ± 5%, respectively, in the healthy volunteers, whereas a large differential in pulmonary artery blood flow was noted in the group of patients with CHD. The results of this study suggest an application of VEC MRI to assess differential flow in the pulmonary arteries, which occurs in various forms of CHD.

Pulmonary arterial hypertension changes the elastic nature of pulmonary arteries, so that the compliance and thus the distensibility of the vessel wall are affected. Distensibility of the main, left, and right pulmonary arteries can be calculated from changes in volume (systolic volume minus diastolic volume divided by systolic volume) on end-diastolic and end-systolic images. Bogren and colleagues (58), stressing the potential of VEC MRI to estimate pulmonary vascular resistance, measured in normal main pulmonary arteries a mean distensibility of 23%, whereas in patients with pulmonary artery hypertension, the distensibility was only 8%. No age-related differences were found.

Several studies investigated flow patterns in the main pulmonary artery in normal persons and in patients with pulmonary hypertension (58,59). In normal subjects, retrograde flow accounted for 2% of total flow and occurred mainly along the posterior wall toward the end of systole through early diastole, serving to close the pulmonic valve. In patients with pulmonary hypertension, retrograde flow

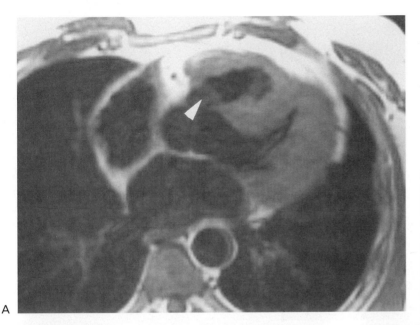

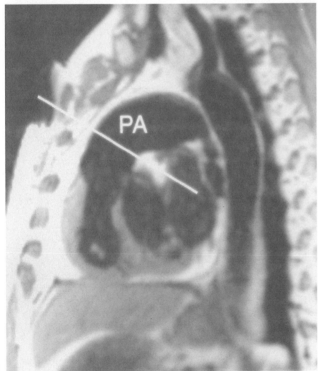

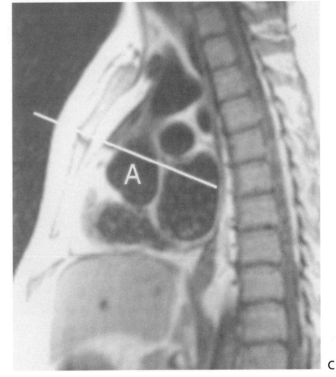

FIGURE 4.3. Shunt quantification. **A:** Transverse electrocardiogram-gated spin-echo T1-weighted MR image demonstrates a supracristal ventricular septal defect *(arrowhead)*. **B–E:** Pulmonary-to-systemic flow ratio (Q_p/Q_s) can be derived by acquiring velocity-encoded cine (VEC) MRI flow measurements in the planes indicated by lines through the pulmonary artery *(PA)* and ascending aorta *(A)*. **B,C:** Sagittal spin-echo T1-weighted images are used to prescribe imaging planes *(indicated by lines)* for VEC MRI through the main pulmonary artery and ascending aorta. *(continued)*

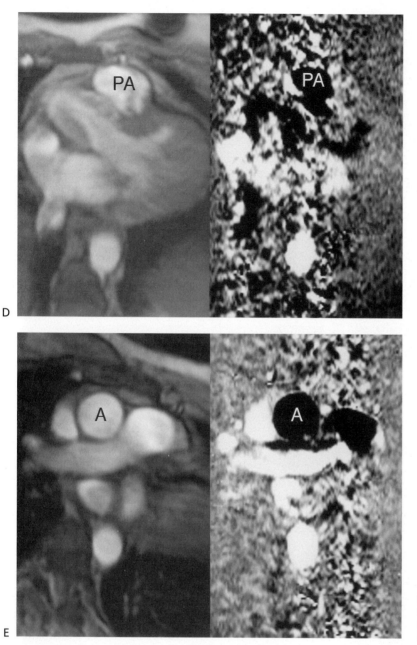

FIGURE 4.3. *(continued)* **D,E:** VEC MRI through the main pulmonary artery and aorta. Magnitude images are on the left, and phase images are on the right. In this patient, Q_p/Q_s was 1.7:1.

accounted for 26% of the total flow, a finding that might be attributed to changes in resistance, impedance, compliance, capacitance, and shape of the vessel (58). When Kondo et al. (59) compared velocity patterns in normal persons and patients with pulmonary hypertension, a significantly lower peak systolic velocity was reached much earlier in systole in the patients with pulmonary hypertension.

Tetralogy of Fallot

Tetralogy of Fallot accounts for approximately 5.5% of cases of CHD (60). The features of tetralogy of Fallot are RV outflow obstruction, malalignment ventricular septal defect, RV hypertrophy, and overriding aorta, which is caused by underdevelopment of the infundibulum with superior and leftward displacement of the parietal band (crista supraventricularis). This displacement is responsible for narrowing of the RV outflow tract and leads to underdeveloped pulmonary arteries and pulmonary valves and to the overriding aorta. Associated anomalies are a right aortic arch (25%) and abnormal origin and course of the coronary arteries.

After right ventriculoplasty or Rastelli procedure to repair tetralogy of Fallot, pulmonic regurgitation is frequently a residual abnormality. VEC MRI has been used to measure the volume of pulmonic regurgitation in this setting (61,62)

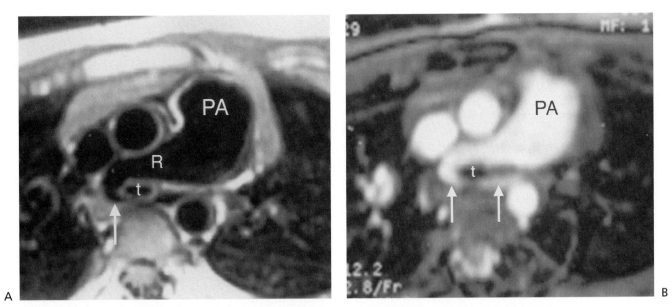

FIGURE 4.4. Differential pulmonary artery flow determination in a child with pulmonary sling. **A:** Transverse electrocardiogram-gated spin-echo T1-weighted MR image. The anomalous left pulmonary artery *(arrow)* arises from the right pulmonary artery, passing behind the trachea *(t)*. The left pulmonary artery is much smaller than the right pulmonary artery. **B:** Transverse segmented k-space cine gradient-echo images also demonstrate the left pulmonary artery *(arrows)* coursing posterior to the trachea *(t)*. The velocity-encoded cine MRI (not shown) demonstrated diminished flow in the left pulmonary artery that accounted for only 20% of pulmonary blood flow. *PA,* main pulmonary artery.

(Fig. 4.5). The volume of pulmonic regurgitation measured by VEC MRI is closely correlated with the difference in stroke volume indices of the two ventricles and with the RV end-diastolic volume (62).

Postoperative Evaluation of Congenital Heart Disease

One of the most useful applications of VEC MRI in CHD is in monitoring patients after surgery (61). Studies can be performed repeatedly with an operator-independent technique and without the need for radiation exposure or iodinated contrast media; furthermore, VEC MRI can display morphology in addition to function, so that catheterization and angiography are unnecessary. Indications are the assessment of ventricular and valvular function as important prognostic parameters of long-term morbidity in postoperative patients with CHD, and evaluation of surgical conduits (61–65).

VEC MRI has also been applied to assess late complications of the venoatrial pathways after the Mustard operation for transposition of the great arteries (65). VEC MRI enabled accurate measurement of the peak velocity of a jet at the site of an obstruction and the direction of the jet; these measurements made it possible to distinguish obstruction from atrial baffle leak because the direction of a jet caused by obstruction is different from that caused by a baffle leak.

In CHD with diminished flow to the pulmonary circulation, several types of palliative shunts can be used to increase blood flow to the pulmonary arteries (61). Currently, those most commonly used are the Glenn shunt, connecting the superior cava to the pulmonary arteries, and the modified Blalock-Taussig shunt, connecting the subclavian artery to the pulmonary circulation. The most frequently encountered complication after shunt placement is stenosis or obstruction of the shunt (66). To evaluate shunt patency, a combination of spin-echo MRI and gradient-echo MRI has been shown to be superior to transthoracic echocardiography (67,68). VEC MRI can be used to measure blood flow in the shunt and estimate the pressure gradient across a site of stenosis (61).

A different type of extracardiac shunt is the connection between the RV and the pulmonary circulation, used in the Rastelli operation. With the use of phase-contrast MRI, a reliable estimation of the pressure gradient within the obstructed conduit can be obtained (61,63). Martinez et al. (63) used VEC MRI to detect obstruction in extracardiac ventriculopulmonary conduits in 52 patients. Calculated gradients in obstructed conduits derived from VEC MRI correlated well with results of continuous-wave Doppler echocardiography ($r = .95$) and accurately localized the site of obstruction, in addition to measuring its severity. Rebergen et al. (62) demonstrated a high degree of accuracy for VEC MRI in quantifying the volume of pulmonary regurgitation after surgical repair of tetralogy of Fallot. The VEC MRI measurements of forward and regurgitant flow volume in the main pulmonary artery corresponded closely to the values acquired by ventricular volumetric studies ($r = .93$).

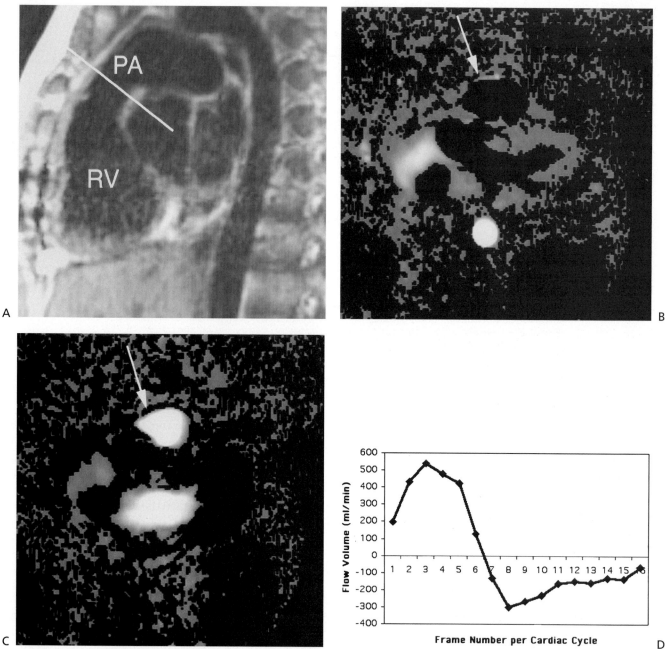

FIGURE 4.5. Pulmonary regurgitation in postoperative tetralogy of Fallot. This patient had previously undergone right ventriculoplasty. **A:** Sagittal electrocardiogram-gated spin-echo T1-weighted MR image was used to prescribe velocity-encoded cine (VEC) MRI through the main pulmonary artery *(PA). RV,* right ventricle. **B:** VEC MRI phase image during systole demonstrates dark signal in the pulmonary artery, indicating forward flow. **C:** VEC MRI phase image during diastole shows bright signal in the pulmonary artery, representing regurgitant flow. **D:** The flow curve demonstrates regurgitant (negative) flow during the entire diastolic period. Integration of the area under the antegrade flow curve (positive values) represents stroke volume, and integration of the area delineated by the retrograde flow curve (negative values) during diastole represents regurgitant volume. Regurgitant fraction is the regurgitant volume divided by the stroke volume. In this patient, the regurgitant fraction was 39%.

ACQUIRED HEART DISEASE

Major clinical indications of blood flow measurements in acquired heart disease include the quantification of valvular heart disease, coronary blood flow, and flow within coronary bypass grafts (69).

Valvular Heart Disease

Volume overload of the ventricles in valvular heart disease can lead to congestive heart failure, myocardial dysfunction, and sometimes sudden death. Therefore, one of the main questions in the management of these patients is whether the disease is severe enough that surgical intervention is warranted (70). Noninvasive methods for an accurate and reproducible quantification of the severity of valvular heart disease and of ventricular dimensions and function may improve patient management. Several MRI techniques may be valuable in monitoring patients with valvular heart disease (70).

Most prosthetic heart valves are not ferromagnetic and can be evaluated with MRI, although the prosthetic valve shows low signal and the metal material shows local image defect. MRI may be used to detect dysfunction in prosthetic valves, and cine gradient-echo imaging has been shown to have an accuracy rate of 96% in detecting pathologic leakage flow in comparison with transesophageal Doppler echocardiography (71). In addition, velocity distribution downstream from a prosthetic aortic valve (72) may provide meaningful information about the function of the prosthetic valve (70).

Valvular stenosis and regurgitation cause jet flow and produce a signal-void area on gradient-echo images. For instance, mitral regurgitation is identified as an area of signal loss extending from the incompetent valve into the left atrium during ventricular systole, whereas aortic regurgitation is shown as an area of signal loss extending from the incompetent valve into the LV during ventricular diastole. However, the major use of noninvasive imaging is to assess the severity of valvular regurgitation in as quantitative a manner as possible.

The three primary methods for assessing the severity of the valvular regurgitation are the following: (a) measurement of the signal-void area at cine MRI, (b) calculation of the regurgitant volume with ventricular volumetric studies, and (c) use of the VEC MRI technique to quantify the regurgitant blood flow (14). To evaluate the severity of valvular stenosis, two methods are available: (a) evaluation of the flow jet and associated findings, and (b) quantification of the transvalvular pressure gradient and valve area with VEC MRI (14).

To calculate the regurgitant volume with VEC MRI, antegrade and retrograde flow can be discriminated during the cardiac cycle and retrograde flow can be measured directly to quantify regurgitation (Fig. 4.6). For example, the ascending aorta contains bright signal during systole, indicating antegrade flow, whereas voxels are dark in diastole, indi-cating the retrograde flow caused by aortic regurgitation (73). Dulce et al. (74) assessed 10 patients with chronic aortic regurgitation and used VEC MRI to measure the regurgitant volume and regurgitant fraction. The VEC MRI-derived data correlated closely with volumetric cine MR measurements ($r > .97$), indicating the high potential of this technique for serial follow-up and monitoring of the therapeutic response. Globits et al. (75) used VEC MRI to evaluate the hemodynamic response to angiotensin-converting enzyme (ACE) inhibitor therapy in nine patients with chronic aortic regurgitation. Three months after the initiation of ACE inhibitor therapy, six patients responded with a significant decrease in regurgitation fraction and a slight increase in forward stroke volume when these factors were compared with those of a reference group of 10 untreated patients with chronic aortic regurgitation.

Alternatively, regurgitant volume can be determined from the difference between LV stroke volume measured with VEC MRI in the ascending aorta and RV stroke volume measured in the main pulmonary artery. In 10 patients with isolated aortic regurgitation, Sondergaard et al. (76) showed an excellent correlation between the difference in stroke volumes calculated by ventricular volumetric cine MRI and regurgitant volume quantified by VEC MRI ($r = .97$). Furthermore, they found a significant correlation between LV end-diastolic volume and regurgitant volume by VEC MRI ($r = .80$) and between regurgitant volume by MRI and angiographic grade ($r = .80$). Fujita et al. (77) demonstrated the feasibility of using VEC MRI to estimate mitral regurgitant volume and regurgitant fraction as the difference between mitral inflow and aortic outflow with imaging planes positioned at the level of the mitral and aortic annuli, respectively. The regurgitant fraction correlated well with the echocardiographic severity of mitral regurgitation ($r = .87$).

Coronary Flow Measurement

MRI is uniquely capable of evaluating coronary blood flow noninvasively in the major epicardial coronary arteries. Roentgenographic angiography has been used for many years to identify coronary artery stenoses. However, visual inspection of the anatomic severity of a coronary stenosis does not adequately determine the functional significance of the lesion (78). Quantitative coronary angiography, which was designed to minimize interpretation variability, cannot reliably predict the physiologic significance of a stenosis of intermediate severity. Assessment of the functional significance of a stenosis is particularly important when the lesion is of intermediate severity because how such lesions are interpreted has a significant influence on patient management. The functional significance of a coronary arterial stenosis can be evaluated by measuring the coronary flow reserve, which is the ratio of the maximal hyperemic coronary flow to the baseline coronary flow.

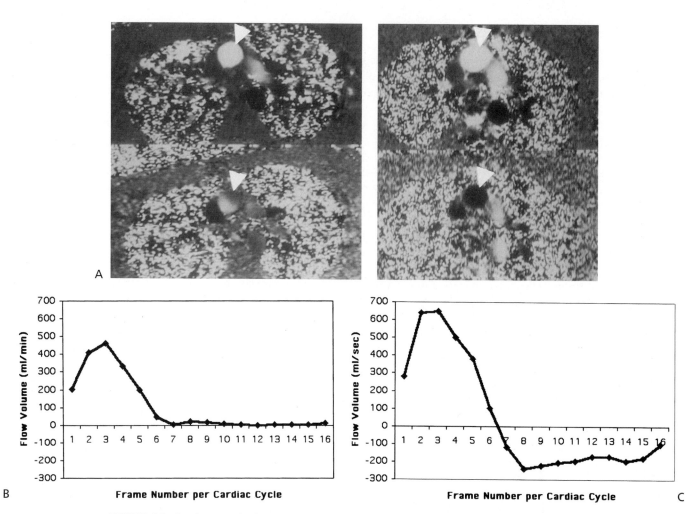

FIGURE 4.6. Aortic regurgitation. **A:** Velocity-encoded cine MRI in a normal person *(left)* and in a patient with aortic regurgitation *(right)*. Velocity of flow in a cranial direction is represented by *white coloration,* and velocity in a caudal direction is represented by *black coloration.* In the normal person, bright voxels are present within the ascending aorta *(arrowheads)* during systole. However, during diastole, the intraaortic voxels show a coloration similar to that of the chest wall (nonmobile structures). This indicates little blood flow during diastole in the normal person. In contradistinction, *black coloration* is seen throughout the ascending aorta during diastole in the patient with aortic regurgitation, representing retrograde blood flow within the aorta at this phase of the cardiac cycle. This is represented graphically in the flow curves for the normal person **(B)** and for the patient with aortic regurgitation **(C).** (From Higgins CB. Acquired heart disease. In: Higgins CB, Hricak H, Helms CA, eds. *Magnetic resonance imaging of the body,* 3rd ed. Philadelphia: Lippincott–Raven Publishers, 1997:409–460, with permission.)

Several different methods have been used in the past to quantify coronary artery blood flow with MRI, including the TOF method (79), MR bolus tagging (80), and phase-contrast technique (VEC MRI) (81). Currently, VEC MRI is the MRI method most frequently used to quantify coronary artery flow. VEC MRI can provide coronary blood flow measurements at multiple phases throughout the cardiac cycle. Volumetric blood flow in the coronary arteries can be quantified by integrating the product of the mean velocity and the cross-sectional area of the vessel from the multiple phase images acquired during the cardiac cycle (82). The normal coronary flow reserve with volumetric MRI flow measurement was 4.2 ± 1.8 according to Grist et al. (83) and 5.0 ± 2.6 according to Davis et al. (84).

VEC MRI can assess coronary blood flow and flow reserve in patients with coronary stenosis (85). In significant coronary stenosis, the distal parts of the coronary arteries are nearly maximally dilated at rest to maintain myocardial perfusion, and during physical or pharmacologic stress, less reserve is available for further dilation. The coronary flow reserve, defined as the ratio of flow during stress to flow at baseline, can therefore be used to determine the significance of a stenosis (86).

VEC MRI measurements of coronary flow and coronary flow reserve have been performed in the left anterior descending and right coronary arteries (82–87) and validated in both animals and humans (88,89). Sakuma et al. (88) used VEC MRI to quantify coronary flow in dogs at rest and during stress (dipyridamole-induced hyperemia). These results were validated by placing epicardial Doppler flow meters in the left anterior descending coronary artery. Mean coronary flow reserve was 2.51 ± 1.06 by VEC MRI and 2.73 ± 1.41 by Doppler flow meter, with a mean proportional difference of 8.7% between the two methods. Regression analysis demonstrated a linear relationship ($r = .95$) between MRI and Doppler flow meter measurements over a wide range of perfusion conditions. Hundley et al. (89) measured coronary flow reserve in humans with VEC MRI and validated the results with intracoronary Doppler flow wires. They found good correlation ($r = .89$) between the two methods for the quantification of coronary flow at rest and during pharmacologically induced hyperemia. In another study, Sakuma et al. (86) measured coronary flow before and after dipyridamole injection in normal human volunteers and found an average coronary flow reserve of 3.1 in this group. This value for coronary flow reserve measured by MRI is consistent with normal values achieved with other modalities (90).

Although this technique has proved useful, MRI measurement of blood flow in the coronary arteries can be challenging, and accuracy may suffer because these vessels are relatively small, only 3 to 4 mm in diameter. Moreover, this approach does not measure total coronary flow, which is critical for the evaluation of coronary flow reserve in nonobstructive myocardial disease. Therefore, an alternative method has been developed for assessing coronary blood flow with VEC MRI. Because 96% of the veins arising from the LV wall and the septum drain into the coronary sinus, coronary sinus flow approximates total coronary arterial flow (91). The diameter of the coronary sinus (~10 mm) is larger than that of the coronary arteries; thus, interrogation of the coronary sinus with VEC MRI is technically easier and more straightforward, and results may be more readily reproducible. Recently, a study in which VEC MRI was used was performed in dogs to validate the measurement of coronary sinus flow as an approximation of total coronary arterial blood flow (92) (Fig. 4.7). In that study, coronary si-

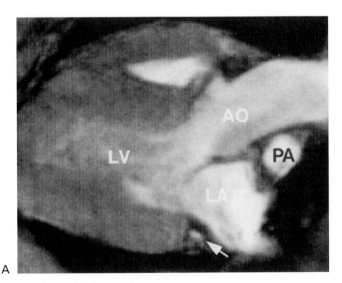

A

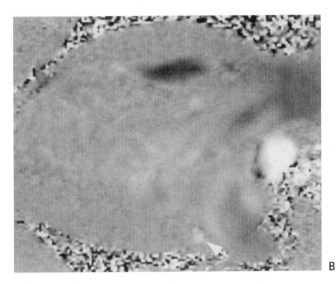

B

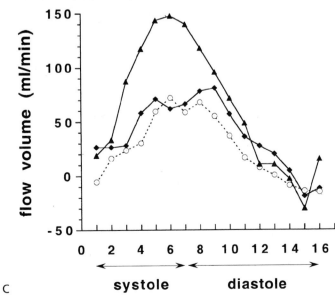

C

FIGURE 4.7. Coronary sinus flow. Magnitude **(A)** and phasic **(B)** velocity-encoded cine MRI of a canine heart in the oblique long-axis view. The coronary sinus *(arrows)* is depicted during late systole with the mitral valve closed and with antegrade flow in the vessel, which is depicted as a bright area on the phasic image. *AO,* ascending aorta; *LA,* left atrium; *LV,* left ventricle; *PA,* right pulmonary artery. **C:** Graph shows phasic coronary sinus flow pattern in a single animal in the basal state *(diamonds),* in the presence of a left circumflex coronary stenosis in the basal state *(open circles),* and during reactive hyperemia *(triangles).* At baseline, a biphasic flow pattern is observed, with a first peak during mid-systole and a second peak during early diastole. Arterial stenosis results in a slight delay in systolic peak flow and loss of the biphasic pattern. During reactive hyperemia, peak flow occurs during late systole and early diastole. (From Lund GK, Wendland MF, Shimakawa A, et al. Coronary sinus flow measurement by means of velocity-encoded cine MR imaging: validation by using flow probes in dogs. *Radiology* 2000;217:487–493, with permission.)

nus flow was measured by VEC MRI at rest and during stress (pharmacologic vasodilation), and results were compared with measurements obtained by placing Doppler flow meters in the epicardial coronary arteries. Coronary sinus flow measured by VEC MRI correlated closely ($r = 0.98$) with total coronary flow measured by Doppler flow probes. This technique also has been used to demonstrate reduced coronary flow reserve in patients with hypertrophic cardiomyopathy (93) and in patients with chronic heart transplant rejection (94).

Coronary Bypass Grafts

The successful long-term results of coronary bypass surgery depend on the maintenance of graft patency (95). About 25% of venous grafts become occluded within 1 year, and half of these within 2 weeks of surgery. In the subsequent 5 years, the annual occlusion rate is approximately 2% per year, increasing to 5% yearly thereafter. Thus, 50% to 60% of venous grafts are occluded after 10 years (96), figures that suggest the need for evaluation of coronary artery bypass graft patency and function during postoperative follow-up. Both noninvasive and semiinvasive methods can be used to determine the patency of coronary bypass grafts, including computed tomography, two-dimensional Doppler echocardiography, and MRI (97).

An important feature of MRI is that blood flow can be measured within the graft. Galjee et al. (98) demonstrated that adequate velocity profiles throughout the cardiac cycle could be obtained in 85% of angiographically patent vein grafts with VEC MRI. Graft velocity was characterized by a biphasic pattern, with one peak in systole and a second peak in diastole. Similar findings have been obtained with invasive Doppler guidewire approaches and transthoracic Doppler echocardiography (97). VEC MRI can also be used to determine the adequacy of flow in internal mammary artery and saphenous vein bypass grafts (98–100). The normal flow pattern in grafts and native coronary arteries is characteristically biphasic, with substantial flow velocity in diastole. Loss of the phasic pattern or loss of vasodilator reserve may indicate an obstructed coronary bypass conduit. Ishida et al. (99) studied internal mammary artery-to-coronary artery bypass grafts with VEC MRI. Obstructed internal mammary artery bypass conduits demonstrated a diastolic-to-systolic peak velocity ratio of 0.61 ± 0.44, which was significantly lower than the ratio in nonobstructed grafts ($1.88 \pm .96$). The sensitivity and specificity of VEC MRI for predicting significant stenosis were 86% and 94%, respectively.

A possible indication for MRI may be to assess the patency of grafts that are not visualized at conventional angiography (100). Another indication for bypass graft MRI may be to evaluate patients who have chest pain shortly after coronary artery bypass surgery. Noninvasive monitoring of the flow parameters may then be useful to detect a grad-

ual increase in graft stenosis and to reach a decision to proceed to x-ray angiography and stent placement before the onset of total occlusion.

SUMMARY

In current clinical practice, VEC MRI is a frequently used technique for quantifying blood flow in congenital and acquired cardiovascular disease. Important clinical applications of VEC MRI include the measurement of collateral circulation in coarctation of the aorta, quantification of intracardiac shunts, differentiation of blood flow in the left and right pulmonary arteries, quantitative evaluation of the postoperative patient with CHD, measurement of valvular stenosis or regurgitation, and appraisal of flow in the coronary circulation and in coronary bypass grafts.

REFERENCES

1. Higgins CB, Sokuma H. Heart disease: Functional evaluation with MR imaging. *Radiology* 1996;199:307–315.
2. Singer JR, Crooks LE. Blood flow rates by nuclear magnetic resonance measurements. *Science* 1959;130:1652–1653.
3. Carr HY, Purcell EM. Effects of diffusion on free precession in nuclear magnetic resonance experiments. *Physiol Rev* 1954;94:630–638.
4. Moran PR. A flow velocity zeugmatographic interlace for NMR imaging in humans. *Magn Reson Imaging* 1982;1:197–203.
5. Van Dijk P. Direct cardiac NMR imaging of the heart wall and blood flow velocity. *J Comput Assist Tomogr* 1983;8:429–436.
6. Bryant DJ, Payne JA, Finnin DN, et al. Measurement of flow with NMR imaging using a gradient pulse and phase difference technique. *J Comput Assist Tomogr* 1984;8:588–593.
7. Singer JR, Crooks LE. Nuclear magnetic resonance blood flow measurements in the human brain. *Science* 1983;221:654–656.
8. Axel L. Blood flow effects in magnetic resonance imaging. *AJR Am J Roentgenol* 1984;143:1157–1166.
9. Wehrli FW, Shimakawa A, Gullberg GT, et al. Time-of-flight MR flow imaging: selective saturation recovery with gradient refocusing. *Radiology* 1986;160:781–785.
10. Nayler GL, Firmin DN, Longmore DB. Blood flow imaging by cine magnetic resonance. *J Comput Assist Tomogr* 1986;10:715–722.
11. Bogren HG, Klipstein RH, Firmin DN, et al. Quantitation of antegrade and retrograde blood flow in the human aorta by magnetic resonance velocity mapping. *Am Heart J* 1989;117:1214–1222.
12. Underwood SR, Firrnin DN, Klipstein RH, et al. Magnetic resonance velocity mapping: clinical application of a new technique. *Br Heart J* 1987;57:404–412.
13. Mohiaddin RH. Clinical application of MR flow mapping in acquired heart disease. In: *Book of abstracts: International Society of Magnetic Resonance in Medicine.* London, 1999:14(abst).
14. Didier D, Ratib O, Lerch R, et al. Detection and quantification of valvular heart disease with dynamic cardiac MR imaging. *Radiographics* 2000;20:1279–1299.
15. Mostbeck GH, Caputo GR, Higgins CB. MR measurements of blood flow in the cardiovascular system. *AJR Am J Roentgenol* 1992;159:453–461.

16. Bogren HG, Buonocore MH. Blood flow measurements in the aorta and major arteries with MR velocity mapping. *J Magn Reson Imaging* 1994;4:119–130.

17. Higgins CB, Caputo G, Wendland MF, et al. Measurement of blood flow and perfusion in the cardiovascular system. *Invest Radiol* 1992;27(Suppl 2):66–71.

18. Mohiaddin RH, Pennell DJ. MR blood flow measurement: clinical application in the heart and circulation. *Cardiol Clin* 1998;16:161–187.

19. Duerinckx AJ, Higgins CB. Valvular heart disease. *Radiol Clin North Am* 1994;32:613–630.

20. Brenner LD, Caputo GR, Mostbeck G, et al. Quantification of left to right atrial shunts with velocity-encoded cine nuclear magnetic resonance imaging. *J Am Coll Cardiol* 1992;20:1246–1250.

21. Axel L. Overview of MR blood flow imaging techniques. In: *Book of abstracts: International Society of Magnetic Resonance in Medicine*. London, 1999:24(abst).

22. Edelman RR, Mattle HP, Kjeefield J, et al. Quantification of blood flow with dynamic MR imaging and presaturation bolus tracking. *Radiology* 1989;171:551–556.

23. Szolar DH, Sakuma H, Higgins CB. Cardiovascular applications of magnetic resonance flow and velocity measurements. *J Magn Reson Imaging* 1996;6:78–89.

24. Mohiaddin RH, Longmore DB. Functional aspects of cardiovascular nuclear magnetic resonance imaging: techniques and application. *Circulation* 1993;88:264–281.

25. Reddy G, Higgins CB. Congenital heart disease: measuring physiology with MRI. *Semin Roentgenol* 1998;33:228–238.

26. Speilman RP, Schneider O, Thiele F, et al. Appearance of poststenotic jets in MRI: dependence on flow velocity and on imaging parameters. *Magn Reson Imaging* 1991;9:67–72.

27. Underwood R. Blood flow measurements. In: Higgins CB, Hricak H, Helms CA, eds. *Magnetic resonance imaging of the body,* 3rd ed. Philadelphia: Lippincott–Raven Publishers, 1997:555–565.

28. Firmin DN, Nayler GL, Kilner PJ, et al. The applications of phase shifts in NMR for flow measurements. *Magn Reson Med* 1990;14:230–241.

29. Pelc JN, Bernstein MA, Shimakawa A, et al. Encoding strategies for three direction phase-contrast MR imaging of flow. *J Magn Reson Imaging* 1991;1:405–413.

30. Kilner PJ, Firmin DN, Rees RS, et al. Valve and great vessel stenosis: assessment with MR jet velocity mapping. *Radiology* 1991;178:229–235.

31. Axel L, Morton D. Correction of phase wrapping in magnetic resonance imaging. *Med Phys* 1989;16:284–287.

32. Mostbeck GH, Caputo GR, Madjumdar S, et al. Assessment of vascular stenoses with MR jet phase velocity mapping at 1.5 T: *in vitro* validation. *Radiology* 1991;181:264(abst).

33. Kilner PJ, Mancara CC, Mohiaddin RH, et al. Magnetic resonance jet velocity mapping in mitral and aortic valve stenosis. *Circulation* 1993;87:1239–1248.

34. Sondergaard L, Hildebrandt P, Lindvig K, et al. Valve area and cardiac output in aortic stenosis: quantification by magnetic resonance velocity mapping. *Am Heart J* 1993;126:1156–1164.

35. Heidenreich PA, Steffens JC, Fujita N, et al. Evaluation of mitral stenosis with velocity-encoded cine MRI. *Am J Cardiol* 1995;75:365.

36. Kondo C, Caputo GR, Semelka R, et al. Right and left ventricular stroke volume measurements with velocity-encoded cine NMR imaging: *in vitro* and *in vivo* validation. *AJR Am J Roentgenol* 1992;157:9–16.

37. van Rossum AC, Sprenger M, Visser FC, et al. An *in vivo* validation of quantitative blood flow imaging in arteries and veins using magnetic resonance phase-shift techniques. *Eur Heart J* 1991;12:117–126.

38. Myreng Y, Smiseth OA. Assessment of left ventricular relaxation by Doppler echocardiography. Comparison of isovolumic relaxation time and transmittal flow velocities with time constant of isovolumic relaxation. *Circulation* 1990;81:260–266.

39. Mohiaddin RH, Amanuma M, Kilner PJ, et al. MR phase-shift velocity mapping of mitral and pulmonary venous flow. *J Comput Assist Tomogr* 1991;15: 237–243.

40. Hartiala JJ, Mostbeck GH, Foster E, et al. Velocity-encoded cine MRI in the evaluation of left ventricular diastolic function: measurement of mitral valve and pulmonary vein flow volume across the mitral valve. *Am Heart J* 1993;125:1054–1066.

41. Hartiala JJ, Foster E, Fujita N, et al. Evaluation of left atrial contribution to left ventricular filling in aortic stenosis by velocity-encoded cine MRI. *Am Heart J* 1994;127:593–600.

42. Hoit BD, Dalton N, Bhargava V, et al. Pericardial influences on right and left ventricular dynamics. *Circ Res* 1991;68:197–208.

43. Suzuki JI, Caputo GR, Masui T, et al. Assessment of right ventricular diastolic and systolic function in patients with dilated cardiomyopathy using cine magnetic resonance imaging. *Am Heart J* 1991;122:1035–1040.

44. Mostbeck GH, Hartiala JJ, Foster E, et al. Right ventricular diastolic filling: evaluation with velocity encoded cine MRI. *J Comput Assist Tomogr* 1993;17: 245–252.

45. Snoep G, Sanders DGM, Smeets J, et al. Cardiac inflow in right ventricular dysplasia assessed by MR velocity mapping. In: *Book of abstracts: Society of Magnetic Resonance in Medicine*. Berkeley, CA: Society of Magnetic Resonance in Medicine, 1994:115 (abst).

46. Higgins CB, Byrd BF III, Farmer DW, et al. Magnetic resonance imaging in patients with congenital heart disease. *Circulation* 1984;70:851–860.

47. Fletcher BD, Jacobstein MD, Nelson AD, et al. Gated magnetic resonance imaging of congenital cardiac malformations. *Radiology* 1984;150:137–140.

48. Didier D, Ratib O, Beghetti M, et al. Morphologic and functional evaluation of congenital heart disease by magnetic resonance imaging. *J Magn Reson Imaging* 1999;10:639–655.

49. Higgins CB. Congenital heart disease. In: Higgins CB, Hricak H, Helms CA, eds. *Magnetic resonance imaging of the body*, 3rd ed. Philadelphia: Lippincott–Raven Publishers, 1997:461–518.

50. Gross GW, Steiner RM. Radiographic manifestations of congenital heart disease in the adult patient. *Radiol Clin North Am* 1991;29:293–317.

51. Didier D, Higgins CB, Fisher MR, et al. Congenital heart disease: gated MR imaging in 72 patients. *Radiology* 1986;158: 227–235.

52. Krinsky GA, Rofsky NM, DeCorato DR, et al. Thoracic aorta: comparison of gadolinium-enhanced three-dimensional MR angiography and conventional MR imaging. *Radiology* 1997; 202:183–193.

53. Mohiaddin RH, Kilner PT, Rees S, et al. Magnetic resonance volume flow and jet velocity mapping in aortic coarctation. *J Am Coll Cardiol* 1993;22:1515–1521.

54. Steffens JC, Bourne MW, Sakuma H, et al. Quantitation of collateral blood flow in coarctation of the aorta by velocity-encoded cine magnetic resonance imaging. *Circulation* 1994;90:937–943.

55. Summers P, Razavi R, Haworth C, et al. MR imaging and flow in the follow-up of coarctation repair. In: *Book of abstracts: International Society of Magnetic Resonance in Medicine*. London, 1999:32(abst).

56. Sechtem U, Pflugfelder P, Cassidy MC, et al. Ventricular septal defect: visualization of shunt flow and determination of shunt size by cine magnetic resonance imaging. *AJR Am J Roentgenol* 1987;149:689–691.

57. Caputo GR, Kondo C, Masui T, et al. Right and left lung per-

fusion: *in vitro* and *in vivo* validation with oblique-angle, velocity-encoded cine MR imaging. *Radiology* 1991;180:693–698.

58. Bogren HG, Klipstein RH, Mohiaddin RH, et al. Pulmonary artery distensibility and blood flow patterns: a magnetic resonance study of normal subjects and of patients with pulmonary arterial hypertension. *Am Heart J* 1990;118:990–999.

59. Kondo C, Caputo GR, Masui T, et al. Pulmonary hypertension: pulmonary flow quantification and flow profile analysis with velocity-encoded cine MR imaging. *Radiology* 1992;183:751–758.

60. Murphy JG, Gersh BJ, Mair DD, et al. Long-term outcome in patients undergoing surgical repair of tetralogy of Fallot. *N Engl J Med* 1993;329:593–599.

61. Roest A.W, Helbing W, van der Wall E. Postoperative evaluation of congenital heart disease by magnetic resonance imaging. *J Magn Reson Imaging* 1999;10:656–666.

62. Rebergen SA, Chin JGJ, Ottenkamp J, et al. Pulmonary regurgitation in the late postoperative follow-up of tetralogy of Fallot: volumetric quantitation by nuclear magnetic resonance velocity mapping. *Circulation* 1993;88:2257–2266.

63. Martinez JE, Mohiaddin RH, Kilner PJ, et al. Obstruction in extracardiac ventriculo-pulmonary conduits: value of nuclear magnetic resonance imaging with velocity mapping and Doppler echocardiography. *J Am Coll Cardiol* 1992;20:338–344.

64. Rebergen SA, Ottenkamp J, Doombos J, et al. Postoperative pulmonary flow dynamics after Fontan surgery: assessment with nuclear magnetic resonance velocity mapping. *J Am Coll Cardiol* 1993;21:123–131.

65. Sampson C, Filner PD, Hirsch R, et al. Venoatrial pathways after the Mustard operation for transposition of the great arteries: anatomic and functional MR imaging. *Radiology* 1994;193:211–217.

66. Agarwal KC, Edwards WD, Feldt RH, et al. Clinicopathological correlates of obstructed right-sided porcine-valve extracardiac conduits. *J Thorac Cardiovasc Surg* 1981;81:591–601.

67. Jacobstein MD, Fletcher BD, Nelson AD, et al. Magnetic resonance imaging: evaluation of palliative systemic–pulmonary artery shunts. *Circulation* 1984;70:650–656.

68. Bornemeier RA, Weinberg PM, Fogel MA. Angiographic, echocardiographic, and three-dimensional magnetic resonance imaging of extracardiac conduits in congenital heart disease. *Am J Cardiol* 1996;78:713–717.

69. Higgins CB. Acquired heart disease. In: Higgins CB, Hricak H, Helms CA, eds. *Magnetic resonance imaging of the body*, 3rd ed. Philadelphia: Lippincott–Raven Publishers, 1997:409–460.

70. Sondergaard L, Stahlberg F, Thomsen C. Magnetic resonance imaging of valvular heart disease. *J Magn Reson Imaging* 1999;10:627–638.

71. Deutsch HJ, Bachman R, Sechtum U, et al. Regurgitant flow in cardiac valve prostheses: diagnostic value of gradient echo nuclear magnetic resonance imaging in reference to transesophageal two-dimensional color Doppler echocardiography. *J Am Coll Cardiol* 1992;19:1500–1507.

72. Houlind K, Eschen O, Pederson EM, et al. Magnetic resonance imaging of blood velocity distribution around St. Jude medical aortic valves in patients. *J Heart Valve Dis* 1996;5:511–517.

73. Caputo GR, Steiinan D, Funari M, et al. Quantification of aortic regurgitation by velocity-encoded cine MR. *Circulation* 1991;84(Suppl II):II-203 (abst).

74. Dulce M, Mostbeck GH, O'Sullivan M, et al. Severity of aortic regurgitation: interstudy reproducibility of measurements with velocity-encoded cine MR imaging. *Radiology* 1992;185:235–240.

75. Globits S, Blake L, Bourne M, et al. Assessment of hemodynamic effects of angiotensin-converting enzyme inhibitor therapy in chronic aortic regurgitation by using velocity-encoded cine nuclear magnetic resonance imaging. *Am Heart J* 1996;131:289–293.

76. Sondergaard L, Lindvig K, Hildebrandt P, et al. Quantification of aortic regurgitation by magnetic resonance velocity mapping. *Am Heart J* 1993;125:1081–1090.

77. Fujita N, Chazouilleres AF, Hartiala JJ, et al. Quantification of mitral regurgitation by velocity-encoded cine nuclear magnetic resonance imaging. *J Am Coll Cardiol* 1994;23:951–958.

78. White CW, Wright CB, Doty DB, et al. Does visual interpretation of the coronary angiogram predict the physiological importance of a coronary stenosis? *N Engl J Med* 1984;310:819–824.

79. Poncelet BP, Weisskoff RM, Wedeen WJ, et al. Time-of-flight quantification of coronary flow with echo-planar MRI. *Magn Reson Med* 1993;30:447–457.

80. Chao H, Burstein D. Multibolus-stimulated echo imaging of coronary artery flow. *J Magn Reson Imaging* 1997;7:603–605.

81. Edelman RR, Manning WJ, Gervino E, et al. Flow velocity quantification in human coronary arteries with fast breath-hold MR angiography. *J Magn Reson Imaging* 1993;3:699–703.

82. Clarke GD, Eckels R, Chaney C, et al. Measurement of absolute epicardial coronary artery flow and flow reserve with breath-hold cine phase-contrast magnetic resonance imaging. *Circulation* 1995;91:2627–2634.

83. Grist TM, Polzin JA, Bianco JA, et al. Measurement of coronary blood flow and flow reserve using magnetic resonance imaging. *Cardiology* 1997;88:80–89.

84. Davis CP, Liu P, Hauser M, et al. Coronary flow and coronary flow reserve measurements in humans with breath-hold magnetic resonance phase contrast velocity mapping. *Magn Reson Med* 1997;37:537–544.

85. Sakuma H, Kawada N, Takeda K, et al. MR measurement of coronary blood flow. *J Magn Reson Imaging* 1999;10:728–733.

86. Sakuma H, Blake LM, Amidon TM, et al. Noninvasive measurement of coronary flow reserve in humans using breath-hold velocity-encoded cine MR imaging. *Radiology* 1996;198:745–750.

87. Hofman MBM, van Rossum AC, Sprenger M, et al. Assessment of flow in the right human coronary artery by magnetic resonance phase contrast velocity measurement: effect of cardiac and respiratory motion. *Magn Reson Med* 1996;35:521–531.

88. Sakuma H, Saeed M, Takeda K, et al. Quantification of coronary artery volume flow rate using fast velocity-encoded cine MR imaging. *AJR Am J Roentgenol* 1997;168:1363–1367.

89. Hundley WG, Lange RA, Clarke GD, et al. Assessment of coronary arterial flow and flow reserve in humans with MRI. *Circulation* 1996;93:1502–1508.

90. Hutchinson SJ, Shen A, Soldo S, et al. Transesophageal assessment of coronary artery flow velocity reserve during "regular"- and "high"-dose dipyridamole stress testing. *Am J Cardiol* 1996;77:1164–1168.

91. Hood WB. Regional venous drainage of the human heart. *Br Heart J* 1968;30:105–109.

92. Lund GK, Wendland MF, Shimakawa A, et al. Coronary sinus flow measurement by means of velocity-encoded cine MR imaging: validation by using flow probes in dogs. *Radiology* 2000;217:487–493.

93. Kawada N, Sakuma H, Yamakado T, et al. Hypertrophic cardiomyopathy: MR measurement of coronary blood flow and vasodilator flow reserve in patients and healthy subjects. *Radiology* 1999;211:129–135.

94. Schwitter J, DeMarco T, Kneifel S, et al. Magnetic resonance-based assessment of global coronary flow and flow reserve and its relation to left ventricular functional parameters: a comparison with positron emission tomography. *Circulation*. 2000;101:2696–2702.

95. Chesebro JH, Clements IP, Fuster V, et al. A platelet-inhibitor-drug trial in coronary artery bypass operations. Benefit of perioperative dipyridamole and aspirin therapy on early post-operative vein graft patency. *N Engl J Med* 1982;307:73–78.

96. Henderson WG, Goldman S, Copeland JS, et al. Antiplatelet or anticoagulant therapy after coronary artery bypass surgery. A meta-analysis of clinical trials. *Ann Intern Med* 1989;111:743–750.

97. Fusejima K, Takahara Y, Sudo Y, et al. Comparison of coronary hemodynamics in patients with internal mammary artery and saphenous vein coronary bypass grafts: a noninvasive approach using combined two-dimensional and Doppler echocardiography. *J Am Cardiol* 1990;15:131–139.

98. Galjee MA, Van Rossum AC, Doesburg T, et al. Value of magnetic resonance imaging in assessing patency and function of coronary artery bypass grafts: an angiographically controlled study. *Circulation* 1996;93:660–666.

99. Ishida N, Sakuma H, Cruz BP, et al. MR flow measurement in the internal mammary artery to coronary artery bypass graft: a comparison with graft stenosis on X-ray angiography. *Radiology* 2001;220:441–447.

100. von Rossum AC, Bedaux WL, Hofman MB. Morphologic and functional evaluation of coronary artery bypass conduits. *J Magn Reson Imaging* 1999;10:734–740.

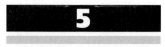

QUANTIFICATION IN CARDIAC MRI

ROB J. VAN DER GEEST
JOHAN H. C. REIBER

MRI offers several acquisition techniques for evaluating the cardiovascular system. The combined use of various MR scanning techniques in a single examination allows the accurate quantification of ventricular dimensions and mass and of global ventricular function. The accuracy and precision of volumetric measurement with cardiovascular MR (CMR) have been demonstrated in many experimental and clinical research studies. The three-dimensional (3D) nature of MRI also provides detailed information on the cardiac system at a regional level. Among others, regional end-diastolic wall thickness and systolic wall thickening are useful in the assessment of the location, extent, and severity of ventricular abnormalities in ischemic heart disease. Velocity-encoded cine MRI (VEC MRI) makes it possible to quantify blood flow through the planes of the aortic, pulmonary, and atrioventricular valves, and this information has been shown to be clinically valuable in the evaluation of patients with complex congenital heart disease.

A typical CMR examination yields a vast amount of image data, so that dedicated software solutions are essential for optimal visual and quantitative analysis. Quantitative image analysis requires the definition of contours describing the inner and outer boundaries of the ventricles; this is a laborious and tedious task when based on the manual tracing of contours. Reliable automated or semiautomated image analysis software is required to overcome these limitations. The large amount of quantitative data that becomes available also creates a need for optimized techniques of graphic display to facilitate clinical diagnosis. This chapter focuses on state-of-the-art CMR postprocessing techniques used in the quantitative assessment of global and regional ventricular function.

R. J. van der Geest and J. H. C. Reiber: Department of Radiology, Division of Image Processing, Leiden University Medical Center, Leiden, The Netherlands.

QUANTIFICATION OF VENTRICULAR DIMENSIONS AND GLOBAL FUNCTION

Accuracy and Reproducibility of Volume Measurements from Multislice Short-Axis MRI

As a 3D tomographic technique, MRI allows the imaging of anatomic objects in multiple parallel sections, enabling volumetric measurements according to the Simpson rule, which states that the volume of an object can be estimated by taking the sum of the cross-sectional areas in each section and multiplying it by the section thickness. Any gap between slices must be corrected for, and the formula for volume becomes $V = \Sigma \{area_i \times (thickness + gap)\}$, where V is the volume of the 3D object and $area_i$ is the area of the cross-section in section i.

The short-axis image orientation is the one most commonly applied in the assessment of left ventricular (LV) size and mass. This image orientation has advantages over other slice orientations in that it yields cross-sectional slices almost perpendicular to the myocardium for the largest part of the LV. As a result, partial volume effects at the myocardial boundaries are minimal, so that an optimal depiction of the myocardial boundaries is provided. However, the curvature of the LV at the apical level leads to significant partial volume averaging. The image voxels in this area simultaneously intersect with blood and myocardium, yielding indistinct myocardial boundaries. By minimizing the slice thickness while keeping a sufficient signal-to-noise ratio, it is possible to reduce this partial volume effect at the apex. Given the relatively small cross-sectional area of the LV in the apical section, the error introduced by the partial volume effect is minimal. At the base of the heart, partial volume averaging is of much greater significance because the cross-sectional

Overestimation   Underestimation

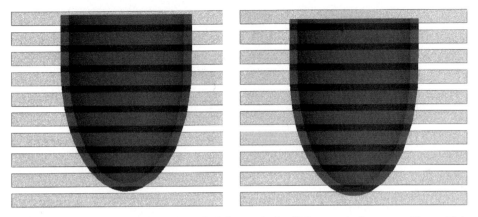

FIGURE 5.1. Schematic representation of a left ventricular (LV) geometry intersected by multiple parallel short-axis sections. Given the same section thickness and intersection gap, LV volume can be either overestimated or underestimated depending on the position of the LV with respect to the imaging slices. **A:** In this situation, the most basal slice will be included in the volumetric assessment. **B:** Here, the most basal slice will not be taken into account because it intersects with the LV myocardium by less than 50%.

area of the LV is largest at this level. The base of the LV exhibits a through-plane motion in the apical direction during systole on the order of 1.3 cm (1,2). Therefore, the significance of partial volume varies over the cardiac cycle. Additional long-axis views may prove helpful in determining more accurately how a basal short-axis slice intersects with the various anatomic regions.

Impact of Slice Thickness and Slice Gap

For an accurate assessment of ventricular volume, it is essential that the stack of short-axis slices cover the ventricle completely from base to apex. Typically, a section thickness between 6 and 10 mm is used, and the gap between slices varies from no gap (consecutive slices) to 4 mm. Quantification of volume and mass requires that contours in the images describing the endocardial and epicardial boundaries of the myocardium be defined in several phases of the cardiac cycle. Although an image voxel may contain several tissues (because of the partial volume effect), it is assumed that the traced contours represent the geometry of the ventricle at the center of the imaged section. As shown in Figure 5.1, the partial volume effect may lead to both overestimation and underestimation of the ventricular volume.

With a simple experiment in which synthetically created LV shapes and short-axis cross-sections are used, it can be shown how the partial volume problem may affect the accuracy and reproducibility of measurements. For this purpose, a computer-generated average LV geometry with a fixed size was constructed and short-axis cross-sections were automatically derived while the position of the ventricular geometry was varied along the long axis. The shape used and its dimensions are presented in Figure 5.2. In this experiment, it

is assumed that the contours in a short-axis slice will be drawn only if more than 50% of the slice thickness intersects with myocardium. The results of the simulations, depicted in Figure 5.3, show that the measurement precision (or measurement variability) decreases as the distance between slices increases. For typical imaging parameters (section thickness, 6 mm; gap, 4 mm), the measurement variability is between 4% and 5%. The measurement accuracy does not depend on the slice thickness or slice gap used; a section thickness of 10 mm with no gap results in the same variability as a section thickness of 6 mm with a gap of 4 mm.

The results of this experiment have two important implications. First, variations between successive scans of the

30 mm   Ø 60 mm

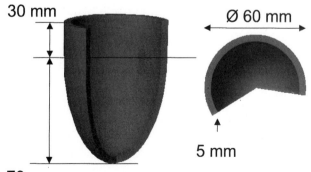

5 mm

70 mm

FIGURE 5.2. Schematic representation of the left ventricular geometry used for the simulation experiments. The phantom consists of a half-ellipsoid with a length of 70 mm and an outer diameter at the base of 60 mm; at the base, the shape is extended with a cylinder having a diameter of 60 mm and a length of 30 mm. The thickness of the phantom was set to 5 mm. In the experiments, the size of the object was varied between the dimensions shown and 80% of this size.

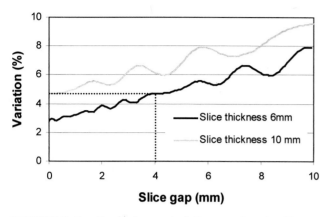

FIGURE 5.3. Results of volume calculation experiments with synthetically constructed left ventricular (LV) geometries. The variability of LV volume estimates increases with increasing slice thickness and slice gap. For a setting of the imaging parameters, such as a thickness of 6 mm and a gap of 4 cm, the measurement variability is 5%. The same variability occurs when consecutive sections having a thickness of 10 mm are used.

same patient may result in volumetric differences of up to 5%, which are inherent to the imaging technique used. Second, because the base of the heart has a significant through-plane motion component, the measurement variability of up to 5% will be present over the cardiac cycle. Therefore, measurements of the ejection fraction will also be affected. By reducing the section thickness and the intersection gap, the variability in volumetric measurements can be reduced.

Myocardial Mass

The measurement of heart muscle weight is of clinical importance in diagnosing and understanding a patient's illness and condition correctly, and in estimating the effects of treatment. If small changes in mass are to be detected, it is of paramount importance to use an accurate and reproducible measurement technique. Several validation studies have been performed comparing estimates of mass derived from MR with postmortem measurements of mass. In a study by Florentine et al. (3), a stack of axial slices was used to quantify LV mass according to the Simpson rule. In this early study, they found good agreement [$r = .95$, standard error of estimate (SEE) = 13 g]. Maddahi et al. (4) carried out extensive studies in a dog model to compare several slice orientations and measurement techniques for quantifying LV mass (4). It was shown that *in vivo* estimates of LV myocardial mass are most accurate when the images are obtained in the short-axis plane ($r = .98$, SEE = 4.9 g).

Left Ventricular Mass

For the LV, it is generally believed and also supported by literature that the short-axis orientation is the most appropriate imaging plane. Although spin-echo images normally

provide better visualization of the myocardial boundaries than do cine gradient-echo techniques, it is current practice to use the latter technique because a stack of cine gradient-echo images provides additional information about LV and RV function. To obtain maximum accuracy and reproducibility, it is important to cover the ventricle completely from apex to base with a sufficient number of slices. Quantification of mass requires that contours describing the endocardial and epicardial boundaries in the stack of images be defined. The muscle volume is assessed from these contours by applying the Simpson rule. The myocardial mass is derived by multiplying the muscle volume by the specific density of myocardium (1.05 g/cm^3).

Typically, a section thickness between 6 and 10 mm is used, with a 0- to 4-mm gap between sections. Significant partial volume averaging will occur at the apical and basal sections because of the section thickness used, and tracing of the myocardial boundaries may not be trivial. Similarly, partial volume averaging will cause significant difficulty in the interpretation of sections with a highly trabeculated myocardial wall and papillary muscles (5). No general consensus has been reached on whether to include or exclude the papillary muscles and trabeculae in the LV mass. Although it is evident that inclusion of these structures results in more accurate measurements of myocardial mass, in an analysis of regional wall thickening, it is important to exclude these structures to avoid artifacts in the quantification. Whether to use an end-diastolic or end-systolic time frame for the measurement is also a subject of ongoing debate. Most likely, optimal accuracy and reproducibility are obtained by averaging multiple time frames, but practical objections will arise in case the contours are derived by manual tracing.

Right Ventricular Mass

For the RV and also for any LV with a geometrically abnormal shape, an accurate assessment of volume requires multiple sections (6). MRI experiments with different slice orientations in phantoms and ventricular casts have shown no significant difference in accuracy and reproducibility between slice orientations (7). However, in a clinical situation, the choice of slice orientation also depends on the availability of a clear depiction of the anatomic features needed to define the myocardial boundaries. It may be better to base volumetric quantification of the RV on axial views. This view provides greater anatomic detail and better differentiates between the RV and right atrial lumen. Nevertheless, for practical reasons, the RV mass is often measured with a stack of short-axis slices, which is also used to measure the LV dimensions.

Quantification of Ventricular Volumes and Global Function

For an assessment of global ventricular function, volumetric measurement of the ventricular cavities is required during at least two phases of the cardiac cycle—end-diastole and end-systole. Numerous reports have described the applicability of various MRI strategies in accurately and reproducibly quantifying LV and RV volumes (3,8). Sufficient temporal resolution is required to capture the end-systolic phase properly. Generally, a temporal resolution, or phase interval, on the order of 40 to 50 milliseconds is assumed to be sufficient. For geometrically normal LVs, one can rely on geometric models to derive the volumes from one or two long-axis imaging sections. In a group of 10 patients with LV hypertrophy and 10 healthy subjects, Dulce et al. (9) demonstrated good agreement between biplane volumetric measurements based on the modified Simpson rule of an ellipsoid model and true 3D volumetric measurements obtained with a multislice MRI approach. In another study, Chuang et al. (10) evaluated 25 patients with dilated cardiomyopathies with both a biplane and a 3D multislice approach. They reported a poor correlation between the two measurement methods.

At present, a single section with sufficient temporal resolution can be acquired during a single breath-hold on most available systems. The total time taken to acquire the 8 to 12 sections needed to image the entire ventricular cavity is about 5 minutes (11,12). All sections should be acquired at the same end-expiration or end-inspiration phase; otherwise, reliable 3D quantification of volumes from the obtained images is not possible. Quantitative analysis starts with manual or semiautomated segmentation of the myocardium and blood pool in the images.

Once contours have been defined in the stack of images describing the endocardial and epicardial boundaries of the myocardium, volumetric measurements, including stroke volume and ejection fraction, can be obtained by applying the Simpson rule. Normal values for global ventricular function and mass have been reported by several investigators (13–15).

Although cine MRI techniques provide good contrast between the myocardium and blood pool because of inflow enhancement, image quality near the apex is often less than optimal because of low flow and partial volume averaging. At the basal imaging sections, a clear visual separation between LV and left atrium is often absent because the imaging sections may contain both ventricular and atrial muscle. It is important to realize that although the imaging sections are fixed in space, the LV annulus exhibits motion in the apical direction on the order of 1.3 cm in normal hearts (16). Consequently, myocardium that is readily visible in an end-diastolic time frame may be replaced by left atrium in an end-systolic time frame. Additional long-axis views may be helpful to analyze the most basal and apical slice levels of a multislice short-axis study more reliably (2). End-diastolic and end-systolic time frames in a long-axis view and three basal short-axis sections obtained during a single MR examination are shown in Figure 5.4. The white lines, indicating the intersection lines of the imaging planes, provide helpful additional information for interpreting the structures seen in the short-axis images.

End-diastole   End-systole

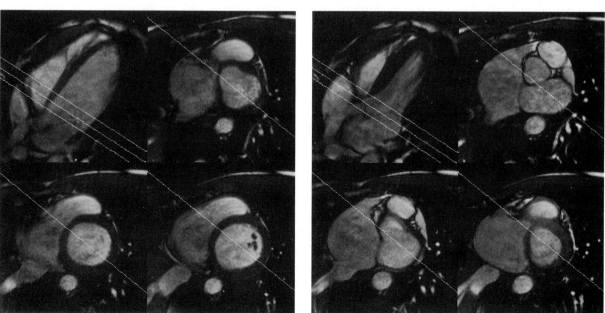

A   B

FIGURE 5.4. Four-chamber long-axis view and three basal level short-axis views acquired within the same examination. The *white lines* show how the short-axis and long-axis imaging planes intersect with each other. The movement of the base toward the apex in systole can easily be appreciated. The use of displays showing how long-axis and short-axis planes intersect may facilitate the interpretation of basal level short-axis images and may be valuable during tracing of the contours.

slices—the actual algorithm should be fast to increase the time efficiency of the operator.

In the next paragraphs, we provide a short description of the underlying methods and validation results of the algorithms developed at our laboratory, which have been integrated in a software package, MASS (MEDIS Medical Imaging Systems, Leiden, The Netherlands)(35). Our contour detection method follows a model-based approach and is directed to defining the endocardial and epicardial contours in all the phases and slices of an imaging study. The amount of user interaction required to obtain reliable contours is limited and is minimal when the images are of good quality. The algorithm accommodates anatomic and MRI-related variations in image appearance by providing a certain learning behavior. Manually traced or edited contours are assumed to be correct, and the contour detection algorithm was designed to generate a consistent set of contours for the total image data set by using the manually defined contours as models. The contour detection starts with a search for circular objects in the imaging slices to find the approximate long axis of the

LV, so that an approximate LV center point is obtained in each image. Based on this center point, epicardial contours are found in the first phase and subsequently in the remaining phases in a frame-to-frame contour detection procedure. The frame-to-frame epicardial contour detection procedure is based on the matching of line profiles that are positioned perpendicular to the model contour (derived from the first phase) and then automatically positioned at the corresponding tissue transitions in other phases within the same slice level. With this approach, the algorithm can accommodate the fact that the epicardial boundary of the myocardium is adjacent to regions with different gray value characteristics. A first estimate of the endocardial contour is found by means of an optimal thresholding technique within the region described by the epicardial contour. The final endocardial contour is found by means of a model-based edge detection technique known as the *minimum cost algorithm* (42). The steps carried out in the algorithm to detect an endocardial contour in an image with an available epicardial contour are illustrated in Figure 5.6.

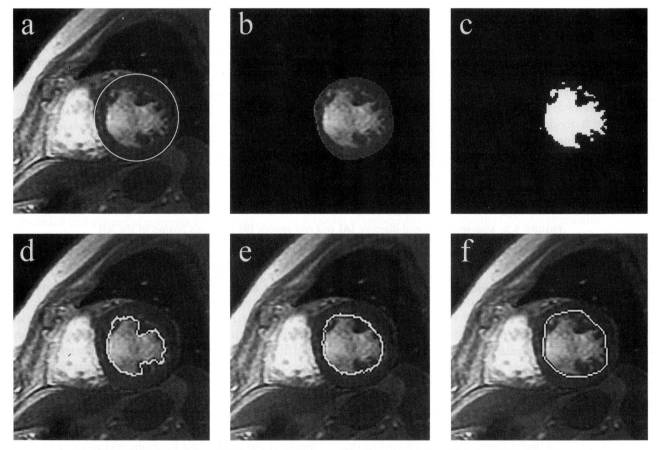

FIGURE 5.6. Automated detection of the endocardial contour. **A:** Original image with epicardial contour. **B:** Search region for the endocardial contour. The region outside the epicardial contour and a small region at the inside of the epicardial contour are masked out from the original image. **C:** Result after determination of the optimal threshold. **D:** Contour around the threshold region serves as a starting contour for the subsequent edge-based contour detection. **E:** When papillary muscled must be excluded from the myocardium, a smooth convex hull contour around the initial contour is determined. **F:** Final result after minimum cost contour detection.

The automated contour detection algorithm was evaluated on MRI studies acquired with two different MRI systems from 10 patients with infarct and 10 healthy volunteers. In each of these studies, the endocardial and epicardial contours were obtained by manual tracing and by using the semiautomated contour detection algorithm. The user was allowed to correct obvious failures of the automated contour detection, which was required for two *epicardial* contours per study on average. Manual editing of automatically detected *endocardial* contours was not allowed. In addition, the contours in the most basal slice were obtained by manual tracing. Manual tracing or editing of a contour was followed by a new iteration of contour detection such that a consistent series of contours was obtained. Manual tracing of the endocardial and epicardial contours in all the phases and slices of an imaging study required 2 to 3 hours; the analysis time was reduced to less than 20 minutes by using the semiautomated approach. In Table 5.1, the random and systematic differences are reported for a number of parameters of global LV function. Some underestimation of ventricular volumes can be observed in the group of normal volunteers. No statistically significant differences between the two analysis methods were found in the group of patients with infarct. The random differences, on the other hand, are relatively small and of the same order of magnitude for both study populations.

New Automated Segmentation Methods

Reliable, fully automated contour detection, not requiring any user interaction, would clearly be an important step in further improving the clinical utility of CMR. Despite a great deal of research in this area, two major problems have limited the success of many of the previously described contour detection strategies for cardiovascular structures. First, because of the presence of noise and image acquisition artifacts, image information can be poorly defined, unreliable, or missing. In these cases, a human observer is still capable of tracing the myocardial contours in the image data based on experience and prior knowledge, whereas many automated techniques fail. Second, a contour as drawn by an expert human observer may not always correspond to the location indicated by the strongest local image evidence. In particular, in short-axis MR images, the papillary muscles and trabeculae pose a problem. For example, many experts prefer to draw the LV endocardial border as a convex hull around the blood pool at a location somewhat "outside" the strongest edge (43,44). A second example is the epicardial boundary, which may be embedded in fatty tissue, as a result of which the edge is strongest at the fat–air transitions. However, the contour often should be drawn on the inside of this fatty layer, an intensity transition that is marked only by a faint edge. Therefore, a decision about the exact location of the contour cannot always be based on the strongest image evidence but should be determined from the examples and preferences provided by expert observers.

To overcome these problems, prior knowledge about image appearance, spatial organ embedding, characteristic organ shape, and anatomic and pathologic variations in shape should form an integral part of a contour detection approach. Moreover, the approach should be adaptable to accommodate the preferences of an observer and easily adjustable to image the characteristics of various pulse sequences and MR systems.

Recently, Cootes et al. (45) introduced the concept of active appearance models (AAMs), which are trainable mathematical models that can learn the shape and appearance of an imaged object from a set of example images. This method was originally developed for facial recognition and later optimized for detection of the LV in CMR (46). An AAM consists of a statistical model of the *shape* of an object combined with a statistical model of the *image appearance* of the object in a set of example images. The combined model is trained to learn the shape and image structure of an organ from a representative set of example images from different subjects. The AAM can be automatically matched to a new study im-

TABLE 5.1. COMPARISON OF SEMIAUTOMATED AND MANUAL IMAGE ANALYSIS

Parameter	Normals (*n* = 10)		Patients (*n* = 10)		Overall (*n* = 20)	
	Mean	SD	Mean	SD	Mean	SD
EDV (mL)	−13.4[a]	5.7	2.4	5.7	−5.5	9.7
ESV (mL)	−5.9[a]	4.9	−1.4	7.1	−3.6[a]	6.5
SV (mL)	−7.5[a]	4.4	3.8	7.6	−1.9[a]	8.4
EF (%)	1.4	3.0	2.1	4.9	1.7[a]	4.1
Mass (g)	22.8[a]	10.2	−8.2	16.2	7.3[a]	20.6

Systematic and random differences (auto vs. manual) in the assessment of left ventricular dimensions and function parameters with either semiautomated or manual image analysis.
[a] Statistically significant difference between semiautomated and manually determined parameter (*p* < .05).
EDV, end-diastolic volume; ESV, end-systolic volume; SV, stroke volume; EF, ejection fraction; SD, standard deviation.

age by minimizing an error function expressing the difference between the model and the underlying image evidence. During this matching process, the model is constrained to resemble only statistically plausible shapes and appearances. Consequently, AAMs are able to capture the association between observer preference and the underlying image evidence, so that they are highly suitable to model an expert observer's analysis behavior. Moreover, AAMs can model multiple objects (in our case, the left and right cardiac ventricles) in their spatial embedding. In a study by Mitchell et al. (47), the AAM technique showed excellent agreement with manually defined contours for both the LV and RV simultaneously. Examples of automatically detected contours for the LV and RV obtained with this new approach are shown in Figure 5.7.

MRI FLOW QUANTIFICATION

VEC MRI also plays an important role in the evaluation of global ventricular function. The accuracy of this imaging technique has been demonstrated in experiments *in vitro* by means of flow phantoms and comparisons with other imaging techniques, such as Doppler echocardiography and invasive oximetry (48,49).

Because flow measurements are obtained at high temporal resolution over the complete cardiac cycle, VEC MRI is especially useful in the evaluation of parameters of LV and RV diastolic function by measuring flow over the atrioventricular valves. The application of this technique to the proximal portion of the ascending aorta or pulmonary artery allows assessment of LV and RV systolic function. After the cross-section of a vessel has been identified in an image by manual or automated contour detection, the instantaneous flow rate within the vessel cross-section is obtained by multiplying the average velocity within the contour by its area. Measurements of ventricular stroke volume are derived by integrating the flow over a complete cardiac cycle (50). Aortic or pulmonary regurgitation can be easily identified and quantified from the derived flow curve. VEC MRI has an established role in the evaluation of patients with congenital heart disease (51,52).

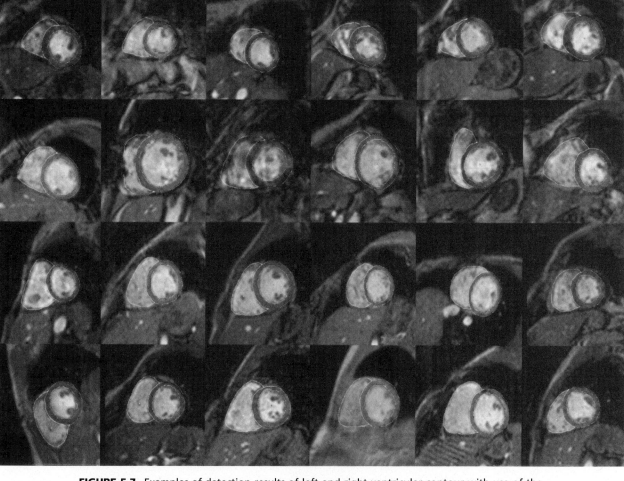

FIGURE 5.7. Examples of detection results of left and right ventricular contour with use of the active appearance model contour detection method.

Automated Quantification of Aortic Flow

The application of VEC MRI to the proximal portion of the ascending aorta allows assessment of LV systolic function by evaluating the flow over a complete cardiac cycle. Such a study requires a VEC MRI acquisition in the transverse plane crossing the ascending aorta. The LV stroke volume can be measured by integrating the flow over a complete cardiac cycle. For an accurate assessment of volume flow, contours describing the lumen of the vessels must be obtained in the images. The in-plane motion of the greater vessels and changes in shape of the vessel cross-section over the cardiac cycle would require the user to trace the luminal border of the vessel in each individual phase of the MR examination. To overcome these practical limitations, an automated analysis method was developed in our department to detect the required contours in each of the cardiac phases automatically (53). This contour detection algorithm has been integrated in the FLOW software package (MEDIS Medical Imaging Systems, Leiden, The Netherlands).

The only user interaction required is the manual definition of an approximate center in one of the available images. In this first image, an initial model contour is detected by means of gray value and edge information. The position of the same vessel at another time frame can be estimated by shifting the model contour in a limited region around the initial location and examining the edge values measured in the modulus image along the contour points. An algorithm was developed to find the most likely contour position for each time frame, with the restriction that a contour be allowed to displace only two pixels (1.6 mm) from phase to phase, so that a temporal continuity of motion would be imposed. After the correct contour location was found, a final optimized contour was detected by allowing small deformations of the model contour such that it would follow the edges in the modulus image. For this purpose, a 2D graph-searching technique was used (minimum cost algorithm). The resulting contour was dilated by one pixel to make sure the entire region was encompassed by flowing blood. The total contour detection process takes less than 10 seconds for a study with 30 cardiac phases.

Validation was performed on flow velocity maps from a study population of 12 healthy volunteers. Two independent observers performed manual and automated image analyses. The first observer repeated the automated and manual analyses after a 2-week interval to avoid learning effects. The time required for manual analysis was 5 to 10 minutes. During automated analysis, the user had to identify the approximate location of the center of the aorta in one of the available images. The total time required for automated analysis was less than 10 seconds. Stroke volume measurements were obtained by integrating the flow over the complete cardiac cycle. The mean LV stroke volume obtained by VEC MRI in the group of 12 volunteers was 86.4 mL (standard deviation, 13.6 mL). No statistically signifi-

cant differences were found between the results of manual and automated analyses. The mean difference between automated and manually assessed stroke volume was 0.78 mL (standard deviation, 1.99 mL). The intraobserver variability was 0.65 mL for manual analysis and 0.58 mL for automated analysis; the interobserver variability was 0.99 mL for manual analysis and 0.90 mL for automated analysis. From this study, it can be concluded that the automated contour detection algorithm performs as well as the manual method in the determination of LV stroke volume based on VEC MRI studies of the ascending aorta.

SUMMARY

Cardiovascular MRI has unique capabilities for noninvasively quantifying global and regional ventricular function. For MRI to become a valuable and routinely applicable imaging modality, the time required for quantifying and interpreting the many images should be reduced considerably. In this chapter, methods of analyzing LV function and measuring vascular flow based on automated contour detection approaches have been described. Validation studies of these methods have confirmed their accuracy, precision, robustness, and usefulness for clinical research studies. Fully automated contour detection methods that operate reliably in a routine clinical environment are needed and may become available in the near future.

REFERENCES

1. Rogers WJ, Shapiro EP, Weiss JL, et al. Quantification and correction for left ventricular systolic long-axis shortening by magnetic resonance tissue tagging and slice isolation. *Circulation* 1991;84:721–731.
2. Marcus JT, Götte MJW, de Waal LK, et al. The influence of through-plane motion on left ventricular volumes measured by magnetic resonance imaging: implications for image acquisition and analysis. *J Cardiovasc Magn Reson* 1998;1:1–6.
3. Florentine MS, Grosskreutz CJ, Chang W, et al. Measurement of left ventricular mass *in vivo* using gated nuclear magnetic resonance imaging. *J Am Coll Cardiol* 1986;8:107–112.
4. Maddahi J, Crues J, Berman DS, et al. Noninvasive quantitation of left ventricular mass by gated proton magnetic resonance imaging. *J Am Coll Cardiol* 1987;10:682–692.
5. Matheijssen NAA, Baur LHB, Reiber JHC, et al. Assessment of left ventricular volume and mass by cine-magnetic resonance imaging in patients with anterior myocardial infarction: intra-observer and inter-observer variability on contour detection. *Int J Card Imaging* 1996;12:11–19.
6. Niwa K, Uchishiba M, Aotsuka H, et al. Measurement of ventricular volumes by cine magnetic resonance imaging in complex congenital heart disease with morphologically abnormal ventricles. *Am Heart J* 1996;131:567–575.
7. Jauhiainen T, Järvinen VM, Hekali PE, et al. MR gradient echo volumetric analysis of the human cardiac casts: focus on the right ventricle. *J Comp Assist Tomogr* 1998;22:899–903.
8. Semelka RC, Tomei E, Wagner S, et al. Normal left ventricular

dimensions and function: interstudy reproducibility of measurements with cine MR imaging. *Radiology* 1990;174:763–768.

9. Dulce MC, Mostbeck GH, Friese KK, et al. Quantification of left ventricular volumes and function with cine MR imaging: comparison of geometrical models with three-dimensional data. *Radiology* 1993;188:371–376.

10. Chuang ML, Hibberd MG, Salton CJ, et al. Importance of imaging method over imaging modality in noninvasive determination of left ventricular volumes and ejection fraction: assessment by two- and three-dimensional echocardiography and magnetic resonance imaging. *J Am Coll Cardiol* 2000;35:477–484.

11. Sakuma H, Fujia N, Foo TKF, et al. Evaluation of left ventricular volume and mass with breath-hold cine MR imaging. *Radiology* 1993;188:377–380.

12. Lamb HJ, Singleton RR, van der Geest RJ, et al. MR imaging of regional cardiac function: low-pass filtering of wall thickness curves. *Magn Reson Med* 1995;34:498–502.

13. Lorenz CH, Walker ES, Morgan VL, et al. Normal human right and left ventricular mass, systolic function and gender differences by cine magnetic resonance imaging. *J Cardiovasc Magn Reson* 1999;1:7–21.

14. Rominger MB, Bachmann GF, Pabst W, et al. Right ventricular volumes and ejection fraction with fast cine MR imaging in breath-hold technique: applicability, normal values from 52 volunteers, and evaluation of 325 adult cardiac patients. *J Magn Reson Imaging* 1999;10:908–918.

15. Marcus JT, de Waal LK, Götte MJW, et al. MRI-derived left ventricular function parameters and mass in healthy young adults: relation with gender and age. *Int J Card Imaging* 1999;15:411–419.

16. Rogers WJ, EPS, Weiss JL, Buchalter MB, et al. Quantification and correction for left ventricular systolic long-axis shortening by magnetic resonance tissue tagging and slice isolation. *Circulation* 1991;84:721–731.

17. Lieberman AN, Weiss JL, Jugdutt BI, et al. Two-dimensional echocardiography and infarct size: relationship of regional wall motion and thickening to the extent of myocardial infarction in the dog. *Circulation* 1981;63:739–746.

18. Azhari H, Sideman S, Weiss JL, et al. Three-dimensional mapping of acute ischemic regions using MRI: wall thickening versus motion analysis. *Am J Physiol* 1990;259(5 Pt 2):H1492–H1503.

19. van Rugge FP, van der Wall EE, Spanjersberg SJ, et al. Magnetic resonance imaging during dobutamine stress for detection of coronary artery disease: quantitative wall motion analysis using a modification of the centerline method. *Circulation* 1994;90:127–138.

20. Haag UJ, Maier SE, Jakob M, et al. Left ventricular wall thickness measurements by magnetic resonance: a validation study. *Int J Card Imaging* 1991;7:31–41.

21. Baer FM, Smolarz K, Voth E, et al. Regional ^{99m}Tc-methoxy-isobutyl-isonitrile uptake at rest in patients with myocardial infarcts: comparison with morphological and functional parameters obtained from gradient-echo magnetic resonance imaging. *Eur Heart J* 1994;15:97–107.

22. Holman ER, Vliegen HW, van der Geest RJ, et al. Quantitative analysis of regional left ventricular function after myocardial infarction in the pig assessed with cine magnetic resonance imaging. *Magn Reson Med* 1995;34:161–169.

23. Sheehan FH, Bolson EL, Dodge HT, et al. Advantages and applications of the centerline method for characterizing regional ventricular function. *Circulation* 1986;74:293–305.

24. von Land CD, Rao SR, Reiber JHC. Development of an improved centerline wall motion model. *Comput Cardiol* 1990: 687–690.

25. Holman ER, Buller VGM, de Roos A, et al. Detection and quantification of dysfunctional myocardium by magnetic resonance imaging: a new three-dimensional method for quantitative wall-thickening analysis. *Circulation* 1997;95:924–931.

26. Buller VGM, van der Geest RJ, Kool MD, et al. Assessment of regional left ventricular wall parameters from short-axis MR imaging using a 3D extension to the improved centerline method. *Invest Radiol* 1997;32:529–539.

27. Guttman MA, Prince JL, McVeigh ER. Tag and contour detection in tagged MR images of the left ventricle. *IEEE Trans Med Imaging* 1993;13:74–88.

28. Moore CC, McVeigh ER, Zerhouni EA. Quantitative tagged magnetic resonance imaging of the normal human left ventricle. *Top MRI* 2000;11:359–371.

29. Pelc NJ, Drangova M, Pelc LR, et al. Tracking of cyclic motion with phase-contrast cine MR velocity data. *J Magn Reson Imaging* 1995;5:339–345.

30. Hennig J, Schneider B, Peschl S, et al. Analysis of myocardial motion based on velocity measurements with a black blood prepared segmented gradient-echo sequence: methodology and applications to normal volunteers and patients. *J Magn Reson Imaging* 1998;8:868–877.

31. McInerney T, Terzopoulos D. A dynamic finite element surface model for segmentation and tracking in multidimensional medical images with application to cardiac 4D image analysis. *Comput Med Imaging Graph* 1995;19:69–83.

32. Matsumura K, Nakase E, Haiyama T, et al. Automatic left ventricular volume measurements on contrast-enhanced ultrafast cine magnetic resonance imaging. *Eur J Radiol* 1995;20:126–132.

33. Goshtasby A, Turner DA. Segmentation of cardiac cine MR images for right and left ventricular chambers. *IEEE Trans Med Imaging* 1995;14:56–64.

34. Baldy C, Doueck P, Croisille P, et al. Automated myocardial edge detection from breath-hold cine-MR images: evaluation of left ventricular volumes and mass. *Magn Reson Imaging* 1994;12:589–598.

35. van der Geest RJ, Buller VGM, Jansen E, et al. Comparison between manual and automated analysis of left ventricular volume parameters from short-axis MR images. *J Comput Assist Tomogr* 1997;21:756–765.

36. Butler SP, McKay E, Paszkowski AL, et al. Reproducibility study of left ventricular measurements with breath-hold cine MRI using a semiautomated volumetric image analysis program. *J Magn Reson Imaging* 1998;8:467–472.

37. Kaushikkar SV, Li D, Haacke EM, et al. Adaptive blood pool segmentation in three dimensions: application to MR cardiac evaluation. *J Magn Reson Imaging* 1996;6:690–697.

38. Singleton HR, Pohost GM. Automatic cardiac MR image segmentation using edge detection by tissue classification in pixel neighborhoods. *Magn Reson Med* 1997;37:418–424.

39. Furber A, Balzer P, Cavaro-Menárd C, et al. Experimental validation of an automated edge-detection method for a simultaneous determination of the endocardial and epicardial borders in short-axis cardiac MR images: application in normal volunteers. *J Magn Reson Imaging* 1998;8:1006–1014.

40. Nachtomy E, Vaturi M, Bosak E, et al. Automatic assessment of cardiac function from short-axis MRI: procedure and clinical evaluation. *Magn Reson Imaging* 1998;16:365–376.

41. Lalande A, Legrand L, Walker PM, et al. Automatic detection of left ventricular contours from cardiac cine magnetic resonance imaging using fuzzy logic. *Invest Radiol* 1999;34:211–217.

42. Amini AA, Weymouth TE, Jain RC. Using dynamic programming for solving variational problems in vision. *IEEE Trans PAMI* 1990;12:855–867.

43. Pattynama PMT, Lamb HJ, van der Velde EA, et al. Left ventricular measurements with cine and spin-echo MR imaging: a study of reproducibility with variance component analysis. *Radiology* 1993;187:261–268.

44. Lamb HJ, Doornbos J, van der Velde EA, et al. Echo-planar MRI of the heart on a standard sytem: validation of measurement of left ventricular function and mass. *J Comput Assist Tomogr* 1996;20:942–949.

45. Cootes TF, Beeston C, Edwards GJ, et al. A unified framework for atlas matching using active appearance models. Proceedings of Information Processing in Medical Imaging 1999. *Lecture Notes in Computer Science* 1999;1613:322–333.

46. Mitchell SC, Lelieveldt BPF, van der Geest RJ, et al. Multistage hybrid active appearance model matching: segmentation of left and right ventricles in cardiac MR images. *IEEE Trans Med Imaging* 2001;20:415–423.

47. Mitchell SC, Lelieveldt BPF, van der Geest RJ, et al. Multistage hybrid active appearance model matching: segmentation of left and right ventricles in MR images. *IEEE Trans Med Imaging* 2001;20:415–423.

48. Karwatowski SP, Brecker SJD, Yang GZ, et al. Mitral valve flow measured with cine MR velocity mapping in patients with ischemic heart disease: comparison with Doppler echocardiography. *J Magn Reson Imaging* 1995;5:89–92.

49. Beerbaum P, Körperich P, Barth P, et al. Noninvasive quantification of left-to-right shunt in pediatric patients. Phase-contrast cine magnetic resonance imaging compared with invasive oximetry. *Circulation* 2001;103:2476–2482.

50. Kondo C, Caputo GR, Semelka R, et al. Right and left ventricular stroke volume measurements with velocity-encoded cine MR imaging: *in vitro* and *in vivo* validation. *AJR Am J Roentgenol* 1991;157:9–16.

51. de Roos A, Helbing WA, Niezen RA, et al. Magnetic resonance imaging in adult congenital heart disease. In: Higgins CB, Inwall JS, Pohost GM, eds. *Current and future applications of magnetic resonance in cardiovascular disease*. Armonk, NY: Futura Publishing, 1988:163–172.

52. Powel AJ, Geva T. Blood flow measurement by magnetic resonance imaging in congenital heart disease. *Pediatr Cardiol* 2000; 21:47–58.

53. van der Geest RJ, Niezen RA, van der Wall EE, et al. Automated measurement of volume flow in the ascending aorta using MR velocity maps: evaluation of inter- and intraobserver variability in healthy volunteers. *J Comp Assist Tomogr* 1998;22:904–911.

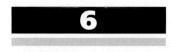

6

CONTRAST MEDIA

**MAYTHEM SAEED
NORBERT WATZINGER
GABRIELE A. KROMBACH
CHARLES B. HIGGINS**

The role of MR in evaluating cardiovascular diseases is expanding rapidly. It is becoming clear that MRI and MRA can safely provide a comprehensive evaluation of patients with cardiovascular diseases. In many of the potential applications of MRI and MRA in cardiovascular diseases, MR contrast media are employed. This chapter provides an overview of the various types of MR contrast media and the possible uses of these agents in cardiovascular diseases.

FEATURES OF CONTRAST MEDIA

Magnetic Properties

The recognition of the importance of magnetic materials and their effects on the relaxation times of resonating protons occurred almost simultaneously with the discovery of the MR process in 1946 (1). In the 1950s, Solomon (2,3) and Bloembergen and Morgan (4,5) outlined the framework of the effect of paramagnetic transition metals. Lauterbur (6) was responsible not only for the seminal development of MRI technique but also for the conception and subsequent development of MR contrast media. In 1978, Lauterbur et al. (7) demonstrated the first use of manganese ions as an MR agent in canine models of myocardial infarction. The development of the first commercial contrast medium, gadopentetate dimeglumine (Gd-DTPA), commenced in 1981, and its first reported use in humans was in 1984. This MR contrast agent received U.S. Food and Drug Administration (FDA) approval in 1988.

M. Saeed and C. B. Higgins: Department of Radiology, University of California San Francisco, San Francisco, California.

N. Watzinger: Departments of Medicine and Cardiology, University of Graz, Graz, Austria.

G. A. Krombach: Department of Radiology, University of Technology (RWTH-Aachen), Aachen, Germany.

MR contrast media have unpaired electrons that generate large fluctuating magnetic fields within the MRI environment. These agents have incorporated magnetic ions such as gadolinium (III), manganese (II), iron (III), and dysprosium (III). The relaxation effect is proportional to the square of the magnetic moment of the paramagnetic ion, which varies with the number of unpaired electrons. Paramagnetic and superparamagnetic ions have different numbers of unpaired electrons (e.g., seven unpaired electrons in gadolinium, five unpaired electrons in iron, and five unpaired electrons in manganese). Unlike other radiographic contrast media, MR contrast media are not directly measurable on imaging; rather, they are measured by their effect on adjacent nuclei. The active moieties of most MR contrast media contain no protons; however, these agents act by shortening the relaxation time of water protons that are close to the contrast agent. The efficacy of these agents in enhancing proton relaxation rates in tissues is related to the magnetic moment of unpaired electrons, electron spin relaxation rate of the metal ion, and number of coordination sites available for water ligation.

Effects on Signal Intensity

The effect of MR contrast media on signal intensity is described in terms of T1 and T2 relaxivities, referred to as *R1* and *R2 relaxivities*. The relaxivity of a contrast agent is defined as the slope of the curve of 1/T1 or 1/T2 plotted against the concentration of a contrast agent. However, the effect of MR contrast agents on tissue or blood signal intensity is not a pure T1 or T2 effect. The relaxivity ratio, R2/R1, can be used to determine whether the agent is causing predominantly T2 shortening with loss of signal on T2-weighted images (R2 significantly greater than R1) or T1 shortening with increased signal on T1-weighted images (R1 significantly greater than R2). It should be noted that efficient T1-enhancing agents have a high magnetic susceptibility effect and can potentially be used to exert susceptibility under appropriate dose and imaging sequences. The dominant effect of MR contrast media determines the increase or decrease in signal intensity in the region-of-interest (8–18).

Specific MR sequences can be employed to exploit the T1-, T2-, and T2*-shortening effects of MR contrast media. The contrast between blood and tissue or between healthy and diseased tissue can be manipulated by combining the administration of agents having the desired contrast properties (T1 or T2*) with MR pulse sequences (e.g., spin-echo, gradient-echo, or echo-planar imaging) that are sensitive to the contrast mechanism (19–31). For example, gadolinium chelates at low doses are potent T1-enhancing agents and cause signal enhancement on T1-weighted sequences with inversion recovery pulse or short TR/TE, whereas at higher doses, susceptibility effects become dominant and can be detected as signal loss on T2*-weighted sequences. The same behavior can be seen with superparamagnetic iron oxide particles (8–11,32).

Distribution and Types

The differences between MR contrast media are based on the compartmentalization, distribution, and residence times of the pharmaceuticals in the blood or tissue (33–50). Thus, they have been classified as extracellular, intravascular, targeted, or intracellular agents (Table 6.1). The molecular weight is a major factor in the distribution and elimination of MR contrast agents in the body. Intravascular MR contrast media have higher molecular weights (>50 kd) than do extracellular agents (<2 kd); therefore, they remain longer (>1 hour vs. <15 minutes) in the blood pool (33–43). The other important factor that determines the distribution of the contrast medium in the body is the shape of MR contrast media (33,42,43). For example, the superparamagnetic iron oxide particle SH L643 (Schering AG, Berlin, Germany) has an actual molecular mass of 17 kd, but because of the globular shape of the molecule, the apparent molecular mass is 35 kd. The higher apparent molecular weight of this agent acts to delay diffusion into interstitial space (43).

The delivery and distribution of MR contrast media occur by a combination of convection (arterial flow, venous flow, and lymphatic drainage) and diffusion through the myocardial matrix. The distribution of extracellular MR contrast media in normal (~18%) and in moderately (~30%) and severely (~90%) ischemically injured myocardium is shown in Figure 6.1. The distribution of extracellular MR contrast media increases as the number of dam-

TABLE 6.1. CONTRAST MEDIA FOR MRI AND MRA

Target	Active Moiety	Contrast Agent	Trade Name (Manufacturer)
Extracellular space	Gadolinium	Gadopentetate dimeglumine (Gd-DTPA)	Magnevist[a] (Berlex, Schering)
		Gadodiamide injection (Gd-DTPA-BMA; nonionic)	Omniscan[a] (Nycomed Amersham)
		Gadoterate meglumine (Gd-DOTA)	Dotarem[a] (Guerbet)
		Gadoteridol injection (Gd-HP-DO3A, nonionic)	ProHance[a] (Bracco Diagnostics)
		Gadobutrol	(Schering)[b]
		Gadobenate dimeglumine (Gd-BOPTA)	MultiHance[a] (Bracco Diagnostics)
Inracellular space	Manganese	Mangafodipir trisodium (Mn-DPDP)	Teslascan[a] (Nycomed Amersham)
Intravascular space	Iron (ultrasmall particles)	NC100150 injection	Clariscan[b] (Nycomed Amersham)
		Ferumoxtran (AMI-227)	Combidex[b] (Advanced Magnetics)
		AG-USPIO (BMS 180549)	Sinerem[b] (Guerbet)
		SH U555A	Resovist[b] (Schering)
	Gadolinium-macromolecules	MS-325	AngioMARK[b] (Epix)
		Gd-DTPA-dextran	(Nycomed Amersham)[c]
		Gadomer-17	(Schering)[c]
		Gd-DTPA-polylysine	(Schering)[c]
		Gd-DTPA-carboxy-methyldextran	(Guerbet)[c]
Targeted agents	Gadolinium-porphyrin	Mesoporphyrin	(Schering)[c]

[a]MR contrast media approved for clinical use.
[b]MR contrast media different phases of clinical trials.
[c]MR contrast media in preclinical phase.
DTPA, diethylene triamine pentaacetic acid; Gd-DTPA-BMA, gadolinium diethylene triamine pentaacetic acid-bis-methyamide; Gd-DOTA, gadolinium tetraazacyclododecane tetraacetic acid; Gd-HP-DO3A, gadolinium 10-(2-hydroxypropyl)-1,4,10-tetraazacyclododecane-1,4,7-triacetic acid.

Ischemia (min)

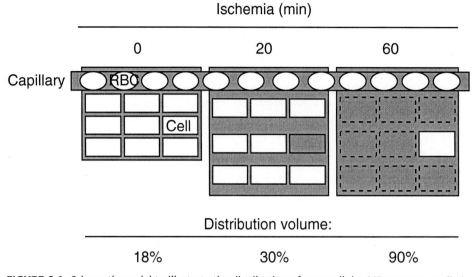

FIGURE 6.1. Schematic model to illustrate the distribution of extracellular MR contrast media in normal and reperfused ischemically injured myocardium. Extracellular MR contrast media are distributed exclusively in the extracellular space in normal myocardium *(left panel)*. In rats subjected to moderate ischemia (20 minutes), the distribution volume increases from 18% to 30% *(center panel)* because of expansion of the extracellular space and the presence of few necrotic cells. In regions with severe myocardial ischemia *(right panel)*, the distribution volume of these agents increases tremendously, to more than 90%, because of the loss of cellular integrity and interstitial edema.

aged cells in the ischemic territory increases. The volume of distribution of intravascular MR contrast media in myocardium primarily depends on the integrity of microvessels. In normal myocardium, it reflects myocardial blood volume (8% to 12%). The interaction between the contrast agent and large molecules in the body (e.g., plasma proteins) converts extracellular agent to intravascular agent, as with MS-325 (Epix, Cambridge, Massachusetts). Such interaction causes a significant increase in the relaxivity of these agents in situ.

Extracellular MR Contrast Media

The widely used extracellular gadolinium chelates enhance the blood and normal myocardium in a homogeneous fashion. Peak enhancement can be achieved 1 minute after intravenous injection of these agents, reflecting the high concentration of the agent in the tissue. Extracellular agents diffuse out of the capillaries into the interstitium but do not enter the intracellular space of viable tissue. During the first pass, approximately 30% to 50% of the agent diffuses into the interstitium. The enhancement produced by these agents is of large magnitude but brief in comparison with the enhancement produced by intravascular agents because they have larger distribution volumes and faster excretion rates.

In MRA, extracellular MR contrast media shorten the T1 of the blood according to the following formula: $1/T1 = (1/1,200) + R [Gd]$, in which R = relaxivity of the gadolinium chelate, [Gd] = concentration of gadolinium in the blood, and 1,200 milliseconds = T1 of the blood before

administration of the contrast medium. To differentiate vascular blood signal from tissue signal, it is necessary to inject contrast media to make the blood T1 shorter than the T1 of surrounding fat, the brightest background tissue, with a T1 of 270 milliseconds. The magnitude of arterial blood enhancement is related to three important factors, including the rate of infusion of the contrast medium, cardiac output, and imaging parameters such as repetition time (TR), echo time (TE), and flip angle. During a constant infusion rate, the arterial blood concentration of the contrast medium is determined as follows: [Gd] = infusion rate/cardiac output.

Gadolinium chelates with extracellular distribution have been used to measure the partition coefficient as a marker of myocardial viability (44–48). The feasibility of measuring the partition coefficient in normal and injured myocardium by extracellular T1-enhancing agents was first described by Diesbourg et al. (44). Measurement of the fractional distribution volume of extracellular agents in tissues from MR images rests on best assumptions pertaining to contrast agent properties, including the following: (a) sufficient blood flow in the region (>30% of baseline flow), (b) rapid exchange of contrast agent between blood and tissue compartments, (c) constant T1 relaxivity of contrast agent in tissue (no binding to tissue proteins or membranes) and blood, and (d) passive distribution in all tissue compartments (48,49). Loss of membrane integrity permits entry of the contrast medium into the intracellular space.

Measurement of the T1 relaxation rate has shown the kinetics of distribution of extracellular, intravascular, and intracellular MR contrast media in normal and infarcted myocardium (49). Unlike the other agents, extracellular MR contrast media provide accurate values of the partition coefficient in normal and infarcted myocardium. This study illustrates that most extracellular MR contrast media (e.g., Gd-DTPA and Gd-DTPA-BMA) have no binding affinity to plasma protein in the blood, interstitium, or myocardial cells; therefore, they are suitable for measuring myocardial viability.

The partition coefficients of extracellular gadolinium chelates were recently measured in 12 healthy volunteers, five patients with acute infarction, and five patients with chronic myocardial infarction (51). Investigators found that the magnitude of the partition coefficient in normal myocardium is uniform over the entire myocardium (0.56 mL/g $\pm$ 0.10). The values of the partition coefficient in patients with acute (0.91 mL/g $\pm$ 0.11, $p < .001$) or chronic (0.78 mL/g $\pm$ 0.09, $p < .001$) infarction were significantly elevated in comparison with those of healthy volunteers. They suggested that a 20% elevation in the partition coefficient, in comparison with the mean value of the corresponding normal circumferential segment, allows the identification of chronically (sensitivity, 88%; specificity, 96%) or acutely (sensitivity, 100%; specificity, 98%) infarcted segments.

Extracellular magnetic susceptibility MR contrast agents (e.g., Dy-DTPA-BMA) have also been used to demonstrate the breakdown of cellular membranes in reperfused infarction (52,53). It was found that reperfused infarction, which appears hyperintense on Gd-DTPA-BMA–enhanced T1-weighted spin-echo images, was also hyperintense on Dy-DTPA-BMA–enhanced T2-weighted spin-echo images. Because the susceptibility agent causes signal loss when distributed heterogeneously in myocardium by virtue of extracellular but not intracellular distribution, the lack of the expected signal loss evident in the infarcted region was considered to result from a more even tissue distribution (extracellular as well as intracellular), signifying that the agent had penetrated the cellular spaces (52,53).

Intravascular MR Contrast Media

These nondiffusible agents are also called *blood pool, macromolecular,* or *nondiffusible* MR contrast media. Distribution of these agents to the intravascular space is achieved by conjugating the paramagnetic ligand to albumin, liposomes, and polymers, which prevent extravasation of these large molecules through the microvessels for some period of time. These agents have a high molecular weight (>50 kd) or globular shape.

The potential advantages of intravascular agents include a long plasma half-life with minimal leakage into the interstitial space and significantly higher relaxivity (R1) values, which allow decreased molar dosing. The T1 relaxivity of these agents is greater than that of extracellular media because multiple paramagnetic ions are attached to each polymeric molecule, and the molecular rotational correlation times of each paramagnetic subunit are slower. For this reason, intravascular agents may more effectively provide prolonged vascular enhancement in MRA. However, their signal-enhancing capacity in tissue is lower than that of extracellular agents because their distribution volume is smaller (vascular space). Gd-DTPA-albumin has been employed as an intravascular agent in experimental animals to study blood volume, microvascular permeability, angiogenesis, and antiangiogenesis drugs in different types of tumor (34). Other intravascular MR contrast media have been used to estimate myocardial blood volume, blood flow, and perfusion (54).

Currently, no intravascular agents have been approved by the FDA. However, clinical trials are being performed with the paramagnetic MS-325 (AngioMARK; Epix, Cambridge, Massachusetts) and superparamagnetic NC100150 injection (Clariscan; Nycomed Amersham, Oslo, Norway) (55,56). MS-325 is a small-molecular-weight gadolinium chelate that is reversibly bound to plasma albumin to form a blood pool MR agent. In baboons, this agent has plasma half-life of 174 minutes. The relaxivity of MS-325 is about 10-fold greater than that of Gd-DTPA (57). Thus far, no important allergic reaction has been attributed to MS-325, but the risk for allergic reactions after repeated administration is a concern. Nevertheless, intravascular MR contrast media are an attractive alternative to extracellular contrast media for MRA of the coronary and peripheral arteries (56–63).

NC100150 injection (Clariscan) consists of very small ferromagnetic particles. Each particle is a single crystal with a single magnetic domain. Within each domain, the magnetic moments of all unpaired electrons are aligned together, and the sum of the electron magnetic moments can be considered a single permanent magnetic dipole. The crystalline symmetry and nature of the coating determine the T1, T2, and T2* relaxivities of these agents. The relaxivity ratio of iron oxide particles is positively correlated with the size of the core particle, so that larger particles demonstrate greater T2/T2* effects. For example, AMI-25, a large crystal aggregate (80 nm) with a dextran coating, has a high R2/R1 ratio of 4.45, whereas NC100150 injection, composed of smaller particles (5 to 7 nm) with a carbohydrate-polyethylene glycol coat, has an R2/R1 ratio of 1.8. The smaller size of superparamagnetic iron oxide particles prolongs the plasma half-life because the particles are not quickly phagocytized by the reticuloendothelial system; this feature is advantageous in MRA. An advantage of another experimental superparamagnetic intravascular MR agent, SH U555A (Schering AG), is that it causes T1 enhancement with homogeneous distribution in blood, and signal loss with heterogeneous distribution in tissues (64). A reduction in signal intensity in tissue was pronounced on T2-weighted sequences but was also observed on T1-weighted sequences, so that signal from the liver was lower than that from blood vessels.

farction size defined by triphenyltetrazolium chloride stain. Both methods correlated well with histopathologic standards. Although contrast-enhanced MRI can detect regions of microvascular obstruction with blood flow less than 40% of remote myocardium, the threshold for microvascular obstruction by echocardiography is less than 60%. The investigators concluded that myocardial and microvascular damages occur during the first 48 hours of reperfusion. In another study of patients by the same investigators (161), microvascular injury remained a strong prognostic marker, even after infarction, when contrast-enhanced MRI was used. Furthermore, microvascular status predicted the occurrence of cardiovascular complications, and the risk for adverse events increased with size of the infarct.

Lima et al. (139) studied 22 patients with acute myocardial infarction treated by a combination of thrombolytic therapy and angioplasty. Four days after reperfusion, patients were examined by rapid T1-weighted MRI to monitor contrast distribution patterns during the first 10 minutes after injection. In 21 of 22 cases, an abnormal MRI signal time profile was observed in some regions. These regions were characterized by a rapid initial rise in signal followed by a slower rise, whereas normal regions exhibited a rapid initial rise followed by a rapid decline. In 10 cases with large infarction, an additional abnormal subregion could be identified in the subendocardium. This region exhibited a much slower initial rise in signal, such that it appeared relatively hypointense in the first minutes after contrast administration. Presumably, this low-intensity core exhibited the no-reflow phenomenon.

A loss of vascular integrity plays a major role in the development of the no-reflow phenomenon. Previous studies have shown that the no-reflow phenomenon can be best identified on a contrast-enhanced MR perfusion map because of the delay in bolus arrival (139,161,165). The evolution of the no-reflow phenomenon as a function of time after reperfusion is shown in Figure 6.7. Schwitter et al. (117) were able to delineate and size the no-reflow zone in reperfused infarction with the use of intravascular MR contrast media. They found that the size of the no-reflow zone progressively increased as the duration of ischemia increased. Rochitte et al. (166) prepared dogs with 90 minutes of coronary artery occlusion followed by reperfusion. Perfusion MRI was performed at 2, 6, and 24 hours after occlusion. They found on contrast-enhanced MRI that the size of the hypoenhanced no-reflow zone progressively increased as a function of time from 3.2% $\pm$ 1.8% at 2 hours to 9.9% $\pm$ 3.2 % at 48 hours.

Gerber et al. (164) used MRI to examine whether the extent of microvascular obstruction directly alters the mechanical properties of reperfused infarction in dogs. MRI and three-dimensional (3D) tagging were performed 4 to 6 hours, 48 hours, and 10 days after reperfusion. An early increase in LV end-diastolic volume (from 42 $\pm$ 9 to 54 $\pm$ 14

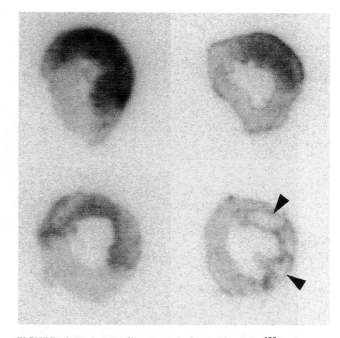

FIGURE 6.7. Autoradiograms enhanced with ^{123}I-Gd-DTPA (gadolinium diethylenetriamine pentaacetic acid)-albumin show evolution of the no-reflow phenomenon in reperfused infarction. This figure also shows distribution of the intravascular agent ^{123}I-Gd-DTPA-albumin in hearts subjected to 1 hour of coronary artery occlusion followed by varying periods of reperfusion. The ^{123}I-Gd-DTPA-albumin was administered at 3 minutes before reperfusion, and imaging was performed at 3 minutes after reperfusion *(top left)*, 30 minutes after reperfusion *(top right)*, 1 hour after reperfusion *(bottom left)*, and 24 hours after reperfusion *(bottom right)*. Accumulation of the contrast medium in the reperfused infarcted myocardium suggests loss of vascular integrity and the presence of residual blood flow, whereas its absence in the infarcted region indicates presence of the no-reflow phenomenon *(arrowheads)*.

mL, $p < .05$) at 4 to 6 and at 48 hours after reperfusion was predictable by both the extent of microvascular obstruction ($r = .89$, $p < .01$) and infarct size ($r = .83$, $p < .01$). A strong inverse relationship was found between the magnitude of the first principal strain ($r = -.80$, $p < .001$) and the relative extent of microvascular obstruction within infarcted myocardium. Also, infarcted myocardium involved by extensive areas of microvascular obstruction demonstrated reductions of circumferential ($r = -.61$, $p < .01$) and longitudinal ($r = -.53$, $p < . 05$) stretching. The investigators concluded that in the early healing phase of acute myocardial infarction, the extent of microvascular obstruction in infarcted tissue is correlated with reduced local myocardial deformation and dysfunction of noninfarcted adjacent myocardium.

Determination of Myocardial Perfusion

The measurement of myocardial perfusion with the use of MR contrast media differs from the original indicator dilution method because MR techniques cannot directly measure the concentration of the contrast medium in myocardium or blood; rather, they measure signal intensity (17,167,168). Wilke et al. (169) used MR contrast media and a methodology validated in animals (54,167,168,170, 171) to estimated absolute (milliliters per gram per minute) myocardial perfusion in humans. Under ideal experimental conditions, they obtained perfusion values in dogs of 1.2 ± 0.5 mL/min per gram and 1.3 ± 0.3 mL/min per gram with contrast-enhanced MRI and microspheres, respectively. Excellent correlation was found between the mean transit time obtained by fitting the perfusion curve with a gamma variate function and myocardial perfusion obtained by microspheres (54). However, Cullen et al. (170) claimed that an injection slower than bolus injection and a temporal resolution (every six R-R intervals) lower than every beat proved more practical in measuring myocardial perfusion reserve in patients with ischemic heart disease.

Pharmacologic stress has been used in nuclear imaging and PET for more than two decades to determine imbalances in myocardial perfusion in patients with coronary artery disease (171). Pharmacologic stress (dobutamine, dipyridamole, or adenosine) has also been used with contrast-enhanced MRI to detect potentially ischemic myocardium (31,54,111,112,115,167–170,172–176). Like nuclear medicine and PET, contrast-enhanced perfusion MRI in the vasodilated state demonstrates hypoperfused myocardium in the presence of a hemodynamically significant coronary arterial stenosis. The hypoperfused region is recognizable as a dark region in comparison with normal myocardium on contrast-enhanced MRI in the vasodilated state, but not at baseline (Fig. 6.8). In addition, it is possible to size the area at risk in the territory of a stenotic or occluded coronary artery by using contrast-enhanced MRI in the vasodilated state (31,114–116). A recent preliminary study (116) has suggested that intravascular contrast media are superior to extracellular agents in providing a longer period for delineating hypoperfused myocardium.

Contrast-enhanced stress-perfusion MRI with and without cine MRI has been applied in the simultaneous evaluation of regional function in several studies of patients with coronary artery disease. Higgins et al. (176) demonstrated the relationship between regional myocardial wall thickening, using functional MRI, and extent of perfusion deficit, using contrast-enhanced MRI and thallium scintigraphy, in patients with ischemic heart disease (Fig. 6.9). Most of these studies showed a delay in regional enhancement, a reduction in peak enhancement, or a diminution in the upward slope of the intensity–time curve in the area at risk in patients with coronary disease (170,172–176). Wilke et al. (173) addressed the issue of the sensitivity and specificity of perfusion MRI. In 22 studies including 559 patients, the average sensitivity was 82% ± 9%, and the average specificity was 88% ± 9.6%.

CONTRAST MEDIA FOR MRA

The 3D spoiled gradient-echo sequence is well suited to T1-enhancing MR contrast agents. The sequence can be performed before and after the administration of extracellular MR contrast media. Contrast-enhanced MRA studies do not rely on blood motion to create signal; rather, the contrast medium reduces the T1 (spin lattice) relaxation time of the blood such that it is significantly different from that of surrounding tissue.

Currently available extracellular contrast agents provide limited imaging time windows for the acquisition of MRA data. As the concentration of the contrast medium equilibrates with interstitium (~3 minutes) and the background signal increases, the contrast-to-noise ratio rapidly decreases. Alternatively, intravascular MR contrast media have a longer intravascular residence time, a higher relaxivity, and a better contrast-to-noise ratio than do extracellular agents (Fig. 6.10). Therefore, they potentially offer greater MRA flexibility, versatility, and accuracy. A disadvantage of intravascular contrast media is the enhancement of both venous and arterial systems. Furthermore, with intravascular contrast media, the timing of the contrast injection becomes less significant because the optimal imaging window is measured in tens of minutes rather than seconds. Some intravascular MR contrast media (e.g., NC100150 and MS-350) are currently being evaluated for MRA in human clinical trials (55–58,177,178).

In the United States, Europe, and Japan, substantial interest has been shown in using extracellular and intravascular contrast media for MRA of the coronary artery (59,60,161,179–185). Coronary images have been acquired during the bolus phase of extracellular and blood pool agents and during the equilibrium phase of blood pool agents (180). Li et al. (59) used fast gradient-echo imaging to collect 3D MR images of the coronary arteries after the administration of MS-325. In another study in pigs (60), they used the same contrast agent with a navigator-echo sequence to improve the images of coronary arteries and suppress myocardial signal.

MR contrast media have been used in imaging pulmonary vessels and perfusion of the lung (184–186). MRA performed with MR contrast media has also been used to assess pulmonary perfusion (161,186–188).

In a study in dogs, NC100150 injection was effective in delineating vessels in the lower extremities for at least 30 minutes (61). The intravascular agent MS-325 was successfully used for MRA of the lower extremities in normal volunteers (55). Investigators were able to distinguish between arteries and veins. One major limitation of steady-state MRA is that venous enhancement may confound the definition of arteries. This problem can be minimized with the appropriate use of currently available viewing techniques, such as targeted maximum intensity projection and multiplanar refor-

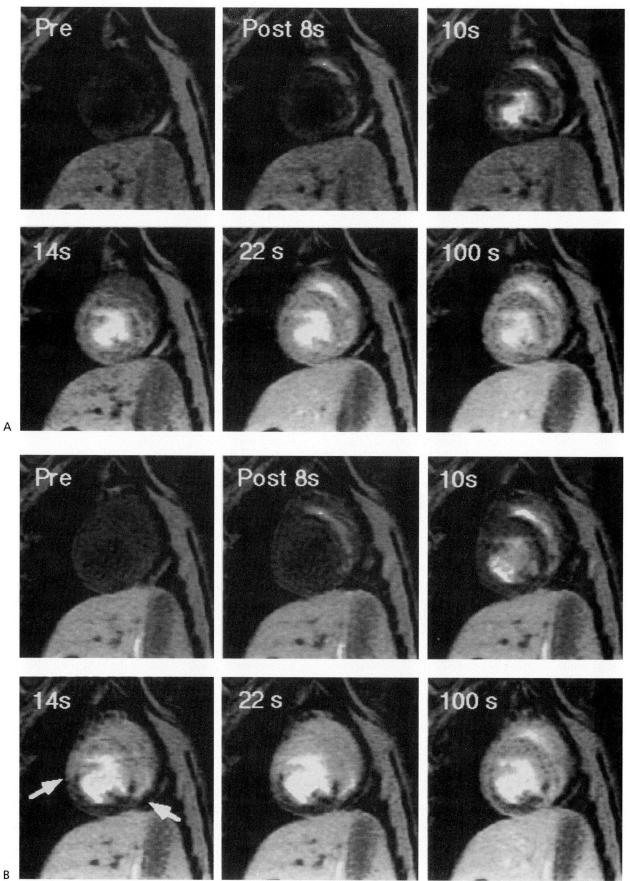

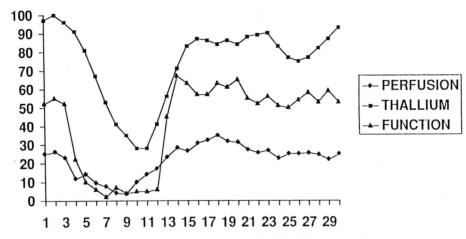

FIGURE 6.9. Comparison of thallium perfusion with MR perfusion as shown on contrast-enhanced MR perfusion images and regional wall thickening as shown by cine MRI in a patient with a fixed thallium defect of the inferior segment of the left ventricle (LV). The values were obtained from 30 segments (x-axis) of the horizontal view of the LV. Data are shown as a percentage of normal myocardium (y-axis).

mation technology. This problem seems to be most effectively managed by using a venous subtraction strategy (55). In the future, newer contrast media having different activities at different pH levels or oxygen tensions may further reduce or completely eliminate venous enhancement (189).

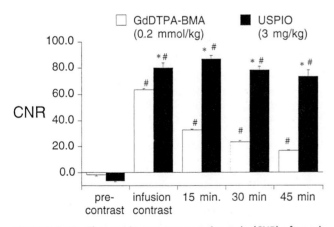

FIGURE 6.10. Changes in contrast-to-noise ratio (CNR) after administration of the extracellular MR contrast medium Gd-DTPA-BMA (gadolinium diethylenetriamine pentaacetic acid-bis-methyamide) (0.2 mmol/kg) and the intravascular ultrasmall particle iron oxide NC100150 (3 mg/kg). All CNR measurements were obtained from maximum intensity projection images of the femoral artery. On MRA of the peripheral circulation, intravascular agents are superior to extracellular agents. *, $p < 0.05$ for CNR values after administration of the contrast media compared to precontrast CNR values; #, $p < 0.05$ for blood pool agent values compared to extracellular agent values.

SUMMARY

The inherent contrast between the blood and myocardium on MR depends largely on proton concentration and on longitudinal (T1) and transverse (T2) relaxation times. The inherent contrast can be manipulated by using specific MR pulse sequences and contrast media. The effects of MR contrast media on signal intensity are described in terms of T1 and T2 relaxivities, referred to as *R1* and *R2 relaxivities*. The R2/R1 ratio can be used to determine whether an agent is causing predominantly T2 shortening (loss of signal) on T2-weighted images or T1 shortening (increased signal) on T1-weighted images. MR contrast media are safe and well tolerated as intravenous agents in patients. The differences between MR contrast media are based on their distribution and residence times in tissue. MR contrast media are distributed initially within the intravascular compartment (arterial and venous compartments) and diffuse rapidly into the extravascular compartment, as do water-soluble iodinated contrast media. Images obtained during the arterial phase are useful for MRA and studies of tissue perfusion, microvascular integrity, and angiogenesis, whereas images obtained during the equilibrium phase are useful for tissue MRI. MR contrast media enhance the role of MRI in detecting and sizing area at risk, infarction, periinfarction zone, and no-reflow zone. The assessment of blood volume, capillary integrity, and angiogenesis in different tissues requires the use of intravascular agents. Intravascular contrast

---

FIGURE 6.8. Contrast-enhanced perfusion MR images acquired before and after the infusion of dipyridamole (0.56 mg/kg) in a dog subjected to critical coronary artery stenosis. Before the infusion of dipyridamole **(A)**, the area at risk is not visible on contrast-enhanced perfusion MRI. Conversely **(B)**, the administration of dipyridamole allows visualization of the area at risk distal to the stenosis *(arrows)*.

media may be important for MRA of some regions of the body, such as the coronary arteries. The further development of targeted MR contrast agents may be helpful in organ- or tissue-specific MRI.

REFERENCES

1. Bloch F. Nuclear induction. *Phys Rev* 1946;70:460.
2. Solomon I. Relaxation processes in a system of two spins. *Phys Rev* 1955;99:559.
3. Solomon I, Bloembergen N. Nuclear magnetic interactions in the HF molecule. *J Chem Phys* 1956;25:261.
4. Bloembergen N. Proton relaxation times in paramagnetic solutions. *J Chem Phys* 1957;27:572.
5. Bloembergen N, Morgan LO. Proton relaxation times in paramagnetic solutions. Effects of electron spin relaxation. *J Chem Phys* 1961;34:842.
6. Lauterbur PC. Image formation by induced local interactions: examples employing nuclear magnetic resonance. *Nature* 1973; 242:19.
7. Lauterbur PC, Mendonca-Dias MH, Rudin AM. Augmentation of tissue water proton spin-lattice relaxation rate by *in vivo* addition of paramagnetic ions. In: Dutton PL, Leigh LS, Scarpa A, eds. *Frontiers of biological energetics.* New York: Academic Press, 1978:752.
8. Saeed M, Wendland MF, Masui T, et al. Dual mechanisms for change in myocardial signal intensity by means of a single MR contrast medium: dependence on concentration and pulse sequence. *Radiology* 1993;186:175.
9. Canet E, Revel D, Forrat R, et al. Superparamagnetic iron oxide particles and positive enhancement for myocardial perfusion studies assessed by subsecond T1-weighted MRI. *Magn Reson Imaging* 1993;11:1139.
10. Yu KK, Saeed M, Wendland MF, et al. Real-time dynamics of an extravascular magnetic resonance contrast medium in acutely infarcted myocardium using inversion recovery and gradient-recalled echo-planar imaging. *Invest Radiol* 1992;27:927.
11. Saeed M, Wendland MF, Yu KK, et al. Dual effects of gadodiamide injection in depiction of the region of myocardial ischemia. *J Magn Reson Imaging* 1993;3:21.
12. Lauffer RB. Paramagnetic metal complexes as water proton relaxation agents for NMRI: theory and design. *Chem Rev* 1987;87:901.
13. Kowalewski J, Nordenskiöld L, Benetis N, et al. Theory of nuclear relaxation in paramagnetic systems in solution. *Prog NMR Spectrosc* 1985;17:141.
14. Kennan RP, Zhong J, Gore JC. Intravascular susceptibility contrast mechanisms in tissues. *Magn Reson Med* 1994;31:9.
15. Albert MS, Huang W, Lee JH, et al. Susceptibility changes following bolus injections. *Magn Reson Med* 1993;29:700.
16. Chu SC, Xu Y, Balschi JA, et al. Bulk magnetic susceptibility shifts in NMR studies of compartmentalized samples: use of paramagnetic reagents. *Magn Reson Med* 1990;13:239.
17. Bauer WR, Schulten K. Theory of contrast agents in magnetic resonance imaging: coupling of spin relaxation and transport. *Magn Reson Med* 1992;26:16.
18. Rosen BR, Belliveau JW, Vevea JM, et al. Perfusion imaging with NMR contrast agents. *Magn Reson Med* 1990;14:249.
19. Geschwind JF, Saeed M, Wendland MF, et al. Depiction of reperfused myocardial infarction using contrast-enhanced spin echo and gradient echo magnetic resonance imaging. *Invest Radiol* 1998;33:386.
20. Rocklage SM, Watson AD. Chelates of gadolinium and dysprosium as contrast agents for MR imaging. *J Magn Reson Imaging* 1993;3:167.
21. Wehrli FW, MacFall JR, Glover GH, et al. The dependence of nuclear magnetic resonance (NMR) imaging contrast on intrinsic and pulse sequence timing parameters. *Magn Reson Imaging* 1984;2:3.
22. Fullerton GD. Physiologic basis of magnetic relaxation. In: Stark DD, Bradley WG, eds. *Magnetic resonance imaging,* 2nd ed. St. Louis: Mosby–Year Book, 1992:88–108.
23. Nelson TR, Hendrick RE, Hendee WR. Selection of pulse sequences producing maximum tissue contrast in magnetic resonance imaging. *Magn Reson Imaging* 1984;2:285.
24. Hendrick RE, Nelson TR, Hendee WR. Optimizing tissue contrast in magnetic resonance imaging. *Magn Reson Imaging* 1984;2:193.
25. Bradley WG, Waluch V. Blood flow: magnetic resonance imaging. *Radiology* 1985;154:443.
26. Schwitter J, Sakuma H, Saeed M, et al. Very fast cardiac imaging. *MRI Clin North Am* 1996;4:419.
27. Haase A. Snapshot FLASH MRI. Application to T1, T2, and chemical-shift imaging. *Magn Reson Med* 1990;13:77.
28. Mathaei D, Haase A, Heinrich D, et al. Cardiac and vascular imaging with an MR snapshot technique. *Radiology* 1990;177: 527.
29. Buxton RB, Edelmann RR, Rosen BR, et al. Contrast in rapid MRI: T1- and T2-weighted imaging. *J Comput Assist Tomogr* 1987;11:7.
30. Moran PR. A general approach to T1, T2 and spin-density discrimination sensitivities in MR imaging sequences. *Magn Reson Imaging* 1984;2:17.
31. Saeed M, Wendland MF, Lauerma K, et al. Detection of myocardial ischemia using first pass contrast-enhanced inversion recovery and driven equilibrium fast GRE imaging. *J Magn Reson Imaging* 1995;5:515.
32. van Beers BE, Gallez B, Pringot J. Contrast enhanced MRI of the liver. *Radiology* 1996;203:297.
33. Roberts HC, Saeed M, Roberts TPL, et al. MRI of acute myocardial ischemia: comparing a new contrast agent, Gd-DTPA-24-cascade-polymer, with Gd-DTPA. *J Magn Reson Imaging* 1999;9:204.
34. Brasch RC. New directions in the development of MR imaging contrast media. *Radiology* 1992;183:1.
35. Schmiedl U, Brasch RC, Ogan MD, et al. Albumin labeled with Gd-DTPA. An intravascular contrast-enhancing agent for magnetic resonance blood pool and perfusion imaging. *Acta Radiol* 1990;374(Suppl):99.
36. Vexler VS, Clement O, Schmitt-Willich H, et al. Effect of varying the molecular weight of the MR contrast agent Gd-DTPA-polylysine on blood pharmacokinetic and enhancement patterns. *J Magn Reson Imaging* 1994;4:381.
37. Wang SC, Wikstrom MG, White DL, et al. Evaluation of Gd-DTPA-labeled dextran as an intravascular MR contrast agent: imaging characteristics in normal rat tissues. *Radiology* 1990; 175:483.
38. Wiener EC, Brechbiel MW, Brothers H, et al. Dendrimer-based metal chelates: a new class of magnetic resonance imaging contrast agents. *Magn Reson Med* 1994;31:1.
39. Adam G, Neuerburg J, Spüntrup E, et al. Gd-DTPA-cascade-polymer: potential blood pool contrast agent for MR imaging. *J Magn Reson Imaging* 1994;4:462.
40. Schmiedl U, Sievers RE, Brasch RC, et al. Acute myocardial ischemia and reperfusion: MR imaging with albumin-Gd-DTPA. *Radiology* 1989;170:351.
41. Prince MR. Gadolinium-enhanced MR aortography. *Radiology* 1994;191:155.

42. Kroft LJM, Doornbos J, van der Geest RJ, et al. Blood pool contrast agent CMD-A2-Gd-DOTA-enhanced MR imaging of infarcted myocardium in pigs. *J Magn Reson Imaging* 1999;10:170.

43. Clarke SE, Weinmann HJ, Dai E, et al. Comparison of two blood pool contrast agents for 0.5-T MR angiography: experimental study in rabbits. *Radiology* 2000;214:787.

44. Diesbourg LD, Prato FS, Wisenberg G, et al. Quantification of myocardial blood flow and extracellular volumes using a bolus injection of Gd-DTPA: kinetic modeling in canine ischemic disease. *Magn Reson Med* 1992;23:239.

45. Tong CY, Prato FS, Wisenberg G, et al. Measurement of the extraction efficiency and distribution volume for Gd-DTPA in normal and diseased canine myocardium. *Magn Reson Med* 1993;30:337.

46. Wendland MF, Saeed M, Lauerma K, et al. Alterations in T1 of normal and reperfused infarcted myocardium after Gd-BOPTA versus Gd-DTPA on inversion recovery EPI. *Magn Reson Med* 1997;37:448.

47. Arheden H, Saeed M, Higgins CB, et al. Reperfused rat myocardium subjected to various durations of ischemia: estimation of the distribution volume of contrast material with echo-planar MRI. *Radiology* 2000;215:520.

48. Wendland MF, Saeed M, Lund G, et al. Contrast-enhanced MRI for qualification of myocardial viability. *J Magn Reson Imaging* 1999;10:694.

49. Saeed M, Higgins CB, Geschwind JF, et al. T1-relaxation kinetics of extracellular, intracellular, and intravascular MR contrast agents in normal and acutely reperfused infarcted myocardium using echo-planar MR imaging. *Eur Radiol* 2000;10:310.

50. Saeed M, Wendland MF, Masui T, et al. Myocardial infarctions on T1- and susceptibility-enhanced MRI: evidence for loss of compartmentalization of contrast media. *Magn Reson Med* 1994;31:31.

51. Flacke SJ, Fisher SE, Lorenz CH. Measurement of the gadopentetate dimeglumine partition coefficient in human myocardium *in vivo*: normal distribution and elevation in acute and chronic infarction. *Radiology* 2001;218:703.

52. Geschwind JF, Wendland MF, Saeed M, et al. Identification of myocardial cell death in reperfused myocardial injury using dual mechanisms of contrast enhanced magnetic resonance imaging. *Acad Radiol* 1994;1:1.

53. Nilsson S, Wikstorm M, Martinussen HJ, et al. Dy-DTPA-BMA as indicator of tissue viability in MR imaging. *Acta Radiol* 1995;36:338.

54. Wilke N, Kroll K, Merkle H, et al. Regional myocardial blood volume estimated with MR first pass imaging and polylysine-Gd-DTPA in the dog. *J Magn Reson Imaging* 1995;5:227.

55. Grist T, Korosec F, Peters D, et al. Steady-state and dynamic MR angiographic imaging with MS-325: initial experience in humans. *Radiology* 1998;207:539.

56. Taylor AM, Panting JR, Keegan J, et al. Safety and preliminary findings with the intravascular contrast agent NC100150 Injection for MR coronary angiography. *J Magn Reson Imaging* 1999;9:220.

57. Lauffer RB, Parmelle DJ, Dunham SU, et al. MS-325: albumin-targeted contrast agent for MR angiography. *Radiology* 1998;207:529.

58. Stillman AE, Wilke N, Li D, et al. Ultrasmall superparamagnetic iron oxide to enhance MRA of the renal and coronary arteries: studies in human patients. *J Comput Assist Tomogr* 1996;20:51.

59. Li D, Dolan B, Walovitch RC, et al. Three-dimensional MRI of coronary arteries using an intravascular contrast agent. *Magn Reson Med* 1998;39:1014.

60. Li D, Zheng J, Bae KT, et al. Contrast enhanced magnetic resonance imaging of the coronary arteries. *Invest Radiol* 1998;33:578.

61. Bremerich J, Roberts TP, Wendland MF, et al. Three-dimensional MR imaging of pulmonary vessels and parenchyma with NC100150 Injection (Clariscan™). *J Magn Reson Imaging* 2000;11:622.

62. Englbrecht M, Saeed M, Wendland MF, et al. Contrast-enhanced 3D-TOF MRA of peripheral vessels: intravascular versus extravascular MR contrast media. *J Magn Reson Imaging* 1998;8:616.

63. Saeed M, Wendland MF, Engelbrecht M, et al. Value of blood pool contrast agents in magnetic resonance angiography of the pelvis and lower extremities. *Euro Radiol* 1998;8:1047.

64. Hamm B, Staks T, Taupitz M, et al. Contrast enhanced MR imaging of liver and spleen: first experience in humans with a new superparamagnetic iron oxide. *J Magn Reson Imaging* 1994;4:659–668.

65. Renshaw PF, Owen CS, Evans AE, et al. Immunospecific NMR contrast agents. *Magn Reson Imaging* 1986;4:351–357,

66. Gerdan Loetscher HR, Kuennecke B, et al. Monoclonal antibody-coated magnetic particles as contrast agents in magnetic resonance imaging of tumors. *Magn Reson Med* 1989;12:151–163.

67. Go KG, Bulte JWM, de Lay, et al. Our approach towards developing a specific tumor-targeted MRI contrast agent for the brain. *Eur J Radiol* 1993;16:171–175.

68. Reimer P, Weissleder R, Shen T, et al. Pancreatic receptors: initial feasibility studies with a targeted contrast agent for MR imaging. *Radiology* 1994;193:527–531.

69. Schaffer BK, Linker C, Papisov M, et al. MION-ASF: biokinetics of an MR receptor agent. *Magn Reson Imaging* 1993;11:411–417.

70. Enochs WS, Weissleder R. MR imaging of the peripheral nervous system. *J Magn Reson Imaging* 1994;4:241–257.

71. Reimer P, Weissleder R, Wittenberg J, et al. Receptor-directed contrast agents for MR imaging: preclinical evaluation with affinity assays. *Radiology* 1992;182:565–569.

72. Lee AS, Weissleder R, Brady TJ, et al. Lymph nodes: microstructural anatomy at MR imaging. *Radiology* 1991;178:519–522.

73. Bethenze Y, Vexler V, Jerome H, et al. Differentiation of capillary leak and hydrostatic pulmonary edema with macromolecular MR imaging contrast agent. *Radiology* 1991;181:773–777.

74. Unger UC, Shen D, Fritz TA. Status of liposomes as MR contrast agents. *J Magn Reson Imaging* 1993;3:195–198.

75. Yeh T, Zhang W, Ilstad ST, et al. Intracellular labelling of T-cells with superparamagnetic contrast agents. *Magn Reson Imaging* 1994;4:381–388.

76. Bulte JWM, Ma LD, Magin RL, et al. Selective MR imaging of labeled human peripheral blood mononuclear cells by liposome mediated incorporation of dextran-magnetite particles. *Magn Reson Med* 1993;20:32–37.

77. Khaw BA, Gold H, Yasuda T, et al. Scintigraphic quantification of myocardial necrosis in patients after intravenous injection of myosin specific antibody. *Circulation* 1986;74:501.

78. Khaw BA, Fallon JT, Beller G, et al. Specificity of localization of myosin-specific antibody fragments in experimental myocardial infarction. *Circulation* 1979;60:1527.

79. Weissleder R, Lee A, Khaw B, et al. Detection of myocardial infarction with MION-antimyosin. *Radiology* 1992;182:381.

80. Gupta H, Weissleder R. Targeted contrast agents in MR imaging. *MRI Clin North Am* 1996;4:171.

81. Ni Y, Marchal G, Yu J, et al. Localization of metalloporphyrin induced specific enhancement in experimental liver tumor:

comparison of MRI, microangiographic and histologic findings. *Acad Radiol* 1995;2:697.

82. Marchal G, Ni Y, Herijgers P, et al. Paramagnetic metallo-porphyrins: infarct avid contrast agents for diagnosis of acute myocardial infarction by MRI. *Eur Radiol* 1996;6:2.

83. Hilger C, Maier F, Ebert W, et al. Patent DE 42 32 925 A1. Berlin, Germany, 1992.

84. Weinmann HJ, Brasch RC, Press WR, et al. Characteristics of gadolinium-DTPA complex: a potential NMR contrast agent. *AJR Am J Roentgenol* 1984;142;619.

85. Saeed M, Bremerich J, Wendland MF, et al. Reperfused myocardial infarction as seen with use of necrosis-specific versus standard extracellular MR contrast media in rats. *Radiology* 1999;213:247.

86. Saeed M, Lund G, Wendland MF, et al. Magnetic resonance characterization of the peri-infarction zone of reperfused myocardial infarction with necrosis-specific and extracellular nonspecific contrast media. *Circulation* 2001;103:871.

87. Choi SII, Choi SH, Kim ST, et al. Irreversibly damaged myocardium at MR imaging with a necrosis tissue-specific contrast agent in a cat model. *Radiology* 2000;215:863.

88. Pislaru SV, Ni Y, Pislaru C, et al. Noninvasive measurements of infarct size after thrombolysis with a necrosis-avid MRI contrast agent. *Circulation* 1999;99:690.

89. Saeed M, Watzinger N, Lund GK, et al. The potential of extracellular and necrosis specific Gd-mesoporphyrin MR contrast media for predicting left ventricular remodeling. International Society for Magnetic Resonance in Medicine 2002, May 18–24; Honolulu, HI.

90. Weissleder R. Molecular imaging: exploring the next frontier. *Radiology* 1999;212:609.

91. Li WH, Fraser SE, Meade TJ. A calcium-sensitive magnetic resonance imaging contrast agent. *J Am Chem Soc* 1999;121:1413.

92. Moats RA, Fraser SE, Meade TJ. A "smart" magnetic resonance imaging contrast agent that reports on specific enzyme activity. *Agnew Chem Int Edu Engl* 1977;726.

93. Aime S, Botta M, Fasanom M, et al. Lanthanide (III) chelates for NMR biomedical applications. *Chem Soc Rev* 1998;27:19.

94. Louie AY, Huber MM, Ahrens ET, et al. *In vivo* visualization of gene expression using magnetic resonance imaging. *Nat Biotechnol* 2000;18:321.

95. Wunderbaldinger P, Bogdanov A, Weissleder R. New approaches for imaging in gene therapy. *Eur J Radiol* 2000;34:156.

96. Bhorade R, Weissleder R, Nakakoshi T, et al. Macrocyclic chelators with paramagnetic cations are internalized into mammalian cells via an HIV-tat derived membrane translocation peptide. *Bioconjug Chem* 2000;11:301.

97. Lewin M, Carlesso N, Tung Ch, et al. Tat peptide-derived magnetic nanoparticles allow *in vivo* tracking and recovery of progenitor cells. *Nature* 2000;18:410.

98. Weissleder R, Moore A, Mahmood U, et al. *In vivo* magnetic resonance imaging of transgene expression. *Nature* 2000;6:351.

99. Lewin M, Bredow S, Sergeyev N, et al. *In vivo* assessment of vascular endothelial growth factor-induced angiogenesis. *Int J Cancer* 1999;83:798.

100. Bogdanov A Jr, Weissleder R. The development of *in vivo* imaging systems to study gene expression. *Trends Biotechnol* 1998;16:5.

101. Wolf GL, Baun L. Cardiovascular toxicity and tissue proton T1 response to manganese injection in the dog and rabbit. *AJR Am J Roentgenol* 1983;141:193.

102. Bremerich J, Saeed M, Arheden H, et al. Differentiation between normal and infarcted myocardium by myocardial cellular uptake of manganese. *Radiology* 2000;216:524.

103. van der Elst L, Colet JM, Muller RN. Spectroscopic and metabolic effects of MnCl2 and MnDPDP on the isolated and perfused rat heart. *Invest Radiol* 1997;32:581.

104. Brurok H, Schjott J, Berg K, et al. Effects of MnDPDP, DPDP, and MnCl2 on cardiac energy metabolism and manganese accumulation. An experimental study in the isolated perfused rat heart. *Invest Radiol* 1997;32:205.

105. Wendland MF, Saeed M, Geschwind JF, et al. Distribution of intracellular, extracellular, and intravascular MR contrast agents for magnetic resonance imaging in hearts subjected to reperfused myocardial infarction. *Acad Radiol* 1996;3:S402

106. Gallez B, Bacic G, Swartz H. Evidence for the dissociation of the hepatobiliary MRI contrast agent Mn-DPDP. *Magn Reson Med* 1996;35:14.

107. Runge VM. Safety of approved MR contrast media for intravenous injection. *J Magn Reson Imaging* 2000;12:205.

108. Wyttenbach R, Saeed M, Wendland MF, et al. Detection of acute myocardial ischemia using first-pass dynamic of MN-DPDP on inversion recovery echo-planar imaging. *J Magn Reson Imaging* 1999;9:209.

109. Wilke N, Simm C, Zhang J, et al. Contrast-enhanced first pass myocardial perfusion imaging: correlation between myocardial blood flow in dogs at rest and during hyperemia. *Magn Reson Med* 1993;29:485.

110. Saeed M, Wendland MF, Lauerma K, et al. Detection of myocardial ischemia using first pass contrast-enhanced inversion recovery and driven equilibrium fast GRE imaging. *J Magn Reson Imaging* 1995;5:515.

111. Schwitter J, Saeed M, Wendland MF, et al. Assessment of myocardial function and perfusion in a canine model of non-occlusive coronary artery stenosis using fast magnetic resonance imaging. *J Magn Reson Imaging* 1999;9:101.

112. Kraitchman DL, Wilke N, Hexeberg, et al. Myocardial perfusion and function in dogs with moderate coronary stenosis. *Magn Reson Med* 1996;35:771.

113. Bremerich J, Buser P, Bongartz G, et al. Noninvasive stress testing of myocardial ischemia: comparison of MRI perfusion and wall motion analysis to 99mTcMIBI SPECT, relation to coronary angiography. *Eur Radiol* 1997;7:990.

114. Szolar DH, Saeed M, Wendland MF, et al. MR imaging characterization of postischemic myocardial dysfunction ("stunned myocardium"): relationship between functional and perfusion abnormalities. *J Magn Reson Imaging* 1996;6:615.

115. Saeed M, Wendland MF, Szolar D, et al. Quantification of the extent of area at risk with fast contrast-enhanced magnetic resonance imaging in experimental coronary artery stenosis. *Am Heart J* 1996;132:921.

116. Gerber BL, Bluemke DA, Chin BB, et al. Comparison between gadomer-17 and gadolinium DTPA for the assessment of myocardial perfusion using first pass MRI in a swine model of single vessel coronary artery stenosis. *Radiology* 2000;217:130.

117. Schwitter J, Saeed M, Wendland MF, et al. Influence of the severity of myocardial injury on the distribution of macromolecules: extra versus intra-vascular gadolinium-based MR contrast agents. *J Am Coll Cardiol* 1997;30:1086.

118. Yu KK, Saeed M, Wendland MF, et al. Comparison of T1-enhancing and magnetic susceptibility magnetic resonance contrast agents for demarcation of the jeopardy area in experimental myocardial infarction. *Invest Radiol* 1993;28:1015.

119. Eichstadt WH, Felix F, Dougherty RC. Magnetic resonance imaging at different stages of myocardial infarction using contrast agent gadolinium DTPA. *Clin Cardiol* 1986;9:527.

120. de Roos A, van Voorthuisen AE. Magnetic resonance imaging of the heart: perfusion, function, and structure. *Curr Opin Radiol* 1991;3:525.

121. Johnson DL, Thompson RC, Liu P, et al. Magnetic resonance imaging during acute myocardial infarction. *Am J Cardiol* 1986;57:1059.

122. Been M, Smith MA, Ridgway P. Serial changes in the T1 magnetic relaxation parameter after myocardial infarction in man. *Br Heart J* 1988;59:1.

123. Thompson RC, Liu P, Brady TJ, et al. Serial magnetic resonance imaging in patients following acute myocardial infarction [see Comments]. *Magn Reson Imaging* 1991;9:155.

124. McNamara MT, Higgins CB. Magnetic resonance imaging of chronic myocardial infarcts in man. *AJR Am J Roentgenol* 1984;143:1135.

125. Dulce MC, Duerinckx AJ, Hartiala J, et al. MR imaging of the myocardium using nonionic contrast medium: signal-intensity changes in patients with subacute myocardial infarction. *AJR Am J Roentgenol* 1993;160:963.

126. Matsunaga N, Hayashi K, Sakamoto I, et al. Serial assessment of contrast enhancement of myocardial infarction with Gd-DTPA-enhanced MR imaging. *Radiology* 1995;197:521.

127. van Dijkman PRM, van der Wall A, de Roos A, et al. Acute, subacute, and chronic myocardial infarction: quantitative analysis of gadolinium-enhanced MR imaging. *Radiology* 1991;180:147.

128. de Roos A, van Rossum AC, van der Wall, et al. Reperfused and non-reperfused myocardial infarction: diagnostic potential of Gd-DTPA-enhanced MRI. *Radiology* 1989;172:717.

129. Lim TH, Lee JH, Kim YH, et al. Occlusive and reperfused myocardial infarction: detection by using MR imaging with gadolinium polylysine enhancement. *Radiology* 1993;189:765.

130. Saeed M, Wendland MF, Masui T, et al. Myocardial infarction: assessment with an intravascular MR contrast medium. *Radiology* 1991;180:153.

131. Kim RJ, Fieno DS, Parrish TB, et al. Relationship of MRI delayed contrast enhancement to reversible injury, infarct age and contractile function. *Circulation* 1999;100:1992.

132. Kim RJ, Hillenbrand HB, Judd RM. Evaluation of myocardial viability by MRI. *Herz* 2000;25:417.

133. Judd RM, Lugo-Olivieri CH, Arai M, et al. Physiological basis of myocardial contrast enhancement in fast magnetic resonance images of 2-day-old reperfused canine infarcts. *Circulation* 1995;92:1902.

134. de Roos A, Doornbos J, van der Wall EE, et al. MRI of acute myocardial infarction: value of Gd-DTPA. *AJR Am J Roentgenol* 1988;150:531.

135. van Rossum AC, Visser FC, Van Eenige MJ, et al. Value of gadolinium-diethylene-triamine pentaacetic acid dynamics in magnetic resonance imaging of acute myocardial infarction with occluded and reperfused coronary arteries after thrombolysis. *Am J Cardiol* 1990;65:845.

136. Dendale P, Franken P, Meusel M, et al. Distinction between open and occluded infarct-related arteries using contrast-enhanced magnetic resonance imaging. *Am J Cardiol* 1997;80:334.

137. Yakota C, Nonogi H, Miyazakis, et al. Gadolinium-enhanced magnetic resonance imaging in acute myocardial infarction. *Am J Cardiol* 1995;75:577.

138. Fedele F, Montesanto T, Ferro-Luzzi M, et al. Identification of viable myocardium in patients with chronic coronary artery disease and left ventricular dysfunction: role of magnetic resonance imaging. *Am Heart J* 1994;94:484.

139. Lima JA, Judd RM, Bazille A, et al. Regional heterogeneity of human myocardial infarcts demonstrated by contrast-enhanced MRI. Potential mechanisms. *Circulation* 1995;92:1117.

140. Sandestede JJW, Lipke C, Baer M, et al. Analysis of first-pass and delayed contrast-enhancement patterns of dysfunctional myocardium on MR imaging: use for the prediction of myocardial viability. *AJR Am J Roentgenol* 2000;174:1737.

141. Rogers WJ, Kramer CM, Geskin G, et al. Early contrast-enhanced MRI predicts late functional recovery after reperfused myocardial infarction. *Circulation* 1999;99:744.

142. Kramer CM, Rogers WJ, Mankad S, et al. Contractile reserve and contrast uptake pattern by magnetic resonance imaging and functional recovery after reperfused myocardial infarction. *J Am Coll Cardiol* 2000;36:1834.

143. Kim RJ, Wu E, Rafael A, et al. The use of contrast-enhanced magnetic resonance imaging to identify reversible myocardial dysfunction. *N Engl J Med* 2000;343;1445.

144. Wu E, Judd RM, Vargas JD, et al. Visualization of presence, location, and transmural extent of healed Q-wave and non–Q-wave myocardial infarction. *Lancet* 2001;357:21.

145. Lim T-H, Choi SH. MRI of myocardial infarction. *J Magn Reson Imaging* 1999;10:686.

146. Fienno DS, Kim RJ, Chen EL, et al. Contrast enhanced MRI of myocardium at risk: distinction between reversible injury throughout infarct healing. *J Am Coll Cardiol* 2000;36:1985.

147. Schaefer S, Malloy CR, Katz J, et al. Gadolinium-DTPA-enhanced nuclear magnetic resonance imaging of reperfused myocardium: identification of the myocardial bed at risk. *Am J Cardiol* 1988;12:1064.

148. Dendale P, Franken PR, Block P, et al. Contrast enhanced and functional magnetic resonance imaging for the detection of viable myocardium after infarction. *Am Heart J* 1998;135:875.

149. Simonetti O, Kim RJ, Fieno DS, et al. An improved MR imaging technique for the visualization of myocardial infarction. *Radiology* 2001;218:215.

150. Ramani K, Judd RM, Holly TA, et al. Contrast magnetic resonance imaging in the assessment of myocardial viability with stable coronary artery disease and left ventricular dysfunction. *Circulation* 1998;98:2687.

151. Hillenbrand HB, Kim RJ, Parker MA, et al. Early assessment of myocardial salvage by contrast-enhanced magnetic resonance imaging. *Circulation* 2000;102:1678.

152. Saeed M, Wendland MF, Yu KK, et al. Identification of myocardial reperfusion with echo planar magnetic resonance imaging: discrimination between occlusive and reperfused infarctions. *Circulation* 1994;90:1492.

153. Saeed M, Wagner S, Wendland MF, et al. Occlusive and reperfused myocardial infarcts: differentiation with Mn-DPDP-enhanced MR imaging. *Radiology* 1989;172:59.

154. Saeed M, Wendland MF, Takehara Y, et al. Reperfusion and irreversible myocardial injury: identification with a nonionic MR imaging contrast medium. *Radiology* 1992;182:675.

155. Saeed M, Wendland MF, Watzinger N, et al. MR contrast media for myocardial viability, microvascular integrity and perfusion. *Eur J Radiol* 2000;34:179.

156. Kondo M, Nakano A, Siato D, et al. Assessment of microvascular no-reflow phenomenon using technetium-99m macro-aggregated albumin scintigraphy in patients with acute myocardial infarction. *Circulation* 1998;97:898.

157. Bremerich J, Wendland MF, Arheden H, et al. Microvascular injury in reperfused infarcted myocardium: noninvasive assessment with contrast-enhanced echo-planar magnetic resonance imaging. *J Am Coll Cardiol* 1998;32:787.

158. Bolognese L, Cerisano G, Buonamici P, et al. Influence of infarct-zone viability on left ventricular remodeling after acute myocardial infarction. *Circulation* 1997;96:3353.

159. Ito H, Tomooka T, Sakai N, et al. Lack of myocardial perfusion immediately after successful thrombolysis. A predictor of poor recovery of left ventricular function in anterior myocardial infarction. *Circulation* 1992;85:1699.

160. Jeremy RW, Links JM, Becker LC. Progressive failure of coronary flow during reperfusion of myocardial infarction: documentation of the no-reflow phenomenon with positron emission tomography. *J Am Coll Cardiol* 1990;16:695.

161. Wu KC, Zerhouni E, Judd RM, et al. Prognostic significance of microvascular obstruction imaging in patients with acute myocardial infarction. *Circulation* 1998;97:765.

162. Asanuma T, Tanabe K, Ochiai K, et al. Relationship between progressive microvascular damage and intramyocardial hemorrhage in patients with reperfused anterior myocardial infarction. *Circulation* 1997;96:448.

163. Ochiai K, Shimada T, Murakami Y, et al. Hemorrhagic myocardial infarction after coronary reperfusion detected *in vivo* by magnetic resonance imaging in humans: prevalence and clinical implications. *J Cardiovasc Magn Reson* 1999;1:247.

164. Gerber BL, Rochitte CE, Melin JA, et al. Microvascular obstruction and left ventricular remodeling early after acute myocardial infarction. *Circulation* 2000;101:2734.

165. Wu KC, Kim RJ, Bluemke DA, et al. Quantification and time course of microvascular obstruction by contrast-enhanced echocardiography and magnetic resonance imaging following acute myocardial infarction and reperfusion. *J Am Coll Cardiol* 1998;32:1756.

166. Richitte CE, Lima JA, Blumke DA, et al. Magnitude and time course of microvascular obstruction and tissue injury after acute myocardial infarction. *Circulation* 1998;98:1006.

167. Kroll K, Wilke N, Jerosch-Herold M, et al. Accuracy of modeling of regional myocardial flows from residue functions of an intravascular indicator. *Am J Physiol* 1996;271:H1643.

168. Wilke N, Jerosch-Herold M, Stillman AE, et al. Concepts of myocardial perfusion imaging in magnetic resonance imaging. *Magn Reson Q* 1994;10:249.

169. Wilke N, Machnig T, Engels G, et al. Dynamic perfusion studies by ultrafast MRI: initial clinical results from cardiology. *Electromedica* 1990:58:102.

170. Cullen JHS, Horsefield MA, Reek CR, et al. A myocardial perfusion reserve index in humans using first-pass contrast-enhanced magnetic resonance imaging. *J Am Coll Cardiol* 1999; 33:1386.

171. Gould KL. PET perfusion imaging and nuclear cardiology. *J Nucl Med* 1991;32:579.

172. Eichenberger AC, Schuiki E, Kochli VD, et al. Ischemic heart disease: assessment with gadolinium-enhanced ultrafast MR imaging and dipyridamole stress. *J Magn Reson Imaging* 1995; 4:425.

173. Wilke N, Jerosch-Herold M, Zenovich A, et al. Magnetic resonance first-pass myocardial perfusion: clinical validation and future applications. *J Magn Reson Imaging* 1999;10:676.

174. Manning WJ, Atkinson DJ, Grossman W, et al. First-pass nuclear magnetic resonance imaging studies using gadolinium-DTPA in patients with coronary artery disease. *J Am Coll Cardiol* 1991;18:959.

175. Schaefer S, van Tyen R, Saloner D. Evaluation of myocardial perfusion abnormalities with gadolinium-enhanced snapshot MR imaging in humans. *Radiology* 1992;185:795.

176. Higgins CB, Saeed M, Wendland MF, et al. Evaluation of myocardial function and perfusion in ischemic heart disease. *MAGMA* 1994;2:177.

177. Meaney JFM. MR angiography of the peripheral arteries. In: Ferris EJ. Waltman AC, Fishman EK, et al., eds. *Categorical course in diagnostic radiology. Vascular imaging RSNA syllabus.* Oak Brook, IL: Radiological Society of North America, 1998:201.

178. Ho KYJAM, de Haan MW, Kessels AGH, et al. Peripheral vascular tree stenosis: detection with subtracted and non-subtracted MR angiography. *Radiology* 1998;206:673.

179. Goldfarb JW, Edelman RR. Coronary arteries: breath-hold, gadolinium-enhanced, three-dimensional MR angiography. *Radiology* 1998;206:830.

180. Woodrad PK, Li D, Zheng J, et al. Current developments and future direction of coronary magnetic resonance angiography. *Coron Artery Dis* 1999;10:135.

181. Danias PG, Stuber M, Edelman RR, et al. Coronary MRA: a clinical experience in the United States. *J Magn Reson Imaging* 1999;10:713.

182. Bunce NH, Pennell DJ. Coronary MRA—a clinical experience in Europe. *J Magn Reson Imaging* 1999;10:721.

183. Nitatori T, Yoshino H, Yokoyama K, et al. Coronary MR angiography—a clinical experience in Japan. *J Magn Reson Imaging* 1999;10:709.

184. Woodrad PK, Li D, Zheng J, et al. Coronary MR angiography. *Appl Radiol* 2000;29:55–64.

185. Lorenz CH, Johansson LOM. Contrast-enhanced coronary MRA. *J Magn Reson Imaging* 1999;10:703.

186. Hatabu H, Gaa J, Kim D, et al. Pulmonary perfusion and angiography: evaluation with breath hold enhanced three dimensional fast imaging steady state precession MR imaging with short TR and TE. *AJR Am J Roentgenol* 1996;161: 635.

187. Steiner P, McKinnon GC, Romanowski B, et al. Contrast enhanced, ultrafast 3D pulmonary MR angiography in a single breath hold: initial assessment of imaging performance. *J Magn Reson Imaging* 1997;7:177.

188. Hatabu H, Gaa J, Kim D, et al. Pulmonary perfusion: qualitative assessment with dynamic contrast enhanced MRI using ultrashort TE and inversion recovery turbo FLASH. *Magn Reson Med* 1996;36:503.

189. Knopp MV, von Tengg-Kobligk H, Floemer F, et al. Contrast agents for MRA: future direction. *J Magn Reson Imaging* 1999;10:314.

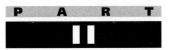

ACQUIRED HEART DISEASE

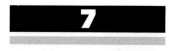

MYOCARDIAL AND PERICARDIAL DISEASES

GABRIELE A. KROMBACH
MAYTHEM SAEED
CHARLES B. HIGGINS

CARDIAC MRI FOR THE EVALUATION OF MYOCARDIAL AND PERICARDIAL DISEASE

MRI is not simply another among several techniques from which to choose in an evaluation of heart disease; rather, it has specific properties that make it desirable for this application. The high degree of spatial resolution obtained with MRI, and the inherently high level of contrast between tissue and flowing blood, provide a sharp delineation of the cardiac anatomy without the administration of contrast media. MRI offers an unlimited choice of imaging planes, so that it is especially suited for a comprehensive evaluation of cardiac anatomy and function. Regional anatomy that is not readily visualized with echocardiography, such as the apex or anterior wall of the right ventricle (RV), is readily examined by MRI. Because pulse sequences are easily synchronized with the cardiac cycle, it is possible to acquire images at precise phases of the cardiac cycle. Cine MRI can evaluate regional wall thickening and wall motion as expressions of regional ventricular function, and it can be used to measure ventricular volumes. Because three-dimensional (3D) volume data sets are acquired, geometric assumptions can be avoided, so that measurements are highly accurate and reproducible (1–3).

G. A. Krombach: Department of Radiology, University of Technology (RWTH-Aachen), Aachen, Germany.

M. Saeed and C. B. Higgins: Department of Radiology, University of California San Francisco, San Francisco, California.

TECHNIQUES

The first step in the MRI evaluation of a patient for myocardial disease is an electrocardiogram (ECG)-gated T1-weighted multislice spin-echo sequence encompassing the entire heart; this is used to assess the anatomy and structural changes (4). The acquisition is performed in either the transaxial or the short-axis plane, which is orthogonal to the long axis of the heart (5). Imaging planes that are aligned to the reference structures of the heart [long axis of the left ventricle (LV)] rather than to the thorax provide a more reproducible display of the anatomy and render the images comparable with the standard views of echocardiography (6).

Cine MR images are acquired for the purpose of quantifying ventricular volumes, mass, and global function. Cine MR images are obtained with standard gradient-echo, interleaved gradient-echo, or interleaved echo-planar sequences. A set of these images at multiple levels encompassing the heart provides a volumetric data set for the direct measurement of the end-diastolic, end-systolic, and stroke volume, mass, and ejection fraction of both ventricles. The blood pool appears bright on gradient-echo images. Contrast between bright blood and ventricular myocardium is excellent with newer rapid gradient-echo sequences, such as true fast imaging with steady-state precession (FISP) and balanced fast-field echo sequences (Fig. 7.1). An abnormal flow pattern, such as high-velocity jet flow at stenotic valves or regurgitation through insufficient valves, may produce a sig-

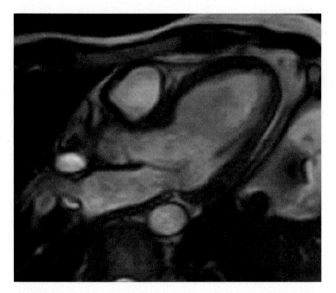

FIGURE 7.1. Balanced fast-field echo image. The contrast between the blood pool and myocardium is better than in conventional gradient-echo images.

nal void within the bright blood, depending on the duration of the echo time (TE).

Velocity-encoded (phase-contrast) cine MRI is based on velocity-induced phase shifts of moving protons in the presence of magnetic field gradients. This technique can be used to measure blood flow into the aorta or pulmonary artery to quantify the LV or RV stroke volume, respectively (7–9). It has also been used for direct measurement of the volume of valvular regurgitation, which may accompany some cardiomyopathies.

CARDIOMYOPATHIES

Classification

According to the consensus of the World Health Organization and the International Society and Federation for Cardiology (10), cardiomyopathies are defined as diseases of the myocardium associated with cardiac dysfunction. Based on pathophysiologic features, they have been divided into four main categories: dilated, hypertrophic, restrictive, and arrhythmogenic RV cardiomyopathy (10,11). In addition, diseases of the myocardium that are associated with specific cardiac or systemic disorders are termed *specific cardiomyopathies* (10).

Dilated cardiomyopathy is characterized by dilation and deteriorated contractile function of the LV or both ventricles. End-systolic and end-diastolic volumes are increased, whereas stroke volume and ejection fraction are decreased. Mild to moderate mitral regurgitation and tricuspid regurgitation are frequently associated with the ventricular enlargement. The wall thickness of the LV is usually within the normal range, so that an overall increase in LV mass results. The most common cause of dilated cardiomyopathy is myocar-

dial ischemia secondary to coronary artery disease in which the degree of myocardial dysfunction is frequently not explained by the obvious extent of myocardial infarction (10). Hypertension, viral diseases, alcoholism, diabetes, obesity, several toxins, and hereditary factors also frequently lead to dilated cardiomyopathy. Findings on histologic analysis of the myocardial tissue are nonspecific (12). The most common clinical feature of dilated cardiomyopathy is LV failure.

In hypertrophic cardiomyopathy, a variety of distribution patterns of inappropriate myocardial hypertrophy develop in the absence of an obvious functional trigger, such as aortic stenosis or systemic hypertension. The disease is genetically transmitted in about half of the cases and follows an autosomal-dominant inheritance pattern with variable penetrance. Possible manifestations are symmetric involvement of the entire LV or both ventricles or asymmetric hypertrophy of the upper septum, midportion of the ventricular septum, or apex. Nonobstructive and obstructive HCM can be distinguished by the associated hemodynamic alterations. Each type carries a different prognosis and requires a specific treatment strategy. Asymmetric septal HCM, which can cause obstruction of the LV outflow tract, is common in the United States and Europe. The hallmark is dynamic subvalvular aortic stenosis. During diastole, the LV outflow tract appears normal or slightly narrowed because of the presence of upper septal hypertrophy. Increasing stenosis develops during systole as the anterior leaflet of the mitral valve moves in an anterior direction toward the septum, thereby narrowing the outflow tract. Although uncommon in the Western world, apical hypertrophy is highly prevalent in Japan. This type of HCM does not cause obstruction of the outflow tract. HCM has a variable natural history and can cause sudden death secondary to arrhythmias.

Restrictive cardiomyopathy is characterized by hampered ventricular filling secondary to myocardial stiffness and a reduced diastolic ventricular volume. Flow into the ventricles is rapid during early diastole; it then plateaus, and little filling takes place in late diastole. End-diastolic pressure is elevated in both ventricles, whereas systolic function is normal or only slightly reduced. Endomyocardial fibrosis and Loeffler endocarditis are now classified as types of restrictive cardiomyopathy. Loeffler endocarditis is associated with hypereosinophilia. Degranulation of endomyocardial eosinophils is suspected to be responsible for focal necrosis and subsequent fibrosis and for the formation of mural thrombus. Increased stiffness of the ventricular walls and reduction of the cavity by organized thrombus contribute to the restrictive filling pattern. Endomyocardial fibrosis, a different entity with a peak geographic distribution in equatorial Africa, is not coupled with hypereosinophilia. In this disease, idiopathic fibrosis of the apex and subvalvular regions lead to restrictive cardiomyopathy. Glycogen storage diseases, radiation fibrosis, and certain infiltrative diseases, such as amyloidosis and sarcoidosis, can also cause restrictive cardiomyopathy. Many cases of restrictive cardiomyopathy are idiopathic.

Specific cardiomyopathies are myocardial diseases that are associated with a specific cardiac or systemic disease. Hemochromatosis, sarcoidosis, amyloidosis, and hypertensive or metabolic cardiomyopathy are examples of specific cardiomyopathies. This category also includes inflammatory cardiomyopathy, which is caused by myocarditis. Idiopathic, infectious, or autoimmune forms of inflammatory cardiomyopathy have been distinguished.

Several classifications also consider infiltrative cardiomyopathy as an additional category. The definition of infiltrative cardiomyopathy refers solely to the histopathologic mechanism of infiltration of myocardial tissue, and the diseases in this group may cause either restrictive or dilated cardiomyopathy. Hemochromatosis is an example of an infiltrative cardiomyopathy in which the cardiomyopathy is of the dilated type, whereas amyloidosis and sarcoidosis usually cause a restrictive pattern.

Dilated Cardiomyopathy

The anatomic abnormalities in dilated cardiomyopathy are easily recognized with either ECG-gated spin-echo MRI or cine MRI (13–15). Morphologic changes include enlargement of the LV (Fig. 7.2) and frequently also of the RV and both atria. The thickness of the LV wall usually remains normal. The MRI features in dilated cardiomyopathy are frequently nonspecific, so that the various underlying causes cannot be distinguished. However, it is usually possible to distinguish between ischemic and nonischemic forms of dilated cardiomyopathy. In most cases of nonischemic dilated cardiomyopathy, the wall thickness of the LV is uniform,

and no regional wall thinning is present. If the cardiac dilation is caused by myocardial ischemia, usually one or more regional areas of conspicuous wall thinning and sometimes ventricular aneurysm are seen. The trabeculae may be decreased in number and size after repeated myocardial infarctions (16). MRI may demonstrate localized ventricular dilation after occlusion of the supplying vessel rather than global dilation, which is characteristic of dilated cardiomyopathy (17). Isolated dilation of the RV has been found to be a sign of ischemic cardiomyopathy secondary to occlusion of the right coronary artery (18).

Ventricular mass, ventricular wall thickness, and ventricular volumes can be quantified with cine MRI to determine the severity of dilated cardiomyopathy (3,19,20). Cine MRI measurements of LV volumes, mass, and ejection fraction in dilated cardiomyopathy have been shown to be highly reproducible between studies (3). In a recent study, MRI provided the most reliable data for LV volumes and ejection fraction in patients with chronic stable heart failure in comparison with other modalities (21). The 3D approach of MRI is especially advantageous in the assessment of nonuniformly dilated or hypertrophic ventricles because no assumed geometric models are applied in calculating volumes. Three-dimensional echocardiography is also highly reliable but is subject to technical limitations, such as a limited acoustic window, and does not provide adequate image quality in approximately 14% of patients (21). Because of its high degree of accuracy and reproducibility, MRI can be used to monitor the effect of treatment in individual patients and in clinical studies to assess the efficacy of new therapeutic interventions. For example, significant decreases in LV systolic volume, wall stress, and mass and an increase in ejection fraction have been shown in dilated cardiomyopathy after angiotensin-converting enzyme inhibitor treatment (22). New therapeutic approaches in dilated cardiomyopathy, such as growth hormone therapy, have also been monitored with MRI (23).

Cine MRI has been used to assess parameters of LV and to a certain degree RV function, such as systolic wall thickening, ejection fraction, and stroke volume. These parameters can be obtained from repeated measurements of wall thickness and ventricular volume in short-axis cine MRI data sets throughout the cardiac cycle. Furthermore, myocardial wall stress can be calculated from ventricular dimensions derived from cine MR images. If the blood pressure and carotid pulse tracing are recorded during the MRI study, this parameter can be calculated from indices of LV end-systolic diameter (ESD) and end-systolic wall thickness (ESWT) as follows:

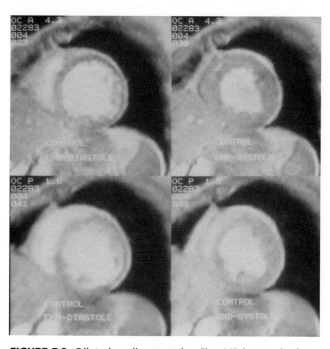

FIGURE 7.2. Dilated cardiomyopathy. Cine MR images in short-axis plane at midventricular level at end-diastole *(left panels)* and end-systole *(right panels).* The diameter of the left ventricle is increased in comparison with normal.

$$\text{end systolic wall stress} = \frac{1.35 \times \overset{\text{end systolic}}{\text{pressure}} \times \text{ESD}}{4\text{ESWT}\left(1 + \dfrac{\text{ESWT}}{\text{ESD}}\right)}$$

With this technique, wall stress has been shown to be elevated in patients with dilated cardiomyopathy (24).

In addition to decreases in stroke volume and ejection fraction, several other signs of deteriorated systolic function of the LV have been demonstrated on cine MRI. In comparison with that in normal subjects, LV wall thickening is significantly less homogeneous (25). The normal ventricle shows an increase in wall thickening from base to apex, but in patients with dilated cardiomyopathy, this gradient is absent (1,26). Myocardial tagging has revealed a severe reduction of cross-fiber shortening in patients with dilated cardiomyopathy in comparison with healthy subjects (27).

Although the LV mass has been shown to be slightly greater in a series of patients with dilated cardiomyopathy than in normal volunteers, the RV mass is not altered (18). Although the RV is usually less dilated and its systolic function is less severely deteriorated, RV diastolic abnormalities, such as an increased time to peak filling rate, have been found (20). The profile of diastolic inflow velocity measured in the region of the tricuspid valve is flattened in comparison with that in healthy volunteers (28). It is suspected that the altered morphology and function of the LV cause functional changes of RV filling.

The signal intensity on spin-echo and gradient-echo images has not been found to be consistently altered in dilated cardiomyopathy. However, hemochromatosis represents an exception. Drastic shortening of relaxation rates was found on spin-echo and gradient-echo images of myocardium overloaded with iron (29). In some patients with dilated cardiomyopathy, Gd-DTPA (gadolinium diethylenetriamine pentaacetic acid) has produced hyperenhancement of regional myocardium on T1-weighted images (30). However, hyperenhancement is a nonspecific finding that can be caused by ischemia, inflammatory infiltration, edema, and other changes.

Hypertrophic Cardiomyopathy

MRI enables a precise delineation of the location and extent of hypertrophic myocardium in persons with hypertrophic cardiomyopathy (Figs. 7.3 and 7.4). Echocardiography is the method of choice for diagnosing this condition and monitoring most patients. However, it may not provide complete information in some cases. With echocardiography, delineation of the anterior and inferior wall and of the apex is difficult to attain, even in patients with adequate acoustic windows, because these regions are located in the near field of the ultrasonic beam (31). In contrast, MRI visualizes possible sites of hypertrophy with equal fidelity. In a recent study performed in patients with hypertrophic cardiomyopathy, wall thickness could be assessed in 67% of ventricular segments with echocardiography, and in 97% with MRI (32). The major clinical role of MRI is to evaluate unusual forms of hypertrophy that are difficult to assess with echocardiography. Another indication for MRI is sequential monitoring of the LV mass.

A comprehensive examination, which also addresses the functional impact of the hypertrophy, includes measurement of the LV mass, volume, and ejection fraction by means of cine MRI (33–35). In hypertrophic cardiomyopathy, the end-systolic and end-diastolic wall thickness is increased (Fig. 7.5). The mean ratio of septal thickness to free-wall thickness was reported to be higher than 1.5 ± 0.8 in the asymmetric septal type of hypertrophic cardiomyopathy, compared with 0.9 ± 0.3 in healthy volunteers and 0.8 ± 0.2 in concentric LV hypertrophy (36). A ratio of end-diastolic septal thickness to free-wall thickness of 1.3:1 is considered highly suggestive of septal hypertrophic cardiomyopathy (Fig. 7.6). The total LV mass is substantially

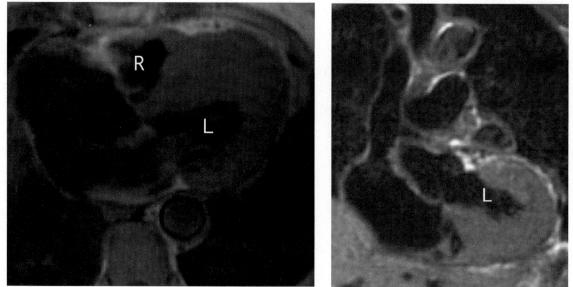

FIGURE 7.3. Hypertrophic cardiomyopathy. Axial **(A)** and coronal **(B)** T1-weighted spin-echo images show increased thickness of the left ventricular myocardium, predominantly involving the septum, apex, and anterior wall. *L,* left ventricle; *R,* right ventricle.

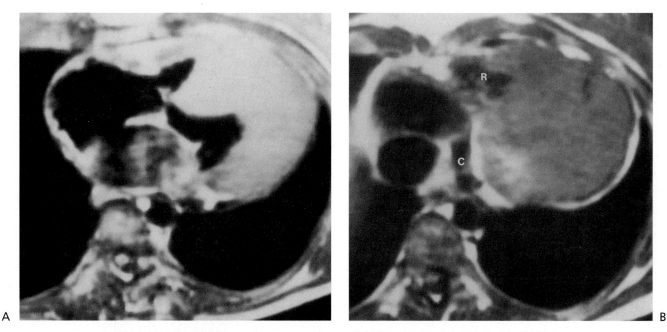

FIGURE 7.4. Hypertrophic cardiomyopathy. Transaxial spin-echo images at the level of the ventricle **(A)** and apex **(B).** The ventricle is symmetrically thickened. The left ventricular cavity is obliterated at the level of the apex because of the severe myocardial hypertrophy. *R,* right ventricle; *C,* coronary sinus.

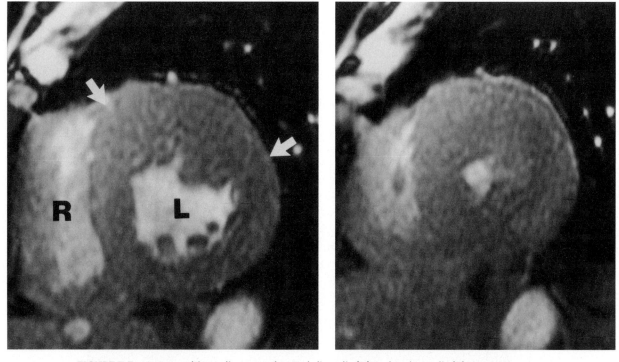

FIGURE 7.5. Hypertrophic cardiomyopathy. End-diastolic **(A)** and end-systolic **(B)** cine MR images in the short-axis plane of a patient with hypertrophic cardiomyopathy. *R,* right ventricle; *L,* left ventricle. The thickness of the myocardium is abnormal in both phases of the cardiac cycle. Hypertrophy is present in all regions but is greatest in the anterior region *(arrows).* The left ventricular cavity is small.

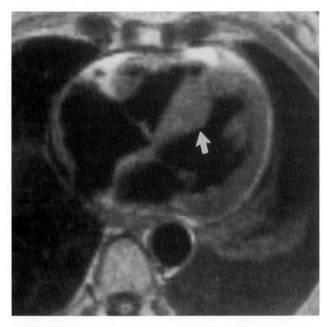

FIGURE 7.6. Hypertrophic cardiomyopathy. Transaxial spin-echo image of a patient with an asymmetric form of hypertrophic cardiomyopathy demonstrates thickening of the cranial portion of the ventricular septum *(arrow)*.

increased in hypertrophic cardiomyopathy. MRI has been used to differentiate among three types of the apical form of hypertrophic cardiomyopathy: the true apical form, a type with additional asymmetric involvement of the ventricular wall segments, and a type with symmetric involvement of the ventricular wall segments (37). It has been demonstrated that the typical "spade form" of the ventricle, which is considered to be a characteristic sign of apical hypertrophic cardiomyopathy, is not present in the early stage of the disease but develops later (38).

Cine MRI measurements of the peak filling rate and time to peak filling rate in both ventricles during diastole have revealed decreased values in comparison with those of healthy volunteers; these reflect reduced compliance of the thickened myocardium (39,40). Systolic wall thickening is decreased and fractional wall thickening is related inversely to regional wall thickness (41,42).

Regional hyperenhancement with gadolinium contrast media has been studied in hypertrophic cardiomyopathy (43). Signal enhancement has been found to be significantly greater in the most hypertrophic regions than in other regions of the ventricle (43). The increased signal intensity is most likely caused by regional myocardial ischemic injury, fibrosis, or both.

A recent study in which velocity-encoded cine MRI (VEC MRI) was used demonstrated a decrease in blood flow per unit of myocardium at rest and in response to a vasodilator (dipyridamole). Coronary blood flow to the LV myocardium was measured in the coronary sinus by means of VEC MRI and normalized by the ventricular mass to express flow as milliliters per minute per gram of LV myocardium. The ratio of vasodilator-induced to resting coronary flow (coronary flow reserve) was 1.72 ± 0.49 in hypertrophic cardiomyopathy and 3.01 ± 0.75 ($p < .01$) in normal subjects (44).

In addition to defining the location and severity of hypertrophy, MRI can differentiate between obstructive and nonobstructive hypertrophic cardiomyopathy. In the obstructive form, a jet flow in the narrowed outflow tract causes a signal void on gradient-echo images (45). A possible outflow tract gradient can be quantified by means of velocity mapping at sites proximal and distal to the stenosis. Additionally, mitral regurgitation, which is frequent in hypertrophic cardiomyopathy, can be detected by cine MRI. It causes a signal void that projects into the left atrium during systole on cine MR images. The volume of mitral regurgitation can be quantified either by calculating the difference in stroke volumes of the ventricles or by measuring the difference in the inflow and outflow volumes of the LV by means of VEC MRI (46).

Myocardial tagging has shown a profound disturbance of the regional contraction pattern of the LV in hypertrophic cardiomyopathy. Wall motion in the hypertrophic septum and cardiac rotation in the posterior region of the LV are markedly reduced (47). The longitudinal and circumferential shortening of the ventricles is also reduced (48). At the same time, ventricular torsion is increased and thickening of the myocardium is more heterogeneous than in healthy volunteers (49).

Because of its high accuracy and reproducibility in quantifying LV mass, MRI has the potential to monitor the response to therapy in hypertrophic cardiomyopathy. In a recent study in which septal ablation was performed in patients with obstructive hypertrophic cardiomyopathy to cause infarction of the hypertrophic tissue and thereby reduce the gradient in the LV outflow tract, MRI defined the size of the infarction and demonstrated a continuous improvement in the size of the outflow tract area during the 12-month follow-up period (50).

Restrictive Cardiomyopathy

The main purpose of MRI in patients with restrictive cardiomyopathy is to differentiate this diagnosis from constrictive pericarditis, which presents with essentially the same clinical picture. Because the hemodynamic features of both entities are similar, distinction solely on clinical grounds is problematic. However, the differential diagnosis is essential because constrictive pericarditis can be treated effectively with surgical resection of the pericardium, whereas restrictive cardiomyopathy is frequently fatal. In constrictive pericarditis, the pericardium is usually thickened, whereas restrictive cardiomyopathy does not have this feature. Spin-echo MRI can demonstrate pericardial thickening reliably. The diagnostic accuracy of MRI for differentiating between these two diseases was 93% in a series of symptomatic patients (51).

The MRI features of restrictive cardiomyopathy, which are characteristic but nonspecific, are caused by impaired diastolic filling of the ventricles. Impaired diastolic expansion

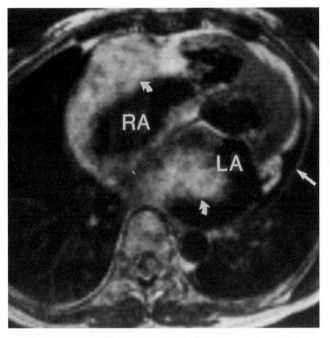

FIGURE 7.7. Restrictive cardiomyopathy. Spin-echo images at the atrial level. Both atria are enlarged. The bright signal of the blood pool *(curved arrows)* is caused by slow flow. There is a small pericardial effusion *(arrow)*. *LA,* left atrium; *RA,* right atrium.

of the ventricles causes dilation of the atria, inferior and superior venae cavae, and hepatic veins. Furthermore, stasis of blood in the atria leads to a high signal intensity in the atrial lumina on spin-echo images (Fig. 7.7). The protons within the atrial lumen do not change their position between both radiofrequency pulses of the spin-echo sequence, so that they are exposed to both pulses and a signal is generated. The restrictive filling pattern of the ventricles can be quantified and monitored during therapy by measuring the diastolic flow across the mitral and tricuspidal valves with VEC MRI (52–54). Evaluation of possible atrioventricular valve regurgitation is also important in patients with restrictive cardiomyopathy and can be performed with cine MRI or VEC MRI, as mentioned earlier.

In endomyocardial fibrosis, areas of circumscribed myocardial fibrosis have been detected as areas of low signal intensity on T1- and T2-weighted images (55). The ventricular walls may be severely thickened by the deposition of subendocardial fibrotic tissue, which causes a narrowing of the cavities and contributes further to the decreased diastolic ventricular filling.

Several specific cardiomyopathies can result in a restrictive filling pattern. The typical imaging findings of these diseases are covered in the following section.

Specific Cardiomyopathies

Amyloidosis

An interstitial deposition of amyloid fibrils causes concentric thickening of the atrial and ventricular walls and the atrioventricular valve leaflets. Severe amyloid deposition in the ventricular myocardium may produce features simulating those of hypertrophic cardiomyopathy (56). However, these two entities can be differentiated by divergent ventricular contraction. In contrast to the hyperdynamic ventricular contraction seen in hypertrophic cardiomyopathy, the systolic contraction is variably diminished in amyloidosis. Ejection fraction and systolic wall thickening are depressed. Amyloidosis most commonly leads to restrictive cardiomyopathy with dilated atria. Because of the deposition of amyloid, the atrial walls and atrioventricular valves may be thickened. Alterations in the T1 and T2 relaxation rates of the myocardium may be detectable, a finding that is evident especially on fat-saturated images (57). The signal intensity of the myocardium has been found to be reduced on T1- and T2-weighted images in patients with amyloidosis in comparison with that in healthy volunteers and in patients with hypertrophic cardiomyopathy (58).

Sarcoidosis

Sarcoidosis can be manifested in the myocardium with typical granulomas and can cause restrictive cardiomyopathy. Only 5% of patients with systemic sarcoidosis have clinical evidence of cardiac involvement, but it is found at autopsy in 20% to 30% of such patients (59). Cardiac symptoms are highly suggestive of myocardial involvement in patients with systemic sarcoidosis. However, in patients with clinical manifestations of myocardial sarcoidosis who do not have systemic disease, the diagnosis is challenging, and myocardial biopsy is usually required for confirmation. Because distribution of the infiltration is patchy, nondirected biopsy is associated with false-negative results. MRI has displayed sarcoid granulomas as nodules of high signal intensity on T2-weighted images with fat suppression, and as focal areas of hyperenhancement on T1-weighted images after the administration of Gd-DTPA (59,60). These findings are not specific and can be observed in other inflammatory diseases. However, they can aid in guiding myocardial biopsies and have been used to monitor the response to steroid therapy (61). After the granulomas have regressed, postinflammatory scars may persist. These can be delineated as regions of diminished or absent wall thickening or as regions of diastolic wall thinning (61).

Hemochromatosis

Hemochromatosis may be primary or secondary. Primary hemochromatosis is an inherited autosomal-recessive disease. Secondary hemochromatosis develops mainly when repeated blood transfusions are required to treat thalassemia and hemolytic anemias. Other common causes are chronic alcohol abuse and long-term hemodialysis. In primary hemochromatosis, iron is deposited in the liver and pancreas, but the spleen remains normal. This characteristic distinguishes primary from secondary hemochromatosis, in which iron is also deposited in the spleen. Increased iron deposition in the cardiac myocytes in hemochromatosis causes diastolic and systolic cardiac dysfunction. After an initial asymptomatic period, cardiopathy caused by iron overload presents as diastolic dysfunction with a restrictive filling pattern (62). When the iron overload reaches a critical level, systolic functional abnormalities occur, and the disease takes the form of a dilated cardiomyopathy.

Iron reduces the T1 and T2 relaxation rates by introducing local magnetic field inhomogeneities (Fig. 7.8). The amount of signal decrease on T2-weighted images correlates with the iron level in tissue (62). MRI is a valuable tool for noninvasively measuring the iron concentration in the heart and for monitoring therapy (62,63).

Arrhythmogenic Right Ventricular Cardiomyopathy

This disease may have characteristic features on spin-echo and cine MRI (see Chapter 8). Typical findings are transmural fatty deposition in the RV free wall (Fig. 7.9). T1-weighted spin-echo images may demonstrate the focal deposition of fat in the myocardial wall as bright spots surrounded by the medium signal intensity of myocardium (64). Another feature is regional or general thinning of the RV free wall, which is not always evidently abnormal because the thickness of the free wall varies among normal persons (65). Cine MRI can demonstrate regional or global RV contractile dysfunction. It has also demonstrated regional dyskinesis and aneurysms. In advanced cases, severe RV dilation and tricuspid regurgitation may be present.

HEART TRANSPLANTATION AND TRANSPLANT REJECTION

The integrity and function of a newly transplanted heart can be monitored by measuring the ventricular volume, myocardial mass, and ejection fraction with cine MRI. In a recent study, at 2 months after successful transplantation,

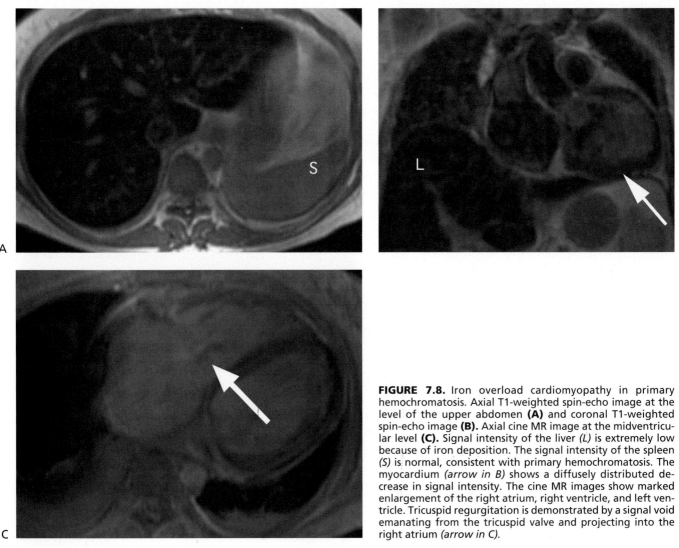

FIGURE 7.8. Iron overload cardiomyopathy in primary hemochromatosis. Axial T1-weighted spin-echo image at the level of the upper abdomen **(A)** and coronal T1-weighted spin-echo image **(B).** Axial cine MR image at the midventricular level **(C).** Signal intensity of the liver *(L)* is extremely low because of iron deposition. The signal intensity of the spleen *(S)* is normal, consistent with primary hemochromatosis. The myocardium *(arrow in B)* shows a diffusely distributed decrease in signal intensity. The cine MR images show marked enlargement of the right atrium, right ventricle, and left ventricle. Tricuspid regurgitation is demonstrated by a signal void emanating from the tricuspid valve and projecting into the right atrium *(arrow in C).*

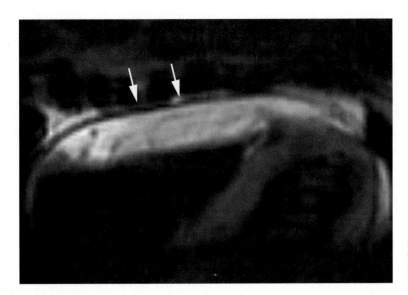

FIGURE 7.9. Right ventricular dysplasia. Axial T1-weighted spin-echo image with saturation band placed dorsal to the ventricular septum. Transmural fat is seen in the right ventricular wall *(arrows)*.

MRI demonstrated an increase of the LV mass coupled with a decrease in the ratio of end-systolic wall stress to volume in comparison with normal volunteers. These changes were interpreted as a sign of early remodeling of the LV (66).

Acute rejection is one of the main causes of death during the first year after transplantation. Currently, RV endomyocardial biopsy represents the gold standard for evaluating this condition. To reduce the need for biopsy, a modality that could replace this invasive test or efficiently guide its timing would be desirable. MRI as a noninvasive imaging modality has been considered for this purpose, and three different approaches have been assessed: (a) tissue characterization by evaluation of T2-relaxivity, (b) evaluation of changes in signal intensity after administration of contrast media, and (c) evaluation of changes in myocardial wall thickness.

Because the onset of acute rejection is characterized by myocardial interstitial edema, the signal intensity on T2-weighted images should increase as a consequence of prolonged T2 relaxation rates. The first results, obtained in animal studies, were encouraging in this regard. With the onset of graft rejection, the myocardial T2 relaxation time was prolonged and increased gradually as the rejection progressed. A linear correlation between myocardial water content and T2 relaxation rate could be demonstrated (67,68). In humans, several investigators reported increases in signal intensity on T2-weighted images during periods of acute rejection, but others could not reproduce their results (69). With conventional spin-echo sequences, the T2 relaxation rates measured on MR images varied widely. The mean values in healthy volunteers and in patients without and with early stages of heart rejection were only slightly different, and the overlap of T2 relaxation rates among the different groups was large (69). Moreover, the measurement of T2 relaxation rates with conventional MR sequences is subject to error related to motion artifacts and artifacts caused by the

flow of blood from the cavities projecting into the myocardium. The application of modern sequences, such as inversion recovery black blood spin-echo sequences, has made it possible to obtain more reliable data. In a recent study, the distinction between patients with moderate rejection and patients without rejection was feasible (70). Because of the lack of a universally applicable threshold T2 value for the diagnosis of rejection, acquisition of a baseline study shortly after surgery is recommended to improve the reliability of MRI in the assessment of rejection (71). However, the increased T2 relaxation rate observed during acute rejection may be nonspecific because acute inflammatory changes can be caused by the transplantation process itself. Consequently, it has been recommended that the baseline study be performed after these changes have subsided, approximately 4 weeks after surgery (71).

The second approach is based on shortening of the T1 relaxation time after the administration of extracellular contrast material. Areas of myocardial hyperenhancement seen after the administration of Gd-DTPA on T1-weighted spin-echo images are associated with allograft rejection (72). These hyperenhanced areas correspond histologically to regions of cellular infiltration and edema (72). However, early and advanced stages of transplant rejection could not be differentiated by measuring the degree of hyperenhancement in humans (73).

The third approach is based on measurement of the wall thickness. During acute rejection, cine MRI demonstrates an increase in LV wall thickness. This change is most likely caused by edematous swelling and cellular infiltration. Wall thickness declines to normal values during successful therapy of an episode of acute rejection (74). However, this approach has not yet been adopted for routine clinical use. Currently, MRI does not offer a reliable parameter for the early detection of chronic rejection, which is characterized by the slow progression of interstitial fibrosis (75).

The transplanted heart is not only at risk for rejection but also prone to the side effects of immunosuppressive drug therapy. For example, ventricular hypertrophy can be caused by cyclosporine. Therefore, if overall long-term success rates are to improve, not only the regular follow-up of individual transplant recipients but also the evaluation of new therapeutic approaches will be necessary. For this purpose, MRI is preferable to other imaging modalities because of its accuracy and interstudy reproducibility in quantifying ventricular volume and mass (3,21). For instance, felodipine, a calcium channel blocker, was shown to be capable of reversing cyclosporine-induced hypertrophy as assessed by cine MRI (74).

MYOCARDITIS

In the early stages of myocarditis, the clinical symptoms are often dominated by nonspecific complaints, such as fatigue, weakness, and palpitations. Profound dysfunction of the ventricles can be ascertained at later stages of the disease, after acute myocarditis has resulted in dilated cardiomyopathy. Most cases of myocarditis are caused by viral infections; the agents are cytomegalovirus in 45% and coxsakievirus B in 30% of cases (76). Currently, a tentative diagnosis of myocarditis must be confirmed by endomyocardial biopsy, which typically shows interstitial edema, lymphocyte infiltration, and necrosis of myocytes (77). MRI has been proposed as a noninvasive test for diagnosing myocarditis and monitoring the response to therapy. Because of the interstitial edema, the T2 relaxation time is increased, so that the signal may be increased on T2-weighted images. Although this characteristic has been demonstrated in small series of patients (78,79), conventional T2-weighted sequences are frequently of poor quality and prone to motion artifacts. The advent of fast imaging sequences that are performed during a breath-hold has substantially improved image quality, and recent evaluations of such sequences in patients with myocarditis have shown promising results (80).

Another approach to the evaluation of myocardial inflammation is to assess tissue enhancement on T1-weighted images after the administration of Gd-DTPA. A recent study sequentially monitored patients with contrast-enhanced T1-weighted spin-echo imaging (80). Focal hyperenhanced myocardium was recognized early after the onset of myocarditis. After 2 weeks, the inflammation had spread, and a disseminated pattern was observed. The relative myocardial hyperenhancement correlated with LV function and with the clinical functional status (80). However, contrast enhancement of the myocardium and an increased T2 relaxation rate are nonspecific findings that can also be encountered in idiopathic dilated and hypertrophic cardiomyopathy, amyloidosis, and myocardial infarction. When a patient with a presumptive diagnosis of myocarditis is assessed, the imaging findings must be interpreted in relation to the clinical situation. Verification of the diagnosis by endomyocardial biopsy remains indispensable for the initial diagnosis.

In Lyme disease, which is caused by the spirochete *Borrelia burgdorferi*, MRI demonstrates signs of myopericarditis. Characteristic features are ventricular wall thickening coupled with regional or global hypokinesia, areas of increased signal intensity in the ventricular wall, and pericardial effusion (81). The changes of the ventricular wall are located predominantly in the anterolateral wall and the apical region of the septum (82).

Chagas disease is caused by the protozoan *Trypanosoma cruzi*. This infection is characterized by an acute, intermediate, and chronic phase. In chronic Chagas disease, the heart is the most frequently affected organ, and lymphocytic infiltration can be observed. Regions of focal inflammation have been shown to enhance strongly on T1-weighted images after the administration of Gd-DTPA (83). In a recent study, MRI showed the infiltration to be distributed most often in the inferolateral wall of the LV (84).

PERICARDIAL DISEASE
Normal Pericardium

The pericardium is composed of fibrous tissue and appears dark on T1- and T2-weighted images (85). In the area of the RV, it is located between the bright mediastinal and subepicardial fat, which provides a natural high level of contrast, so that the sensitivity for visualization of the pericardium in this region is 100%. In regions adjacent to the lung, the natural contrast is lower, so that the sensitivity for visualization in the area of the lateral wall of the LV is only 61% (86). The average thickness of the pericardium on MR images ranges from 1.2 mm in diastole to 1.9 mm in systole (86). Anatomic studies have shown the thickness of the pericardium to be in the range of 0.4 to 1 mm. The overestimation on MRI has been presumed to result from motion-induced signal loss of the pericardial fluid, which cannot be distinguished from the pericardium itself (87). Pericardial thickness depends also on the anatomic level and increases toward the diaphragm (88). This effect results from the ligamentous insertion of the pericardium into the diaphragm and from its tangential direction to the imaging plane. Consequently, the measurement of pericardial thickness is most reliable at the midventricular level. The pericardium extends approximately to the middle of the ascending aorta and the bifurcation of the pulmonary artery. It forms a tube that encloses both vessels. A second, more posterior pericardial tube surrounds the vena cava and pulmonary veins. Both compartments are connected by the transverse sinus, which is visible on MRI in 80% of cases (89,90). The oblique sinus is the second major pericardial recess, located behind the left atrium (91). Knowledge of the anatomy of the superior pericardial recesses is essential to avoid misinterpreting them as lymph nodes or aortic dissection (92).

Pericardial Effusion

MRI is very sensitive for the detection of generalized or loculated pericardial effusions. The pericardial space normally contains 10 to 50 mL of fluid. MRI can detect a pericardial effusion as small as 30 mL, and in most normal subjects, fluid can be seen in the superior pericardial recess. MRI provides information on the location of a pericardial effusion (Fig. 7.10). In 70% of cases, the fluid is posterolateral to the LV (93). Freely flowing fluid collects at this region when patients are placed in a supine position to undergo MRI. Because of this uneven distribution, the total fluid volume cannot be calculated from the width of the pericardial space by applying a simple formula. However, a semiquantitative estimation can be obtained by measuring the width of the pericardial space in front of the RV. A moderate effusion is associated with a width of more than 5 mm (94). Loculated effusion occurs when fluid is trapped by adhesions between the parietal and visceral pericardium. MRI is more sensitive than echocardiography in detecting loculated effusion because of its wide field of view.

Hemorrhagic effusion can be distinguished from nonhemorrhagic effusion by its characteristic signal intensity. Hemorrhagic effusion and hemopericardium are typically characterized by a short T1 relaxation rate and appear bright on T1-weighted spin-echo images (93). Nonhemorrhagic effusions have low signal intensity on T1-weighted images and high signal intensity on T2-weighted images. Further differentiation of nonhemorrhagic effusion as either transudative or exudative is not reliable by differences in signal intensity. Movement of the fluid during the cardiac cycle introduces flow-void effects that make an accurate assessment of the signal intensity impossible. However, the signal intensity of exudative effusions is typically reported to be higher than that of normal pericardium (93).

Pericardial Thickening and Acute Pericarditis

Pericardial thickening is defined as an increase in the pericardial thickness to more than 4 mm (94). It appears as a widening of the low-signal pericardial line if it is caused by an increase of fibrous tissue. In these cases, it cannot be differentiated from a small rim of pericardial effusion by its signal intensity. However, the distribution of pericardial effusion differs considerably from the pattern of pericardial thickening. The accumulation of fluid is typically posterolateral to the LV or in the superior recess, as mentioned earlier. If the fluid is not trapped by pericardial adhesions, its distribution changes during the cardiac cycle.

In acute pericarditis, fibrinous exudate and edema rather than an increase of fibrous tissue cause pericardial thicken-

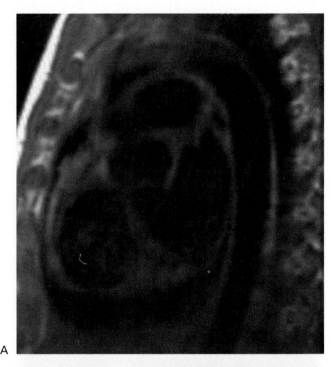
A

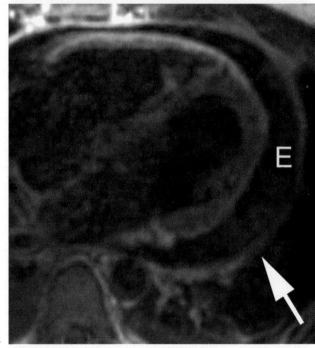
B

FIGURE 7.10. Pericardial effusion. Sagittal **(A)** and transaxial **(B)** T1-weighted spin-echo images at the midventricular level demonstrate a large pericardial effusion *(E)*. The thickened parietal pericardium is clearly visible *(arrow)*.

ing. Therefore, the pericardium exhibits intermediate signal intensity and can readily be distinguished from a pericardial effusion, which is often present in these cases (95) (Fig. 7.11). A thickened pericardium caused by acute or subacute inflammation demonstrates considerable enhancement after the administration of Gd-DTPA.

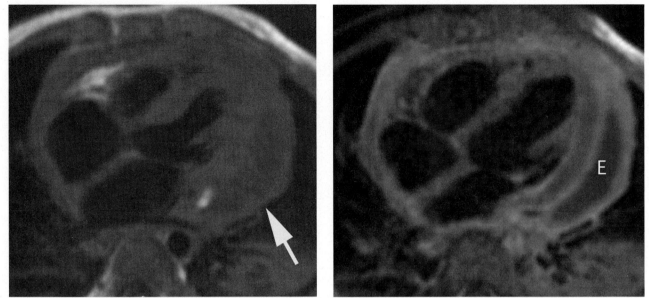

A   B

FIGURE 7.11. Acute pericarditis. Axial T1-weighted spin-echo images before **(A)** and after **(B)** administration of Gd-DTPA (gadolinium diethylenetriamine pentaacetic acid). Thickening of the pericardium *(arrow)* and pericardial effusion *(E)* are seen. After administration of contrast material, the pericardium enhances.

Constrictive Pericarditis

Constrictive pericarditis is associated with progressive pericardial fibrosis, which causes the pericardium to shrink and so limit diastolic ventricular expansion. It is a nonspecific reaction to various conditions, such as infectious pericarditis, connective tissue disease, neoplasm, trauma, long-term renal dialysis, cardiac surgery, and radiation therapy. Currently, constrictive pericarditis is most often a sequela of cardiac surgery in Europe and North America. However, tuberculous pericarditis remains a leading cause of constrictive pericarditis in third world countries. The diagnostic features of constrictive pericarditis are a thickened pericardium (Figs. 7.12–7.14) coupled with signs of impaired diastolic filling of the RV, such as dilation of the venae cavae, hepatic veins, and right atrium. The volume of the RV is frequently normal or reduced. Sometimes, the RV is elongated and narrowed so that it appears tubular, and the ventricular septum may be have a sigmoid shape (96). Thickening of the pericardium is often localized and is most frequently observed in the region of the RV (Fig. 7.12) (97). The diagnostic accuracy of MRI in constrictive pericarditis is 93% (51). As mentioned above, MRI effectively distinguishes between constrictive pericarditis and restrictive cardiomyopathy. In this context, measurement of the pericardial thickness is most significant in the diagnosis of constrictive pericarditis. Localized forms of constrictive pericarditis may cause unusual anatomic and functional abnormalities. Pericardial constriction of the right atrioventricular groove has appeared on MRI as pericardial thickening limited to this region along with right atrial enlargement and a normal or small RV (Figs. 7.13–7.14).

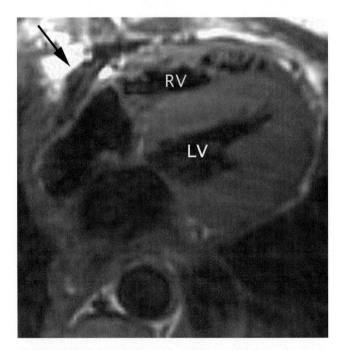

FIGURE 7.12. Constrictive pericarditis. T1-weighted spin-echo image demonstrates pericardial thickening, most pronounced over the right ventricle and right atrium *(arrow)*. The right ventricle *(RV)* has a tubular shape. In addition, hypertrophy of the left ventricle *(LV)* is present.

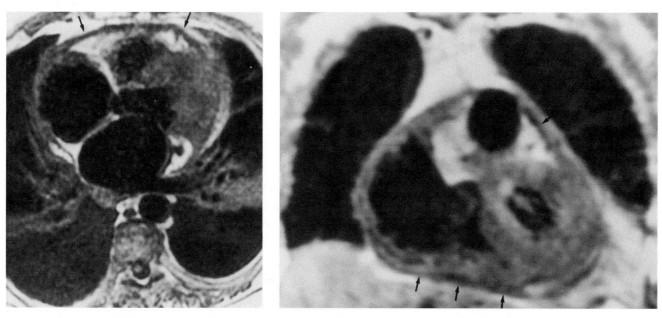

FIGURE 7.13. Constrictive pericarditis. Transaxial **(A)** and coronal **(B)** spin-echo images show marked thickening of the pericardium *(arrows)*. The coronal image shows the thickened pericardium extending over the pulmonary artery *(single arrow)*.

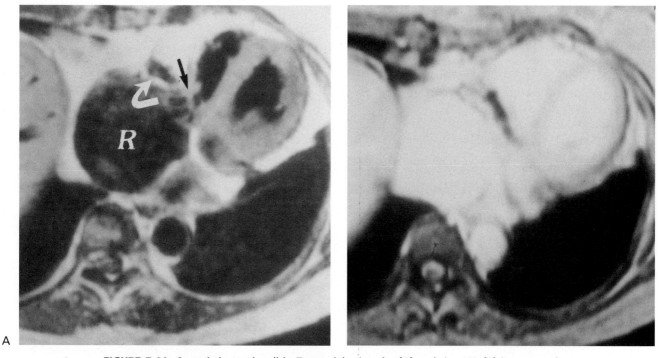

FIGURE 7.14. Constrictive pericarditis. Transaxial spin-echo **(A)** and cine MR **(B)** images at the midventricular level. Focal pericardial thickening is present in the atrioventricular groove *(curved arrow)*. The focal pericardial constriction compresses the tricuspid annulus *(black arrow)*. The right atrium *(R)* is enlarged, whereas the right ventricle is small and has a tubular shape.

Absence of Pericardium

Congenital absence of the pericardium results from abnormalities of the vascular supply to the developing pericardium during embryogenesis. It is relative rare and usually remains asymptomatic but may cause chest pain. In 30% of cases, absence of the pericardium is associated with other abnormalities, such as congenital heart disease, bronchogenic cysts, and hiatus hernia (98). Agenesis of the pericardium is circumscribed in approximately 91% of cases, occurring on the left side in 70%, inferior side in 17%, and right side in 4% (98). Absence of the pericardium on the left side often leads to a leftward shift of the heart. Attachment of the pericardium to the sternum and diaphragm stabilizes the position of the heart within the thorax. Consequently, absence of the pericardium on the left side is associated with leftward displacement of the heart because this stabilizing structure is missing (99). A characteristic finding on transaxial MRI is an interposition of lung parenchyma between the aortic

knob and the main pulmonary artery (99) (Fig. 7.15). Absence of the low-signal pericardial line is an additional characteristic finding.

Pericardial Cysts and Diverticula

Pericardial cysts are caused by developmental abnormalities and are suspected to occur when a small portion of the pericardium is pinched during embryonic development. Ninety percent of pericardial cysts are located in the cardiophrenic angle (70% on the right and 20% on the left side). However, they can occur anywhere in the pericardium, and a pericardial cyst at an unusual location sometimes cannot be distinguished from a thymic or bronchogenic cyst. Pericardial cysts usually do not communicate with the pericardial cavity. A nonhemorrhagic cyst filled with low protein fluid appears dark on T1-weighted and bright on T2-weighted images (Fig. 7.16). If the cyst is filled with blood or pro-

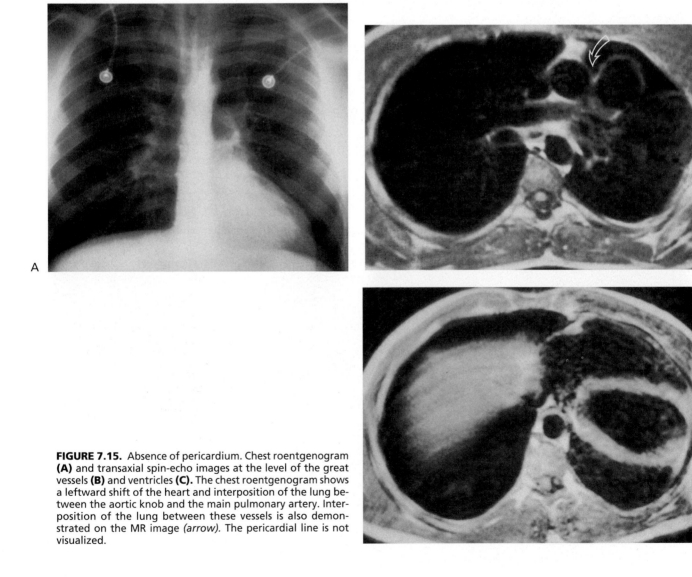

FIGURE 7.15. Absence of pericardium. Chest roentgenogram **(A)** and transaxial spin-echo images at the level of the great vessels **(B)** and ventricles **(C)**. The chest roentgenogram shows a leftward shift of the heart and interposition of the lung between the aortic knob and the main pulmonary artery. Interposition of the lung between these vessels is also demonstrated on the MR image *(arrow)*. The pericardial line is not visualized.

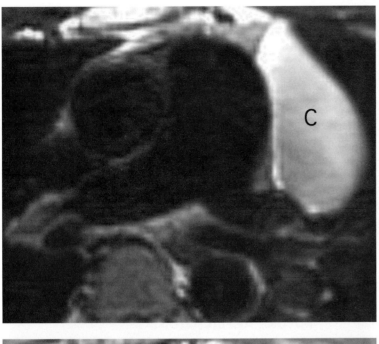

A

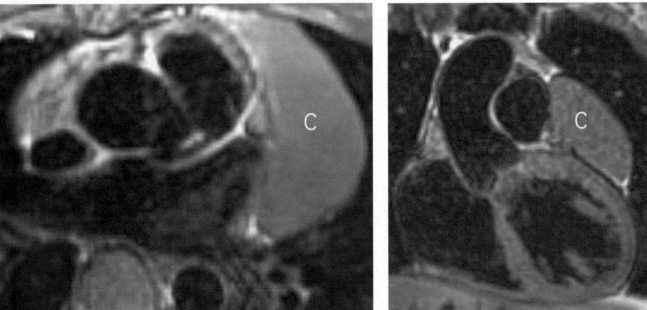

B

C

FIGURE 7.16. Pericardial cyst. Transaxial T2-weighted **(A)** and T1-weighted **(B)** spin-echo images and coronal T1-weighted spin-echo image **(C).** A cystic mass *(C)* conforms to the contour of the heart and main pulmonary artery. The cyst has a homogeneous low to intermediate signal intensity on the T1-weighted images and a high signal intensity on the T2-weighted images.

teinaceous fluid, it is bright on T1-weighted images (100) (Fig. 7.17). The pericardial rim is visible with the characteristic low signal intensity of the pericardium. In contrast to pericardial cysts, diverticula communicate with the pericardial cavity. They correspond to a congenital or acquired defect in the parietal pericardium (101). MRI may demonstrate variations in the size of a diverticulum during changes in body position.

Pericardial Tumors

Primary pericardial tumors occur less frequently than secondary tumors. Mesothelioma is the most common primary malignant tumor of the pericardium. Fibrosarcoma, angiosarcoma, and teratoma also occur in the pericardium. Characterization of the tumor entity is possible only for lipoma and liposarcoma, which show high signal intensity on T1-weighted images. However, the extent of the lesions, their relation to the cardiac structures and great vessels, and their effects on the cardiac function can be evaluated.

Secondary tumors occur either by extension from mediastinal or lung tumors or by metastasis. Pericardial metastases have been found in 22% of cancer patients at autopsy (102). They are most frequently caused by lung and breast carcinoma, leukemia, and lymphoma. Metastasis often causes a hemorrhagic effusion. In such cases, it may be dif-

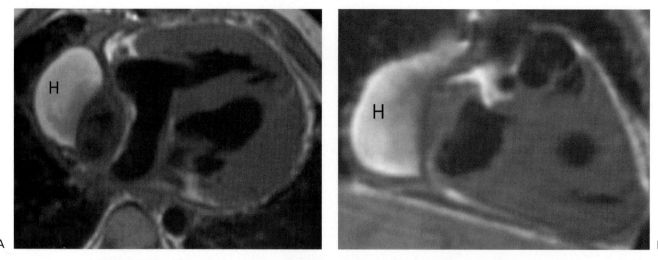

A   B

FIGURE 7.17. Pericardial hematoma. Axial **(A)** and coronal **(B)** T1-weighted spin-echo images demonstrate high signal intensity of a loculated fluid collection *(H)* adjacent to the right atrium. High signal intensity on T1-weighted images is characteristic of hematoma.

ficult to distinguish the tumor itself from the surrounding fluid because of the high signal intensity of the hemorrhagic fluid. Visualization of metastatic deposits can be improved by hyperenhancement after the administration of gadolinium contrast media.

MRI can be used to assess tumor infiltration of the pericardium. Interruption of the pericardial line can be used to distinguish a mass that infiltrates the pericardium from a lesion that reaches the pericardium but has not exceeded this boundary. If the pericardium is visible adjacent to a mass, pericardial invasion is unlikely (103) (Fig. 7.18).

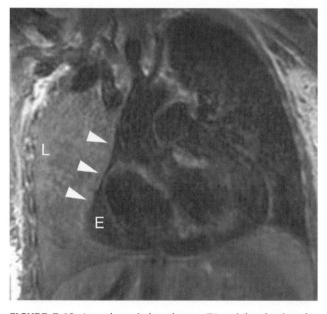

FIGURE 7.18. Intrathoracic lymphoma. T1-weighted spin-echo image after administration of Gd-DTPA (gadolinium diethylene-triamine pentaacetic acid) shows a mass filling the right side of the thorax *(L)*. The mass reaches the pericardium *(arrowheads)*. Pericardial effusion is present *(E)*.

FUTURE APPLICATIONS

Further improvements in pulse sequences will permit a more comprehensive evaluation of morphology and function by providing better spatial and temporal resolution. Examples are nearly real-time or real-time imaging techniques, such as the reduced field-of-view technique coupled with spiral sequences (104) or sensitivity-encoded imaging (SENSE); these reduce the acquisition time of a single image to 13 milliseconds (105). The combination of faster imaging techniques and automated postprocessing will make it possible to investigate various aspects of cardiac function during a single comprehensive examination.

In addition, MRI will offer the option of therapeutic interventions in patients with cardiac diseases. Real-time imaging is the basic requisite for interventional procedures and therapeutic applications, such as biopsy, deployment of intravascular devices, and local delivery of drugs.

REFERENCES

1. Semelka RC, Tomei E, Wagner S, et al. Normal left ventricular dimensions and function: interstudy reproducibility of measurements with cine MR imaging. *Radiology* 1990;174:763.
2. Dulce MC, Mostbeck GH, Friese KK, et al. Quantification of the left ventricular volume and function with cine MR imaging: comparison of geometric models with three-dimensional data. *Radiology* 1993;188:371.
3. Semelka RC, Tomei E, Wagner S, et al. Interstudy reproducibility of dimensional and functional measurements between cine magnetic resonance studies in the morphologically abnormal left ventricle. *Am Heart J* 1990;119:1367.
4. Ehman RL, McNamara MT, Pallack M, et al. Magnetic resonance imaging with respiratory gating: techniques and advantages. *AJR Am J Roentgenol* 1984;143:1175.
5. Dinsmore RE, Wismer GL, Levine RA, et al. Magnetic resonance imaging of the heart: positioning and gradient angle se-

lection for optimal imaging planes. *AJR Am J Roentgenol* 1984; 143:1135.

6. Higgins CB, Stark D, McNamara M, et al. Multiplane magnetic resonance imaging of the heart and major vessels: studies in normal volunteers. *AJR Am J Roentgenol* 1984;142:661.

7. Mostbeck GH, Caputo GR, Higgins CB. MR measurements of blood flow in the cardiovascular system. *AJR Am J Roentgenol* 1992;159:453.

8. Szolar DH, Sakuma H, Higgins CB. Cardiovascular applications of magnetic resonance flow and velocity measurements. *J Magn Reson Imaging* 1996;6:78.

9. Mohiaddin RH, Longmore DB. Functional aspects of cardiovascular magnetic resonance imaging. Techniques and application. *Circulation* 1993;88:264.

10. Report of the 1995 World Health Organization/International Society and Federation of Cardiology task force on the definition and classification of cardiomyopathies. *Circulation* 1996;93:841.

11. Report of the WHO/ISFC task force on the definition and classification of cardiomyopathies. *Br Heart J* 1980;44:672.

12. Schaper J, Froede R, Hein S, et al. Impairment of the myocardial ultrastructure and changes in the cytoskeleton in dilated cardiomyopathy. *Circulation* 1991;83:504.

13. Higgins CB, Byrd BF, McNamara MT, et al. Magnetic resonance imaging of the heart: a review of the experience in 172 subjects. *Radiology* 1985;155:671.

14. Buser PT, Auffermann W, Holt WW, et al. Noninvasive evaluation of global left ventricular function with cine nuclear magnetic resonance. *J Am Coll Cardiol* 1989;13:1294.

15. Caputo GR, Suzuki J, Kondo C, et al. Determination of left ventricular volume and mass with use of biphasic spin-echo MR imaging: comparison with cine MR. *Radiology* 1990;177:773.

16. Imai H, Kumai T, Sekiya M, et al. Left ventricular trabeculae evaluated with MRI in dilated cardiomyopathy and old myocardial infarction. *J Cardiol* 1992;22:83.

17. Wagner S, Auffermann W, Buser P, et al. Functional description of the left ventricle in patients with volume overload, pressure overload, and myocardial disease using cine nuclear magnetic resonance imaging. *Am J Card Imaging* 1991;5:87.

18. Fujita N, Hartiala J, O'Sullivan M, et al. Assessment of left ventricular diastolic function in dilated cardiomyopathy with cine magnetic resonance imaging: effect of an angiotensin converting enzyme inhibitor, benazepril. *Am Heart J* 1993;125:171.

19. Doherty N, Fujita N, Caputo GR, et al. Measurement of right ventricular mass in normal and dilated cardiomyopathic ventricles using cine magnetic resonance imaging. *Am J Cardiol* 1992;69:1223.

20. Suzuki J, Caputo GR, Masui T, et al. Assessment of right ventricular diastolic and systolic function in patients with dilated cardiomyopathy using cine magnetic resonance imaging. *Am Heart J* 1991;122:1035.

21. Bellenger NG, Burgess MI, Ray SG, et al. Comparison of left ventricular ejection fraction and volumes in heart failure by echocardiography, radionuclide ventriculography and cardiovascular magnetic resonance: are they interchangeable? *Eur Heart J* 2000;21:1387.

22. Doherty NE, Seelos KC, Suzuki J, et al. Application of cine nuclear magnetic resonance imaging for sequential evaluation of response to angiotensin-converting enzyme inhibitor therapy in dilated cardiomyopathy. *J Am Coll Cardiol* 1992;19:1294.

23. Friedrich MG, Strohm O, Osterziel KJ, et al. Growth hormone therapy in dilated cardiomyopathy monitored with MRI. *MAGMA* 1998;6:152.

24. Fujita N, Duerinekx AJ, Higgins CB. Variation in left ventricular regional wall stress with cine magnetic resonance imaging: normal subjects versus dilated cardiomyopathy. *Am Heart J* 1993;125:1337.

25. Buser PT, Wagner S, Aufferman W, et al. Three-dimensional analysis of the regional contractility of the normal and the cardiomyopathic left ventricle using cine-magnetic resonance imaging [in German].*Z Kardiol* 1990;79:573.

26. Dong SJ, Crawley AP, MacGregor JH, et al. Regional left ventricular systolic function in relation to the cavity geometry in patients with chronic right ventricular pressure overload. A three-dimensional tagged magnetic resonance study. *Circulation* 1995;91:2359.

27. MacGowan GA, Shapiro EP, Azhari H, et al. Noninvasive measurement of shortening in the fiber and cross-fiber directions in the normal human left ventricle and idiopathic dilated cardiomyopathy. *Circulation* 1997;96:535.

28. Nakagawa Y, Fujimoto S, Nakano H, et al. Magnetic resonance velocity mapping of transtricuspid velocity profiles in dilated cardiomyopathy. *Heart Vessels* 1998;13:241.

29. Blankenberg F, Eisenberg S, Scheinman MN, et al. Use of cine gradient echo (GRE) MR in the imaging of cardiac hemochromatosis. *J Comput Assist Tomogr* 1994;18:136.

30. Koito H, Suzuki J, Ohkubo N, et al. Gadolinium-diethylenetriamine pentaacetic acid enhanced magnetic resonance imaging of dilated cardiomyopathy: clinical significance of abnormally high signal intensity of left ventricular myocardium. *J Cardiol* 1996;28:41.

31. Devlin AM, Moore NR, Ostman-Smith I. A comparison of MRI and echocardiography in hypertrophic cardiomyopathy. *Br J Radiol* 1999;72:258.

32. Pons-Llado G, Carreras F, Borras X, et al. Comparison of morphologic assessment of hypertrophic cardiomyopathy by magnetic resonance versus echocardiographic imaging. *Am J Cardiol* 1997;79:1651.

33. Higgins CB, Byrd BF III, Stark D, et al. Magnetic resonance imaging in hypertrophic cardiomyopathy. *Am J Cardiol* 1985; 55:1121.

34. Suzuki J-I, Sakamoto T, Takenaka K, et al. Assessment of the thickness of the right ventricular free wall by magnetic resonance imaging in patients with hypertrophic cardiomyopathy. *Br Heart J* 1988;60:440.

35. Park JH, Kim YM, Chung JW, et al. MR imaging of hypertrophic cardiomyopathy. *Radiology* 1992;185:441.

36. Been M, Kean D, Smith MA, et al. Nuclear magnetic resonance in hypertrophic cardiomyopathy. *Br Heart J* 1985;54:48.

37. Soler R, Rodriguez E, Rodriguez JA, et al. Magnetic resonance imaging of apical hypertrophic cardiomyopathy. *J Thorac Imaging* 1997;12:221.

38. Suzuki J, Shimamoto R, Nishikawa J, et al. Morphologic onset and early diagnosis in apical hypertrophic cardiomyopathy: a long-term analysis with nuclear magnetic resonance imaging. *J Am Coll Cardiol* 1999;33:146.

39. Suzuki J, Chang JM, Caputo GR, et al. Evaluation of right ventricular early diastolic filling by cine nuclear magnetic resonance imaging in patients with hypertrophic cardiomyopathy. *J Am Coll Cardiol* 1991;18:120.

40. Yamanari H, Kakishita M, Fujimoto Y, et al. Effect of regional myocardial perfusion abnormalities on regional myocardial early diastolic function in patients with hypertrophic cardiomyopathy. *Heart Vessels* 1997;12:192.

41. Arrive L, Assayag P, Russ G, et al. MRI and cine MRI of asymmetric septal hypertrophic cardiomyopathy. *J Comput Assist Tomogr* 1994;18:376.

42. Dong SJ, MacGregor JH, Crawley AP, et al. Left ventricular wall thickness and regional function in patients with hypertrophic cardiomyopathy: a three-dimensional tagged magnetic resonance imaging study. *Circulation* 1994;90:1200.

43. Koito H, Suzuki J, Nakamori H, et al. Clinical significance of abnormal high signal intensity of left ventricular myocardium

by gadolinium-diethylenetriaminepenta-acetic acid enhanced magnetic resonance imaging in hypertrophic cardiomyopathy. *J Cardiol* 1995;25:163.

44. Kawada N, Sakuma H, Yamakado T, et al. Hypertrophic cardiomyopathy: magnetic resonance measurement of coronary blood flow and vasodilator flow reserve in patients and healthy subjects. *Radiology* 1999;211:129.

45. Di Cesare E, Marsili L, Chichiarelli A, et al. Characterization of hypertrophic cardiomyopathy with magnetic resonance imaging. *Radiol Med* (Torino) 1994;87:614.

46. Didier D, Ratib O, Lerch R, et al. Detection and quantification of valvular heart disease with dynamic cardiac MR imaging. *Radiographics* 2000;20:1279.

47. Maier SE, Fischer SE, McKinnon GC, et al. Evaluation of left ventricular segmental wall motion in hypertrophic cardiomyopathy with myocardial tagging. *Circulation* 1992;86:1919.

48. Kramer CM, Reichek N, Ferrari VA, et al. Regional heterogeneity of function in hypertrophic cardiomyopathy. *Circulation* 1994;90:186.

49. Young AA, Kramer CM, Ferrari VA, et al. Three-dimensional left ventricular deformation in hypertrophic cardiomyopathy. *Circulation* 1994;90:854.

50. Schulz-Menger J, Strohm O, Waigand J, et al. The value of magnetic resonance imaging of the left ventricular outflow tract in patients with hypertrophic obstructive cardiomyopathy after septal artery embolization. *Circulation* 2000;101:1764.

51. Masui T, Finck S, Higgins CB. Constrictive pericarditis and restrictive cardiomyopathy: evaluation with MR imaging. *Radiology* 1992;182:369.

52. Hartiala JJ, Mostbeck GH, Foster E, et al. Velocity-encoded cine MRI in the evaluation of left ventricular diastolic function: measurement of mitral valve and pulmonary vein flow velocities and flow volumes across the mitral valve. *Am Heart J* 1993;125:1054.

53. Mostbeck GH, Hartiala JJ, Foster E, et al. Right ventricular diastolic filling: evaluation with velocity-encoded cine MRI. *J Comput Assist Tomogr* 1993;17:245.

54. Chandra M, Pettigrew RI, Eley JW, et al. Cine-MRI-aided endomyocardectomy in idiopathic hypereosinophilic syndrome. *Ann Thorac Surg* 1996;62:1856.

55. D'Silva SA, Kohli A, Dalvi BV, et al. MRI in right ventricular endomyocardial fibrosis. *Am Heart J* 1992;123:1390.

56. Siqueira-Filho AG, Cunha CLP, Tajik AJ, et al. M-mode and two-dimensional echocardiographic features in cardiac amyloidosis. *Circulation* 1981;63:188.

57. Benson L, Hemmingsson A, Ericsson A, et al. Magnetic resonance imaging in primary amyloidosis. *Acta Radiol* 1987;28:13.

58. Fattori R, Rocchi G, Celletti F, et al. Contribution of magnetic resonance imaging in the differential diagnosis of cardiac amyloidosis and symmetric hypertrophic cardiomyopathy. *Am Heart J* 1998;136:824.

59. Riedy K, Fisher MR, Belic N, et al. MR imaging of myocardial sarcoidosis. *AJR Am J Roentgenol* 1988;151:915.

60. Chandra M, Silverman ME, Oshinski J, et al. Diagnosis of cardiac sarcoidosis aided by MRI. *Chest* 1996;110:562.

61. Doherty MJ, Kumar SK, Nicholson AA, et al. Cardiac sarcoidosis: the value of magnetic resonance imaging in diagnosis and assessment of response to treatment. *Respir Med* 1998;92:697.

62. Liu P, Olivieri N, Sullivan H, et al. Magnetic resonance imaging in beta-thalassemia: detection of iron content and association with cardiac complications. *J Am Coll Cardiol* 1993;21:491.

63. Blankenberg F, Eisenberg S, Scheinman MN, et al. Use of cine GRASS MR in the imaging of cardiac hemochromatosis. *J Comput Assist Tomogr* 1994;18:136.

64. Marcus FI, Fontaine G, Guiraudon G, et al. Right ventricular dysplasia: a report of 24 adult cases. *Circulation* 1982;65:384.

65. White RD, Trohman RG, Flamm SD, et al. Right ventricular arrhythmia in the absence of arrhythmogenic dysplasia: MR imaging of myocardial abnormalities. *Radiology* 1998;207:743.

66. Globits S, De Marco T, Schwitter J, et al. Assessment of early left ventricular remodeling in orthotopic heart transplant recipients with cine magnetic resonance imaging: potential mechanisms. *J Heart Lung Transplant* 1997;16:504.

67. Tscholakoff D, Aherne T, Yee ES, et al. Cardiac transplantations in dogs: evaluation with MR. *Radiology* 1985;157:697.

68. Aherne T, Tscholakoff D, Finkbeiner W, et al. Magnetic resonance imaging of cardiac transplants: the evaluation of rejection of cardiac allografts with and without immunosuppression. *Circulation* 1986;74:145.

69. Doornbos J, Verwey H, Essed CE, et al. MR imaging in assessment of cardiac transplant rejection in humans. *J Comput Assist Tomogr* 1990;14:77.

70. Marie PY, Angioi M, Carteaux JP, et al. Detection and prediction of acute heart transplant rejection with the myocardial T2 determination provided by a black-blood magnetic resonance imaging sequence. *J Am Coll Cardiol* 2001;37:825.

71. Smart FW, Young JB, Weilbaecher D, et al. Magnetic resonance imaging for assessment of tissue rejection after heterotopic heart transplantation. *J Heart Lung Transplant* 1993;12:403.

72. Konstam MA, Aronovitz MJ, Runge VM, et al. Magnetic resonance imaging with gadolinium-DTPA for detecting cardiac transplant rejection in rats. *Circulation* 1988;78:87.

73. Mousseaux E, Farge D, Guillemain R, et al. Assessing human cardiac allograft rejection using MRI with Gd-DOTA. *J Comput Assist Tomogr* 1993;17:237.

74. Schwitter J, De Marco T, Globits S, et al. Influence of felodipine on left ventricular hypertrophy and systolic function in orthotopic heart transplant receptions: possible interaction with cyclosporine medication. *J Heart Lung Transplant* 1999;18:1003.

75. Revel D, Chapelon C, Mathieu D, et al. Magnetic resonance imaging of human orthotopic heart transplantation: correlation with endomyocardial biopsy. *J Heart Lung Transplant* 1989;8:139.

76. Maisch B, Trostel-Soeder R, Stechemesser E, et al. Diagnostic relevance of humoral and cell-mediated immune reactions in patients with acute viral myocarditis. *Clin Exp Immunol* 1982;48:533.

77. Aretz HT, Billingham ME, Edwards WD, et al. Myocarditis: a histopathologic definition and classification. *Am J Cardiovasc Pathol* 1987;1:3.

78. Gagliardi MG, Bevilacqua M, Di Renzi P, et al. Usefulness of magnetic resonance imaging for diagnosis of acute myocarditis in infants and children, and comparison with endomyocardial biopsy. *Am J Cardiol* 1991;68:1089.

79. Shen CT, Jeng CM, Lin YM, et al. Intensification of relative myocardial T2-weighted magnetic resonance signals in patients with acute viral myocarditis (report of one case). *Acta Paediatr Sin* 1993;34:405.

80. Friedrich MG, Strohm O, Schulz-Menger J, et al. Contrast-media enhanced magnetic resonance imaging visualizes myocardial changes in the course of viral myocarditis. *Circulation* 1998;97:1802.

81. Bergler-Klein J, Sochor H, Stanek G, et al. Indium 111-monoclonal antimyosin antibody and magnetic resonance imaging in the diagnosis of acute Lyme myopericarditis. *Arch Intern Med* 1993;153:2696.

82. Globits S, Bergler-Klein J, Stanek G, et al. Magnetic resonance imaging in the diagnosis of acute Lyme carditis. *Cardiology* 1994;85:415.

83. Kalil-Filho R, de Albuquerque CP. Magnetic resonance imaging in Chagas' heart disease. *Rev Paul Med* 1995;113:880.

84. Bellotti G, Bocchi EA, de Moraes AV, et al. *In vivo* detection of

Trypanosoma cruzi antigens in hearts of patients with chronic Chagas' heart disease. *Am Heart J* 1996;131:301.

85. Stark DD, Higgins CB, Lanzer P, et al. Magnetic resonance imaging of the pericardium: normal and pathologic findings. *Radiology* 1984;150:469.

86. Sechtem U, Tscholakoff DT, Higgins CB. MRI of the normal pericardium. *AJR Am J Roentgenol* 1986;147:239.

87. Pope CF, Gore JC, Sostman D, et al. The apparent pericardium on cardiac NMR images. *Circulation* 1985;72(Suppl III):124.

88. Silverman PM, Harell GS. Computed tomography of the normal pericardium. *Invest Radiol* 1983;18:141.

89. Ferrands VJ, Ishihara T, Roberts WC. Anatomy of the pericardium. In: Reddy PS, Leon DF, Shaver JA, eds. *Pericardial disease.* New York: Raven Press, 1982;77–92.

90. Im JG, Rosen A, Webb WR, et al. MR imaging of the transverse sinus of the pericardium. *AJR Am J Roentgenol* 1988;150:79.

91. McMurdo KK, Webb WR, von Schulthess GK, et al. Magnetic resonance imaging of the superior pericardial recesses. *AJR Am J Roentgenol* 1985;145:985.

92. Solomon SL, Brown JJ, Glazer HS, et al. Thoracic aortic dissection: pitfalls and artifacts in MR imaging. *Radiology* 1990;177:223.

93. Mulvagh SL, Rokey R, Vick GWD, et al. Usefulness of nuclear magnetic resonance imaging for evaluation of pericardial effusions, and comparison with two-dimensional echocardiography. *Am J Cardiol* 1989;64:1002.

94. Sechtem U, Tscholakoff D, Higgins CB. MRI of the abnormal pericardium. *AJR Am J Roentgenol* 1986;147:245.

95. White CS. MR evaluation of the pericardium. *Top Magn Reson Imaging* 1995;7:258.

96. Soulen RL, Stark DD, Higgins CB. Magnetic resonance imaging of constrictive pericardial disease. *Am J Cardiol* 1985;55:480.

97. Sechtem U, Higgins CB, Sommerhoff BA, et al. Magnetic resonance imaging of restrictive cardiomyopathy. *Am J Cardiol* 1987;59:480.

98. Letanche G, Gayer C, Souquet PJ, et al. Agenesis of the pericardium: clinical echocardiographic and MRI aspects. *Rev Pneumol Clin* 1988;44:105.

99. Gutierrez FR, Shackelford GD, McKnight RC, et al. Diagnosis of congenital absence of left pericardium by MR imaging. *J Comput Assist Tomogr* 1985;9:551.

100. Vinée P, Stover B, Sigmund G, et al. MRI of the paracardial cyst. *J Magn Reson Imaging* 1992;2:593.

101. Higgins CB. Pericardial cysts and diverticula. In: Higgins CB, ed. *CT of the heart and the great vessels.* Mount Kisco, NY: Futura Publishing, 1983:296.

102. Hanock EW. Pericardial disease in patients with neoplasm. In: Reddy PS, Leon DF, Shaver JA, eds. *Pericardial disease.* New York: Raven Press, 1982;325.

103. Lund JT, Ehman RL, Julsrud PR, et al. Cardiac masses: assessment by MR imaging. *AJR Am J Roentgenol* 1989;152:469.

104. Madore B, Fredrickson JO, Alley MT, et al. A reduced field-of-view method to increase temporal resolution or reduce scan time in cine MRI. *Magn Reson Med* 2000;43:549.

105. Weiger M, Pruessmann KP, Boesinger P. Cardiac real-time imaging using SENSE. *Magn Reson Med* 2000;43:177.

8

RIGHT VENTRICULAR DYSPLASIA AND OUTFLOW TRACT TACHYCARDIA

LAWRENCE M. BOXT
ANNA ROZENSHTEIN

In arrhythmogenic right ventricular dysplasia (ARVD), a rare disease occurring in young adults, ventricular arrhythmias are associated with a predominantly right-sided cardiomyopathy. Interest in the disease has increased because of a better awareness of its incidence, a more complete understanding of its pathophysiology, and a better appreciation of its association with other right ventricular (RV) arrhythmogenic cardiomyopathies. Furthermore, the diagnostic sensitivity has been improved by the application of MRI techniques, so that earlier detection and medical intervention are possible.

ARVD is the most common of a group of diseases classified by the World Health Organization (1) as *arrhythmogenic right ventricular cardiomyopathy.* This term encompasses a wide spectrum of cardiac diseases, all of which feature ventricular arrhythmia of RV origin and a similar basic histologic structure. Despite these similarities, the diseases vary greatly in clinical presentation and outcome. Naxos disease (2) is a variant that presents with clinical symptoms and electrocardiographic (ECG) changes similar to those of ARVD (3) but is also associated with a particular palmar and plantar keratosis. Persons with this disease seem to be clustered on the Greek island of Naxos. The demographic pattern may have resulted from inbreeding, like

that of the particular cardiomyopathy seen in Suffolk, England (4). Venetian cardiomyopathy (originally referred to as *right ventricular cardiomyopathy*) (5), a peculiar cardiomyopathy seen in northern Italy, exhibits a familial incidence reaching nearly 50% in the Veneto region of Italy (6). It is interesting that Naxos was occupied by Venetian merchants between 1207 and 1556. The incidence of sudden death is increased among the relatives of patients with the Venetian variant, and a larger number of patients have left ventricular (LV) involvement (6). RV outflow tachycardia and benign extrasystoles of RV outflow tract origin are two other variants of ARVD that are of clinical significance despite their relatively benign course, and their identification and differential diagnosis are discussed below.

In this chapter, we describe the clinical and pathologic features of an apparently large family of diseases. Because it has become apparent that MRI plays such an important role in the evaluation of these patients, we emphasize a diagnosis based on the identification of characteristic morphologic features. We also describe our technique for MR evaluation, again emphasizing methods that allow a confident and reliable identification of characteristic morphologic findings that can be used to establish or exclude the diagnosis.

HISTORICAL PERSPECTIVE

Isolated instances of young persons dying suddenly have been observed and reported in the medical literature since

L. M. Boxt: Department of Radiology, Beth Israel Medical Center, New York, New York.

A. Rozenshtein: Department of Radiology, St. Luke's-Roosevelt Hospital Center, New York, New York.

time immemorial. Osler was the first to describe the postmortem examination of the heart of a 40-year-old man who had died suddenly; he noted thinning and dilatation of all four chambers and a "parchment-like" appearance of the RV myocardium (7). He commented that the right side of the heart was more seriously involved than the left, and that no abnormality or obstruction of the coronary arteries was apparent that might have been responsible for the observed loss of myocardium. Uhl (8) reported his postmortem examination of the heart of a 7-month-old girl with severe right-sided congestive heart failure. He stated that although the RV free-wall myocardium was nearly completely absent, the musculature of the interventricular septum and the papillary muscles of the tricuspid valve were normal. Since then, many case reports have appeared of persons with ventricular tachyarrhythmia and sudden death associated with diffuse or localized abnormalities of the RV. The term *arrhythmogenic right ventricular dysplasia* was first used by Frank et al. in 1978 (9) to describe this syndrome, characterized by progressive fibrofatty replacement of the RV free wall that is manifested as ventricular arrhythmia. Marcus et al. (10) reported the first large series of patients with ARVD. They found a male-to-female ratio of 2.7:1, and the mean age at hospitalization was 39 years. Of the 24 patients in their series, 22 presented with ventricular tachycardia, supraventricular arrhythmias, and right-sided heart failure. Only 2 of the 24 subjects presented with asymptomatic cardiomegaly. These workers described a characteristic left bundle branch block appearance of the ECG, an increased RV size on echocardiography, and RV dilatation in 22 of their 24 patients. Furthermore, they reported unusual abnormalities on contrast right ventriculography, including deep fissuring of the RV free wall and nonopacified areas in the RV outflow tract. The results of selective coronary angiography were negative in all but one patient, in whom the LV myocardium supplied by this solitary vessel appeared to contract normally. Morphologic findings were obtained in 12 patients at surgery and in one additional patient at autopsy. The authors found that the RV cavity was always enlarged, and that usually one or more areas of oblong or dome-shaped dilatations were present over the anterior surface of the RV infundibulum, at the RV apex, and on the inferior wall of the RV. They called these areas the *triangle of dysplasia*. The areas were frequently covered with abundant subepicardial fat, usually replaced by fibrofatty tissue. Histologic examination revealed a paucity of myocardium and a variable amount of histiocytic and lymphocytic infiltration.

Since the publication of this report, the term *arrhythmogenic right ventricular dysplasia* has been used increasingly often, replacing other descriptive terms that include *adipose dysplasia of the right ventricle*, *right ventricular cardiomyopathy*, and *arrhythmogenic right ventricular adiposis*. References to an etiologic association between ARVD and Uhl's anomaly have also decreased.

Familial cases of ventricular tachycardia with a left bundle branch configuration were first reported by Waynberger et al. (11). However, Marcus et al. (10) were the first to note a familial occurrence of ARVD. Since then, cases of familial occurrence with autosomal inheritance, variable incomplete penetrance, and polymorphic phenotype expression have been reported (6,12–18). Nava et al. (6) studied 72 subjects from nine families in which cases of juvenile death with autopsy evidence of massive fibrofatty replacement of the RV myocardium had occurred. Of the 72 subjects studied, 56 were alive, and 15 died suddenly. One subject died of heart failure. They found that at least two family members in eight of the nine families studied had RV structural and dynamic abnormalities. In the two families in which three generations were studied, members of all three generations were affected. In the two youngest members of one of these families, results of echocardiographic evaluation of the RV were normal at 11 years of age. At follow-up examination 4 years later, a typical echocardiographic picture of ARVD was found.

In a follow-up review of 365 subjects in 37 families with ARVD, Nava et al. (19), using standardized criteria for the diagnosis of ARVD (20), found that 151 (41.3%) of subjects were affected, 157 (43%) were unaffected, and the diagnosis was uncertain in 40 (11%). Furthermore, 17 (5%) of the subjects had no clinical disease. Because it was felt that the latter subjects could potentially transmit the disease, they were considered healthy carriers. Members of all the families were affected by the disease; the percentage of affected persons among clinically evaluated subjects in each family ranged from 33% to 75%. Among the 132 living affected patients, the disease was never diagnosed in infancy, and only twice under the age of 10 years. The mean age at diagnosis was 31 ± 13 years. Among the 19 probands who died suddenly, the mean age at death was 27 ± 10.5 years. Nine (47%) had a previous history of syncope, and of the 13 (68%) who died during effort, six had had a previous syncopal episode.

ETIOLOGY

The etiology of ARVD is unknown. A few comments concerning several interesting theories that have been proposed (21) to explain the morphologic and clinical characteristics of this disease are in order. In the disontogenic theory, congenital aplasia or hypoplasia of the RV free wall leads to the parchment-like appearance reported by Osler (7), Uhl (8), and others (9,22,23). Thus, the disease may be regarded as a gross cardiac structural defect present at birth and should be considered among other congenital malformations. Use of the term *dysplasia* ("maldevelopment") seems appropriate.

A degenerative theory suggests that the loss of ventricular myocardium is the consequence of progressive myocyte death secondary to some unknown metabolic or ultrastructural defect. The familial occurrence (6,12–15) of this disease has always strongly suggested a genetic basis with variable expression and penetration. However, recent demonstration of a specific gene defect mapped to chromosome 14q23-q24 in a large family (24) favors the idea of a genetically determined myocardial atrophy. The 14q23-q24 region includes the genes for β-spectrin and α-actinin. The myocardial dystrophy observed in ARVD and the skeletal muscular dystrophy seen in the Duchenne and Becker diseases are similar in appearance. Moreover, the structural homology between the α-actinin gene and the amine terminal domain of dystrophin are highly suggestive of a defective α-actinin gene (24). Nevertheless, no skeletal muscular involvement similar to that found in the skeletal muscle of patients with the Duchenne or Becker disease was found in patients with ARVD, nor was any erythrocyte or skeletal muscle abnormality found that might reflect a defective β-spectrin gene.

An inflammatory theory raises the possibility that ARVD may be the result of an infectious or immune myocardial reaction (25). It treats the fibrofatty replacement seen in ARVD as the result of a healing process in the setting of myocardial necrosis in chronic myocarditis (16,25–27). Support for this idea does not conflict with the significant familial occurrence of ARVD. In experimental coxsackievirus myocarditis in mice, selective RV perimyocarditis was obtained (28). In later stages, ventricular aneurysms similar to those of ARVD were found. Furthermore, a genetic predisposition to viral infection eliciting immune reactions cannot be excluded. Genetic factors may play a role in both susceptibility to infection and the site of cardiac involvement in these patients.

It has been proposed that ARVD may represent an example of programmed myocardial cell death (apoptosis) (29). In a manner similar to the involution of RV myocardium seen in normal postnatal RV remodeling, ARVD may be caused by abnormal bouts of recurring or continued apoptosis leading to progressive myocardial disappearance and fibrofatty replacement. Furthermore, the apoptotic bouts may enhance the electrical vulnerability of the ventricular myocardium, possibly causing the characteristic life-threatening arrhythmias seen in this disease.

PATHOLOGY

The pathologic features of ARVD are striking. Gross evaluation of the hearts of patients with ARVD usually reveals RV dilatation with focal bulging of the infundibulum and the apical and subtricuspid areas (the triangle of dysplasia of Marcus). RV dilatation is usually mild to moderate but occasionally severe. Most of the RV free-wall myocardium is replaced by fat. Typically, the midmural or external layers of the RV myocardium are replaced. Although LV involvement may be found, the LV myocardium is usually spared.

Basso et al. (21) reviewed the pathologic examination findings of 30 hearts with ARVD. The age range of the hearts was 15 to 65 years (mean, 28 years). Among the 27 autopsy cases studied (the other three hearts were explanted at the time of cardiac transplantation), the mode of death was sudden death in 24 and congestive heart failure in three. RV free-wall thickness ranged from 2 to 7 mm (mean, 3.5 mm). RV aneurysms were found in 15 (50%) of the hearts. The aneurysms were inferior in four; inferior and apical in three; inferior, apical, and infundibular in three; infundibular in three; and inferior and infundibular in two. Thus, 12 (80%) of the aneurysms were inferior in location. The subendocardial muscular trabeculae were occasionally shrunken but were mostly spared. The corresponding intertrabecular spaces were enlarged. The endocardium in the ventricular aneurysms was thickened, and the wall was thinner. LV involvement was observed in 14 (47%) of the hearts, and in six (20%), changes were found to extend to the interventricular septum. Extensive LV involvement may occur (30), and LV dysfunction may be latent (31).

Histologic evaluation of these hearts showed two types of myocardial replacement: fibrofatty in 18 (60%) and fatty in 12 (40%). Transmyocardial atrophy was found in both patterns. Fatty or fibrofatty infiltration was more extensive on the epicardial side. Residual myocytes were scattered within the fibrofatty tissue. It is important to clarify the nature of the fatty and fibrofatty replacement found in the hearts of patients with ARVD. In normal subjects, epicardial fat is distributed about the anterior atrioventricular ring and RV free wall (32). Significant fatty infiltration occurs in more than 50% of normal hearts in elderly persons (33,34). Furthermore, an analysis of RV biopsy specimens from patients with ARVD showed a greater amount of fibrous tissue in young patients and a greater prevalence of fatty tissue in adults (35).

Burke et al. (36) investigated the relationship between the appearance of the RV in patients with ARVD and that in persons with pure RV fat replacement. These workers found that the primary features of ARVD were replacement fibrosis and myocyte atrophy, which could occur in virtually any area of the RV; these usually resulted in myocardial thinning. In comparison with control hearts, intramyocardial fat infiltration was most extensive in the RV outflow tract and lateral ventricular apex. They found no significant increase in the amount of epicardial fat in patients with ARVD except in the region of the outflow tract. They point out that the site of fat measurement influences the significance of increased ventricular fat composition. In other words, although a 15% fat replacement would be abnormal in the RV outflow or posterior walls, such a finding would be normal in the anterior wall or near the ventricular apex. Furthermore, these workers demonstrated an intermingling of both fibrous and fatty tissue (not merely the presence of fat) in patients with ARVD. This finding was noted near the endocardial surface in nearly 72% of RV sites investigated. Fatty infiltration of both ventricles without associated fibrous scarring has been anecdotally associated with sudden cardiac death (37). However, this is not considered a form of ARVD.

Comparing the hearts of patients with ARVD and hearts with fatty replacement without fibrosis, Burke et al. (36) found significant differences in the male-to-female ratio (20:5 vs. 2:5 in patients with fatty replacement), history of arrhythmia (40% vs. none with fatty replacement), family history of sudden death (28% vs. none with fatty replacement), family history of arrhythmia (56% vs. none with fatty replacement), and death during exercise (56% vs. none with fatty replacement). In comparison with patients with fibrofatty ARVD, the patients with fatty replacement had a significant increase in the epicardial fat thickness in all areas of the RV except the posterior base. Furthermore, they found inflammatory infiltrates with myocyte necrosis in the myocardium in 20 of 25 cases of fibrofatty ARVD. The infiltrates were isolated to the RV in 14 cases, biventricular in five cases, and isolated to the LV in one case. Such inflammatory infiltrates were found in the RV in only one case of fatty replacement. No LV was involved. These stark differences between the hearts with fibrofatty ARVD and those with pure fatty replacement are not nearly so obvious as the differences reported by Basso et al. (21). In the latter series, the authors found no difference in the incidence of previous symptoms, ECG changes, or mode of death or heart failure between fibrofatty and fatty RV replacement. However, they also found that RV free-wall thickness was significantly less (2.9 ± 1.0 vs. 4.3 ± 1.2 mm, $p <.0001$) in the fibrofatty hearts, and that the incidence of patchy inflammatory infiltrates (100% vs. 17%, $p <.001$) was significantly greater in the fibrofatty hearts. How can we reconcile these similarities and differences? Geographic variations may exist. Basso et al. (21) reported cases from Padua, Italy; Burke et al. (36) reviewed cases from the Armed Forces Institute of Pathology in Washington, D.C. The selection of cases was biased toward sudden death in the Italian series. The American study was a review of a large series of consecutive deaths. More extensive sampling of the RV myocardium in the American series may have revealed small areas of fibrosis that could have been overlooked in the Italian series. Nevertheless, the significant differences in sex distribution, frequency of inflammation, presence of myocardial aneurysms, LV involvement, exertion-related sudden death, and frequency of arrhythmias may mean that pure fatty myocardial replacement is not part of the pathologic spectrum of ARVD. Might this be a morphologic variant of normal? Pathologic evidence of fibrosis may be necessary for a conclusive diagnosis of ARVD.

CLINICAL PRESENTATION

The diagnosis of ARVD is most commonly made in males. However, the male-to-female ratio in the literature is variable (19,21,26,36,38), as is the clinical presentation of patients with ARVD. The spectrum of clinical presentations includes, at one end, those children and adolescents who are entirely asymptomatic and are investigated only because they are relatives of symptomatic persons. At the other end of the spectrum are those who present for the first time with sudden cardiac death, which usually occurs during exercise (39,40). In fact, ventricular tachyarrhythmia associated with morphologic and histologic changes of the RV is the most common cause of sudden cardiac death in young males in Europe (5). The typical patient is a youth or middle-aged man who presents with palpitations, tachycardia, or syncope. Other common symptoms include lightheadedness or dizziness (predominantly related to exercise). These symptoms are probably all related to hemodynamic compromise caused by ventricular arrhythmia.

The physical examination findings are surprisingly normal. A prominence of the left precordium may be present, indicating long-standing enlargement of the right side of the heart. A fourth and even a third heart sound may be audible. The ECG in patients with ARVD is usually in regular sinus rhythm. The most frequent abnormalities on resting ECG are ventricular tachycardia with a left bundle branch pattern, T-wave inversion in the anterior precordial leads (V_1 to V_4), a QT interval of more than 110 milliseconds, a characteristic sharp spike in the ST segment (the so-called postexcitation or epsilon wave), and, if Holter monitoring is performed, ventricular ectopic beats in excess of 1,000 per day (41).

DEFINITIVE DIAGNOSIS

The definitive diagnosis of ARVD is a challenge. Clinical signs may be absent, and ECG findings may be inconclusive. Conventional echocardiographic and RV angiographic imaging may not yield characteristic or reproducible changes in patients with milder forms of the disease (42,43). Endomyocardial biopsy may provide explicit data for a definitive diagnosis. However, the disease may be sporadic in the RV free wall, so that the diagnostic sensitivity is lowered. In addition, for safety reasons, RV free-wall biopsy is rarely attempted. Most RV endomyocardial biopsy specimens are obtained from the interventricular septum, a region uncommonly involved by the disease (44). For these reasons, confusion arose concerning the diagnosis of ARVD, and differentiating that diagnosis from the other arrhythmia-associated RV diseases. An accurate diagnosis of ARVD was limited by the wide array of results of the history, physical examination, and testing in these patients, and the need for objective diagnostic criteria was evident (45).

A task force of the European Society of Cardiology and the International Society and Federation of Cardiology established criteria for the diagnosis of ARVD (20). Major and minor criteria had to be identified, including structural abnormalities, fatty or fibrofatty replacement of the RV myocardium, ECG changes, arrhythmias of RV origin, and familial disease (Table 8.1). Analogous to the diagnosis of rheumatic heart disease, the diagnosis of ARVD is based on the identification of two major criteria, one major plus two minor criteria, or four minor criteria. Traditional studies—radionuclide scintigraphy, echocardiography, and contrast right ventriculography—will now be enhanced by the application of MRI to detect ventricular dysfunction and structural alterations. Although such a scheme for diagnosis does not eliminate ambiguity in terms of identifying re-

gional RV wall motion abnormalities or structural changes, it does provide a common approach for analyzing the phenotypic expression of ARVD. In addition, it suggests a potential role for MRI in the evaluation of these patients. MR examination may be useful for explicitly demonstrating abnormal right (and left) ventricular myocardium, areas of fatty infiltration, regional thinning, and regional akinesia.

MRI OF ARRHYTHMOGENIC RIGHT VENTRICULAR DYSPLASIA

The complex shape of the RV and the ubiquitous epicardial fat pad along the RV free wall make it difficult to visualize the chamber in its entirety and evaluate regional changes by conventional imaging techniques. The large field of view afforded by MR scanners allows detailed visualization of the entire RV with evaluation of the shape and internal morphology of the chamber (46,47). The high contrast resolution of spin-echo and double-inversion recovery images allows a confident differentiation between cavitary blood, ventricular myocardium, and epicardial fat in the analysis of myocardial trabecular structure and wall thickness (48–50). Furthermore, the high temporal resolution of cine gradient reversal acquisition techniques provides a means for evaluating changes in myocardial thickness and cavitary appearance through the cardiac cycle. The MR findings in ARVD are listed in Table 8.2.

The earliest reports of the use of MRI in the evaluation of patients with ARVD emphasized the potential utility of MR examination for demonstrating increased signal intensity in the fat-infiltrated myocardium of the RV free wall and the abnormal contractile function associated with the disease (51–54) (Fig. 8.1). In addition, these studies found that the sites of increased signal intensity on MR examination corresponded to regions that electrophysiologic investigation showed were producing the ventricular tachycardias. These workers appreciated the limitations of spin-echo acquisition and found that it was often difficult or impossible to judge increased signal intensity in the thin RV free wall or differentiate the wall from cavitary blood or signal artifacts caused by turbulent blood flow. In particular, they

TABLE 8.1. CRITERIA FOR DIAGNOSIS OF ARRHYTHMOGENIC RIGHT VENTRICULAR DYSPLASIA

1. **Global or regional dysfunction and structural alterations**
   Major:
   Severe RV dilatation and reduced EF with no (or minimal) LV impairment
   Localized RV aneurysms
   Severe segmental RV dilatation
   Minor:
   Mild global RV dilatation or reduced EF with normal LV
   Mild segmental RV dilatation
   Regional RV hypokinesia

2. **Tissue characterization of the walls**
   Major:
   Fibrofatty myocardial replacement on endomyocardial biopsy

3. **Repolarization abnormalities**
   Minor:
   Inverted T waves in the right precordial leads (V_2 and V_3) (in people >12 years old; in absence of right bundle branch block)

4. **Depolarization/conduction abnormalities**
   Major:
   Epsilon waves or localized prolongation (>110 milliseconds) of the QRS complex in the right precordial leads (V_1 through V_3)
   Minor:
   Late potentials (signal-averaged ECG)

5. **Arrhythmia**
   Minor:
   Left bundle branch block type of ventricular tachycardia (sustained and nonsustained)
   Frequent ventricular extrasystoles (>1,000/24 hours)

6. **Family history**
   Major:
   Familial disease confirmed at autopsy or surgery
   Minor:
   Familial history of premature sudden death (<35 years old) from suspected arrhythmogenic right ventricular dysplasia
   Familial history (based on present criteria)

RV, right ventricle; EF, ejection fraction; LV, left ventricle; ECG, electrocardiogram.
From McKenna WJ, Thiene G, Nava A, et al. Diagnosis of arrhythmogenic right ventricular dysplasia/cardiomyopathy. *Br Heart J* 1994;71:215–218, with permission.

TABLE 8.2. FINDINGS IN ARRHYTHMOGENIC RIGHT VENTRICULAR DYSPLASIA

Increased right ventricular free wall signal intensity
Decreased right ventricular free wall thickness
Decreased right ventricular free wall systolic thickness
Regional wall motion abnormalities
Regional excavations
Regional aneurysms
Right ventricular dilatation
Right atrial dilatation
(Left ventricular involvement)

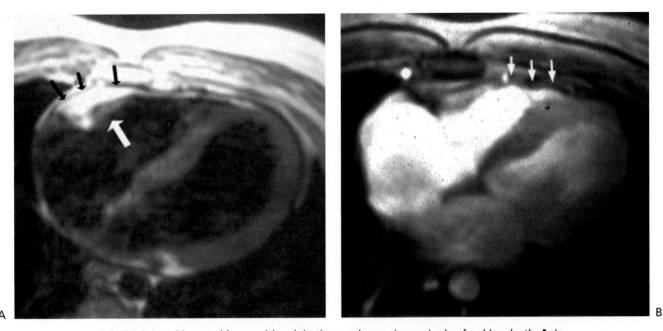

FIGURE 8.1. A 39-year-old man with palpitations and a previous episode of sudden death. **A:** In this axial spin-echo acquisition, the right ventricular (RV) free wall myocardium is not visualized. Myocardium medial to the atrioventricular ring *(long arrow)* and subjacent to the epicardial fat *(short arrows)* is identified. The interventricular septum is flat, indicating RV dilatation. **B:** End-systolic axial cine gradient reversal acquisition obtained at the same anatomic location. The medial RV free-wall myocardium and the left ventricular myocardium are thickened, as expected in systole. Failure of the RV free-wall myocardium to thicken gives the high-signal-intensity RV cavity the appearance of extending to the chest wall *(arrows)*. No local bulge or aneurysm is seen, however.

pointed out the significance of this problem in an evaluation of the apex and subtricuspid regions of the ventricle, which are usually covered with epicardial fat. They found that reaching a diagnosis by the consensus of a group of observers often increased confidence in their observations. The diagnosis of ARVD in the large majority of cases in their small series was based on an analysis of combined spin-echo and cine gradient reversal examination. In patients with ARVD, areas of increased signal intensity correlated with regions of asynergy or focal aneurysm formation (Fig. 8.2). In addition, increases in end-diastolic cavitary volume and decreases in RV ejection fraction were found. The functional abnormality was confirmed in a series of 36 patients with biopsy-proven ARVD in whom the RV ejection fraction was calculated from MRI data (55). In this study, the RV ejection fractions were significantly lower in patients with inducible ventricular tachycardia than in patients in whom ventricular tachycardia was not induced. The investigators found areas of increased signal intensity that corresponded to biopsy-proven regions of fatty replacement.

Midiri et al. (56) studied 30 patients (22 men and 8 women) 12 to 74 years of age (mean age, 42.1 years) with a suspected diagnosis of ARVD. They used five morphologic criteria to make the diagnosis: areas of myocardium with high signal intensity, dilatation of the RV outflow tract, dyskinetic bulges, RV dilatation, and right atrial (RA) di-

latation. RV outflow tract dilatation was present when its diameter was observed to be equal to or greater than that of the LV outflow. An RV end-diastolic dimension (measured from a four-chamber view) greater than 42 mm indicated RV dilatation. RA dilatation was judged to be present when the end-systolic anteroposterior dimension (measured from a four-chamber view) was greater than 41 mm. The diagnosis of ARVD was judged to be highly probable if at least three of these criteria were met. It was judged to be probable if two criteria were met, dubious with one, and negative if none was met.

Using this system based on criteria, the authors found that 12 (40%) of their 30 cases were highly probable or probable and 18 (60%) were dubious or negative for ARVD. In the highly probable or probable group, they were able to demonstrate myocardial fat substitution in 11 of 12, outflow tract dilatation in 7 of 12, regional dyskinesia in 4 of 12, RV dilatation in 7 of 12, and RA dilatation in 6 of 12 (not observed in any probable cases). In comparison, in the group judged dubious or negative for ARVD, they found myocardial fat substitution in 3 of 18 (including 3 of 7 with a dubious diagnosis), outflow tract dilatation in 1 of 18, RV dilatation in 1 of 18, and RA dilatation in 2 of 18. In a review of their cine gradient reversal acquisitions, they found regional dyskinesia in 4 of 12 highly probable or probable cases, and in none of the dubious or negative cases. Al-

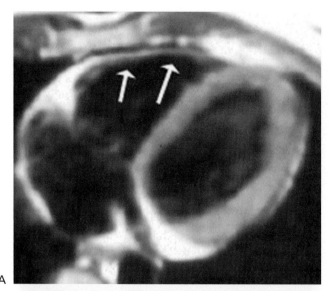

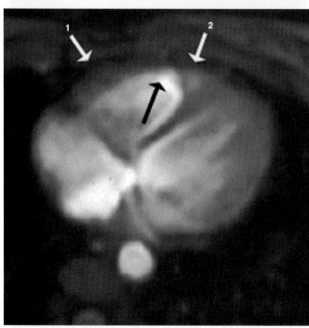

FIGURE 8.2. A 30-year-old man who experienced an episode of sudden death. **A:** Axial spin-echo acquisition shows diffuse thinning and increased signal intensity of the right ventricular (RV) free wall. Epicardial fat cannot be visually separated from the RV free-wall myocardium *(arrows).* **B:** End-systolic axial gradient reversal acquisition obtained at the same anatomic level as in A. The RV myocardium, including the apical portion *(arrow 2),* can be identified or seen to thicken *(arrow 1),* save for the medial akinetic segment *(black arrow).*

though no statistical analysis was performed to test the significance of their findings, they pointed out the variability in appearance of RVs with and without this disease and indicated the need for a combined analysis of static (spin-echo) and dynamic (cine gradient reversal) image acquisition.

Thus, MR examination in patients suspected of having ARVD is a means of demonstrating specific morphologic and functional abnormalities that can be used as diagnostic criteria. The utility of MRI to visualize regions of RV free-wall thinning or increased signal intensity appears to be limited, so that the sensitivity of these observations for providing clear diagnostic criteria is decreased. However, areas of abnormal RV myocardium apparently do not function normally. Thus, global RV size and contractile function, in addition to regional wall motion abnormalities, are very helpful in establishing diagnostic criteria (Fig. 8.3). Combining static with dynamic acquisitions may provide the most sensitive means of establishing this diagnosis.

MRI EVALUATION OF RIGHT VENTRICULAR OUTFLOW TRACT TACHYCARDIA

Evidence is increasing that previously unrecognized morphologic abnormalities of the RV may be the cellular or functional basis of a variety of ventricular arrhythmias of RV origin. In particular, ventricular arrhythmias originating from the RV outflow tract, which had been considered idiopathic in origin (57), may in fact originate from foci of abnormal RV myocardium. Carlson et al. (58) found significant myocardial structural and wall motion abnormalities in 22 consecutive patients with electrocardiographically diagnosed RV outflow tract tachycardia (RVOTT) (Fig. 8.4). Cine gradient reversal MRI demonstrated structural abnormalities of the RV in 21 of 22 patients. The most common finding was regionally decreased systolic wall thickening or areas of abnormal wall motion. In addition, they found regions of fixed focal wall thinning. These regions were seen with and without excavations of the RV free wall or discrete areas of severely diminished wall thickness. Wall thinning was more apparent during systole than in diastole. Both excavated and nonexcavated regions could be distinguished from adjacent regions of the RV with normal wall thickness. None of the focal structural or regional RV wall motion abnormalities seen in the group of patients with tachycardia were found in the group of patients without tachycardia. They emphasized that focal decreased RV wall thickening alone is not diagnostic of RVOTT, but that these findings must be accompanied by morphologic abnormalities localized to the RV outflow tract.

White et al. (59) evaluated 53 patients with arrhythmias originating from the RV. The electrophysiologic diagnosis was idiopathic RVOTT in 35 (66%) and indeterminate in 18 (34%). They found abnormalities of the RV free wall in 25 (71%) of the patients with the diagnosis of RVOTT and in 7 (39%) of the patients with an indeterminate diagnosis, a significant difference. Among the patients with the diagnosis of RVOTT, abnormal regions of the RV free wall, especially in the lower infundibulum, were evident in 33 (94%). No patient with the diagnosis of RVOTT had MRI abnormalities limited to the RV body. These workers were impressed with the similarity in appearance and difference

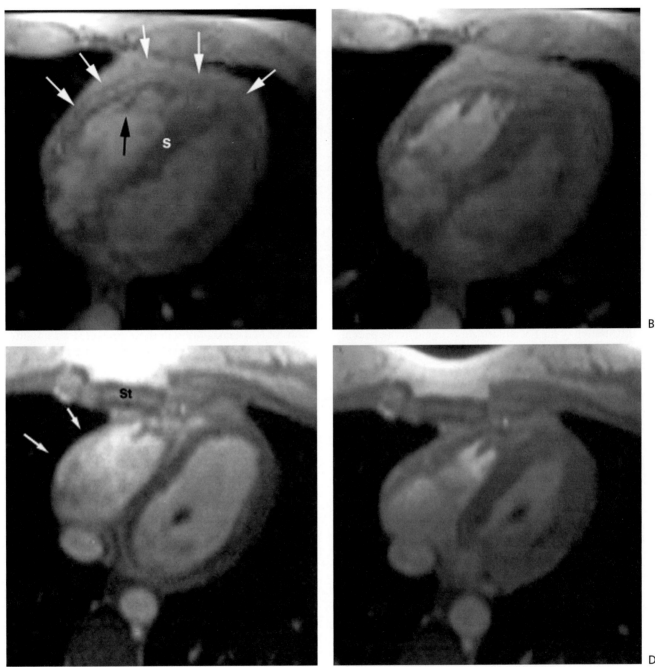

FIGURE 8.3. Two patients with syncope. **A:** A 34-year-old man with characteristic electrocardiographic changes and a family history of sudden death at a young age. Four-millimeter-thick axial k-space segmented breath-hold gradient reversal image acquired at end-diastole. A thick band of epicardial and pericardial fat surrounding the right ventricular (RV) free wall and cardiac apex is separated by the normal pericardial space *(arrows)*. The septum *(S)* is flat. A papillary muscle from the RV free wall *(black arrow)* extends into the ventricular cavity. **B:** Image obtained at the same anatomic level at end-systole. The left ventricular (LV) myocardium, including the interventricular septum, has thickened uniformly. RV free wall thickening is inhomogeneous, and where thickening occurs, it is diminished. Note the papillary muscle. **C:** A 40-year-old woman with syncope and no electrocardiographic abnormality. End-diastolic k-space segmented breath-hold gradient reversal image. The RV is behind the sternum *(St)* in the midline. The RV free-wall myocardium *(arrows)* cannot be visually separated from the cavity. **D:** End-systolic image. Uniform thickening of both the LV and RV myocardium. The substance of the RV free-wall myocardium is easily separated from the cavity.

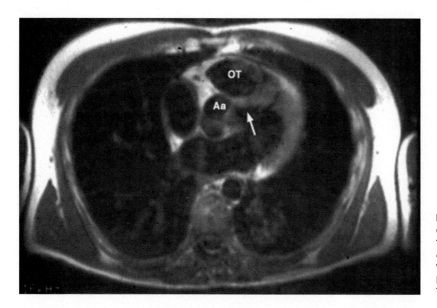

FIGURE 8.4. A 40-year-old man with syncopal episodes. Axial spin-echo image obtained through the anterior aortic sinus of Valsalva *(Aa)* and right ventricular outflow tract *(OT)*. The free wall is thin, and the outflow tract is dilated, displacing the interventricular septum *(arrow)* posteriorly.

in distribution of the RV abnormalities found in this patient population and in patients with ARVD, and they argued that these conditions may be related.

Proclemer et al. (60) prospectively assessed MR examinations in 19 patients (13 male and six female) with a diagnosis of RV outflow premature contractions. They found that the RV outflow tracts in the patients who experienced extrasystolic contractions originating from the RV outflow tract were wider than those in control normal subjects. In addition, they found wall motion abnormalities in 84% of these patients, which were confined to the anterolateral RV wall. Cine gradient reversal acquisitions revealed a very high prevalence of localized regions of decreased systolic wall thickening adjacent to areas of morphologic abnormality. These workers also pointed out the similarity between the abnormalities detected by MR in these patients and the abnormalities in patients with a diagnosis of RVOTT, suggesting a common substrate.

TECHNIQUE OF EXAMINATION

No objective criteria for designating abnormal RV free-wall thickness or signal intensity are available. Therefore, examinations of the highest quality are needed to provide imagery that can be confidently analyzed. A patient with a tentative diagnosis of ARVD or RVOTT can be successfully examined if careful attention is paid to the planning and execution of the examination. A successful examination is one that produces imagery allowing an imager to identify with confidence the regional morphologic and functional changes that are the criteria for a diagnosis of ARVD or RVOTT. Even before the day of the examination, the referring physician should be contacted. It is important that the referring physician understand the advantages and limita-

tions of MR examination in these diseases. Two important issues should be understood by the referring physician and imaging diagnostician.

First, MR examination findings do not diagnose or exclude the diagnosis of ARVD or RVOTT. Rather, they can provide important morphologic or functional criteria for the diagnosis or its exclusion. Second, because the underlying physiologic problem in these cases is ventricular arrhythmia, special care must be taken to ensure cardiac rate control and optimal ECG gating. ARVD is a rate-dependent tachyarrhythmia, which means that in addition to the usual extrasystolic beats, these patients experience further extrasystolic beats if their resting rate is elevated. Therefore, many of them are treated with beta blockers. However, no experimental evidence indicates that the long-term administration of beta blockers or administering them immediately before the examination controls the cardiac rate or minimizes the incidence of extrasystoles and so improves image quality. An additional benefit is that the examination time is usually shortened. Arrhythmia rejection algorithms are written into the gating packages of most MR scanners. The gating software keeps track of the cardiac rhythm by sampling the length of successive R-R intervals. If the length of an R-R interval exceeds tolerances set at the time of examination preparation, then the scanner rejects that R wave and may wait for two or three additional R waves to recommence phase encoding. Although arrhythmia rejection may be helpful in a patient with an occasional extrasystole, it can significantly increase the examination time in a patient with many extrasystoles. Furthermore, if runs of extrasystoles are encountered, the examination may fail.

When the patient arrives for the examination, the procedure should be explained, and the technologist or radiologist should describe the breathing procedure to be utilized during the examination. Although conventional gradient reversal and spin-echo acquisition can be entirely adequate for data collection, more rapid k-space segmented pulse sequences are becoming more prevalent and should be used, if available. Considering that the pioneering work in the MR examination of patients with ARVD was performed on scanners with lower field strengths (51,52,56), one cannot argue that high field and gradient strengths are essential for an adequate examination. On the other hand, a higher gradient strength increases signal and is helpful for differentiating normal RV free-wall myocardium from epicardial fat.

Care must be taken when the ECG leads are applied to the precordium. Skin preparation for good electrical contact and proper placement of the chest wall electrodes are essential for obtaining a clear ECG signal. Whether anterior or posterior chest wall leads are applied, care should be taken to keep the electrodes within a 10- to 15-cm radius and the leads attached to the electrodes parallel to the bore of the magnet. Tuned or simple Helmholz imaging coils increase the signal obtained from the chest and should be used if available. The examination should be performed with the patient in the supine position and the coil applied to the anterior chest wall. Performing an MR examination in the prone position with the patient's arms extended in front is very uncomfortable and should be avoided. Dedicated cardiac coils have their advantages (smaller size, improved patient comfort), but general chest and body imaging coils can be used successfully. When the coil is applied to the anterior chest wall, care should be taken to center the coil over the heart. The heart of a patients with RV disease and RV dilatation is rotated into the left side of the chest, away from the midline. The coil should be centered medial and cephalic to the point of maximum impulse.

After applying the dedicated cardiac imaging coil, we advance the patient into the scanner. Before commencing examination, we evaluate the ECG-gating signal. No matter how sharp the signal may appear before the magnet bore is entered, once the patient is inside the scanner, the tracing deteriorates. In general, if good contact is made between the chest wall and electrodes, and if the course of the leads is parallel to the scanner bore, then a good tracing will be obtained. Not uncommonly, a good tracing is obtained but the superior deflection of the trace is much less than the inferior deflection, so that the accuracy of R-wave detection is limited. In this circumstance, we remove the patient from the scanner and reverse the attachment of the ECG leads. We exchange the cephalic leads with the caudal pair. This changes the polarity of the downward deflection and allows more precise gating. Remember that the ECG tracing is not obtained for diagnostic purposes. Rather, it is obtained so that the scanner can find an R wave for stepping phase encoding during examination. The patient is moved back into the scanner, and after it has been determined that the ECG tracing is adequate, examination is commenced.

Cardiac MR examination is performed to characterize the right side of the heart and the RV myocardium. There-fore, a protocol for examining these patients should be designed to answer specific questions. A good protocol and a successful examination answer these questions, and the examination is not complete until the questions are answered. When we study these patients, our imaging protocol commences with a series of ungated gradient reversal scout images in sagittal section. These low-resolution images provide little diagnostic information but demonstrate the excursion of the local increase in signal intensity subjacent to the cardiac coil. If the heart is not subtended by the coil, then the patient is removed from the scanner, the coil repositioned, and the patient returned to the scanner for examination.

We begin the diagnostic examination with a series of breath-hold k-space segmented gradient reversal acquisitions. We prescribe 4-mm-thick sections without an interslice gap. We choose the sagittal scout demonstrating the RV outflow tract and proximal main pulmonary artery, and slices are prescribed in axial section from the pulmonary valve to below the diaphragm. In general, we obtain images from the pulmonary valve and progress in a caudal direction.

We choose gradient reversal cine acquisition first because differentiation between normal and abnormal myocardium based on differences in signal intensity or thickness on spin-echo acquisition may be ambiguous. Volume averaging between adjacent voxels containing epicardial fat and ventricular myocardium may give the appearance of myocardium replaced by fat (Fig. 8.5). A normal region of RV free-wall myocardium situated between two adjacent muscular trabeculae may have the appearance of an excavation. On the other hand, no matter how the myocardium appears at end-diastole, normal myocardial thickens at end-systole and fat-replaced myocardium does not. With thin-section cine gradient reversal acquisition, more time is required to examine the entire myocardium. However, it has the advantage of interrogating smaller portions of the myocardium at each acquisition. This minimizes the distortion of the RV outflow tract caused by its cephalic and posterior course, and provides a review of smaller regions of the ventricular myocardium. Image analysis is tedious, but the problem of missing skip areas in less pronounced cases is avoided. The decreased signal obtained from the interrogation of thin sections of tissue is augmented by the use of a high gradient strength, if available, and a cardiac coil.

Thin-section acquisition through the entire heart in axial section may necessitate 25 to 30 breath-holds. Even if each acquisition takes between 18 to 24 seconds per breath-hold, between 45 and 60 minutes may be required to complete the acquisition. Unless the patient cannot tolerate further examination, we follow the gradient reversal acquisition with a series of 6- to 8-mm spin-echo or double-inversion recovery images in the same axial plane (no interslice gap). Turbulent blood flow frequently results in a bandlike artifact in an anteroposterior direction through the RV in axial sections. This artifact may be diminished or removed by re-

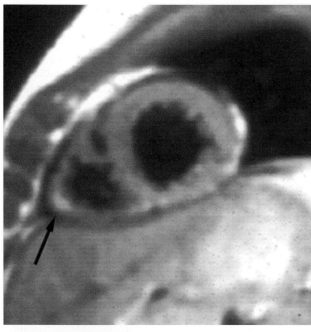

A

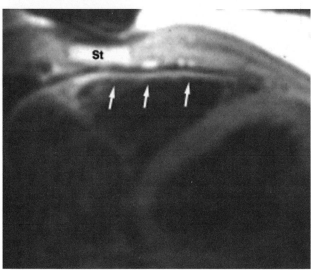

B

FIGURE 8.5. Fat deposition in the right ventricular (RV) free wall. **A:** Short-axis spin-echo acquisition from a 66-year-old woman studied for aortic disease. A discrete deposit of fat *(arrow)* in this otherwise normal-appearing RV appears as an isolated locus of increased signal intensity. **B:** Axial spin-echo acquisition obtained from a 40-year-old woman with runs of ventricular tachycardia. The RV free wall is thin. The entire wall *(arrows)* is infiltrated with fat and exhibits increased signal intensity. RV dilatation is indicated by the position of the RV, rotated to the left of the sternum *(St).*

of myocardial contractile function on gradient reversal acquisition, we acquire additional views with gradient reversal acquisition. The cardiac short axis is oblique to the axial body plane and may be useful for visualizing RV free-wall changes.

The interpretation is made on an anatomic section-by-section basis, and regions of abnormal myocardial thickness, end-systolic thickness, and regional akinesia and dyskinesia are recorded (Fig. 8.6). Increased myocardial signal intensity representing pathologic fatty and fibrofatty infiltration is generally through-and-through the myocardial wall but may be localized and surrounded by apparently normal myocardium (Fig. 8.6). Local excavations (Fig. 8.7) appear as dramatic areas of locally decreased myocardial thickness surrounded by nearly normal myocardium. Abnormal myocardial thickening may be local or diffuse and is characterized by little or no change in the thickness of the RV free-wall myocardium through the cardiac cycle. Often, even in cases of normal RV myocardium, the free wall may not be identified on end-diastolic images. However, normal myocardium thickens, and in the normal RV at end-systole, a band of ventricular myocardium with intermediate signal intensity separates the RV chamber from the pericardium and anterior mediastinum. In patients with ARVD, the RV myocardium may or may not be identifiable on end-diastolic images. However, on systolic images, the abnormal region of nonthickening myocardium is exaggerated when adjacent to normally contracting myocardium and may be identified

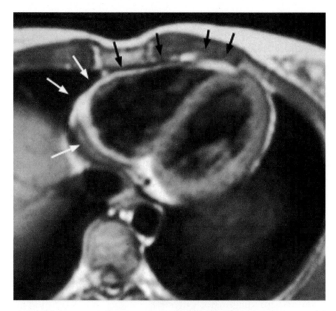

FIGURE 8.6. Axial spin-echo acquisition from a 32-year-old woman with syncope and a family history of episodes of sudden death. An epicardial fat deposit around the anterior border of the heart *(arrows)* cannot be visually separated from the right ventricular (RV) free-wall myocardium. The visualized RV free-wall myocardium is thin and exhibits increased signal intensity. In addition, the RV is dilated, and the heart is rotated toward the left side of the chest.

versing the phase- and frequency-encoding directions (61). Alternatively, one may sandwich the interrogated tissue between a pair of saturation bands (56).

The decision to acquire additional images in other cardiac planes should depend on how well the patient tolerates the examination and on the reasons for the additional acquisition. Because we put greater confidence in our analyses

59

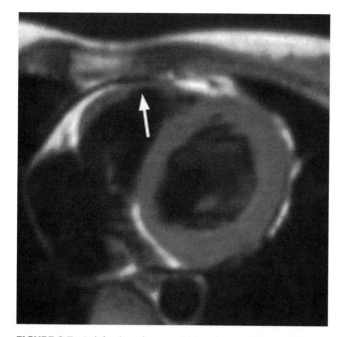

FIGURE 8.7. Axial spin-echo acquisition from a 30-year-old man who collapsed during exercise. An acute change in the thickness of the right ventricular free wall *(arrow)* is seen medial to the insertion of the moderator band. Because of thinning of the myocardium in this region, the epicardial fat pad cannot be visually separated from it, nor can one exclude increased signal intensity secondary to infiltration.

by its lack of change in appearance. Ventricular aneurysms are rarely very large. They often appear as an extension of the high signal intensity of the RV cavity through normal-appearing myocardium toward the pericardial space. In the normal section, a band of myocardium separates ventricular cavity from the pericardium and anterior mediastinum; here, no such boundary is seen, and the cavity seems to extend toward the pericardium. Differentiation between ARVD and RVOTT is based on the localization of RV abnormalities. In ARVD, morphologic and functional abnormalities are found to some extent throughout the RV, whereas in RVOTT, changes are generally more localized to the infundibulum and spare the ventricular body. Limited as these features may be, they provide a means of differentiation in clinical practice.

SUMMARY

ARVD and RVOTT are the two most common primary diseases of the RV. They are characterized by a distinct distribution of areas of abnormal RV myocardium and ventricular tachyarrhythmias. Although the cause of these and other diseases marked by RV morphologic changes and ventricular arrhythmia is unknown, the histologic examination findings, familial incidence, and demonstration of a genetic locus for ARVD suggest potential mechanisms. The mor-

phologic changes reflect areas of fatty and fibrofatty replacement of RV and (in up to 30% of cases) LV myocardium. These changes are manifested as areas of thinning and increased signal intensity on spin-echo and double-inversion recovery imagery. The functional sequelae of these processes are hypokinesia, akinesia, and aneurysmal dilatation. The changes are best demonstrated with cine gradient reversal acquisition. The limitations of the MR technique and the nature of the RV changes in these diseases necessitate a careful examination technique to acquire diagnostic imagery.

REFERENCES

1. Richardson PJ, McKenna WJ, Bristow M, et al. Report of the 1995 World Health Organization/International Society and Federation of Cardiology task force on the definition and classification of cardiomyopathies. *Circulation* 1996;93:841–842.
2. Protonotarios N, Tsatsopoulou A, Patsourakos P, et al. Cardiac abnormalities in familial palmoplantar keratosis. *Br Heart J* 1986;56:321–326.
3. Fontaine G, Protonotarios N, Tsatsopoulou A, et al. Comparisons between Naxos disease and arrhythmogenic right ventricular dysplasia by electrocardiography and biopsy. *Circulation* 1994;90(Suppl I):I-600(abst).
4. Barry M, Hall M. Familial cardiomyopathy. *Br Heart J* 1962;24:613–624.
5. Thiene G, Nava A, Corrado D, et al. Right ventricular cardiomyopathy and sudden death in young people. *N Engl J Med* 1988;318:129–133.
6. Nava A, Thiene G, Canciani B, et al. Familial occurrence of right ventricular dysplasia: a study involving nine families. *J Am Coll Cardiol* 1988;12:1222–1228.
7. Segall HN. Parchment heart (Osler). *Am Heart J* 1950;40:948–950.
8. Uhl HS. A previously undescribed congenital malformation of the heart: almost total absence of the myocardium of the right ventricle. *Bull Johns Hopkins Hosp* 1952;91:197–209.
9. Frank R, Fontaine G, Vedel J, et al. Electrocardiologie de quatre cas de dysplasie ventriculaire droite arythmogène. *Arch Mal Coeur Vaiss* 1978;71:963–972.
10. Marcus FI, Fontaine GH, Guiraudon G, et al. Right ventricular dysplasia: a report of 24 adult cases. *Circulation* 1982:65:384–398.
11. Waynberger M, Courtadon M, Peltier JM, et al. Tachycardies ventriculaires familiales: à propos de 7 observations. *Nouv Presse Med* 1974;30:1857–1860.
12. Rakover C, Rossi L, Fontaine G, et al. Familial arrhythmogenic right ventricular disease. *Am J Cardiol* 1986;58:377–378.
13. Nava A, Scognamiliglio R, Thiene G, et al. A polymorphic form of familial arrhythmogenic right ventricular dysplasia. *Am J Cardiol* 1987;59:1405–1409.
14. Buja GF, Nava A, Daliento L, et al. Right ventricular cardiomyopathy in identical and nonidentical young twins. *Am Heart J* 1993;126:1187–1193.
15. Miani D, Pinamonti B, Bussani R, et al. Right ventricular dysplasia: a clinical and pathological study of two families with left ventricular involvement. *Br Heart J* 1993;69:151–157.
16. Sabel KG, Blomstrom-Lundqvist C, Olsson MB, et al. Arrhythmogenic right ventricular dysplasia in brother and sister: is it related to myocarditis? *Pediatr Cardiol* 1990;11:113–116.
17. Bloomstrom-Lundqvist C, Enestroem S, Edvarsson N, et al. Ar-

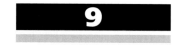

CARDIAC MASSES

GABRIELE A. KROMBACH
MAYTHEM SAEED
CHARLES B. HIGGINS

CARDIAC MRI FOR THE ASSESSMENT OF CARDIAC MASSES

Although primary cardiac tumors are relatively rare, with a reported occurrence of 0.001% to 0.5% in unselected autopsy studies, intracardiac masses are not; tumors of the heart that are metastases or direct extensions of malignant extracardiac tumors are encountered with a 40-fold higher frequency (1–3). The most frequent cardiac mass is intracavitary thrombus. An evaluation of the presence and location of a cardiac mass is an important indication for MRI. Because of its wide field of view, which encompasses the cardiovascular structures, mediastinum, and adjacent lung simultaneously, MRI can vividly display the intracardiac and extracardiac extent of a tumors. In addition, the capability of imaging in multiple planes makes MRI especially suited for the comprehensive delineation of the spatial relationship of a cardiac mass to the various cardiac and mediastinal structures. The multiplanar approach overcomes the volume averaging problem at the diaphragmatic interface encountered with a solely transaxial imaging technique, such as computed tomography. These features permit a clear delineation of the possible infiltration of a mass lesion into cardiac and adjacent mediastinal structures. In addition, MRI allows the assessment of functional parameters, such as ventricular wall thickening, ejection fraction, or flow velocity in adjacent vessels. Therefore, the impact of a tumor on cardiac function can be evaluated.

In clinical practice, MRI is most often used to verify or exclude a possible mass suggested initially by echocardiography. Echocardiography clearly depicts heart morphology and provides an assessment of functional parameters. However, the effectiveness of transthoracic echocardiography is limited by the acoustic window, which varies considerably with patient habitus. Image quality may be severely decreased by obesity or chronic obstructive pulmonary disease. Transesophageal echocardiography overcomes this problem but adds invasiveness. The soft-tissue contrast achieved with echocardiography remains limited in comparison with that obtained with MRI. Usually, pericardial involvement and infiltration of the myocardium can be better visualized with MRI (4,5). Tissue characterization based on specific T1 and T2 relaxation times is possible to a limited degree. Nevertheless, definitive differentiation between benign and malignant tumors is usually not feasible because of the wide overlap of relaxation times among various types of tumor. Most cardiac tumors have low to intermediate signal intensity on T1-weighted images and high signal intensity on T2-weighted images. However, the combination of imaging characteristics of a cardiac mass, such as location, signal intensity on T1- and T2-weighted images, possible hyperenhancement after the administration of paramagnetic contrast agents, and possible suppression of signal with the application of a fat-saturation technique, may render a specific tissue diagnosis highly probable in some cases.

G. A. Krombach: Department of Radiology, University of Technology (RWTH-Aachen), Aachen, Germany.

M. Saeed and C. B. Higgins: Department of Radiology, University of California San Francisco, San Francisco, California.

TECHNIQUES

Electrocardiogram (ECG)-gated transaxial T1-weighted spin-echo images of the entire thorax are initially acquired for the evaluation of suspected cardiac or paracardiac masses. In addition, such images are frequently acquired in the sagittal or coronal plane to delineate the regions that are displayed suboptimally in the transaxial plane, such as the diaphragmatic surface of the heart. Coronal images facilitate the evaluation of masses involving the aortopulmonary window and pulmonary hili, and mediastinal masses that extend through the cervicothoracic junction. Contrast between intramural tumor and normal myocardium may be low on nonenhanced T1-weighted images. Transaxial T2-weighted spin-echo images are acquired to enhance the contrast between myocardium and tumor tissue, which usually has a longer T2 relaxation time, and to delineate possible cystic or necrotic components of a mass. Prolongation of the echo time (TE) causes considerable degradation of MR images of the heart. Because this obstacle is alleviated with fast spin-echo images, they have become standard for the acquisition of T2-weighted images of the heart (6). The comparison of signal intensities of a mass lesion on T1-weighted and T2-weighted images may to a certain degree allow for tissue characterization. For example, lipomas have relatively high signal intensity on T1-weighted images and moderate signal intensity on T2-weighted images. Cystic lesions (filled with simple fluid) have low signal intensity on T1-weighted and high signal intensity on T2-weighted images (4). After T2-weighted images have been obtained, contrast-enhanced images are acquired. The administration of Gd-DTPA (gadolinium diethylenetriamine pentaacetic acid) usually improves the contrast between tumor tissue and myocardium on T1-weighted images and may facilitate tissue characterization (7,8). Hyperenhancement of tumor tissue with MR contrast agents indicates either an enlarged extracellular space of tumor tissue in comparison with normal myocardium or a high degree of vascularization of the mass. Application of a fat-saturation sequence, which vitiates the bright signal of fat, is effective for the tissue characterization of lipomas (9).

Cine MR images are acquired for the purpose of quantifying ventricular volumes, mass, and global function. In patients with cardiac tumors, cine MRI provides valuable information regarding the movement of the cardiac mass relative to the cardiovascular structures. For example, myxomas have been reported to be more mobile and distensible than sarcomas (10). Because cine MR images are acquired with gradient-echo sequences, a different contrast is obtained than with the spin-echo technique. On spin-echo images, flowing blood appears with low signal intensity, whereas gradient-echo images display the blood pool with high signal intensity. As a gradient-echo technique, cine MRI is prone to susceptibility effects, which occur in the presence of paramagnetic substances that cause local magnetic field inhomogeneities. Subacute and chronic thrombus containing substances that induce a magnetic susceptibility effect has low signal intensity on gradient-echo images. This feature can facilitate the delineation of these intraluminal masses, which may have low signal intensity in contrast to the bright signal of intracavitary blood. Rarely, tumors that contain abundant iron or calcium may have low signal intensity and are delineated optimally on cine gradient-echo sequences.

BENIGN PRIMARY CARDIAC TUMORS

Approximately 80% of all primary cardiac tumors are benign (6). Although these tumors do not metastasize or invade locally, they may lead to significant morbidity and mortality by causing arrhythmias, obstruction, or embolism. The clinical presentation is determined by the location of the tumor, which may interfere with normal conduction pathways and produce arrhythmias, obstruct blood flow, or diminish compliance or contractility through replacement of myocardium.

Myxoma

Myxoma, the most common benign cardiac tumor, accounts for 25% of primary cardiac masses. It is located in the left atrium (LA) in 75% and in the right atrium (RA) in 20% of cases (11). This tumor is usually spherical in shape, but the shape may vary during the cardiac cycle because of its gelatinous consistency. LA myxomas are typically attached by a narrow pedicle to the area of the fossa ovalis (Figs. 9.1 and 9.2). Infrequently, myxomas have a wide base of attachment to the atrial septum (10) (Fig. 9.3). However, this shape is more frequently encountered with malignant tumors and must raise the suspicion of such a process. The extent of attachment may be difficult to assess for large tumors, which nearly fill the entire cavity, so that they are compressed against the septum. As a result, the tumor appears to have broad contact with the atrial septum on static MR images. Myxomas can grow through a patent foramen ovale and extend into both atria, a condition that has been described as a "dumbbell" appearance (12). Cine MRI permits an evaluation of tumor motion and may help to identify the site and length of attachment of the tumor to the wall(s) of cardiac chamber(s) (13). With this technique, myxomas have been shown to prolapse into the corresponding ventricle during diastole.

Usually, myxomas display an intermediate signal intensity (isointense to the myocardium) on T1-weighted spin-echo images (7,14). On T2-weighted spin-echo images, myxomas usually have a higher signal intensity than myocardium. However, myxomas with lower signal intensity have also been observed (15,16). This variable appearance is the consequence of a variable content of water-rich myxo-

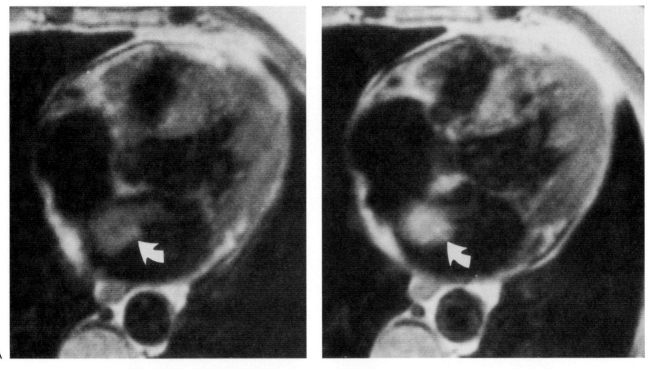

A

B

FIGURE 9.1. Myxoma arising from the septum of the left atrium. Axial T1-weighted spin-echo images before **(A)** and after **(B)** the administration of Gd-DTPA (gadolinium ethylenediamine pentaacetic acid) show a mass in the left atrium *(arrow)*. The mass is isointense to the myocardium on the nonenhanced image. After the administration of contrast medium, the mass enhances.

matous stroma in comparison with the components that have a short T2 relaxation time. Fibrous stroma, calcification, and the deposition of paramagnetic iron following interstitial hemorrhage can reduce the signal intensity of the tumor on T2-weighted spin-echo images (17,18). Rarely, myxomas have been reported to be invisible on spin-echo

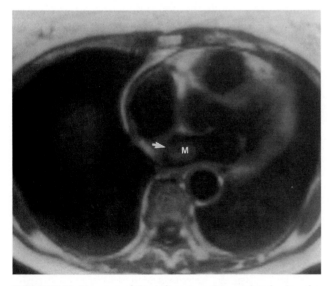

FIGURE 9.2. Myxoma of the left atrium. T1-weighted spin-echo image. The myxoma *(M)* is attached by a narrow pedicle *(arrow)* to the atrial septum.

images because of a lack of contrast with the dark blood pool (15). Such tumors can be delineated with cine MRI, on which they appear with high contrast against the surrounding bright blood. Most myxomas show increased signal intensity after the administration of Gd-DTPA on T1-weighted images, which is most probably secondary to an increased interstitial space and therefore larger distribution volume of the contrast agent within the tumor than in normal tissue (19).

Lipoma and Lipomatous Hypertrophy of the Atrial Septum

Lipomas are reported to be the second most common benign cardiac tumor in adults but may be actually be the most common. They may occur at any age but are encountered most frequently in middle-aged and elderly adults. Lipomas consist of encapsulated mature adipose cells and fetal fat cells. The tumor consistency is soft, and lipomas may grow to a large size without causing symptoms. Lipomas are typically located in the RA (Fig. 9.4) or atrial septum (20). They arise from the endocardial surface and have a broad base of attachment. Lipomas have the same signal intensity as subcutaneous and epicardial fat on all MRI sequences. Because fat has a short T1 relaxation time, lipomas have high signal intensity on T1-weighted images, which can be suppressed with fat-saturating pulse sequences (Figs. 9.4 and 9.5). Usu-

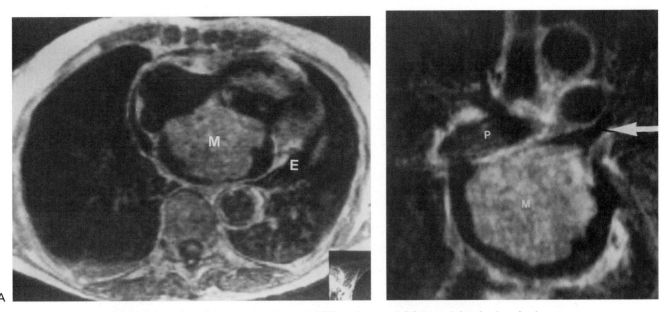

FIGURE 9.3. Left atrial myxoma. Transaxial **(A)** and coronal **(B)** T1-weighted spin-echo images demonstrate the large mass arising from the atrial septum. The tumor is attached by a broad base to the atrial septum. Nearly the entire left atrium is filled by the tumor *(M)*. Pericardial effusion *(E)* is present. *P,* right pulmonary artery; *arrow,* pulmonary vein. (Courtesy of A. Lomonoco, M.D., Tucson, Arizona.)

ally, they appear with homogeneous signal intensity but may have a few thin septations (21). They do not enhance after the administration of contrast material (21). On T2-weighted images, lipomas have intermediate signal intensity.

Lipomas are considered to be distinct from lipomatous hypertrophy of the atrial septum. Lipomatous hypertrophy of the atrial septum is more common and may have a greater

clinical effect, as this lesion can be a cause of supraventricular arrhythmias. It is usually associated with older age, but not with obesity. Lipomatous hypertrophy is defined as a deposition of fat in the atrial septum around the fossa ovalis that exceeds 2 cm in transverse diameter (21). It spares the fossa ovalis, a characteristic feature that is clearly delineated with T1-weighted spin-echo images. Lipomatous hypertro-

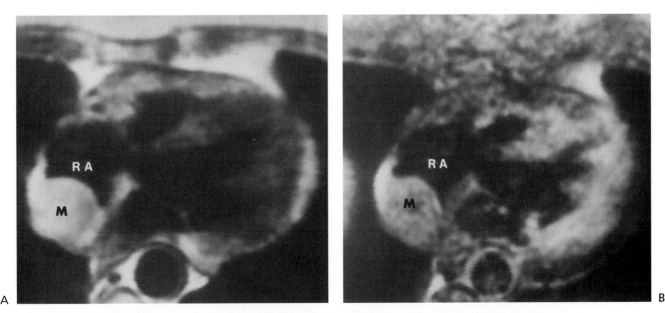

FIGURE 9.4. Lipoma. T1-weighted spin-echo images without **(A)** and with **(B)** fat saturation show a mass *(M)* in the right atrium *(RA)*. The tumor has a sharp border to the myocardium. Signal intensity is decreased after the application of fat saturation.

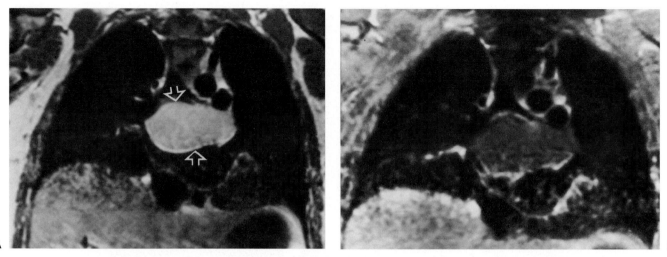

A   B

FIGURE 9.5. Paracardial lipoma. Coronal T1-weighted spin-echo images without **(A)** and with **(B)** fat saturation. The mass is located above the left atrium and demonstrates sharp borders *(arrows).* The bright signal of the tumor is depleted by fat saturation.

phy has the same cellular composition as lipoma but is not encapsulated and infiltrates into the tissue of the atrial septum. It is not a true neoplasm. Fatty tissue may extend from the septum into both atria to a considerable degree. Signal intensity on MRI is similar to that of lipomas (22). MRI is used for tissue characterization, delineation of the extent of the fat, and the evaluation of possible caval obstruction (23).

Papillary Fibroelastoma

Papillary fibroelastomas constitute approximately 10% of benign primary cardiac tumors (10). Fibroelastomas usually present in the seventh decade of life. These tumors consist of avascular fronds of connective tissue lined by endothelium. Papillary fibroelastomas are attached to the valves by a short pedicle in approximately 90% of cases. They usually do not exceed 1 cm in diameter. Papillary fibroelastomas have been found to occur on the aortic (29%), mitral (25%), pulmonary (13%), and tricuspid valves (17%) (24). Right-sided tumors usually remain asymptomatic. Symptoms associated with fibroelastoma typically relate to the embolization of thrombi, which accumulate on the tumor (24). Because of their high content of fibrous tissue, they have low signal intensity on T2-weighted images (25). The diagnosis of these valvular tumors is challenging because of their small size, low contrast relative to the blood pool on spin-echo images, and location on the rapidly moving valves (10). However, with recent advances in fast MR sequences and improved homogeneity of the bright blood pool signal, the visualization of valve motion during the cardiac cycle has become possible (26). Small masses attached to valves have been accurately depicted with MRI (27). In many cases, such lesions can be assessed only with cine MRI. In these cases, signal intensity characteristics after the administration of Gd-DTPA cannot be evaluated, and the differential diag-

nosis between thrombus and tumor may not be feasible (28). Cine MRI can be used to assess the effect of valvular tumors on valve function; it demonstrates jet flow caused by either obstruction or regurgitation (28).

Rhabdomyoma

In children, rhabdomyomas are the most common cardiac tumors, comprising 40% of all cardiac tumors in this age group (10). One-third to one-half of rhabdomyomas are found in patients with tuberous sclerosis. Rhabdomyomas may vary in size and are frequently multiple (Fig. 9.6). They

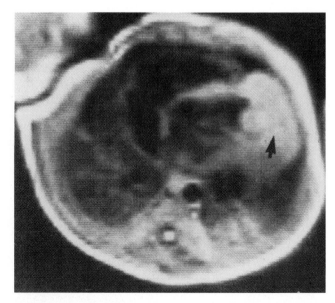

FIGURE 9.6. Rhabdomyoma. T1-weighted spin-echo image demonstrating multiple masses with high signal intensity in the walls of both ventricles. The largest lesion is located in the left ventricle *(arrow).*

are characterized by an intramural location and involve equally the left ventricle (LV) and right ventricle (RV). Small, entirely intramural tumors may be difficult to identify (29). Larger tumors distort the shape of the myocardial wall or may bulge into the cavity. Larger tumors can also distort the epicardial contour of the heart. Rhabdomyomas may have a signal intensity similar to that of normal myocardium on spin-echo images, cine MRI, and contrast-enhanced T1-weighted spin-echo images (13). They also have been reported to have a high signal intensity on T1-weighted spin-echo images and may display hyperenhancement after the administration of gadolinium contrast media (30,31).

Fibroma

Fibroma is the second most common benign cardiac tumor in children. It is a connective tissue tumor that is composed of fibroblasts interspersed among collagen fibers. It arises within the myocardial walls. Unlike most other primary cardiac tumors, fibromas usually do not display cystic changes, hemorrhage, or focal necrosis, but dystrophic calcification is common. Fibromas may cause arrhythmias and have been reported to be associated with sudden death (32). Approximately 30% of these tumors remain asymptomatic and may be discovered incidentally because of heart murmurs, ECG changes, or abnormalities on chest roentgenography (32). Fibromas occur most often within the septum or anterior wall of the RV and can reach a large diameter. On T2-weighted

MR images, they are characteristically hypointense to the surrounding myocardium, which is compatible with the short T2 relaxation time of fibrous tissue. On T1-weighted images, fibromas may appear isointense to the myocardium. Usually, fibromas show little or no contrast enhancement after the administration of Gd-DTPA (6). However, Gd-DTPA has been effectively used to demarcate these intramural tumors more clearly from normal myocardium (7) (Figs. 9.7 and 9.8). Enhancement of normal myocardium has been shown to be as high as 42% ± 17% (12). Hyperenhancement of compressed myocardium at the margin of the tumor facilitates delineation of the borders of the nonenhancing tumor (12).

The differential diagnosis for intramural masses in children is rhabdomyoma. If the tumor is solitary and has low signal intensity on T2-weighted images, fibroma is more likely. If multiple tumors are present, especially in cases of tuberous sclerosis, rhabdomyoma can confidently be diagnosed (33).

Pheochromocytoma

Pheochromocytomas arise from neuroendocrine cells clustered in the visceral paraganglia in the posterior wall of the LA, roof of the RA, and atrial septum, and along the coronary arteries. Pheochromocytomas can be found at each of these locations but are predominantly encountered in and around the LA (Fig. 9.9). Most are paracardial in location (Fig. 9.10). They usually have a broad interface with the

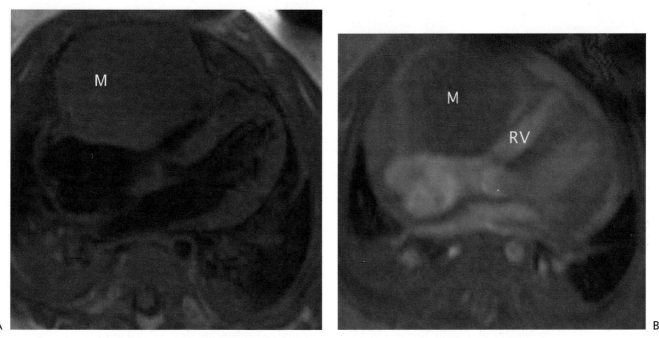

A   B

FIGURE 9.7. Fibroma of the left ventricle. Axial T1-weighted spin-echo **(A)** and cine MR **(B)** images show a large mass *(M)* centered in the right ventricular free wall that narrows the right ventricle *(RV)*. The mass demonstrates intermediate signal intensity on the spin-echo image and low signal intensity on the cine MR image.

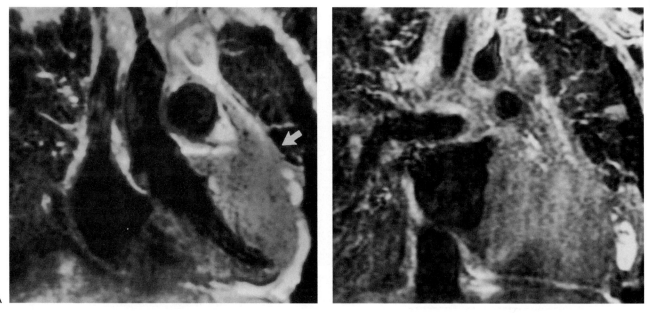

FIGURE 9.11. Left ventricular lymphosarcoma. Coronal T1-weighted spin-echo images at the level of the left ventricle **(A)** and left atrium **(B)** show the mass arising from the left ventricular free wall. The mass invades the pericardium *(arrow)* and extends into the left atrium and left upper lobe pulmonary vein.

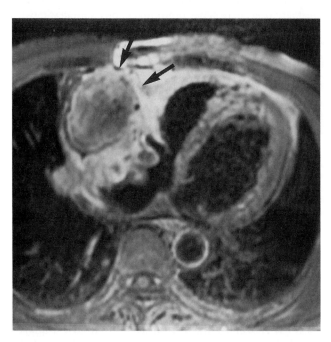

FIGURE 9.12. Right atrial angiosarcoma. Transaxial T1-weighted spin-echo image after the administration of contrast medium demonstrates a mass that fills the right atrium and extends into the mediastinum. There is disruption of the pericardial and mediastinal fat *(arrows)*.

Extension into the mediastinum and metastasis are also clear signs of malignancy. The organs most frequently involved are the lungs, pleurae, mediastinal lymph nodes, and liver. The inherent contrast between pericardium, which is delineated with a low signal intensity, and mediastinal fat, which has a high signal intensity, permits a clear delineation of mediastinal invasion (43).

The rapid growth of malignant cardiac tumors may cause focal necrosis in the central part of the tumor. Necrotic areas are delineated as regions of lower signal intensity within a hyperenhancing mass after the administration of Gd-DTPA (Fig. 9.14).

Angiosarcoma

Angiosarcomas are the most common malignant cardiac tumors in adults and constitute one-third of malignant cardiac tumors. They occur predominantly in men between 20 and 50 years of age. This entity has been divided into two clinicopathologic forms (44). Most frequently, angiosarcomas are found in the RA and usually arise from the atrial septum. In this form, no evidence of Kaposi sarcoma is found. Another form is characterized by evolvement of the epicardium or pericardium in the presence of Kaposi sarcoma. These lesions are usually small, localized, and asymptomatic. This form is associated with the acquired immunodeficiency syndrome (45). Angiosarcomas consist of ill-defined anastomotic vascular spaces that are lined by endothelial cells and avascular clusters of moderately pleomorphic spindle cells surrounded by collagen stroma (44). T1-weighted spin-echo imaging usually demonstrates heterogeneous signal in-

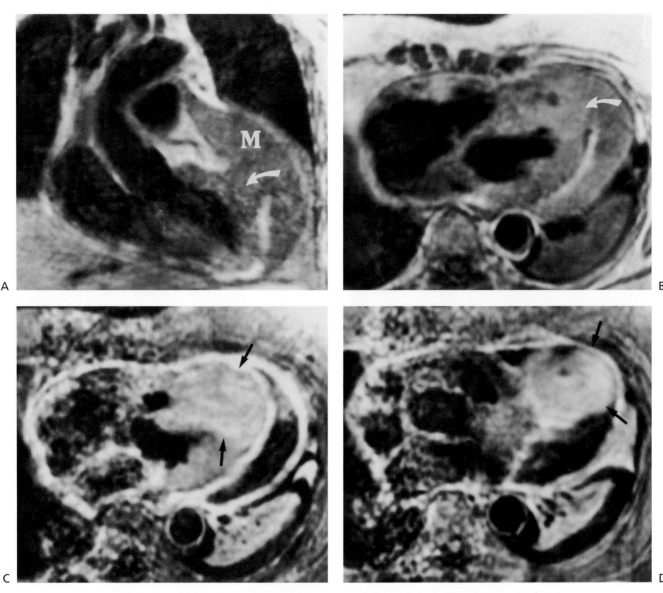

FIGURE 9.13. Angiosarcoma of the left ventricle. T1-weighted spin-echo images in the coronal **(A)** and transaxial **(B)** planes and transaxial images with fat saturation after the administration of contrast medium at the base of the heart **(C)** and near the apex **(D)**. Before the administration of contrast material, the tumor *(M)* cannot readily be distinguished from the pericardial effusion, especially in regions where pericardial fat is absent *(arrows in A and B)*. After the administration of Gd-DTPA (gadolinium diethylenetriamine pentaacetic acid), the tumor and pericardium demonstrate hyperenhancement. Effective differentiation from the surrounding normal myocardium *(arrows in C)* and the pericardial effusion *(arrows in D)* is possible.

tensity of the tumor with focal areas of high signal intensity, which presumably represent hemorrhage (46). However, angiosarcomas can also have homogeneous signal intensity (Fig. 9.15). After the administration of contrast medium, angiosarcomas show hyperenhancement (Fig. 9.16). Some of the tumors show regions of low signal intensity on both T1- and T2-weighted images. These central regions have a high signal intensity on cine gradient-echo images and represent vascular channels. This finding is often described as a "cauliflower" appearance (47). Cases with diffuse pericardial

infiltration have been found to show linear hyperenhancement along vascular spaces (48).

Rhabdomyosarcoma

Rhabdomyosarcomas are the most common malignant cardiac tumors in children. They can arise anywhere in the myocardium. Rhabdomyosarcomas are often multiple. Their signal intensity on MRI is variable. Rhabdomyosarcomas may be isointense to the myocardium on T1- and T2-

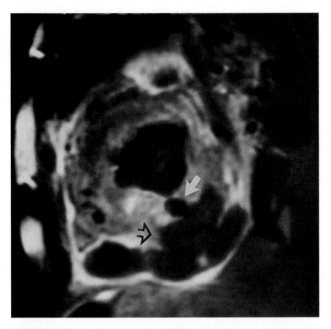

FIGURE 9.14. Left ventricular rhabdomyosarcoma. Sagittal T1-weighted spin-echo image after the administration of contrast medium demonstrates a mass with central necrosis *(arrow)*. A loculated pericardial effusion is adjacent to the necrotic area *(open arrow)*.

weighted images, but areas of necrosis can exhibit heterogeneous signal intensity and patchy hyperenhancement after the administration of Gd-DTPA (29,49) (Fig. 9.14). Extracardiac extension into the pulmonary arteries and descending aorta has been clearly delineated with MRI (50).

Other Sarcomas (Fibrosarcoma, Osteosarcoma, Leiomyosarcoma, Liposarcoma)

Other possible primary sarcomas are fibrosarcomas, osteosarcomas, leiomyosarcomas, and liposarcomas. These all are rare tumors, comprising approximately 4% of primary cardiac masses (10). The signal intensity characteristics of these entities are nonspecific (51,52). On T1-weighted images, signal intensity is isointense to normal myocardium (Fig. 9.17), whereas it is hyperintense on T2-weighted images. Most of these tumors show increased signal intensity on T1-weighted images after the administration of Gd-DTPA (53–55), so that the lesions are more conspicuous and the delineation of the tumor margins is increased. As mentioned previously, findings on MRI that suggest malignancy are involvement of more than one chamber or great vessel, extension to the pericardium or beyond, and necrosis of the tumor (42).

Lymphoma

Primary cardiac lymphoma is less common than secondary lymphoma involving the heart, which usually represents the

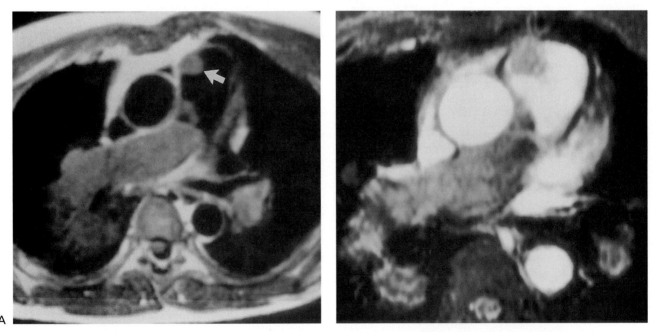

A   B

FIGURE 9.15. Angiosarcoma of the pulmonary artery. T1-weighted spin-echo **(A)** and cine MR **(B)** images at the level of the main and right pulmonary arteries. A mass fills the right pulmonary artery. A tumor nodule is attached to the wall of the main pulmonary artery *(arrow)*. The mass shows intermediate signal intensity on the cine MR image, which indicates tumor rather than subacute or chronic clot.

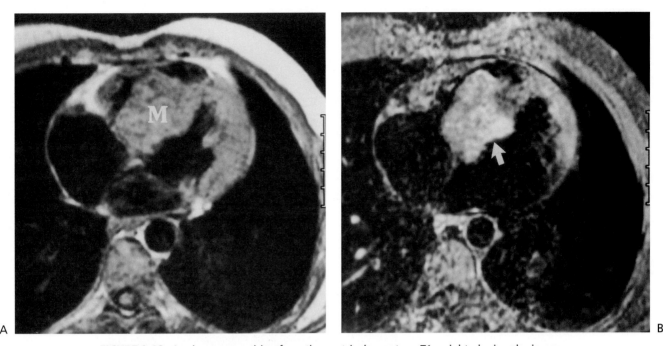

FIGURE 9.16. Angiosarcoma arising from the ventricular septum. T1-weighted spin-echo images before **(A)** and after **(B)** the administration of Gd-DTPA (gadolinium diethylenetriamine pentaacetic acid) and fat saturation. The mass *(M)* shows hyperenhancement *(arrow)* after the administration of contrast material. Hyperenhancement facilitates demarcation from normal myocardium.

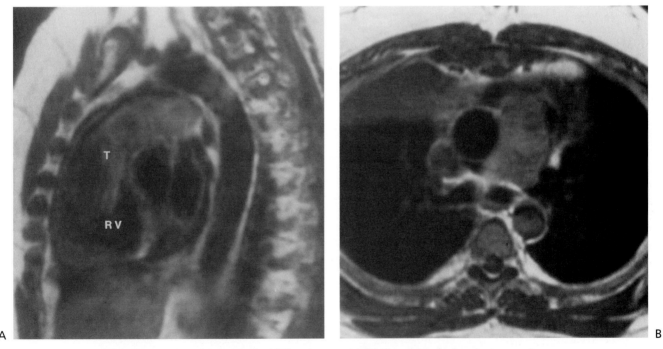

FIGURE 9.17. Liposarcoma. Sagittal **(A)** and transaxial **(B)** T1-weighted spin-echo images demonstrate the tumor *(T)* in the right ventricle *(RV)*. The tumor extends into the right ventricular outflow tract and pulmonary artery.

spread of non-Hodgkin lymphoma (56). Primary lymphoma of the heart most often occurs in immunocompromised patients and is highly aggressive. Almost all primary cardiac lymphomas are B-cell lymphomas (56,57). Although primary cardiac lymphoma is rare, it is mandatory to suspect this entity in the diagnosis because early chemotherapy appears to be effective (58). The tumor arises most often on the right side of the heart, especially in the RA, but has also been found in the other chambers (59). A large pericardial effusion is frequently present. Variable morphology of the masses has been described; both circumscribed polypoid and ill-defined infiltrative lesions have been reported (60). Lymphomas may appear hypointense to the myocardium on T1-weighted and hyperintense on T2-weighted images (59,60). After the administration of Gd-DTPA, homogeneous or heterogeneous enhancement of the tumor, depending on the presence of necrosis, may be seen (61).

SECONDARY CARDIAC TUMORS

Secondary tumors of the heart are 30- to 40-fold more frequent than primary tumors. In patients with malignancies, the reported frequency ranges from 3% to 18% (62). In general, three different patterns of involvement of the heart can be distinguished: (a) direct extension from intrathoracic tumors (mediastinum or lung), (b) spread from the abdomen through the inferior vena cava into the RA, and (c) metastasis.

Direct Extension from Adjacent Tumors

Tumors of the lung and mediastinum can infiltrate the pericardium and heart directly (Fig. 9.18). It is important to recognize invasion of the heart because such a tumor is usually nonresectable. In mediastinal lymphoma, possible invasion of the pericardium can change the staging of the tumor. MRI is especially suited for delineating paracardiac tumors and possible extension into the heart because of its wide field of view. MRI clearly shows extension of these tumors to the cardiac structures and possible evidence of hemorrhagic or nonhemorrhagic pericardial effusion. In studies comparing the accuracy of computed tomography with that of MRI for staging advanced lung cancer invading the cardiac chambers, MRI was more effective in demonstrating invasion of the pericardium and myocardium (63,64).

Metastasis

Melanomas, leukemias, and lymphomas (Figs. 9.19 and 9.20) most frequently metastasize to the heart, but cardiac metastases can arise from almost any malignant tumor in the body. Melanomas have the highest frequency of seeding into the heart and have been found in 64% of patients with this entity at autopsy (65). The mechanism of metastatic

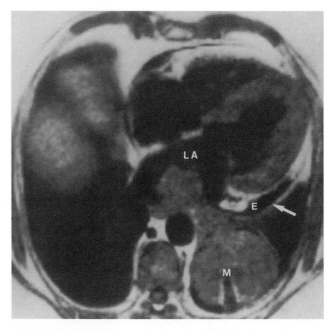

FIGURE 9.18. Pulmonary tumor extending into the left atrium. The T1-weighted spin-echo image demonstrates the mass *(M)* extending into the left atrium *(LA)*. Pericardial effusion *(E)* is present. The pericardium is clearly visible *(arrow)*.

spread to the heart is either direct seeding at the endocardium, passage of tumor emboli through the coronary arteries, or retrograde lymphatic flow through bronchomediastinal lymphatic channels (6). MRI is highly effective for delineating the extent of secondary cardiac tumors (Figs. 9.21 and 9.22) and assessing potential resectability (66).

Transvenous Extension into the Heart

The third pathway for the entry of secondary tumors into the heart is tumor infiltration of vessels connecting with cardiac cambers. Tumor thrombus arising from carcinoma of the kidney or adrenal gland can extend through the inferior vena cava into the RA (Fig. 9.23), and primary carcinoma of the thymus can extend through the superior vena cava into the RA. Carcinoma of the lung can invade pulmonary veins and grow into the LA or invade the superior vena cava (Fig. 9.24). The evaluation of the possible attachment of such tumors to the atrial wall is mandatory for surgical planning. If the atrial walls are not infiltrated, complete resection of the tumor may still be possible.

INTRACARDIAC THROMBUS

Thrombus is the most common intracardiac mass, involving most frequently the LV or LA. Atrial thrombus is most often seen in patients with mitral valve disease or atrial fibrillation. Mural thrombus is associated with akinetic or dyskinetic regions of the ventricle. It is most often located in the

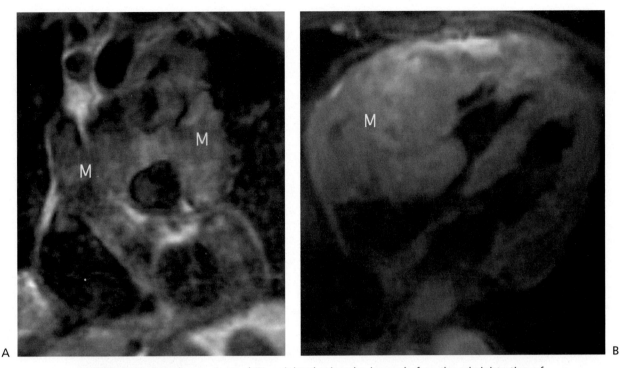

FIGURE 9.19. Lymphoma. Coronal T1-weighted spin-echo image before the administration of contrast material **(A)** and transaxial T1-weighted spin-echo image with fat saturation after the administration of Gd-DTPA (gadolinium diethylenetriamine pentaacetic acid) **(B)**. A large mediastinal mass *(M)* encases the main mediastinal vessels. The mass invades the wall of the right ventricle and extends into the right ventricular chamber. After the administration of Gd-DTPA, the mass enhances.

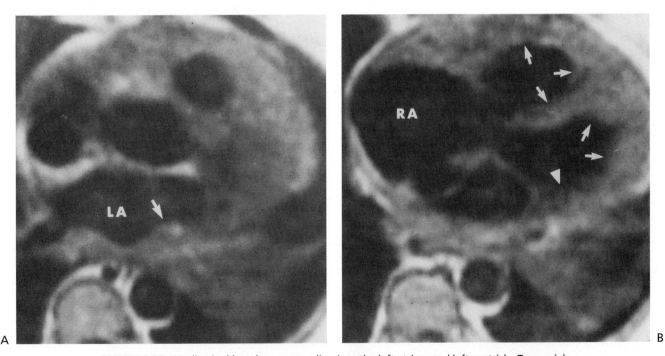

FIGURE 9.20. Mediastinal lymphoma extending into the left atrium and left ventricle. Transaxial spin-echo images at the level of the left atrium **(A)** and left ventricle **(B)** demonstrate the mass infiltrating the pericardium and posterior wall *(arrow in A)* of the left atrium *(LA)*. The mass invades the posterior left ventricular wall *(arrowhead)*. Thickening of the ventricular walls *(arrows in B)* was confirmed at autopsy to be secondary to the spread of lymphoma. *RA,* right atrium.

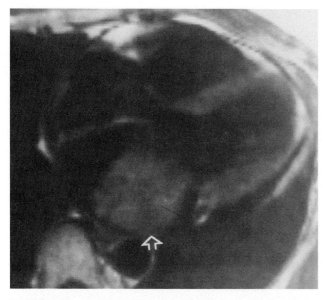

FIGURE 9.21. Metastatic tumor in the left atrium. The spin-echo image demonstrates a mass in the left atrial cavity. The tumor is attached at a narrow point to the left atrial wall *(arrow)*.

LV after myocardial infarction or in dilated cardiomyopathy (Fig. 9.25). However, any region of the ventricular cavity with static blood is prone to thrombus formation. MRI is especially advantageous for detecting thrombus in the LA appendage, which may be difficult to assess by means of transthoracic echocardiography.

On spin-echo images, the signal intensity of thrombus can vary from low to high depending on age-related changes in

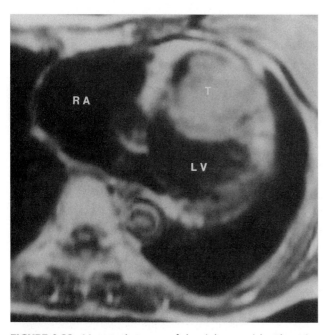

FIGURE 9.22. Metastatic tumor of the right ventricle. The spin-echo image demonstrates the tumor *(T)* in the right ventricle. *RA,* right atrium; *LV,* left ventricle.

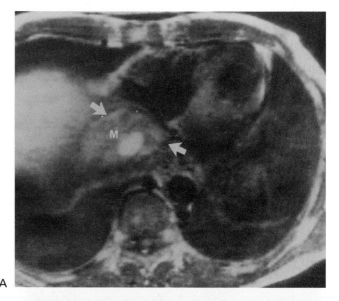

A

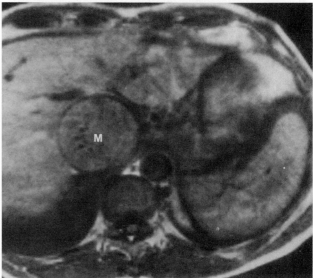

B

FIGURE 9.23. Adrenal tumor with extension through the inferior vena cava into the right atrium. T1-weighted spin-echo images at the level of the right atrium **(A)** and liver **(B)** demonstrate the mass *(M)* extending through the inferior vena cava into the right atrium *(arrows)*. The high signal intensity within the tumor is caused by hemorrhage.

the composition of the thrombus (67). Thrombus can with time acquire paramagnetic hemoglobin breakdown products, such as intracellular methemoglobin and hemosiderin, or superparamagnetic substances, such as ferritin. Fresh thrombus usually shows high signal intensity on T1- and T2-weighted spin-echo images, whereas older thrombus may have low signal intensity on T1- and T2-weighted images (68,69). An intracavitary high signal on spin-echo images caused by slowly flowing blood may be difficult to distinguish from thrombus (70,71). However, this problem can be overcome either by using the spin-echo sequences after inversion recovery pulses to null intracavitary signal or by using cine MRI (72,73).

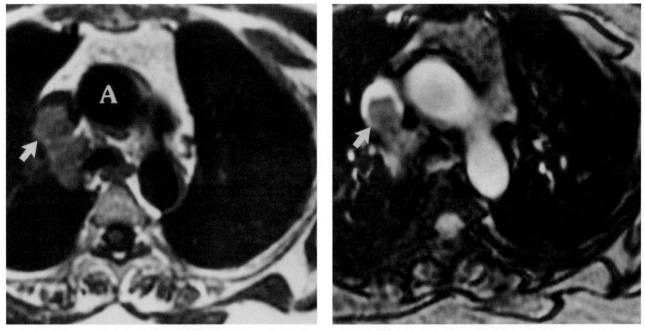

FIGURE 9.24. Pulmonary carcinoma infiltrating the superior vena cava. Transaxial T1-weighted spin echo **(A)** and cine MR **(B)** images show a mass adjacent to the superior vena cava. The mass has infiltrated the vessel and fills it partially *(arrow). A,* aorta.

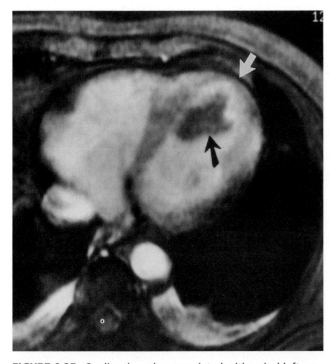

FIGURE 9.25. Cardiac thrombus associated with apical left ventricular aneurysm. Transaxial cine MR image. The thrombus demonstrates low signal intensity *(black arrow).* An apical left ventricular aneurysm is present *(white arrow).*

DIFFERENTIATION BETWEEN TUMOR AND BLOOD CLOT

The distinction between blood clot and tumor is more reliably attained with gradient-echo sequences. The gradient-echo technique is more sensitive to susceptibility and T2* effects than is the spin-echo technique. As the various blood degeneration products pass through the different stages of magnetic susceptibility, they continue to cause shortening of T2* relaxivity; the result is low signal intensity of the thrombus on gradient-echo images (Fig. 9.26). An exception to this generalization is fresh thrombus, which can have high signal intensity (69). Tumor tissue usually is hyperintense in comparison with myocardium and skeletal muscle on T2-weighted spin-echo images. However, some myxomas can produce low signal and so mimic thrombus. Another method for differentiating between tumor and clot is to use Gd-DTPA–enhanced T1-weighted images. Thrombus does not enhance after the administration of Gd-DTPA, whereas tumors show enhancement (7). Tumor can usually be differentiated from thrombus by combining gradient-echo images and T1-weighted spin-echo images after the administration of Gd-DTPA.

PITFALLS: DIFFERENTIATION OF CARDIAC MASSES FROM NORMAL ANATOMIC VARIANTS

Diagnostic difficulties may arise from the misdiagnosis of normal anatomical variants, such as a prominent crista ter-

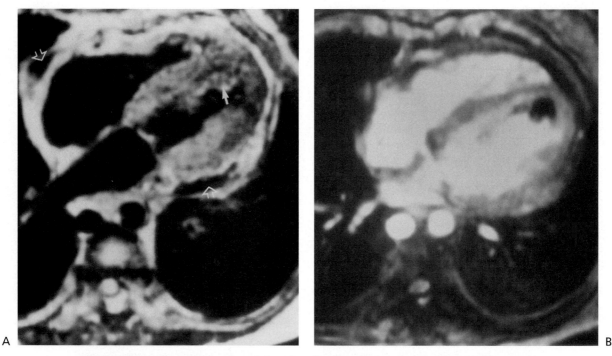

A   B

FIGURE 9.26. Left ventricular thrombus and pericardial effusion. Transaxial T1-weighted spin-echo **(A)** and cine MR **(B)** images. Thrombus is present at the apex of the left ventricle *(arrow).* On cine MR images, the thrombus demonstrates low signal intensity. *Open arrows,* pericardial effusion.

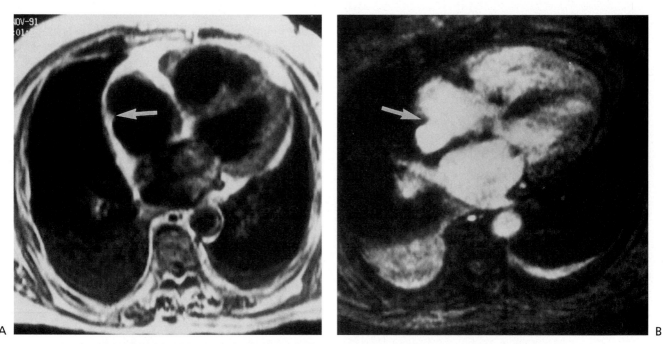

A   B

FIGURE 9.27. Axial spin-echo **(A)** and cine MR **(B)** images demonstrate prominence of crista terminalis projecting into the right atrium *(arrow).* (From Meier RA, Hartnell GG. MRI of right atrial pseudomass: is it really a diagnostic problem? *J Comput Assist Tomogr* 1994;18:398, with permission.)

minalis, eustachian valve, or Chiari network (74). The crista terminalis is a fibromuscular band extending between the ostia of the superior and inferior venae cavae on the posterior RA wall and represents a residuum of the septum spurium where the sinus venosus was incorporated into the RA wall (75). The Chiari network is a reticulum situated in the RA. It is attached to the region of the crista terminalis and extends to the valves of the inferior vena cava and coronary sinus, or sometimes to the floor of the RA near the ostium of the coronary sinus. The Chiari network is derived from the valvulae venosae (75). These structures regress to variable degrees, and nodule-like forms in the RA may be visible on MRI in some patients (Fig. 9.27). Awareness of these variants can prevent misinterpretation as mass lesions.

REFERENCES

1. Lam KJ, Dickens P, Chan AC, et al. Tumors of the heart: a 20-year experience with a review of 12,485 consecutive autopsies. *Arch Pathol Lab Med* 1993;117:1027.
2. Blondeau P. Primary cardiac tumors: French studies of 533 cases [Review]. *Thorac Cardiovasc Surg* 1990;2:192.
3. Arciniegas E, Hakimi M, Farooki ZQ, et al. Primary cardiac tumors in children. *J Thorac Cardiovasc Surg* 1980;79:582.
4. Brown JJ, Barakos JA, Higgins CB. Magnetic resonance imaging of cardiac and paracardiac masses. *J Thorac Imaging* 1989;4:58.
5. Task Force Report of the European Society of Cardiology/Association of European Cardiologists. The clinical role of magnetic resonance in cardiovascular disease. *Eur Heart J* 1998;19:19.
6. Fujita N, Caputo GR, Higgins CB. Diagnosis and characterization of intracardial masses by magnetic resonance imaging. *Am J Card Imaging* 1994;8:69.
7. Funari M, Fujita N, Peck WW, et al. Cardiac tumors: assessment with Gd-DTPA enhanced MR imaging. *J Comput Assist Tomogr* 1991;15:953.
8. Niwa K, Tashima K, Terai M, et al. Contrast-enhanced magnetic resonance imaging of cardiac tumors in children. *Am Heart J* 1989;118:424.
9. Araoz PA, Mulvagh SL, Tazlaar HD, et al. CT and MR imaging of benign primary cardiac neoplasms with echocardiographic correlation. *Radiographics* 2000;20:1303.
10. Araoz PA, Eklund HE, Welch TJ, et al. CT and MR imaging of primary cardiac malignancies. *Radiographics* 1999;19:1421.
11. MacGowan SW, Sidhu P, Aherne T, et al. Atrial myxoma: national incidence, diagnosis and surgical management. *Ir J Med Sci* 1993;162:223.
12. Semelka RC, Shoenut JP, Wilson ME, et al. Cardiac masses: signal intensity features on spin-echo, gradient-echo, gadolinium-enhanced spin-echo and turbo FLASH images. *J Magn Reson Imaging* 1992;2:415.
13. Go RT, O'Donnell JK, Underwood DA, et al. Comparison of gated cardiac MRI and 2D echocardiography of intracardiac neoplasm. *AJR Am J Roentgenol* 1985;145:21.
14. Conces DJ Jr, Vix VA, Klatte EC. Gated MR imaging of left atrial myxomas. *Radiology* 1985;156:445.
15. Pflugfelder PW, Wisenberg G, Boughner DR. Detection of atrial myxoma by magnetic resonance imaging. *Am J Cardiol* 1985;55:242.
16. Scholz TD, Boskis M, Roust L, et al. Noninvasive diagnosis of recurrent familiar left atrial myxoma: observations with echocardiography, ultrafast computed tomography, nuclear magnetic resonance imaging, and *in vitro* relaxometry. *Am J Card Imaging* 1989;3:142.
17. Masui T, Takahashi M, Miura K, et al. Cardiac myxoma: identification of tumoral hemorrhage and calcification on MR images. *AJR Am J Roentgenol* 1995;164:850.
18. Matsuoka H, Hamada M, Honda T. Morphologic and histologic characterization of cardiac myxomas by magnetic resonance imaging. *Angiology* 1996;47:693.
19. Higgins CB. Acquired heart diseases. In: Higgins CB, Hricak H, Helms CA, eds. *Magnetic resonance imaging of the body.* Philadelphia: Lippincott–Raven Publishers, 1997:409–460.
20. Mousseaux E, Idy-Peretti I, Bittoun J, et al. MR tissue characterization of a right atrial mass: diagnosis of a lipoma. *J Comput Assist Tomogr* 1992;16:148.
21. Kaplan KR, Rifkin MD. MR diagnosis of lipomatous infiltration of the intraatrial septum. *AJR Am J Roentgenol* 1989;153:495.
22. Levine RA, Weyman AE, Dinsmore RE, et al. Noninvasive tissue characterization: diagnosis of lipomatous hypertrophy of the atrial septum by nuclear magnetic resonance imaging. *J Am Coll Cardiol* 1986;7:688.
23. Kriegshauser JS, Julsrud PR, Lund JT. MR imaging of fat in and around the heart. *AJR Am J Roentgenol* 1990;155:271.
24. Grinda JM, Couetil JP, Chauvaud S, et al. Cardiac valve papillary fibroelastoma: surgical excision for revealed or potential embolization. *J Thorac Cardiovasc Surg* 1999;117:106.
25. Al-Mohammad A, Pambakian H, Young C. Fibroelastoma: case report and review of the literature. *Heart* 1998;79:301.
26. Atkinson DJ, Edelmann RR. Cineangiography of the heart in a single breath hold with a segmented turbo FLASH sequence. *Radiology* 1991;178:357.
27. Kamata J, Yoshioka K, Nasu M, et al. Myxoma of the mitral valve detected by echocardiography and magnetic resonance imaging. *Eur Heart J* 1995;16:1435.
28. Wintersprenger BJ, Becker CR, Gulbins H, et al. Tumors of the cardiac valves: imaging findings in magnetic resonance imaging, electron beam computed tomography, and echocardiography. *Eur Radiol* 2000;10:443.
29. Rienmüller R, Lloret JL, Tiling R, et al. MR imaging of pediatric cardiac tumors previously diagnosed by echocardiography. *J Comput Assist Tomogr* 1989;13:621.
30. Winkler M, Higgins CB. Suspected intracardiac masses: evaluation with MR imaging. *Radiology* 1987;165:117.
31. Lund JT, Ehman RL, Julsrud PR, et al. Cardiac masses: assessment by MR imaging. *AJR Am J Roentgenol* 1989;152:469.
32. Cina SJ, Smialek JE, Burke AP, et al. Primary cardiac tumors causing sudden death: a review of the literature. *Am J Forensic Med Pathol* 1996;17:271.
33. Beghetti M, Gow RM, Haney I, et al. Pediatric primary benign cardiac tumors: a 15-years review. *Am Heart J* 1997;134:1107.
34. Arai A, Naruse M, Naruse K, et al. Cardiac malignant pheochromocytoma with bone metastases. *Intern Med* 1998;37:940.
35. Cruz PA, Mahidara S, Ticzon A, et al. Malignant cardiac paraganglioma. *J Thorac Cardiovasc Surg* 1984;87:942.
36. Hamilton BH, Francis IR, Gross BH, et al. Intrapericardial paraganglioma (pheochromocytoma): imaging features. *AJR Am J Roentgenol* 1997;168:109.
37. Orr LA, Pettigrew RI, Churchwell AL, et al. Gadolinium utilization in the MR evaluation of cardiac paraganglioma. *Clin Imaging* 1997;21:404.
38. Brodwater B, Erasmus J, McAdams HP, et al. Pericardial hemangioma. *J Comput Assist Tomogr* 1996;20:954.
39. Seline TH, Gross BH, Francis IR. CT and MR imaging of mediastinal hemangiomas. *J Comput Assist Tomogr* 1990;14:766.
40. Schurawitzki H, Stiglbauer R, Klepetko W, et al. CT and MRI in benign mediastinal hemangioma. *Clin Radiol* 1991;43:91.
41. Kemp JL, Kessler RM, Raizada V, et al. MR and CT appearance of cardiac hemangioma. *J Comput Assist Tomogr* 1996;20:482.

Noninvasive methods for accurately and reproducibly quantifying the severity of valvular heart disease and ventricular dimensions and function may improve patient management. Several MRI techniques may be valuable for monitoring valvular heart disease. The purpose of this chapter is to review morphologic and functional MRI methods; we focus especially on validation and potential pitfalls.

MR TECHNIQUES

Volume Measurements

Right ventricular (RV) and left ventricular (LV) dimensions can be quantified by volumetry of a set of contiguous MR slices encompassing the heart. Initially, measurements were performed with a spin-echo technique and the acquisition of a few image frames during the cardiac cycle at each spatial position. To ensure an image at true end-systole (defined as the time in the cardiac cycle when the volume of the ventricular cavity is smallest), a high degree of temporal resolution is required, which is generally provided by cine gradient-echo imaging (18). The use of breath-hold cine gradient-echo imaging (19) or echo-planar imaging (20) substantially reduces both imaging time and respiration artifacts. From an entire image series covering the cardiac cycle, an image is selected at each spatial position at both end-diastole and end-systole, and the ventricular end-diastolic and end-systolic volumes are calculated by adding the planimetrically measured areas of the cavities multiplied by the slice thickness. The ventricular myocardial mass or, more precisely, the myocardial volume can be determined in a similar way (21). Derived parameters, such as stroke volume and ventricular ejection fraction, can be assessed from the end-diastolic and end-systolic volumes. Generally, the imaging plane for the volume measurements is transverse or oriented along the short axis of the heart. With transverse imaging, slices transect the myocardial wall obliquely, so that partial volume effects are created. Obviously, this is a source of error when planimetry is intended to take place along the presumed endocardial or epicardial border. With the use of short-axis slices, it is generally assumed that the partial volume effects are less pronounced. In this direction, however, problems may arise in defining the valvular planes, especially the atrioventricular plane. These may be overcome at least in part by using an end-diastolic horizontal, long-axis view as a base image for the short-axis images and starting the volume measurements with the most basal slice positioned across the atrioventricular valve plane. An additional pitfall in MR volume measurements is defining the endocardial and epicardial borders. Artifacts caused by respiration and blood pulsation and by poor blood–myocardial contrast resulting from slow flow may obscure the border definition. However, displaying the image series in a cine loop can help in the identification of borders by simplifying the differentiation between moving blood and myocardium.

Several studies have validated MR volume measurements of the dimensions and function of the LV (22–29) and RV (24,30–34) with quantitative reference techniques, such as indicator dilution, radionuclide angiography, and studies of postmortem hearts. MR volume measurements, in fact, may be considered as a gold standard for determining ventricular volume, stroke volume, ejection fraction, and myocardial mass, all of which are important measures of the hemodynamic consequences of valvular heart disease. Furthermore, MR volume measurements can be used to quantify valvular insufficiency. In the absence of valvular regurgitation, this method measures LV and RV stroke volumes with a differt of less than 5% (35,36). Consequently, regurgitant volume can be calculated as the difference between LV and RV stroke volumes, whereas the regurgitant fraction is determined as the ratio of regurgitant volume to LV stroke volume. It has been reported that the volume technique measures the regurgitant fraction with an accuracy of 90% when radionuclide ventriculography is used as the reference technique (37). Furthermore, the measurements are in agreement with semiquantitative grading by angiography or Doppler echocardiography (38,39). However, the technique is valid only for patients with a single insufficient valve. In patients with combined left- or right-sided regurgitation, the method assesses the total regurgitation; thus, a left-sided regurgitation is underestimated in the case of a concomitant regurgitant valve on the right side of the heart.

Signal-Void Phenomena

Cine gradient-echo imaging provides rapid imaging of flowing blood with high signal intensity because of the so-called inflow effect. However, the presence of complex flow patterns—including higher-order motion components such as acceleration and jerk and the formation of flow vortices in valvular regurgitant or stenotic lesions—may cause a signal void through an intravoxel dephasing of spins with subsequent cancellation of the net signal (40). This phenomenon can be used to visualize regurgitant and stenotic jets as discrete areas of low signal in image planes in the direction of the jet (41) (Fig. 10.1).

MR signal-void phenomena are valuable tools for valve location and semiquantitative studies of valvular blood flow. The technique has been found to be in concordance with color Doppler echocardiography and cardiac catheterization in the evaluation of aortic regurgitation (42–47) and mitral regurgitation (42,44,45,48–50), with a sensitivity of 90% or higher and a specificity of 93% or higher. Furthermore, the signal-void technique can be used for the semiquantitative grading of aortic stenosis (45,51) (Fig. 10.2) and mitral stenosis (45). However, the use of signal-void phenomena for quantitative measurements is impeded by the fact that the extent of the signal void depends on several parameters, such as echo time, flip angle, alignment between the imaging plane and jet, and display settings, and also hemody-

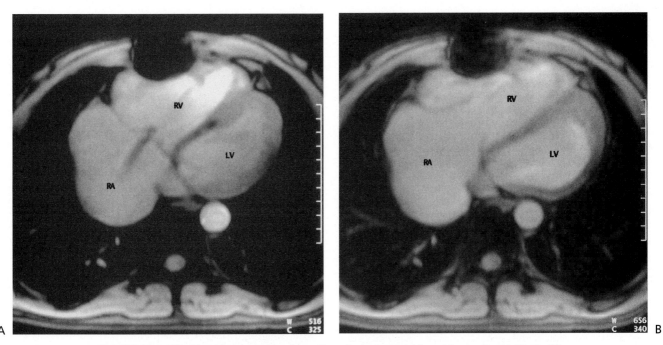

FIGURE 10.1. Signal-void phenomena through an incompetent tricuspid valve in a patient with a dilated right ventricle *(RV)* secondary to free pulmonary regurgitation after repair of tetralogy of Fallot. The complex flow pattern of the tricuspid regurgitant jet causes a discrete area of signal void in the right atrium *(RA)* during systole **(A)**. The tricuspid valve function during diastole is normal **(B)**. *LV,* left ventricle.

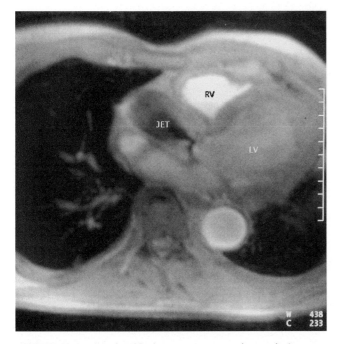

FIGURE 10.2. Signal-void phenomena at peak systole in a patient with severe aortic stenosis. *LV,* left ventricle; *JET,* stenotic jet; *RV,* right ventricle.

namic parameters, including transvalvular pressure gradient, orifice size, and cardiac chamber size (52,53). Moreover, a potential pitfall in the use of the signal-void technique is a naturally decreased signal intensity in normal hearts, such as at the walls of the LV outflow tract and aortic root during early systole, at the valvar leaflet tips just after opening or closure, and along the anterior mitral leaflet in early diastole (54). However, unlike valvular dysfunction, these phenomena are transient in healthy subjects, usually lasting only 50 to 100 milliseconds. Another drawback is that it may be necessary to examine two or more planes to appreciate the extent of the jet fully, particularly in mitral regurgitation, in which eccentric jets are common.

Another suggested application of the signal-void method is in the quantification of aortic regurgitant volume. For jets emerging through a small circular orifice in a flat plate, flow accelerates just proximal to the orifice, converging on the orifice in hemispheric shells of equal velocity. Theoretically, the area of the proximal signal loss, as detected by cinematographic gradient-echo imaging, is related to the degree of regurgitation and may be a better indicator of the grade of aortic regurgitation than is the size of the distal regurgitant jet. However, the technique is associated with several sources of error, such as the above-mentioned imaging and hemodynamic parameters, the relatively small size of the signal void, and the fact that most regurgitant orifices are neither flat nor circular. Despite these drawbacks, the technique has been shown to have a specificity of 100% and a sensitivity of more than 87% in the detection of aortic regurgitation (55,56).

Flow Measurement

Even before the development of MRI, quantitative flow measurements by MR were proposed (57), but the clinical application of MR flow quantification was not reported until the beginning of the 1980s. Flow quantification can be performed in two general approaches, based on either modulus or phase information (Fig. 10.3); examples are the time-of-flight (TOF) technique and the velocity-mapping technique, respectively. Presently, methods based on phase information are used most frequently for flow quantification.

Time-of-Flight Technique

When quantitative blood flow measurements are made with the TOF technique (also called *bolus tracking*), blood is labeled at one position within a vessel, and the distance that the labeled blood has moved in a given amount of time is subsequently determined (58,59). Usually, the labeling is performed with a saturation band (i.e., a radiofrequency pulse); this cancels out the MR signal in a predetermined slice, so that a dark line of low signal appears perpendicular to the vessel. Next, an image is obtained along the center of the vessel to measure how far the labeled blood has moved within a given period of time. One limitation of this technique is that the determination of the two-dimensional velocity profiles is laborious. However, in a study by Ambrosi et al. (60), the TOF technique was used to assess the severity of aortic regurgitation according to the length of the diastolic retrograde movement of a transverse saturation band

in the descending aorta. The results were in reasonable accordance with angiographic and Doppler grades, but the technique is only semiquantitative because aortic compliance and the diameter of the aorta affect the measurements.

Velocity-Mapping Technique

The theoretical framework for velocity mapping with the use of phase information was first described in 1982 by Moran (61), and early *in vivo* demonstrations of the technique were made by Van Dijk (62), Bryant et al. (63), and Nayler et al. (64). According to the Larmour equation (Eq. 1), spins exposed to a magnetic field obtain a resonance frequency proportional to the magnetic field strength and therefore a phase shift proportional to the time integral of the magnitude of the magnetic field.

$$\nu_0 = \gamma \cdot B_0/(2\pi) \qquad [1]$$

where ν_0 is the precession frequency, γ the gyromagnetic ratio specific for each nucleus, and B_0 the intensity of the static magnetic field. Consequently, the application of a magnetic field gradient results in a phase shift according to the location along the gradient. Consider the application of two consecutive magnetic field gradients with the same duration and magnitude, but with opposite signs (Fig. 10.4). When the first magnetic gradient is applied, all stationary spin groups (isochromate groups) accumulate a phase shift determined by their location in proportion to the magnetic field gradient (Fig. 10.4A). Immediately after the first gra-

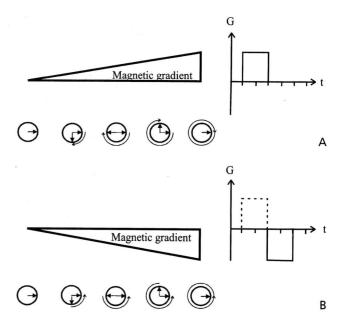

FIGURE 10.4. Application of a magnetic field gradient alters the precession frequency of spins. Thus, each stationary spin group (isochromate group) accumulates an additional phase shift according to its position along the gradient **(A)**. If another gradient with the same magnitude but opposite sign is applied, all spin groups lose their accumulated phase shift **(B)**. *G,* magnetic field gradient amplitude; *t,* time.

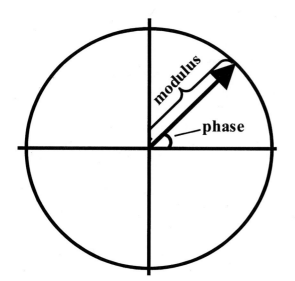

FIGURE 10.3. The information in each voxel of an MR image can be regarded as a vector, described by its magnitude (modulus information) and direction (phase information).

dient, the second magnetic field gradient is applied, and all the stationary spins lose their accumulated phase shift and obtain a net phase shift of zero (Fig. 10.4B). However, spins moving along the magnetic field gradients during their execution experience unequal positive and negative magnetic gradients, and consequently accumulate a net phase shift φ according to the motion (Fig. 10.5). The net phase shift φ can be calculated as follows:

$$\phi \sim \int G(t) \bullet x(t) dt \qquad [2]$$

where G(t) and x(t) describe the magnetic gradient amplitude and the position of the spins, respectively, as a function of time. In the case of a constant velocity v and magnetic gradient, Eq. 1 can be reduced to the following expression:

$$\phi_v \sim v \bullet G \bullet \int t \bullet dt \qquad [3]$$

where the phase shift is proportional to the velocity along the magnetic gradient. Consequently, the phase image can be regarded as a *velocity map* in which the phase shift in each voxel represents a velocity. Theoretically, the phase shift in voxels with stationary tissue should be zero, but additional phase shifts may be caused by factors other than motion. Examples of such factors are magnetic field inhomogeneities, local magnetic field gradients induced by variations in magnetic susceptibility between different tissues and tissue–air interfaces, and eddy currents. These problems may partly be overcome by creating an additional phase image with a different set of gradient amplitudes, which in turn has another

velocity sensitivity or often no velocity sensitivity at all (Fig. 10.6) but has the same phase shift caused by magnetic field inhomogeneities and other factors.

Generally, velocity-sensitive and velocity-insensitive phase images are obtained in an interleaved way and subsequently subtracted voxel-wise to result in a phase image in which the phase shift is determined only by motion (64,65). A pulse sequence for velocity mapping can be designed to have the velocity encoding within or through the imaging plane and also in all three directions. The major advantage of the through-plane technique is the ability to measure volume flow. If the through-plane technique is used perpendicular to, for example, a vessel, the cross-sectional area of

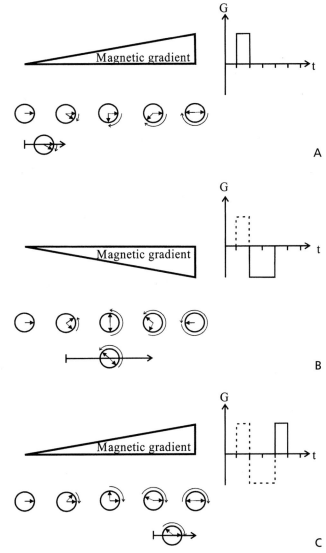

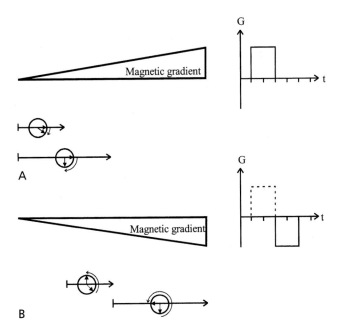

FIGURE 10.5. Schematic illustration shows that the spin groups moving along the magnetic field gradient (with a constant velocity) accumulate a phase shift according to Eq. 2 **(A)**. When the magnetic gradient is inverted, the spin groups overcompensate for the phase shift gained in A, leaving a residual phase shift proportional to the velocity **(B)**. *G,* magnetic field gradient amplitude; *t,* time.

FIGURE 10.6. As in Figure 10.5, but with the application of three consecutive magnetic field gradients, the first **(A)** and third **(C)** spin groups are identical, whereas the second **(B)** has the same magnitude but the opposite sign and double the duration. This combination leaves both stationary spin groups and spin groups with a constant velocity without any residual phase shift. *G,* magnetic field gradient amplitude; *t,* time.

the vessel and the velocity distribution within it can be displayed in a single velocity map, so that the volume flow can be calculated as the product of area and average velocity within the vessel.

MR Velocity Mapping of Complex Flow Patterns

Although MR velocity mapping is based on a linearity between the phase shift and the velocity along a magnetic gradient, one important pitfall is related to complex flow patterns (e.g., in relation to valvular stenosis or regurgitation) (66). Thus, a constriction causes a jet to form. In addition to undergoing a time-dependent acceleration caused by the pulsatility of cardiovascular flow, the blood accelerates as it approaches the constriction. This convective (or spatial) acceleration is generated by the decrease in flow area and can contribute substantially to the phase shift (67). After passing through an abrupt contraction, the jet continues to constrict for a certain length to form a vena contracta, and then it expands radially (68). Consequently, separated flow with a central jet and an annular region of recirculation is observed downstream of the constriction (66). This region with separated flow includes components of higher-order motion, such as acceleration and jerk and the formation of flow vortices. Thus, in the velocity mapping of complex flow patterns, each voxel may contain a spectrum of velocities in addition to higher-order motion components. Such higher-order motion terms give rise to additional phase shifts. Furthermore, temporal and spatial variations in the flow patterns in regions with complex flow cause a further phase incoherence within the voxels (69).

The net flow-induced phase signal within the voxel is obtained from a vectorial summation of all the elementary phase contributions, and when this vectorial summation is made, several situations can occur that affect both phase and modulus information (70). Thus, the average voxel phase is equivalent to the voxel phase derived from the vector sum of isochromate magnetization only when the phase distribution is symmetric and the modulus of each isochromate is identical. Furthermore, phase incoherence results in a decreased net modulus signal, and because of limited signal-to-noise ratio, the net phase signal may be affected by random noise. Consequently, with increasing phase dispersion within the voxel, the linearity between net flow-induced phase and average velocity in the flow-encoding direction may be disturbed even though a non-zero modulus signal is still obtained. In situations with breakdown of the phase–velocity relation, a loss of corresponding modulus information occurs, indicating severe phase dispersion within the voxels.

An efficient way of reducing the influence of higher-order motion components is to decrease the duration of the motion-encoding magnetic gradient field (69,71), as demonstrated by *in vitro* validation of the pulse sequences designed for velocity mapping of complex flow patterns (72,73).

IN VIVO IMPLEMENTATION OF MR VELOCITY MAPPING

Several methodologic variations are possible in designing a measurement protocol for the velocity mapping of valvular flow patterns. However, certain precautions must be taken to avoid pitfalls and erroneous measurements. Below, different methodologic aspects of implementation and evaluation procedures are provided.

Synchronization with Cardiac Phases

Several problems are associated with the MR velocity mapping of pulsatile flow that do not arise in the mapping of steady flow. First, to obtain an MR velocity map at a certain phase of the cardiac cycle, all data used to calculate the image must be related to that specific phase of the cycle. This is generally achieved by synchronizing the data acquisitions with the electrocardiogram (ECG). Second, multiple MR velocity maps are required to elucidate the flow pattern during the entire cardiac cycle. These may be obtained by cine MR (i.e., data used to create different MR velocity maps are acquired consecutively during the cardiac cycle). The result is the acquisition of multiple MR velocity maps at the same spatial position, but with a temporal resolution of typically 20 to 40 milliseconds.

Two strategies are commonly used to synchronize data acquisition with the cardiac cycle: ECG triggering (74) and retrospective gating (75). In the former technique, the R wave in the ECG triggers data acquisition, and the duration of the cine acquisition depends on the chosen number of frames and temporal resolution. In several applications (e.g., quantification of aortic regurgitation or mitral flow), it is essential to measure flow during the entire diastole, and this is usually accomplished by extending the cine data acquisition into the next cardiac cycle. However, the acquisition time is doubled. ECG triggering is also hampered by changes in the patient's heart rate during data acquisition, and velocity maps constructed of both end-diastolic and early systolic data are obtained rather than true end-diastolic velocity maps. Furthermore, the repeated interruption of data acquisition in waiting for a trigger pulse causes variation in modulus information (76), variable phase-shift contribution from eddy currents, and ghosting artifacts (77,78) in the first cine frames.

Most of these problems can be solved by retrospective gating, in which data are acquired continuously and sorted subsequently according to their position in the cardiac cycle. To avoid severe image artifacts, all phase-encoding steps should be represented in each cine frame before image reconstruction. This may be ensured by repeating each phase step for a period extending the mean duration of the cardiac cycle and causing a corresponding extension in the acquisition time. Such oversampling is often accompanied by the interpolation of data from adjacent intervals (79). However, the interpolation algorithm may cause a low-pass filtering in the time domain, so that the determinations of timing and instantaneous velocities in pulsatile flow erroneous are erroneous (80). Although the net volume flow during the pulsatile cycle is unaffected by filtering, problems may arise when volume flow is measured in separate phases of the pulsatile cycle (e.g., cardiac output or regurgitant volume in valvular regurgitation, peak velocity in valvular stenosis). Tailoring the algorithm to use a narrow time window for interpolation can reduce the problems arising from low-pass filtering (80).

Both ECG triggering and retrospective gating require that data be acquired during multiple heart beats; therefore, an irregular heart rhythm (e.g., atrial fibrillation) substantially diminishes image quality. Furthermore, motion of the heart secondary to respiration causes some image artifacts, and although data acquisition can be synchronized with both the cardiac cycle and respiration (81), this process is time-consuming. However, the problems associated with respiration can also be reduced by fast imaging techniques, such as segmented k-space data collection within one breath-hold (82) and real-time imaging (83). An example of the latter technique is echo-planar imaging (84), which has been suggested for flow measurements (85) and has demonstrated a temporal resolution corresponding to that of conventional velocity mapping (86). A further development of real-time imaging methods may also help to solve the problems associated with flow measurements in patients with arrhythmia.

Measurement and Evaluation Procedures

Imaging plane. The position of the imaging plane can be critical to the reliability of MR velocity mapping. In aortic regurgitation, an imaging plane downstream in the ascending aorta may prevent breakdown of the phase–velocity relation in the presence of complex flow patterns, but this position is associated with pitfalls related to coronary flow and aortic compliance (87). The reverse flow to the coronary arteries has been found to account for 6.3% (range, 2.5% to 14%) of the forward flow when a slice position is used in the midportion of the ascending aorta (88). Furthermore, because of aortic compliance, a movement of the imaging plane from a position between the aortic valve and coronary arteries to a position 2 cm distal to the sinotubular junction has been reported to cause a significant underestimation of the regurgitant volume (89,90). Thus, provided that the pulse sequence is robust to complex flow patterns, the imaging plane should be chosen between the aortic valve and the origin of the coronary arteries to obtain accurate quantification of the regurgitation.

In valvular stenosis, the transvalvular pressure gradient ΔP can be estimated from the maximum velocity V_{max} by using the modified Bernoulli equation (9,91):

$$\Delta P = 4 \bullet V_{max^2} \qquad [4]$$

After passing through the stenotic valve, the jet continues to constrict to form a vena contracta. A drawback with the through-plane technique in measuring peak velocity is that the exact location of the vena contracta may not be predicted in advance. However, the centerline velocity of the jet remains constant over a distance typically five times the jet diameter (68), so that a margin is left for positioning the imaging plane. The in-plane technique has been used mainly to measure flow velocities, and the advantage of this technique is that the velocity distribution along a stenotic jet can be displayed in the velocity map, which enables determination of the peak velocity. However, because the voxels are anisometric, with the longest axis through the image plane, partial volume effects may arise as a result of in-plane examinations of narrow stenotic jets. This problem can be avoided by using a thin image slice, although this in turn increases the sensitivity to movement of the flow region out of the image slice in cases of pulsatile flow, respiration, or patient movement (92). The through-plane technique is less sensitive to movement, especially if the flow region is homogeneous along the flow direction.

Spatial misregistration can occur if the blood moves during the time needed for spatial encoding (i.e., during the execution of the magnetic field gradients) (93). The phenomenon may arise with the through-plane technique but is more pronounced when the in-plane technique is used if the flow direction, although still in the image plane, is angulated relative to the motion-encoding direction (69). Consequently, the flow signal is misregistered on the velocity map, and furthermore, when the flow signal overlies stationary tissue, it may cause partial volume effects. Because the total phase shift for the voxel is obtained by vectorial summation, the velocity is measured erroneously, particularly when the stationary tissue has a large modulus signal. Misregistration may also occur when the through-plane technique is used in complex flow areas with in-plane motion components (94). Misregistration can be minimized by ensuring that the motion encoding and flow directions are equal and by reducing the time for spatial encoding (69,94).

Misalignment between the direction of flow and the direction of the motion-encoding magnetic gradients may also lead to erroneous MR velocity measurements. The phenomenon can be avoided in the through-plane technique by carefully angulating the imaging plane perpendicular to the flow direction. Conversely, when the in-plane technique is used, misalignment may occur because rotation of the imaging plane to allow velocity-encoding alignment to the jet direction may be difficult in conventional MR units. However, if the angle ϕ of misalignment is known, then the true flow value F_{true} can theoretically be calculated from the measured flow value F_{meas} as follows:

$$F_{meas} = F_{true} \cdot \cos \phi \qquad [5]$$

Furthermore, in the absence of partial volume errors, a misalignment of as much as 20 degrees will produce only a 6% error, whereas a more realistic misalignment of 5 degrees will cause an error of less than 1% (69).

Partial volume effects at the boundary of a vessel may occur because the voxels contain both intravascular and extravascular spins. This leads to a systematic error in volume flow measurements (70), and consequently the partial volume error is related to the ratio between voxel and vessel size. It has been calculated that approximately 16 voxels must cover the cross-sectional lumen of the vessel to keep this error within 10% (95,96). With smaller vessels, the problem becomes significant, and different techniques have been proposed to correct partial volume effects (97,98). It should be noted that partial volume effects in through-plane velocity measurements increase the angulation error in cases of misalignment.

Even though the influence of random error resulting from a limited signal-to-noise ratio is modest when the peak velocity of, for example, a stenotic jet is measured, it has been suggested that this parameter might be estimated from an average of at least four adjacent voxels in the central jet core region (72). However, because of limited spatial resolution, partial volume effects may lead to an underestimation of the peak velocity, especially when the through-plane technique is used, in which the jet region consists of only few voxels. Another suggestion is to use a jet-recognition algorithm based on assumptions of a spatial and temporal continuum of the jet for automatic selection of the highest voxel phase shift (99).

Velocity sensitivity. The phase is cyclic, giving a natural limit of $\pm \pi$ radians to the maximum angular range that can be measured without phase wrap, so-called aliasing and ambiguity of the velocity data. Furthermore, for signal-to-noise reasons, the velocity-induced phase shift must significantly exceed the random variation of the phase (100). This is in practice accomplished by selecting a suitable gradient combination in the measurement protocol. The sensitivity is chosen by selecting the cutoff velocity value $\pm \pi$ radians such that the predicted peak velocity covers approximately two-thirds of the available phase interval to avoid aliasing the velocity data while retaining adequate sensitivity (72). A general drawback of the velocity-mapping technique is thereby introduced because it is sometimes difficult to know the velocities a priori, and a change in velocity encoding normally requires a second examination. In cases of aliasing, this can be overcome with a general phase shift so long as the total range of velocity-induced phase shifts in one frame is smaller than 2π (101) or with postprocessing algorithms that use spatial continuity to resolve ambiguity (102).

Residual phase offset. Theoretically, the phase in voxels with stationary tissue should be zero after subtraction between velocity-sensitive and velocity-insensitive phase images (64). However, a residual phase generally is present in the velocity map, especially in older systems with suboptimal eddy current compensation. A minor residual phase offset may be neglected when peak velocity is measured, but the same phase offset can cause significant errors when volume flow is quantified (100). Extended postprocessing routines have been proposed to reduce this problem (87,103), and *in vitro* tests have revealed that such routines can overcome the problem, leaving a remaining phase offset of less than 0.3% of the full phase range (87). A simplified way of dealing with background phase is to subtract the average phase in one or more background regions from the average phase in the region-of-interest (ROI) before the velocity is calculated.

Region-of-interest. Generally, the anatomy is better visualized in the modulus image than in the velocity map, and therefore demarcation of an ROI is usually traced on the modulus image and subsequently projected onto the corresponding phase image to measure the mean velocity in the ROI. Under ideal conditions, the volume flow in a vessel can be quantified from a through-plane velocity map, as the average velocity within an ROI multiplied by the cross-sectional area of the ROI. However, a general problem is the size of the chosen ROI. If the ROI is smaller than the cross section of the vessel, then the volume flow is underestimated. On the other hand, if the ROI is much larger than the lumen of the vessel, eventually the flow-related phase shift may vanish within the phase noise from the stationary tissue (104). Therefore, care should be taken to use as small an ROI as possible and yet still enclose the vessel (70). In addition to potential pitfalls in choosing the size of the ROI, the postprocessing and data analysis may be time-consuming; however, robust automated postprocessing routines are becoming available (105,106).

MR VELOCITY MAPPING OF VALVULAR HEART DISEASES

MR velocity mapping in the quantification of valvular flow, pressure gradient, and valve area has been validated in several studies by means of different measurement protocols and reference techniques. To obtain a uniform presentation of results, mean accuracy rates, interstudy reproducibility rates (precision), and intraobserver and interobserver reproducibility rates were calculated from the reported data and are set forth in the discussion below.

Aortic Regurgitation

In aortic regurgitation, the important parameters measured by MR velocity mapping are the LV stroke volume and the regurgitant volume. In the phase map, the velocity in each voxel is displayed on a gray scale. Velocity in one direction

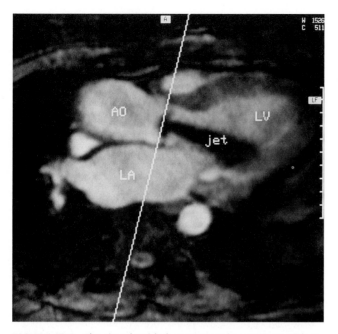

FIGURE 10.7. The signal-void phenomenon in a patient with severe aortic regurgitation. A broad-based regurgitant jet *(JET)* is seen in the left ventricle *(LV)* during diastole and can be used to semiquantify the valvular lesion and to position the imaging plane for MR velocity mapping *(solid line)*. AO, ascending aorta; LA, left atrium.

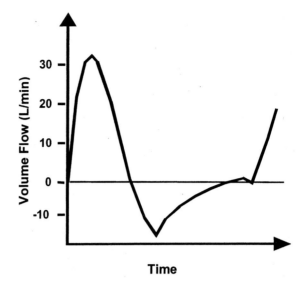

FIGURE 10.9. Volume flow through an incompetent aortic valve during the cardiac cycle as quantified by MR velocity mapping. Areas under the positive and negative parts of the curve represent forward and regurgitant flow, respectively.

along the velocity-encoding gradient appears bright, velocity in the opposite direction is dark, and stationary tissue is gray (Figs. 10.7 and 10.8). A cinematographic velocity-mapping pulse sequence can be used to determine the volume flow rate through the aortic valves during the entire cardiac cycle (Fig. 10.9).

LV stroke volume measured by MR velocity mapping has been validated in both healthy subjects and patients with aortic regurgitation or stenosis by means of classic reference techniques such as the Fick method, indicator dilution, and thermodilution, and an accuracy ranging from 81% to 97% has been revealed (87,88,107–113). The interstudy reproducibility is reported to be 95% for measurements performed on different days (113) and 98% to 99% for consecutive measurements performed during the same examination (112,113), whereas the intraobserver and in-

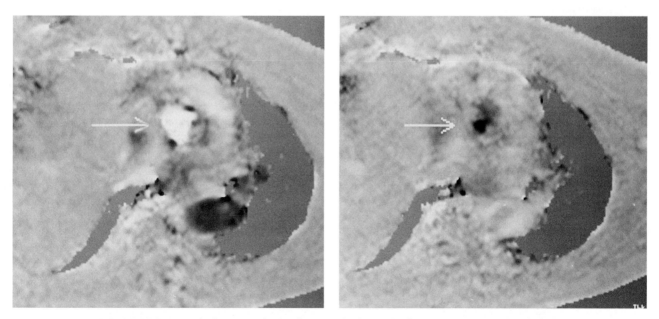

FIGURE 10.8. MR velocity maps obtained perpendicular to the flow direction at the level of the aortic valve *(arrow)* in a patient with aortic regurgitation. The velocities through the imaging plane are displayed on a gray scale, on which systolic forward flow appears bright *(left)* and diastolic regurgitation dark *(right)*.

terobserver reproducibility rates are 97% to 99% (108,111) and 96% to 99% (108,111,112), respectively.

Regurgitant volume and fraction cannot be measured directly by any widely used gold standard technique, so the capability of MR velocity mapping has been evaluated against methods that indirectly assess these parameters. Thus, regurgitation was estimated from the difference between the LV and RV stroke volumes as determined by MR volume measurements made with the assumption that no coexisting regurgitant valve lesion was present (114). In another study, it was shown that MR velocity mapping reliably measures both total and forward cardiac output, and it was therefore assumed that the technique is also capable of measuring the difference between these two parameters, namely regurgitation (87). Thus, the accuracy rates of MR velocity mapping in quantifying the regurgitation volume and fraction were 82% to 93% (87,114) and 89% (114), respectively. Furthermore, regurgitation was compared with the semiquantitative grading of aortic root angiography and color Doppler echocardiography, and despite minor discrepancies, the studies revealed agreement between the techniques (87–90,111,115). The precision rates of MR velocity mapping in quantifying the regurgitant volume in consecutive measurements were 90% to 91% (113,114) and 89% for measurements made on different days (113). The corresponding values for the regurgitation fraction were 91% to 95% (113,114) and 87% (113). Intraobserver and interobserver reproducibility rates of 99% (111) and 95% (114), respectively, for quantifying the regurgitation fraction were reported, whereas the interobserver reproducibility rate for measurement of the regurgitant volume was 96% (114).

Interventional studies. A reduction in systemic afterload may decrease volume overload in the LV and so be beneficial in aortic regurgitation, as shown in several studies (116). However, because of a lack of reliable noninvasive methods, only sparse data regarding the effects on cardiac output and regurgitation are available in previous studies of the hemodynamic effects of vasodilation in these patients. MRI may in this situation be unique in providing noninvasive monitoring of the hemodynamic effects of therapeutic intervention, offering a high level of accuracy and precision in quantifying aortic valvular volume flow and the possibility of monitoring LV volumes, function, and myocardial mass in response to therapy. In this context, two trials of MR velocity mapping have been reported, both demonstrating beneficial effects of vasodilation in chronic aortic regurgitation (113,117).

Aortic Stenosis

Aortic stenosis is a reduction of the valvular orifice, which may increase the transvalvular pressure gradient. However, in severe stenosis, the gradual deterioration in LV function may result in a decreased cardiac output and a paradoxical decline in the transvalvular pressure gradient. Although the

orifice area and cardiac output significantly affect the prognosis, these parameters were previously hard to measure reliably. Consequently, the transvalvular pressure gradient has traditionally been the major parameter used to assess the severity of aortic stenosis. MR velocity mapping in aortic stenosis has primarily been applied in quantifying the pressure gradient, but the abilities of the technique to measure valve area and cardiac output have also been evaluated.

Transvalvular pressure gradient. The peak velocity or estimated pressure gradient across the stenotic aortic valve has been assessed by MR velocity mapping with through-plane velocity encoding (99,118) and in-plane velocity encoding (72,92) using Doppler echocardiography or cardiac catheterization as a reference technique. Most studies have used an imaging plane including the stenotic jet immediately downstream of the valve to measure the peak velocity at the vena contracta. In general, good agreement between MR velocity mapping and the reference techniques was found, indicated by an accuracy exceeding 83% (92,99,118). The interobserver reproducibility was 93% (92).

Valve area in aortic stenosis measured by MR velocity mapping has been evaluated in a single study in which a through-plane technique and an imaging plane at the level of the aortic valve were used (110). Ideally, the orifice area may be determined from the spatially adjoining voxels with phase shift caused by the stenotic jet; the systolic velocity map with the maximum jet velocity is used to increase the signal-to-noise ratio. However, potential pitfalls are encountered in determining the area. First, partial volume effects related to the relatively small orifice area and a limited spatial resolution in the MR velocity maps influence the accuracy of the area measurement. Secondly, the imaging plane may be thick compared with the length of the orifice. Consequently, the phase shift in the voxels in the boundary of the jet arises not only from flow passing through the orifice but also from convergent flow proximal to the stenosis and from divergent flow distal to the orifice. To reduce these partial volume effects, the flow through the stenosis was assumed to have a plug velocity profile, and based on a computer simulation, only voxels with velocities of more than 50% of the maximum jet velocity were included in the determination of the area. Even though the flow profile cannot be considered to be pluglike as the orifice becomes larger, the relative error can be assumed to decrease as the area of the orifice increases (95). The area measurements were found to be reliable *in vitro* in circular orifices of various sizes (73). In patients with aortic stenosis, the valve area was determined with an accuracy of 77% to 80% (110) when the continuity equation (15) and the classic Gorlin formula (14) were used as the best available references.

Cardiac output has been quantified in valvular aortic stenosis by MR velocity mapping; when a simultaneously performed indicator dilution measurement was used as the reference, an accuracy of 93% was revealed (116). It may be argued that because of the pronounced complex flow patterns in aortic stenosis, velocity mapping may be more reliably performed distally in the ascending aorta or pulmonary trunk. However, when an imaging plane at the level of the aortic valve is used, not only can the prognostically important valve area and cardiac output be determined, concomitant aortic regurgitation may also be quantified in a single measurement (84,110).

Mitral Regurgitation

Validation of the velocity mapping of forward volume flow through the mitral annulus has shown an accuracy of more than 90% (109,119,120) and an interobserver reproducibility of 93% (120). However, measurements of regurgitation are associated with at least three problems. First, many patients with severe mitral valve disease have atrial fibrillation, which causes a wide variation in the duration of the cardiac cycle and flow pattern. The problem may be solved by real-time flow measurements, but the impact of this technique has yet to be established. Second, the movement of the atrioventricular valves during systole may cause the peak velocity of the regurgitant jet to be underestimated. However, this error can be reduced by using different imaging planes at different times in the cardiac cycle, so that the slice is always positioned at the annulus (121,122), or by correcting the velocity maps for through-plane motion of the base of the heart (123). Third, in mitral regurgitation, the frequent eccentricity of the regurgitant jet causes misalignment problems. Consequently, the mitral regurgitant volume has been calculated indirectly as the difference between the LV stroke volume, determined by volume measurements, and the forward volume flow through the mitral annulus (119) or in the ascending aorta (124). The reported accuracy rates of this technique in determining the regurgitant volume and regurgitant fraction were 91% and 94% (124), respectively, and the corresponding values for interobserver reproducibility were more than 90% and 85% (119,124), respectively. Furthermore, in the same studies, the regurgitant fraction correlated well with the Doppler echocardiographic grade of severity.

Another method has been suggested for quantifying mitral regurgitation (125). The technique is based on acquiring a number of contiguous slices with all three velocity components measured. A control volume is then selected encompassing the regurgitant orifice. Mass conservation dictates that the net flow into the control volume is equal to the regurgitant flow.

Mitral Stenosis

Both in-plane and through-plane velocity mapping have been used to measure the transmitral peak velocity in mitral stenosis. With Doppler echocardiography used as a reference technique, an accuracy of more than 87% was found (92,126,127), and the interobserver reproducibility was more than 96% (92,127).

Pulmonary Regurgitation

Surgical repair of tetralogy of Fallot frequently includes placement of a transannular patch to relieve the RV outflow tract obstruction and pulmonary stenosis. However, the consequence of the patch is often a severe pulmonary regurgitation that sometimes leads to impaired RV function. When these patients require a pulmonary valve homograft remains controversial, but MRI may facilitate the decision by providing quantitative measurements of both the regurgitation and the RV. The accuracy rates for the velocity mapping of pulmonary regurgitant volume and regurgitant fraction have been reported to be 78% and 76%, respectively (128).

Prosthetic Heart Valves

Most prosthetic heart valves are not ferromagnetic and can be examined in an MRI unit, although the prosthetic material itself causes a localized image artifact (129). Therefore, MRI can be used to detect dysfunctional prosthetic heart valves, and the signal-void phenomena have been shown to have an accuracy of 96% in detecting pathologic leakage flow in comparison with transesophageal Doppler echocardiography (130). In addition, velocity mapping makes it possible to quantify the blood velocity distribution downstream from a prosthetic aortic valve (131–133) and so may provide valuable information on the functioning of the valvular prosthesis. However, the clinical impact of MR on prosthetic heart valves has yet to be established.

FUTURE ASPECTS
Clinical Relevance

MRI can be used to evaluate valvular heart diseases in an integrated approach that offers noninvasive quantification of a valvular lesion and its hemodynamic consequences, reflected by ventricular dimensions, function, and wall stress (134). The clinical relevance of reliably quantifying these parameters in the management of patients with valvular regurgitation or stenosis is obvious. However, despite the increased accessibility of cardiac MRI, the technique is not used routinely in the evaluation of these patients, for at least four possible reasons. First, Doppler echocardiography is a well-established technique within cardiac units. It is applied by the cardiologist and often yields the information required for making a therapeutic decision. Second, at present, only a limited number of radiologists and cardiologists are trained in cardiac MRI, although organized educational courses have recently been introduced. Third, the current inability to provide detailed information on valve leaflets with any consistency is a problem for a subset of patients, primarily those with acute valvular regurgitation. Finally, postprocessing and data analysis may be time-consuming, although this problem may be overcome as robust automated techniques become available.

Nevertheless, several indications can at present be proposed for MRI in the management of patients with valvular heart disease. In a case of poor acoustic windows for transthoracic Doppler echocardiography, MR may be less unpleasant for the patient than transesophageal echocardiography and may provide additional information on the valvular lesion. If it cannot be determined by Doppler echocardiographic examination whether a valvular lesion requires surgical intervention, the patient is generally referred for cardiac catheterization. In such cases, MRI offers a more exact assessment of the disease without risk to the patient. If a valvular lesion does not require surgical intervention at the moment but is sufficiently severe that regular follow-up is required, MRI can be the method of choice for monitoring the patient; its reproducibility is clearly better than that of Doppler echocardiography in the assessment of regurgitation, ventricular dimensions, and function. Finally, MRI must be considered the method of choice for monitoring the hemodynamic effects of medical intervention in patients with valvular heart disease.

Further Technologic Development

Although MRI allows the noninvasive quantification of valvular regurgitation and stenosis and provides information regarding ventricular dimensions, function, and myocardial mass, the technique has some limitations that, until now, have delayed its widespread clinical application.

Valvular morphology. In addition to assessing the severity of valvular heart disease accurately, if management is to be optimal, it may be necessary to establish the cause of valvular disease and the morphology of the valve. For instance, the degree of valvular calcification and the presence of infective endocarditis may affect the therapeutic decision. Calcified valve leaflets are thick and exhibit a restrictive pattern of motion; in general, they are evaluated easily with MRI. Visualization of valvular vegetation (135), aortic root abscess (136), and perivalvular infectious pseudoaneurysm (137,138) has been reported, but the valve leaflets are generally thin in endocarditis, and because of their movement, they are not usually well delineated on MR images. Further technologic developments, including better temporal and spatial resolution, are needed for consistent visualization of the valve leaflets (139). Echo-planar imaging has been proposed (140); however, current MR techniques are inferior to echocardiography in the assessment of valvular morphology, especially in cases of infective endocarditis. However, new techniques with a high degree of temporal resolution, such as true fast imaging with steady-state precession (FISP) and balanced fast-field echo (FFE) MRI, depict valve morphology and motion extremely well.

Coronary arteries. The preoperative assessment of patients with valvular heart disease who are at risk for coronary artery disease usually includes coronary angiography, and evaluation of the coronary arteries is one of the major challenges in cardiovascular MRI. Significant obstacles include small vessel size, vessel motion related to the cardiac and respiratory cycles, complex flow patterns in stenotic vessels, and vessel tortuosity. To depict the coronary arteries, MRI must provide a high degree of spatial resolution, a high signal-to-noise ratio, and rapid or motion-synchronized imaging. The continuing development of MRA may lead to a comprehensive method capable of noninvasively evaluating the anatomy of the coronary arteries. In addition, methods for the measurement of blood flow in the major coronary arteries have been proposed (141), and a method for the noninvasive evaluation of coronary flow reserve has been described (142). Currently, substantial efforts are being made to develop MR units dedicated to cardiovascular imaging; these include gradient systems with increased capabilities in combination with dedicated radiofrequency coil systems and imaging software. With the development of such units, the necessary technologic prerequisites for the more widespread clinical use of cardiovascular MRI may be met.

SUMMARY

MR velocity mapping offers a noninvasive method of flow quantification. The potential breakdown of the phase–velocity relation in the presence of complex flow patterns in valvular heart disease can be overcome by using magnetic field gradients of short duration. *In vitro* and *in vivo* validation studies of MR velocity mapping have revealed high rates of accuracy and reproducibility in measuring volume flow, valve areas, and transvalvular pressure gradients. Several pitfalls are encountered in the clinical application of velocity mapping, but if the investigator is aware of these potential sources of error, the technique offers a reliable means to assess the severity of aortic regurgitation and stenosis. Furthermore, because velocity mapping can be used in an integrated approach with MR volume measurements of LV dimensions and function, MRI may prove to be superior to other imaging techniques in monitoring valvular heart disease and predicting the optimal time for valvular surgery. Despite the capability of MRI, its general acceptance for assessing valvular heart disease has been slow. One obstacle is the lack of availability of MRI units for cardiologists, and cooperation between cardiologists and radiologists should therefore be emphasized, including specific education in cardiovascular MRI for both specialties so that the unique possibilities of the technique may be utilized for the benefit of patients.

REFERENCES

1. Perry GJ, Helmcke F, Nanda NC, et al. Evaluation of aortic insufficiency by Doppler color flow mapping. *J Am Coll Cardiol* 1987;9:952–959.

2. Sahn DJ. Instrumentation and physical factors related to visualization of stenotic and regurgitant jets by Doppler color flow mapping. *J Am Coll Cardiol* 1988;12:1354–1365.

3. Croft CH, Lipscomb K, Mathis K, et al. Limitations of qualitative angiographic grading in aortic or mitral regurgitation. *Am J Cardiol* 1984;53:1593–1598.

4. Rigo P, Alderson PO, Robertson RM, et al. Measurement of aortic and mitral regurgitation by gated cardiac blood pool scans. *Circulation* 1979;60:306–312.

5. Kelbaek H, Aldershvile J, Svendsen JH, et al. Combined first pass and equilibrium radionuclide cardiographic determination of stroke volume for quantitation of valvular regurgitation. *J Am Coll Cardiol* 1988;11:769–773.

6. Carabello BA, Crawford FA. Valvular heart disease. *N Engl J Med* 1997;337:32–41.

7. Ross J, Braunwald E. Aortic stenosis. *Circulation* 1968;38:V-61–V-67.

8. Carabello BA. Timing of surgery in mitral and aortic stenosis. *Cardiol Clin* 1991;9:229–238.

9. Holen J, Aaslid R, Landmark K, et al. Determination of pressure gradient in mitral stenosis with a noninvasive ultrasound Doppler technique. *Acta Med Scand* 1976;199:455–460.

10. Hatle L, Angelsen BA, Tromsdal A. Non-invasive assessment of aortic stenosis by Doppler ultrasound. *Br Heart J* 1980;43:284–292.

11. Griffith MJ, Carey C, Coltart DJ, et al. Inaccuracies in using aortic valve gradients alone to grade severity of aortic stenosis. *Br Heart J* 1989;62:372–378.

12. Turina J, Hess O, Sepulcri F, et al. Spontaneous course of aortic valve disease. *Eur Heart J* 1987;8:471–483.

13. Martin RP, Rakowski H, Kleiman JH, et al. Reliability and reproducibility of two-dimensional echocardiograph measurement of the stenotic mitral valve orifice area. *Am J Cardiol* 1979;43:560–568.

14. Gorlin R, Gorlin SG. Hydraulic formula for calculation of the area of the stenotic mitral valve, other cardiac valves, and central circulatory shunts. *Am Heart J* 1951;41:1–29.

15. Skjaerpe T, Hegrenaes L, Hatle L. Noninvasive estimation of valve area in patients with aortic stenosis by Doppler ultrasound and two-dimensional echocardiography. *Circulation* 1985;72:810–818.

16. Cannon SR, Richards KL, Crawford M. Hydraulic estimation of the stenotic orifice area: a correction of the Gorlin formula. *Circulation* 1985;71:1170–1178.

17. Baumgartner H, Kratzer H, Helmreich G, et al. Determination of aortic valve area by Doppler echocardiography using the continuity equation: a critical evaluation. *Cardiology* 1990;77:101–111.

18. Haase A, Frahm J, Matthaei D, et al. FLASH imaging. Rapid NMR imaging using low flip-angle pulses. *J Magn Reson* 1986;67:258–266.

19. Sakuma H, Fujita N, Foo TK, et al. Evaluation of left ventricular volume and mass with breath-hold cine MR imaging. *Radiology* 1993;188:377–380.

20. Hunter GJ, Hamberg LM, Weisskoff RM, et al. Measurement of stroke volume and cardiac output within a single breath hold with echo-planar imaging. *J Magn Reson Imaging* 1994;4:51–58.

21. Williams RJ, Muir DF, Pathi V, et al. Randomized controlled trial of stented and stentless aortic bioprosthesis: hemodynamic performance at 3 years. *Semin Thorac Cardiovasc Surg* 1999;11(4 Suppl 1):93–97.

22. Møgelvang J, Stockholm KH, Saunamäki K, et al. Assessment of left ventricular volumes by magnetic resonance in comparison with radionuclide angiography, contrast angiography and echocardiography. *Eur Heart J* 1992;13:1677–1683.

23. Markiewicz W, Sechtem U, Kirby R, et al. Measurement of ventricular volumes in the dog by nuclear magnetic resonance imaging. *J Am Coll Cardiol* 1987;10:170–177.

24. Culham JAG, Vince DJ. Cardiac output by MR imaging: an experimental study comparing right ventricle and left ventricle with thermodilution. *Can Assoc Radiol J* 1988;39:247–249.

25. Møgelvang J, Thomsen C, Mehlsen J, et al. Evaluation of left ventricular volumes measured by magnetic resonance imaging. *Eur Heart J* 1986;7:1016–1021.

26. Underwood SR, Klipstein RH, Firmin DN, et al. Magnetic resonance assessment of aortic and mitral regurgitation. *Br Heart J* 1986;56:455–462.

27. Møgelvang J, Thomsen C, Mehlsen J, et al. Left ventricular ejection fraction determined by magnetic resonance imaging and gated radionuclide ventriculography. *Am J Noninvas Cardiol* 1987;1:278–283.

28. Møgelvang J, Thomsen C, Horn T, et al. Determination of left ventricular myocardial volume (mass) by magnetic resonance imaging. *Am J Noninvas Cardiol* 1987;1:231–236.

29. Katz J, Milliken MC, Stray-Gundersen J, et al. Estimation of human myocardial mass with MR imaging. *Radiology* 1988;169:495–498.

30. Markiewicz W, Sechtem U, Higgins CB. Evaluation of the right ventricle by magnetic resonance imaging. *Am Heart J* 1987;113:8–15.

31. Møgelvang J, Stubgaard M, Thomsen C, et al. Evaluation of right ventricular volumes measured by magnetic resonance imaging. *Eur Heart J* 1988;9:529–533.

32. Møgelvang J, Stockholm KH, Stubgaard M, et al. Assessment of right ventricular volumes be magnetic resonance imaging and by radionuclide angiography. *Am J Noninvas Cardiol* 1991;5:321–327.

33. Doherty NE, Fujita N, Caputo GR, et al. Measurement of right ventricular mass in normal and dilated cardiomyopathic ventricles using cine magnetic resonance imaging. *Am J Cardiol* 1992;69:1223–1228.

34. Katz J, Whang J, Boxt LM, et al. Estimation of right ventricular mass in normal subjects and in patients with pulmonary hypertension by magnetic resonance imaging. *J Am Coll Cardiol* 1993;21:1475–1481.

35. Longmore DB, Klipstein RH, Underwood SR, et al. Dimensional accuracy of magnetic resonance in studies of the heart. *Lancet* 1985;1(8442):1360–1362.

36. Lorenz CH, Walker ES, Morgan VL, et al. Normal human right and left ventricular mass, systolic function, and gender differences by cine magnetic resonance imaging. *J Cardiovasc Magn Reson* 1999;1:7–21.

37. Underwood SR, Klipstein RH, Firmin DN, et al. Magnetic resonance assessment of aortic and mitral regurgitation. *Br Heart J* 1986;56:455–462.

38. Sechtem U, Pflugfelder PW, Cassidy MM, et al. Mitral or aortic regurgitation: quantification of regurgitant volumes with cine MR imaging. *Radiology* 1988;167:425–430.

39. Globits S, Frank H, Mayr H, et al. Quantitative assessment of aortic regurgitation by magnetic resonance imaging. *Eur Heart J* 1992;13:78–83.

40. Evans AJ, Blinder RA, Herfkens RJ, et al. Effects of turbulence on signal intensity in gradient echo images. *Invest Radiol* 1988;23:512–518.

41. Sechtem U, Pflugfelder PW, White RD, et al. Cine MR imaging: potential for evaluation of cardiovascular function. *AJR Am J Roentgenol* 1987;148:239–246.

42. Wagner S, Auffermann W, Buser P, et al. Diagnostic accuracy and estimation of the severity of valvular regurgitation from the signal void on cine magnetic resonance images. *Am Heart J* 1989;118:760–767.

43. Pflugfelder PW, Landzberg JS, Cassidy MM, et al. Comparison

of cine MR imaging with Doppler echocardiography for evaluation of aortic regurgitation. *AJR Am J Roentgenol* 1989;152: 729–735.

44. Utz JA, Herfkens RJ, Heinsimer JA, et al. Valvular regurgitation: dynamic MR imaging. *Radiology* 1988;168:91–94.

45. Mitchell L, Jenkins JP, Watson Y, et al. Diagnosis and assessment of mitral and aortic valve disease by cine-flow magnetic resonance imaging. *Magn Reson Med* 1989;12:181–197.

46. Aurigemma G, Reichek N, Schiebler M, et al. Evaluation of aortic regurgitation by cardiac cine magnetic resonance imaging: planar analysis and comparison to Doppler echocardiography. *Cardiology* 1991;78:340–347.

47. Nishimura F. Oblique cine MRI for evaluation of aortic regurgitation: comparison with cineangiography. *Clin Cardiol* 1992; 15:73–78.

48. Pflugfelder PW, Sechtem UP, White RD, et al. Noninvasive evaluation of mitral regurgitation by analysis of left atrial signal loss in cine magnetic resonance. *Am Heart J* 1989;117:1113–1119.

49. Aurigemma G, Reichek N, Schiebler M, et al. Evaluation of mitral regurgitation by cine magnetic resonance imaging. *Am J Cardiol* 1990;66:621–625.

50. Kizilbash AM, Hundley WG, Willett DL, et al. Comparison of quantitative Doppler with magnetic resonance imaging for assessment of the severity of mitral regurgitation. *Am J Cardiol* 1998;81:792–795.

51. de Ross A, Reichek N, Axel L, et al. Cine MR imaging in aortic stenosis. *J Comput Assist Tomogr* 1989;13:421–425.

52. Suzuki J, Caputo GR, Kondo C, et al. Cine MR imaging of valvular heart disease: display and imaging parameters affect the size of the signal void caused by valvular regurgitation. *AJR Am J Roentgenol* 1990;155:723–727.

53. Spielmann RP, Schneider O, Thiele F, et al. Appearance of poststenotic jets in MRI: dependence on flow velocity and on imaging parameters. *Magn Reson Imaging* 1991;9:67–72.

54. Mirowitz SA, Lee JK, Gutierrez FR, et al. Normal signal-void patterns in cardiac cine MR images. *Radiology* 1990;176:49–55.

55. Yoshida K, Yoshikawa J, Hozumi T, et al. Assessment of aortic regurgitation by the acceleration flow signal void proximal to the leaking orifice in cine magnetic resonance imaging. *Circulation* 1991;83:1951–1955.

56. Cranney CB, Benjelloun H, Perry GJ, et al. Rapid assessment of aortic regurgitation and left ventricular function using cine nuclear magnetic resonance imaging and the proximal convergence zone. *Am J Cardiol* 1993;71:1074–1081.

57. Singer JR. Blood flow rates by nuclear magnetic resonance measurements. *Science* 1959;130:1652–1653.

58. Singer JR, Crooks LE. Nuclear magnetic resonance blood flow measurements in the human brain. *Science* 1983;221:654–656.

59. Edelman RR, Mattle HP, Kleefield J, et al. Quantification of blood flow with dynamic MR imaging and presaturation bolus tracking. *Radiology* 1989;171:551–556.

60. Ambrosi P, Faugère G, Desfossez L, et al. Assessment of aortic regurgitation severity by magnetic resonance imaging of the thoracic aorta. *Eur Heart J* 1995;16:406–409.

61. Moran PR. A flow velocity zeugmatographic interlace for NMR imaging in humans. *Magn Reson Imaging* 1982;1:197–203.

62. Van Dijk P. ECG-triggered NMR imaging of the heart. *Diagn Imaging Clin Med* 1984;53:29–37.

63. Bryant DJ, Payne JA, Firmin DN, et al. Measurement of flow with NMR imaging using a gradient pulse and phase difference technique. *J Comput Assist Tomogr* 1984;8:588–593.

64. Nayler GL, Firmin DN, Longmore DB. Blood flow imaging by cine magnetic resonance. *J Comput Assist Tomogr* 1986;10: 715–722.

65. Axel L, Morton D. MR flow imaging by velocity-compensated/uncompensated difference images. *J Comput Assist Tomogr* 1987;11:31–34.

66. Azuma T, Fukushima T. Flow patterns in stenotic blood vessel models. *Biorheology* 1976;13:337–355.

67. Oshinski JN, Ku DN, Bohning DE, et al. Effects of acceleration on the accuracy of MR phase velocity measurements. *J Magn Reson Imaging* 1992;2:665–670.

68. Yoganathan AP, Cape EG, Sung HW, et al. Review of hydrodynamic principles for the cardiologist: applications to the study of blood flow and jets by imaging techniques. *J Am Coll Cardiol* 1988;12:1344–1353.

69. Firmin DN, Nayler GL, Kilner PJ, et al. The application of phase shifts in NMR for flow measurement. *Magn Reson Med* 1990;12:230–241.

70. Wolf RL, Ehman RL, Riederer SJ, et al. Analysis of systematic and random error in MR volumetric flow measurements. *Magn Reson Med* 1993;30:82–91.

71. Schmalbrock P, Yuan C, Chakeres DW, et al. Volume MR angiography: methods to achieve very short echo times. *Radiology* 1990;175:861–865.

72. Kilner PJ, Firmin DN, Rees RS, et al. Valve and great vessel stenosis: assessment with MR jet velocity mapping. *Radiology* 1991;178:229–235.

73. Søndergaard L, Ståhlberg F, Thomsen C, et al. Accuracy and precision of MR velocity mapping in measurement of stenotic cross-sectional area, flow rate, and pressure gradient. *J Magn Reson Imaging* 1993;3:433–437.

74. Van Dijk P. Direct cardiac NMR imaging of heart wall and blood flow velocity. *J Comput Assist Tomogr* 1984;8:429–436.

75. Glover GH, Pelc NJ. A rapid-gated cine MRI technique. *Magn Reson Annu* 1988:299–333.

76. Waterson JC, Jenkins JP, Zhu XP, et al. Magnetic resonance (MR) cine imaging of the human heart. *Br J Radiol* 1985;58: 711–716.

77. Haacke EM, Patrick JL. Reducing motion artefacts in two-dimensional Fourier transform imaging. *Magn Reson Imaging* 1986;4:359–376.

78. Lewis CE, Prato FS, Drost DJ, et al. Comparison of respiratory triggering and gating techniques for the removal of respiratory artifacts in MR imaging. *Radiology* 1986;160:803–810.

79. Lenz GW, Haacke EM, White RD. Retrospective cardiac gating: a review of technical aspects and future directions. *Magn Reson Imaging* 1989;7:445–455.

80. Søndergaard L, Ståhlberg F, Thomsen C, et al. Comparison between retrospective gating and ECG triggering in magnetic resonance velocity mapping. *Magn Reson Imaging* 1993;11:533–537.

81. Runge VM, Clanton JA, Partain CL, et al. Respiratory gating in magnetic resonance imaging at 0.5 tesla. *Radiology* 1984;151: 521–523.

82. Atkinson DJ, Edelman RR. Cineangiography of the heart in a single breath hold with a segmented turboFLASH sequence. *Radiology* 1991;178:357–360.

83. Nayak KS, Pauly JM, Kerr AB, et al. Real-time color flow MRI. *Magn Reson Med* 2000;43:251–258.

84. Mansfield P. Multi-planar image formation NMR spin-echoes. *J Phys C* 1977;10:L55–L58.

85. Firmin DN, Klipstein RH, Hounsfield GL, et al. Echo-planar high-resolution flow velocity mapping. *Magn Reson Med* 1989;12:316–327.

86. Debatin JF, Leung DA, Wildermuth S, et al. Flow quantitation with echo-planar phase-contrast velocity mapping: *in vitro* and *in vivo* evaluation. *J Magn Reson Imaging* 1995;5:656–662.

87. Søndergaard L, Lindvig K, Hildebrandt P, et al. Quantification of aortic regurgitation by magnetic resonance velocity mapping. *Am Heart J* 1993;125:1081–1090.

88. Bogren HG, Klipstein RH, Firmin DN, et al. Quantitation of antegrade and retrograde blood flow in the human aorta by magnetic resonance velocity mapping. *Am Heart J* 1989;117: 1214–1222.

89. Chatzimavroudis GP, Walker PG, Oshinski JN, et al. The importance of slice location on the accuracy of aortic regurgitation measurements with magnetic resonance phase velocity mapping. *Ann Biomed Eng* 1997;25:644–652.

90. Chatzimavroudis GP, Oshinski JN, Franch RH, et al. Quantification of the aortic regurgitant volume with magnetic resonance phase velocity mapping: a clinical investigation of the importance of imaging slice location. *J Heart Valve Dis* 1998;7: 94–101.

91. Hatle L, Brubakk A, Tromsdal A, et al. Noninvasive assessment of pressure drop in mitral stenosis by Doppler ultrasound. *Br Heart J* 1978;40:131–140.

92. Kilner PJ, Manzara CC, Mohiaddin RH, et al. Magnetic resonance jet velocity mapping in mitral and aortic valve stenosis. *Circulation* 1993;87:1239–1248.

93. von Schulthess GK, Higgins CB. Blood flow imaging with MR: spin-phase phenomena. *Radiology* 1985;157:687–695.

94. Ståhlberg F, Thomsen C, Søndergaard L, et al. Pulse sequence design for MR velocity mapping of complex flow: notes on the necessity of low echo times. *Magn Reson Imaging* 1994;12: 1255–1262.

95. Tang C, Blatter DD, Parker DL. Accuracy of phase-contrast flow measurements in the presence of partial-volume effects. *J Magn Reson Imaging* 1993;3:337–385.

96. Hofman MM, Visser FC, van Rossum AC, et al. *In vivo* validation of magnetic resonance blood volume flow measurements with limited spatial resolution in small vessels. *Magn Reson Med* 1995;33:778–784.

97. Hamilton CA. Correction of partial volume inaccuracies in quantitative phase contrast MR angiography. *Magn Reson Imaging* 1994;12:1127–1130.

98. Tang C, Blatter DD, Parker DL. Correction of partial-volume effects in phase-contrast flow measurements. *J Magn Reson Imaging* 1995;5:175–180.

99. Eichenberger AC, Jenni R, Von Schulthess GK. Aortic valve pressure gradients in patients with aortic valve stenosis: quantification with velocity-encoded cine MR imaging. *AJR Am J Roentgenol* 1993;160:971–977.

100. Buonocore MH, Bogren H. Factors influencing the accuracy and precision of velocity-encoded phase imaging. *Magn Reson Med* 1992;26:141–154.

101. Maier SE, Meier D, Boesinger P, et al. Human abdominal aorta: comparative measurements of blood flow with MR imaging and multigated Doppler US. *Radiology* 1989;171:487–492.

102. Axel L, Morton D. Correction of phase wrapping in magnetic resonance imaging. *Med Phys* 1989;16:284–287.

103. Walker PG, Cranney GB, Scheidegger MB, et al. Semiautomated method for noise reduction and background phase error correction in MR phase velocity mapping. *J Magn Reson Imaging* 1993;3:521–530.

104. Conturo TE, Smith GD. Signal-to-noise in phase angle reconstruction: dynamic range extension using phase reference offsets. *Magn Reson Med* 1990;15:420–437.

105. Chwialkowski MP, Ibrahim YM, Li HF, et al. A method for fully automated quantitative analysis of arterial flow using flow-sensitized MR images. *Comput Med Imaging Graph* 1996;20: 365–378.

106. van der Geest RJ, Niezen RA, van der Wall EE, et al. Automated measurement of volume flow in the ascending aorta using MR velocity maps: evaluation of inter- and intraobserver variability in healthy volunteers. *J Comput Assist Tomogr* 1998;22:904–911.

107. Firmin DN, Nayler GL, Klipstein RH, et al. *In vivo* validation of MR velocity imaging. *J Comput Assist Tomogr* 1987;11: 751–756.

108. Kondo C, Caputo GR, Semelka R, et al. Right and left ventricular stroke volume measurements with velocity-encoded cine MR imaging: *in vitro* and *in vivo* validation. *AJR Am J Roentgenol* 1991;157:9–16.

109. Søndergaard L, Thomsen C, Ståhlberg F, et al. Mitral and aortic valvular flow: quantification with MR phase mapping. *J Magn Reson Imaging* 1992;2:295–302.

110. Søndergaard L, Hildebrandt P, Lindvig K, et al. Valve area and cardiac output in aortic stenosis: quantification by magnetic resonance velocity mapping. *Am Heart J* 1993;127:1156–1164.

111. Honda N, Machida K, Hashimoto M, et al. Aortic regurgitation: quantitation with MR imaging velocity mapping. *Radiology* 1993;186:189–194.

112. Hundley WG, Hong FL, Hillis LD, et al. Quantitation of cardiac output with velocity-encoded, phase-difference magnetic resonance imaging. *Am J Cardiol* 1995;75:1250–1255.

113. Søndergaard L, Aldershvile J, Hildebrandt P, et al. Vasodilatation with felodipine in chronic asymptomatic aortic regurgitation. *Am Heart J* 2000;139:667–674.

114. Dulce MC, Mostbeck GH, O'Sullivan M, et al. Severity of aortic regurgitation: interstudy reproducibility of measurements with velocity-encoded cine MR imaging. *Radiology* 1992;185: 235–240.

115. Engels G, Reynen K, Müller E, et al. Quantifizierung der Aortenklappeninsuffizienz in der Magnetresonanztomographie. *Z Kardiol* 1993;82:345–351.

116. Levine HJ, Gaasch WH. Vasoactive drugs in chronic regurgitant lesions of the mitral and aortic valves. *J Am Coll Cardiol* 1996;28:1083–1091.

117. Globits S, Blake L, Bourne M, et al. Assessment of hemodynamic effects of angiotensin-converting enzyme inhibitor therapy in chronic aortic regurgitation by using velocity-encoded cine magnetic resonance imaging. *Am Heart J* 1996;131:289–293.

118. Engels G, Müller E, Reynen K, et al. Phase-mapping technique for the evaluation of aortic valve stenosis by MR. *Eur Radiol* 1992;2:299–304.

119. Fujita N, Chazouilleres AF, Hartiala JJ, et al. Quantification of mitral regurgitation by velocity-encoded cine nuclear magnetic resonance imaging. *J Am Coll Cardiol* 1994;23:951–958.

120. Hartiala JJ, Mostbeck GH, Foster E, et al. Velocity-encoded cine MRI in the evaluation of left ventricular diastolic function: measurement of mitral valve and pulmonary vein flow velocities and flow volume across the mitral valve. *Am Heart J* 1993;125: 1054–1066.

121. Søndergaard L, Fritz-Hansen T, Larsson HBW, et al. Left ventricular diastolic function evaluated by magnetic resonance velocity mapping. Presented at the XVIIth Congress of the European Society of Cardiology, Amsterdam. *Eur Heart J* 1995; 16(Suppl):2200(abst).

122. Walker PG, Houlind K, Djurhuus C, et al. Motion correction for the quantification of mitral regurgitation using the control volume method. *Magn Reson Med* 2000;43:726–733.

123. Kayser HW, Stoel BC, van der Wall EE, et al. MR velocity mapping of tricuspid flow: correction for through-plane motion. *J Magn Reson Imaging* 1997;7:669–673.

124. Hundley WG, Li HF, Willard JE, et al. Magnetic resonance imaging assessment of the severity of mitral regurgitation. Comparison with invasive techniques. *Circulation* 1995;92:1151–1158.

125. Chatzimavroudis GP, Oshinski JN, Pettigrew RI, et al. Quantification of mitral regurgitation with MR phase-velocity mapping using a control volume method. *J Magn Reson Imaging* 1998;8:577–582.

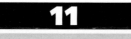

MYOCARDIAL PERFUSION IN ISCHEMIC HEART DISEASE

PENELOPE R. SENSKY
GRAHAM R. CHERRYMAN

In the last decade, the management of ischemic heart disease has become progressively more interventional. The number of patients receiving thrombolysis and undergoing percutaneous and surgical revascularization procedures continues to rise as efforts are made to minimize the deleterious process of myocardial ischemia. Interventions are performed to prevent total coronary occlusion, alleviate symptoms of chronic ischemia, preserve failing left ventricular (LV) function, and improve long-term prognosis (1–5). In addition, new methods of revascularization, such as transmyocardial laser revascularization and targeted gene therapy, are undergoing clinical trials (6–9). The accurate application of interventional strategies requires not only angiographic visualization of the patient's epicardial coronary anatomy but also a detailed knowledge of the effects of coronary atheroma on myocardial perfusion.

Impaired blood flow through a stenosed coronary artery results in reduced perfusion and correspondingly diminished myocardial oxygen delivery. Initially, hypoperfusion is seen in the subendocardial portion of the cardiac muscle (10). As blood flow is further reduced, the perfusion deficit becomes transmural, so that first diastolic and then systolic myocardial function become impaired. These events are precursors to electrocardiographic (ECG) changes and the clinical syndrome of angina pectoris (11). Because myocardial perfusion abnormalities occur early in the pathophysiologic ischemic cascade, the regional heterogeneity of myocardial perfusion is a sensitive marker of ischemia (Fig. 11.1).

P. R. Sensky: Department of Cardiology, Glenfield Hospital, Leicester, United Kingdom.

G. R. Cherryman: Department of Radiology, University of Leicester, Leicester, United Kingdom.

CLINICAL INDICATIONS FOR MYOCARDIAL PERFUSION IMAGING

The clinical indications for myocardial perfusion imaging in patients with known or suspected ischemic heart disease are shown in Table 11.1. In addition to its usefulness as a diagnostic test to confirm initial or recurrent coronary artery disease and myocardial viability, perfusion imaging may be helpful to distinguish patients with symptoms of ischemia but normal findings on coronary angiography (syndrome X) (12–15). Myocardial blood flow has also been evaluated diagnostically in the emergency setting (16,17). A wealth of literature has been published describing the value of nuclear imaging techniques in providing prognostic information. Applications include assessing the risk of patients for future cardiac events, determining the need for further intervention, and elucidating the cardiovascular risk associated with noncardiac surgical procedures (17–20). A clarification of the physiologic effects of single or sequential angiographic stenoses and the collateral circulation is invaluable in planning treatment (21–23). Serial perfusion imaging to evaluate changes in myocardial perfusion following conventional or novel treatment strategies is a useful tool in both clinical and research settings (24–27).

Like all investigational methods for the evaluation of ischemia, perfusion imaging is enhanced by the addition of cardiac stress. This may be in the form of physical exercise or pharmacologic stressors (28). Perfusion deficits may be assessed qualitatively by visual image interpretation and categorized as either reversible (present on stress imaging alone) or fixed (present on stress and rest imaging). In addition, some methods permit a more quantitative estimate of blood flow, and the parameters *coronary flow reserve* (CFR) and

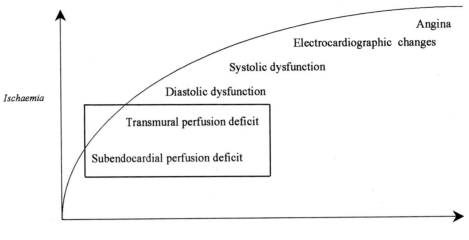

FIGURE 11.1. Schematic demonstrating the sequence of myocardial events in the progression of ischemia. Note the early occurrence of abnormal perfusion.

TABLE 11.1. CLINICAL INDICATIONS FOR MYOCARDIAL PERFUSION IMAGING

Diagnosis	New or recurrent ischemic heart disease
	Myocardial viability
	Syndrome X
	Emergency evaluation of chest pain
Risk stratification	Prognosis for future coronary events
	After myocardial infarction
	Before noncardiac surgery
Treatment planning/ evaluation	Evaluation of the effects of collateral circulation
	Functional significance of known angiographic lesions
	Follow-up after medical or interventional treatment
Research tool	Characterization of novel revascularization strategies

myocardial perfusion reserve (MPR) have been devised to express the quantitative relationship of blood flow at rest to flow during stress (29,30). CFR is defined as the ratio of epicardial arterial blood flow during maximal hyperemia to flow at rest. MPR is the ratio of blood flow within the myocardium during maximal hyperemia to flow in basal conditions.

IMAGING TECHNIQUES FOR THE MEASUREMENT OF MYOCARDIAL PERFUSION

Several techniques are in current clinical use to assess myocardial perfusion (Table 11.2).

Angiography

Angiographic visualization of an epicardial stenosis and estimation of the loss in vessel luminal cross-sectional area are

TABLE 11.2. ADVANTAGES AND DISADVANTAGES OF IMAGING MODALITIES CURRENTLY AVAILABLE TO ASSESS MYOCARDIAL PERFUSION

Imaging Modality	Ionizing Radiation	Function	Spatial Resolution (mm)	Artifact	Contrast Agent	Sensitivity (%)	Specificity (%)
Angiography	+	++	0.5–1	+	Iodinated compounds	–	–
SPECT	+++	+	10–15	+++	Radioactive tracers	79–96	53–76
PET	++	–	6–10	++	Radioactive tracers	82–97	82–100
CT	++	+	1	+	Iodinated compounds	–	–
Contrast echocardiography	–	++	<1 (axial)	+++	Microbubbles	–	–
MRI	–	+++	2–3	+	Gadolinium compounds	60–90	60–100

Sensitivities and specificities given are for the detection of angiographic disease.
SPECT, single photon emission computed tomography; PET, position emission tomography; CT, computed tomography.

frequently used to predict obstruction to arterial blood flow and the likely presence of reversible ischemia. Information regarding the functional effects of specific lesions on the myocardium cannot be obtained objectively by angiographic interpretation alone. In the presence of widespread atheroma, arterial stenoses may have a complex geometry, so that morphologic appearances are misleading (31,32). Quantitative angiographic measurement can be inaccurate, especially when referenced vessel segments are diseased. Coronary artery Doppler flow wires provide a measure of CFR. This invasive technique is limited in the presence of diffuse epicardial atheroma, collateral vessel recruitment, and pathologic myocardial states that directly affect MPR, such as microvascular disease and LV hypertrophy (33).

Single Photon Emission Computed Tomography

Single photon emission computed tomography (SPECT) is the most commonly available clinical method of assessing cardiac perfusion (34,35). The radioisotopes thallium 201 and technetium 99m are taken up by the myocardium in proportion to blood flow. Image analysis requires careful reconstruction into double-oblique imaging planes, and reporting techniques are usually qualitative. This methodology may limit accuracy in the presence of triple-vessel disease and global ischemia. SPECT has poor spatial resolution in comparison with other techniques, and artifacts frequently degrade image quality. Such artifacts include attenuation from breast tissue in the anterior wall and signal loss inferiorly, the latter predominantly in men as a result of respiratory motion and increased distance from the camera. Although diagnostic sensitivities are quite high, specificity is generally lower (12,22).

Positron Emission Tomography

Positron emission tomography (PET) provides the closest clinical method available for absolute quantification of perfusion (36,37). Tracers labeled with radioactive isotopes, such as rubidium and oxygen, are imaged dynamically as they pass through the cardiovascular circulation. Regional blood flow at rest and stress can be quantified with the use of radiotracer biodistribution kinetic modeling. The method is less prone to attenuation than SPECT and its spatial resolution is better, but still not sufficient to delineate minor perfusion deficits or those limited to the subendocardial layer. In addition, PET is expensive and available only in specialized centers.

Computed Tomography

Computed tomography (CT) has recently been shown to have potential for estimating regional myocardial blood flow (38,39). Dynamic imaging of iodinated contrast agents is used, and preliminary results of electron beam CT suggest that a quantitative measure of myocardial blood flow can be obtained. Multislice CT is now replacing this modality and is likely to become the future CT method for perfusion evaluation.

Contrast Echocardiography

The advent of pulsed and power harmonic Doppler modalities has led to considerable advances in contrast echocardiography for myocardial perfusion imaging (40,41). Images are subject to multiple artifacts, including attenuation, contrast blooming, and failure of bubble opacification owing to the inhomogeneous delivery of ultrasound to tissue. Further work must be done to elucidate fully the complex interactions of the varying microbubble contrast agents and ultrasonographic modalities before contrast echocardiography becomes sufficiently robust for clinical application.

MRI

MRI is well established as the gold standard for delineating mediastinal anatomy and assessing cardiac function (42). A combination of the development of high-specification hardware and the implementation of ultrafast imaging sequences has overcome many MRI difficulties created by respiration and cardiac cyclic motion. In recent years, MRI has become a genuine competitor of current clinical methods in the evaluation of myocardial perfusion. In contrast to other techniques, MRI requires no ionizing radiation and is therefore a safe modality for serial patient studies. A high degree of spatial resolution permits discrete visualization of the subendocardial layer. This feature is ideal for detecting subtle pathophysiologic perfusion abnormalities. Available temporal resolution facilitates the rapid tracking and characterization of the first pass of contrast agents and quantitative estimates of myocardial blood flow. In addition, perfusion imaging can be combined with an assessment of anatomy and myocardial wall thickening at rest and during stress in a single examination (43,44).

MRI TECHNIQUES

The MRI technique used in the majority of clinical studies is dynamic imaging of the first pass of a paramagnetic contrast agent, such as a gadolinium chelate, through the heart (15,45–52). To optimize an MR system for imaging cardiac blood flow, a variety of factors should be considered. These include scanner hardware, the imaging sequences and pharmacologic stressors employed, properties of the gadolinium compounds, and postprocessing analytical techniques.

Imager Hardware

Although myocardial perfusion MRI has been successfully performed on conventional whole body imagers, hardware

space) of 300 and 516 milliseconds, respectively, are used. Temporal resolution with this sequence is limited to approximately every two R-R intervals for single-slice acquisition and every six R-R intervals for three-slice acquisition, although this can be doubled by removing the trigger delay and imaging with a constant total repetition time (TR_0) rather than gating to the ECG (62). With the use of high-performance gradients, relatively short TR and TE times can be achieved, and in combination with the inversion time and flip angle, they can be used to maximize image contrast. Under these conditions, T2* dephasing is minimal, and motion and susceptibility artifacts are insignificant, even in nongated cardiac acquisitions.

Saturation Recovery Snapshot Fast Low-Angle Shot

The snapshot FLASH sequence can also be used with a 90-degree saturation recovery prepulse to null the myocardial signal (15,63). Wilke et al. (15) have proposed the subsequent use of a gradient crusher pulse to dephase transverse magnetization and prevent the modulation of image intensity caused by heart rate variability or poor ECG triggering. This technique is referred to as *arrhythmia-insensitive magnetization preparation.* Although it allows imaging every R-R interval and the acquisition of up to five parallel short-axis slices at heart rates of up to 65 beats/min (15), the more rapid image acquisition time (160 to 235 milliseconds) employed necessitates some loss of spatial resolution (image matrix 128 * 60). The sequence is prone to image artifact, and image contrast is considerably less than with inversion recovery preparation because myocardial nulling is less effective with the saturation prepulse. The sequence allows the user only three (TR, TE, flip angle) of the four (TR, TE, flip angle, TI) degrees of freedom with which to manipulate image contrast. Although images within one slice are acquired during the same part of the cardiac cycle, image sequences for further slices are acquired at different points within the R-R interval.

Echo-Planar Imaging

Single-shot echo-planar imaging is one approach that has been used to reduce image acquisition time (64,65). A rapidly oscillating frequency-encoding gradient is used to produce a rapid train of echoes to generate all k-space data following just a single RF excitation pulse. Because image acquisition times are extremely short (50 to 100 milliseconds), coverage of the ventricle is significantly increased without loss of temporal resolution. Up to 10 parallel short-axis slices can be acquired with this sequence. The technique has not been widely used because the images are extremely prone to artifact resulting from by bulk magnetic susceptibility, eddy currents, and chemical shifts producing displacement of fat signal. Spatial resolution and signal-to-

noise ratio are poor. An inversion recovery prepulse can be used to enhance T1 weighting and thus increase image contrast, but the TE required to achieve this is several times longer than that used with the snapshot FLASH sequences, so that T2* effects are exacerbated.

Hybrid Echo-Planar Imaging

Hybrid echo-planar imaging represents a compromise between the single-shot echo-planar approach and inversion recovery-prepared gradient-echo sequences. Sequences with multiple recalled gradient echoes generated per RF excitation and segmented k-space acquisition may retain the image quality of the snapshot FLASH sequences, and scan time is reduced sufficiently to allow multiple imaging slices to be acquired within a given TR (66).

Imaging Planes

Cardiac MRI can be performed in any orientation. Conventionally, however, imaging is performed in the standard double-oblique short-axis views. Following the acquisition of scouting images, the slice is positioned parallel to the plane of the mitral valve (Fig. 11.3). Most institutions use three to seven short-axis views according to the constraints of the imaging sequence. A major limitation to the use of the short-axis plane alone is that partial volume effects hamper evaluation of the true apex of the heart. A long-axis orientation may be useful to overcome this difficulty, but separate image acquisition is required.

Pharmacologic Stressors

Because space is limited within the magnet bore, physical exercise is not a practical form of cardiac stress. Exercise may also produce patient motion artifacts on stress images. Thus,

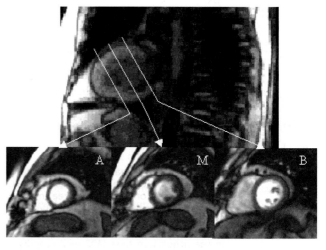

FIGURE 11.3. Localization of short-axis slices of the left ventricle at apical *(A)*, midpapillary *(M)*, and basal *(B)* levels.

pharmacologic stressors are used, most commonly dipyridamole and adenosine, although dobutamine has also been utilized for perfusion imaging (67).

Vasodilators: Adenosine and Dipyridamole

Adenosine is a naturally occurring purine that causes vasodilation. It acts on vascular smooth-muscle cell surface A_1 and A_2 adenosine receptors to produce an increase in intracellular cyclic adenosine monophosphate (cAMP). Dipyridamole causes a rise in interstitial adenosine concentration by inhibiting the cellular uptake and metabolism of adenosine. Both agents give rise to a fourfold or fivefold hyperemia, in contrast to the twofold vasodilator effect of dobutamine. Thus, during stress, a fourfold to fivefold increase in blood flow to normal myocardial territories occurs in comparison with the basal state. In the presence of coronary artery stenosis, vasodilation is impaired and the stress-to-rest ratio is reduced. Subendocardial ischemia may be precipitated by a loss of distal arterial perfusion pressure and by redirection of endocardial blood flow to the epicardial layer. High-resistance collateral flow may also be impaired because of generalized vasodilation.

The standard regime for dipyridamole is $0.56 \, mg \, kg^{-1}$ over 4 minutes. Imaging is commenced at 2 minutes into the infusion. Adenosine is infused at $140 \, \mu g \, kg^{-1} \, min^{-1}$ for 6 minutes and imaging initiated after 3 minutes. Contraindications to these agents include asthma, high-grade atrioventricular block, sinus arrhythmia, stenotic valvular disease, and carotid artery stenosis. Aminophylline, theophylline, and other xanthines, including foods such as coffee, tea, cocoa products, and cola, are competitive antagonists for adenosine. Any medication containing these products should be withdrawn for 24 hours before the scan, and foods containing caffeine should be omitted for 12 hours. Because dipyridamole potentiates the effects of adenosine, it should be omitted for 24 hours before the scan, or the prescribed dose of adenosine reduced. Patients are frequently symptomatic during infusions, reporting flushing, dizziness, nausea, and chest discomfort. Indications to terminate the scan include bronchospasm, ventricular arrhythmias, and the onset of second- or third-degree atrioventricular block and bradycardia. Intravenous aminophylline should be available for immediate administration as an antidote to both dipyridamole and adenosine.

Dobutamine

Dobutamine is a sympathomimetic agonist that acts on cardiac β_1 receptors to increase cardiac output and the oxygen demand of the heart. Initially, the inotropic effect gives rise to an increase in systolic, diastolic, and mean arterial blood pressure. Subsequently, a tachycardia is induced. The rise in the rate–pressure product is indicative of an increased cardiac workload.

A standard dobutamine regimen is commenced at $0.01 \, mg \, kg^{-1} \, min^{-1}$ for 3 minutes, then increased in increments of $0.01 \, mg \, kg^{-1} \, min^{-1}$ every 3 minutes until a maximal infusion rate of $0.04 \, mg \, kg^{-1} \, min^{-1}$ or the desired heart rate is achieved. If an insufficient chronotropic response is achieved, atropine can be added to the protocol (68). Stress imaging can be performed at the maximal dose tolerated, although evidence suggests that maximal vasodilation is achieved with a steady-state moderate-dose infusion of dobutamine (69). Contraindications to dobutamine include unstable ischemia and exercise-induced arrhythmias. Beta blockers must be withheld for 48 hours before the scan. Dobutamine is normally well tolerated, although some patients report nausea, dizziness, tremor, palpitations, dyspnea, and chest pain. Serious side effects include the induction of prolonged ischemia and ventricular arrhythmias. Conduction at the atrioventricular node is enhanced, so that a rapid ventricular response rate may develop in patients with atrial fibrillation or flutter. The half-life of dobutamine is approximately 2 minutes, and side effects usually subside rapidly. Intravenous beta blockade should be available to treat any prolonged or severe adverse events.

The vasodilators are most commonly used for perfusion imaging with MRI. Adenosine is preferred by the authors because although it is expensive, its extremely short half-life of less than 10 seconds ensures that adverse events are short-lived. Dipyridamole has a half-life of 30 minutes, so that prolonged ischemia may be provoked and persist despite aminophylline administration. In addition, its vasodilator effects are less predictable than those of adenosine; a significant proportion of patients (10% to 25%) do not achieve maximal vasodilation with the standard dose (67). Although theoretically a less potent vasodilator, dobutamine has been presented as an alternative stressor for perfusion imaging (70). It is technically more challenging to use because a more pronounced tachycardia is typically induced that gives rise to a greater potential for image blurring from cardiac motion. Results have been less satisfactory with this agent (70).

Contrast Agents

Gadolinium chelates are paramagnetic compounds widely used as contrast agents in MRI. They are composed of stable complexes of organic acids in association with gadolinium metal ions. Although the chemical structures of the varying compounds differ slightly, their properties are essentially similar, and no specific agent is superior to the others for perfusion imaging.

Kinetics

Gadolinium compounds are water-soluble and have relatively low molecular weights. They are therefore able to diffuse rapidly across capillary membranes into tissue extracellular space but are unable to enter cells with intact membranes. Although approximately 30% to 50% of the first-pass bolus enters myocardial interstitium following intravenous administration (71,72), the myocardial gadolinium concentration is determined primarily by coronary perfusion (73). Perfusion deficits are recognized as areas of reduced or delayed signal intensity. These changes in signal intensity form the basis of both qualitative and quantitative methods of image analysis. Because recirculation and bolus dilution lead to rapid equilibration between the vascular and extracellular compartments, gadolinium does not remain fixed in the myocardium in proportion to blood flow (73). The contrast agent accumulates rapidly in the myocardial interstitium, with a loss of any heterogeneity in signal intensity. Images must therefore be acquired during the first pass of the contrast agent. Any mathematical models applied to quantify myocardial blood flow parameters must take these kinetic properties into account.

Mechanism of Action

At clinical doses, gadolinium compounds create image contrast by shortening the T1 relaxation time; in other words, they reduce the time required for tissue longitudinal magnetization to return to equilibrium following an RF pulse application (74). Signal intensity is enhanced in areas of myocardium into which gadolinium is delivered by blood flow. The alteration in signal intensity is not a direct result of changes in tissue gadolinium concentration alone. Dipolar interactions between paramagnetic ions and protons produce an enhancing effect on proton T1 relaxivity (75). These interactions occur not only with protons within the same compartment as the contrast agent but also with protons that can exchange into that tissue compartment. Thus, the change in signal intensity produced by gadolinium also depends on the rate of water exchange between different tissue compartments (76,77).

When quantitative imaging is carried out, a dose of 0.02 to 0.025 mmol kg^{-1} is optimal and ensures that the measured changes in signal intensity are proportional to the changes in gadolinium concentration within the myocardium (45,78–80). Above this concentration, saturation effects occur, and the relationship no longer applies. This fact is particularly important when signal intensity changes of the bolus within the LV are used to normalize myocardial blood flow. Because the gadolinium concentration within the LV is relatively high, the linear relationship threshold may be reached and flow calculations compromised (46,57). Low-dose gadolinium may be suboptimal for qualitative viewing in the clinical setting, and a higher dose (e.g., 0.05 mmol kg^{-1}) may be helpful.

Mode of Delivery

Gadolinium is given as a compact intravenous bolus. Although the authors find peripheral hand injection to be sat-

isfactory, some workers prefer central venous access and the use of mechanical injectors. The quality of the bolus curve is determined by pulmonary and cardiac circulation hemodynamics (81). The central administration of contrast agent in a patient with normal right ventricular (RV) and LV function results in compact bolus delivery to the coronary circulation. Injection in patients with cardiac dysfunction is compromised by any RV impairment, abnormality in LV filling parameters, or valvular incompetence.

Adverse Effects

Gadolinium is a very safe contrast agent with no known contraindications. Approximately 95% of the administered bolus is eliminated by the kidneys within 24 hours. The half-life of gadolinium within normal myocardium is approximately 20 minutes, although this may vary in different pathologic states. Side effects of gadolinium compounds are rare but can include nausea, headache, and dizziness (82).

Image Postprocessing

Image postprocessing refers to the interpretation, analysis, and representation of raw image data. A variety of postprocessing methods have been used to extract information from perfusion images obtained by MRI. These include qualitative image interpretation, semiquantification of blood flow parameters, and the use of complex mathematical models to provide a measure of MPR.

Qualitative Image Assessment

Qualitative evaluation provides a comprehensive and rapid interpretation of perfusion images that is ideal for clinical use. It can be performed either on the imager graphics user interface or at a remote workstation. Images can be scrolled through on screen with the use of a dynamic viewing mode, or printed onto film. The quality of bolus arriving in the LV is evaluated, and then regional myocardial enhancement is considered. Peak enhancement and time to peak enhancement are key criteria for the identification and characterization of perfusion deficits (Table 11.3). Any reduction or delay in regional peak signal intensity suggests hypoperfusion (Fig. 11.4). This can be further categorized as reversible or fixed by a comparison of stress and rest studies.

Qualitative image interpretation requires an experienced reader and may be subject to observer bias. This method relies on the identification of relative signal enhancement characteristics in each region, and therefore ischemia in patients with global hypoperfusion may be masked. The imaging sequence chosen should provide maximal image contrast (e.g., inversion recovery snapshot FLASH), so that small perfusion differences may be appreciated visually.

TABLE 11.3. QUALITATIVE PARAMETERS FOR THE ASSESSMENT OF CONTRAST-ENHANCED MRI AND DEFINITION OF MYOCARDIAL DISEASE STATES

Perfusion Pattern		Perfusion: Rest versus Stress	
Enhancement	Peak Signal	Enhancement	Evaluation
Normal	Satisfactory	Normal at rest and on stress	Normal
Slow	Satisfactory	↑ Delay or hypoenhancement on stress	Reversible
Slow	Low	Impaired, equivalent at rest and on stress	Fixed
None		Absent at rest and on stress	Scar

Quantitative Image Assessment

Semiquantitative and quantitative evaluations require the definition of myocardial regions-of-interest (ROIs), image registration, extraction of signal intensity time curve data, and analysis or mathematical modeling of the contrast agent kinetics to derive chosen parameters.

Delineation of Regions-of-Interest

The extraction of signal intensity changes over time forms the basis of quantitative methods of image analysis. Because ischemic heart disease is a heterogeneous process, regional division of the myocardium is necessary to make clinical sense of data. Defined ROIs are therefore required. A variety of methods for myocardial division have been applied. These include hand-drawn free-form or spherical ROIs placed in areas of myocardium representing blood supply from the different coronary arteries (15,46–49), a circumferential central profile (60), and epicardial and endocardial contouring and subsequent radial division of the myocardium (51,52,56). The latter method requires care to exclude signal intensity data from the LV cavity and adjacent pericardial structures, but this approach is less subjective and more consistent than individual region placement. The most basal short-axis slice is anatomically closest to the coronary ostia and should be used for region assignment to char-

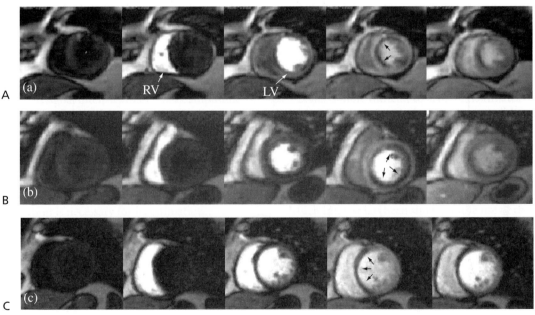

FIGURE 11.4. Sequential contrast-enhanced first-pass perfusion images acquired with an inversion recovery snapshot fast low-angle shot (FLASH) sequence. Myocardial signal is initially nulled. The bolus of gadolinium contrast *(white arrows)* appears first in the right ventricle *(RV)* and then in the left ventricular cavity *(LV)*. Normally, perfused myocardium is enhanced. **A:** *Black arrows* show anteroseptal subendocardial deficit with adenosine in a patient presenting with in-stent restenosis in the left anterior descending artery. *Open arrow* indicates a small artifact produced by the stent. **B:** *Arrows* demonstrate global subendocardial ischemia produced with adenosine in a patient with triple-vessel disease and hypertensive LV hypertrophy. **C:** *Arrows* show extensive septal transmural deficit in a patient with a history of anterior myocardial infarction.

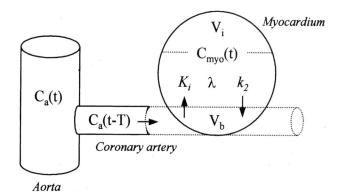

FIGURE 11.6. Graphic depiction of modified two-compartmental Kety model for calculating the unidirectional transfer constant of gadolinium (K_i) over the capillary membrane. $C_a(t)$, input function to myocardium; T, transit time through the coronary arteries; V_b, vascular volume; V_i, intracellular space; $C_{myo}(t)$, gadolinium concentration in the extravascular volume; k_2, back-diffusion of gadolinium into the vascular volume. $C_{myo}(t) = C_a(t - T) \otimes K_i \exp^{-k_2 t}$, where $\otimes$ denotes convolution.

functions. The model is less sensitive to noise and more independent of the separation of first and second passes of the contrast agent than those described above. Thus, it is possible to use peripheral venous injection for bolus delivery, and the technique is potentially applicable in patients with impaired circulatory hemodynamics. K_i is expressed as the product of the contrast agent extraction fraction (E) and flow (F)—that is, $K_i = F \times E$. Determined parameters describe myocardial flow and distribution volume. The Kety model was originally proposed for application to freely diffusible tracers for which E is assumed to be unity. Because gadolinium is barrier-limited, this assumption does not apply. Although K_i alone is related to perfusion, for absolute blood flow quantification, this method is limited by its dependence on E because direct measurement of this factor is not possible in humans. E has been measured in animal studies for small molecular compounds in normal myocardium. It has been found to be 0.5 at rest and 0.4 during dipyridamole stress (72). These parameters could be used to extrapolate absolute values for myocardial flow in normal tissue, but as yet no work has reliably measured E in ischemia. Despite this limitation, values of K_i have been shown to have a linear relationship with blood flow determined by microspheres and with PET (91). K_i has been shown to be sensitive to changes in perfusion induced by vasodilator stress and by the presence of coronary artery stenosis (49,51,62,91). The ratio of vasodilator-induced stress and rest K_i values has been presented as an index of MPR (51,62).

From the heterogeneous approaches to derive indicators of myocardial perfusion, it is clear that perfusion imaging with MRI is still in evolution and that many difficulties remain to be overcome. Qualitative analysis is effective in the clinical workplace but is limited by its subjective nature. Quantification aims to overcome the weaknesses of the lat-

ter. Many parameters presented in the literature have appeared robust when tested in the laboratory. However, transferring these methods to the diverse pathophysiology of ischemic heart disease has proved to be a challenge because any proposed diagnostic test must be applicable to all potential recipients. Most clinical studies have tight inclusion criteria, excluding patients not in sinus rhythm and those with a history of myocardial infarction or LV dysfunction.

No data evaluating the reproducibility of the described techniques in patients have yet been published. The database of perfusion findings in subjects without angiographic coronary artery disease is still very small. Presented data are frequently from patients with suspected coronary disease or with chest pain but angiographically normal coronary vessels, or from normal coronary artery territories in patients with remote arterial lesions. Parameters obtained in this population are likely to be unrepresentative of healthy subjects because a high prevalence of microvascular disease or early endothelial dysfunction with impaired vasodilator response is likely. Myocardial perfusion is influenced by heart rate, myocardial afterload, and contractility and so varies in accordance with patient hemodynamic parameters, metabolic states, and response to pharmacologic interventions. These factors are difficult to keep static within patients, especially in the context of serial examinations. Changes in intramyocardial blood volume, arterial pressure, or LV dysfunction induced by stressors will affect quantitative results. A wide range of normal values for myocardial blood flow have been demonstrated with the use of PET (92). A definite distinction between normal perfusion and ischemia is difficult to define because parameters frequently overlap. A further complexity in identifying a normal range of values is that the autoregulatory mechanisms that govern myocardial perfusion are not homogeneous across the myocardium, so that a natural spatial variation of flow exists (93–95). The degree of flow dispersion is related to the size of the segments examined. ROIs of several grams may be required to detect perfusion differences of less than 20% of mean flow (96).

Interpretation of the indices of MPR derived from quantitative data is not straightforward because variations may occur in both rest and stress components. Deviations from normal resting flow values may produce artificially high or low MPR values. Some pathologic conditions of the LV muscle (e.g., scarring or LV hypertrophy from valvular disease, hypertension, postinfarction remodeling) may exert an effect on MPR independently of angiographic disease. Derivation of an absolute measure of myocardial perfusion with MRI has many potential applications. However, these factors should be borne in mind, especially when measurements are repeated in individuals or compared between patient groups. For clinical use, quantitative analysis is uneconomical in regard to both time and resources, and any additional clinical information gained over qualitative reporting must be established.

APPLICATIONS

Relatively few clinical studies have evaluated rest and stress perfusion MRI (Table 11.4). Most workers have aimed at establishing and evaluating varying quantitative parameters against a chosen "gold standard" imaging modality.

Angiography

The diagnostic potential of perfusion imaging with MR has been evaluated against coronary angiography by several groups. Despite the limitations of angiography as a gold standard, the sensitivities and specificities of MRI for the detection of significant coronary angiographic lesions ranged from 44% to 93% and 60% to 100%, respectively (46,52,58–60,97,98). The variation in results reflects differences in the imaging techniques used and in the definition of a "significant" angiographic lesion. Qualitative analysis is practical for routine clinical work. In patients with chronic ischemic heart disease, we found qualitative assessment to be sensitive but not very specific for the presence of epicardial stenoses. Lack of specificity was likely a consequence of collateral flow effects and difficulty in recognizing areas of normality in patients with severe disease (98). Wolff et al. (99) achieved a higher specificity but a lower sensitivity. Quantitative modes of analysis may enhance the diagnostic accuracy of MRI. In a prospective study by Al-Saadi et al. (52), the use of a predefined perfusion reserve index cutoff of 1.5 gave a sensitivity of 90% and a specificity of 83% for detecting an angiographic cross-sectional area loss of more than 75%. This study demonstrates the need to interpret results in the light of the methodology used; these authors obtained a poorer diagnostic accuracy when they used the same MRI technique but with dobutamine as the stressor rather than adenosine. Here, a perfusion reserve index of 1.2 was found to have the best threshold value, reflecting the poorer vasodilator properties of the inotrope (70).

TABLE 11.4. CLINICAL PERFUSION STUDIES PERFORMED WITH STRESS MRI

Study Ref. No.	MRI Technique (Stressor)	MRI Parameter Evaluated	Inclusion	N	Angiographic Cut Off (%)	Angiograpy Sensitivity (%)	Specificity (%)	SPECT Sensitivity (%)	Specificity (%)
60	IR-TF (D)	Peak SI	(N) CAD	(4) 6	>70	65	76		
59	IR-TF (D)	SI/qualitative	CAD	5	>50	81	100	77 (92[a])	57 (57[a])
46	EPI (D)	Max upslope (/LV upslope)	CAD	10	>75	44	80	56	79
58	IR-TF (D)	Qualitative	CAD	18	>70	83	100	92	100
47	IR-TF (D)	SI increase (linear fit)/ upslope	SVD	10	>75	70		90	
97	IR-TF (D)	Qualitative	Suspected CAD	12	>50	60		88	87
48	IR-TF (D)	SI increase (linear fit)/ defect size	SVD LAD	11	>75			85	86
15	SR-TF (A)	MPR model	(N) Syndrome X	8		$r = .8$[b]			
49	IR-TF (D)	K_i	(N) SVD LAD	(10) 10	>75				
51	IR-TF (A)	K_i	(N) CAD	(5) 20	>50	$r = .81$[c]			
99	EPI	Qualitative	(N) CAD	(14) 33	>70	72	80		
52	IR-TF (D)	Upslope (linear fit)	(N) [SVD] CAD— prospective	(5) [15] 34	>75	90	83		
98	IR-TF (A)	Qualitative	CAD	30	>50	93	60		
56	IR-TF (D)	SI/upslope/ mean transit time	SVD	11	>70			71/77/74	71/61/70

Figure for sensitivity and specificity in the detection of angiographic or SPECT abnormalities are given where appropriate.
[a] Retrospective analysis.
[b] Value of r for myocardial perfusion reserve versus coronary flow reserve.
[c] Value of r for myocardial perfusion reserve versus percentage coronary artery stenosis.
IR-TF, inversion recovery snapshot FLASH (fast low-angle shot); SR-TF, saturation recovery snapshot FLASH; EPI, echo planar imaging; D, dipyridamole; A, adenosine; SI, signal intensity; LV, left ventricle; MPR, myocardial perfusion reserve; K_i, unidirectional transfer constant of gadolinium; N, normal; CAD, coronary artery disease; SVD, single-vessel disease; LAD, left anterior descending artery.

Perfusion MRI is a complementary modality to coronary angiography in the assessment of the physiologic effects of collateral circulation and given angiographic stenoses. Cullen et al. (51) demonstrated an inverse relationship between the MPR index and the severity of coronary artery stenosis as assessed by angiography. Wilke et al. (15) showed an excellent correlation between MPR obtained by MRI and Doppler CFR. In patients with symptoms of myocardial ischemia but angiographically normal coronary arteries (syndrome X), MRI demonstrated a reduced MPR (15). Similar findings were noted in patients with coronary artery disease in myocardial regions supplied by normal remote epicardial vessels (62). Thus, quantitative MRI may be a powerful tool for the diagnosis of microvascular dysfunction and early endothelial arterial abnormalities.

Nuclear Techniques

Sensitivities and specificities for the detection by MRI of perfusion deficits seen on SPECT images range from 56% to 90% and 61% to 90%, respectively (46–48,56,58,59, 97). Although of interest, the findings are difficult to interpret because of inherent differences between the techniques. Disparities are likely to occur because of superior spatial resolution with MRI, difficulties in assessing attenuated areas on scintigraphy, and variations in protocol between centers. In a preliminary study of eight patients with scintigraphic inferior wall attenuation, three were shown to have evidence of subendocardial infarction with MR (100). MRI has the potential to have equivalent if not greater diagnostic value than scintigraphic techniques. As yet, no definitive studies have compared stress perfusion MRI with PET.

Revascularization

Early work by Manning et al. (45) demonstrated the ability of MRI to evaluate the efficacy of revascularization. Lauerma et al. (48) documented a decrease in perfusion deficit size following arterial revascularization that was in reasonable agreement with the decrease seen with thallium scintigraphy. Recovery of the MPR index early following percutaneous transluminal coronary angioplasty (PTCA) has been demonstrated (101). Al-Saadi et al. (102) used MRI to compare perfusion changes following balloon angioplasty with changes after direct stenting. Clinical trials are currently under way to assess whether MRI is of value in the serial follow-up of revascularization techniques such as transmyocardial laser revascularization and gene therapy (103–105).

At present, first-pass MRI does not play a prominent role in the identification of viable myocardium in patients with LV dysfunction. A more promising MRI technique is that of delayed enhancement following gadolinium bolus injection (106).

Prognosis

In contrast to the detailed literature available for nuclear methods, no data have been published regarding the prognostic significance of perfusion MRI findings. Longitudinal studies are required to document adverse cardiac events and mortality rates following imaging in patients with stable symptomatology after myocardial infarction. The role of perfusion MRI in the risk assessment of patients undergoing noncardiac surgical procedures also must be elucidated.

One-Stop Shop

In contrast to other perfusion imaging tools, MRI can offer an integrated examination of cardiac anatomy, function, and perfusion in a single session. MRI protocols to assess cardiac structure and global and regional myocardial function are well established. The diagnostic value of systolic wall thickening in response to inotropic stress is superior to that of conventional echocardiography (107). The addition of perfusion imaging to this armory is likely to make MRI a very powerful tool for imaging the varying myocardial states that stem from ischemia.

Several authors have explored this combined approach (58,63,97). We have developed a dual adenosine–dobutamine stress (DADS) MRI protocol that is designed to provide optimal preoperative assessment (44). The ejection fraction and regional systolic function at rest and during a two-step low-dose dobutamine infusion are measured with standard cine sequences. The presence of any contractile reserve indicative of myocardial hibernation in resting dysfunctional segments can be determined. The transmural extent and reversibility of perfusion defects are demonstrated with first-pass MRI at rest and during adenosine. The protocol, which can be completed in less than an hour, is safe and well tolerated, and it provides valuable and comprehensive information.

FUTURE PERSPECTIVES

The technologic developments of the last few years—dedicated cardiac scanners, improved image quality, and increased speed of imaging—are likely to continue for the foreseeable future.

The production of dedicated cardiac imagers with improved gradient performance, specialized multiple receiver coil systems, and vector ECG monitoring will increase the accuracy and rapidity of image acquisition without a loss of quality. The utilization of ultrafast hybrid echo-planar or parallel imaging sequences will facilitate whole myocardial coverage, so that MRI will have a more equal competitive stance against nuclear techniques.

Intravascular contrast agents would be ideal for the quantitative analysis of myocardial perfusion because the assumptions of the indicator dilution theory would be followed without modification. However, the introduction of such compounds into the clinical workplace has been difficult because they are composed of toxic metal compounds with poor excretion. The myocardial distribution of intravascular agents is only 10%. Thus, the associated signal responses are small and susceptible to noise, and the peak signal intensities are critically dependent on variations in intravascular volume. Alternative forms of contrast specific to MRI have been used. T2-shortening or susceptibility contrast agents produce local magnetic field disturbances that result in signal loss rather than enhancement. Some workers have used intrinsic myocardial contrast to distinguish between normal and ischemic states, exploiting the blood oxygenation level-dependent (BOLD) effect (108,109). However, differences in signal contrast between oxygenated and unoxygenated blood in ischemic and nonischemic regions are small and cannot be differentiated reliably.

The majority of image postprocessing packages remain time-consuming and cumbersome to use. Before the utilization of quantitative analytical parameters can become widespread, better automated edge detection software is needed to reduce analysis time and increase cost-effectiveness.

At present, the clinical application of perfusion MRI is limited by the relatively small number of working centers, scarcity of experienced personnel, and diverse methodology. Varying sequences, contrast agents, modes of injection, comparative imaging methods, and analytic techniques have been utilized. Protocols for perfusion imaging must be standardized and analytic criteria made uniform. Industry, pharmaceutical manufacturers, physicists, and clinicians must cooperate to set up multicenter trials to establish the robustness and reproducibility of the techniques and to create a reference database. This is unlikely to occur until the rapid rate of imager hardware and sequence evolution reaches a plateau. Until then, technologic development is likely to overtake clinical experience. In the light of the current data, this aim is clearly worth pursuing to establish a definitive role for perfusion MRI in the management of patients with ischemic heart disease.

REFERENCES

1. Eagle KA, Guyton RA, Davidoff R, et al. ACC/AHA guidelines for coronary artery bypass graft surgery: a report of the American College of Cardiology/American Heart Association Task Force on Practice Guidelines. *J Am Coll Cardiol* 1999;34:1262–1347.
2. Beanlands RS, Hendry PJ, Masters RG, et al. Delay in revascularization is associated with increased mortality rate in patients with severe left ventricular dysfunction and viable myocardium on fluorine 18-fluorodeoxyglucose positron emission tomography imaging. *Circulation* 1998;98:II51–II56.
3. Goldman L. Cost and quality of life: thrombolysis and primary angioplasty. *J Am Coll Cardiol* 1995;25:38S–41S.
4. Hollman JL. Myocardial revascularization. Coronary angio-
plasty and bypass surgery indications. *Med Clin North Am* 1992; 76:1083–1097.
5. Lieu TA, Gurley RJ, Lundstrom RJ, et al. Primary angioplasty and thrombolysis for acute myocardial infarction: an evidence summary. *J Am Coll Cardiol* 1996;27:737–750.
6. Hughes GC, Abdel-aleem S, Biswas SS, et al. Transmyocardial laser revascularization: experimental and clinical results. *Can J Cardiol* 1999;15:797–806.
7. Owen AR, Stables RH. Myocardial revascularisation by laser. *Int J Cardiol* 2000;72:215–220.
8. Losordo DW, Vale PR, Isner JM. Gene therapy for myocardial angiogenesis. *Am Heart J* 1999;138:S132–S141.
9. Sinnaeve P, Varenne O, Collen D, et al. Gene therapy in the cardiovascular system: an update. *Cardiovasc Res* 1999;44:498–506.
10. Bache RJ, Schwartz JS. Effect of perfusion pressure distal to a coronary stenosis on transmural myocardial blood flow. *Circulation* 1982;65:928–935.
11. Nesto RW, Kowalchuk GJ. The ischemic cascade: temporal sequence of hemodynamic, electrocardiographic and symptomatic expressions of ischemia. *Am J Cardiol* 1987;59:23C–30C.
12. Go RT, Marwick TH, MacIntyre WJ, et al. A prospective comparison of rubidium-82 PET and thallium-201 SPECT myocardial perfusion imaging utilizing a single dipyridamole stress in the diagnosis of coronary artery disease. *J Nucl Med* 1990;31:1899–1905.
13. Bax JJ, Valkema R, Visser FC, et al. Detection of myocardial viability with F-18-fluorodeoxyglucose and single photon emission computed tomography. *Giornale Italiano di Cardiologia* 1997;27:1181–1186.
14. Wieneke H, Zander C, Eising EG, et al. Non-invasive characterization of cardiac microvascular disease by nuclear medicine using single-photon emission tomography. *Herz* 1999;24:515–521.
15. Wilke N, Jerosch-Herold M, Wang Y, et al. Myocardial perfusion reserve: assessment with multisection, quantitative, first-pass MR imaging. *Radiology* 1997;204:373–384.
16. Hilton TC, Thompson RC, Williams HJ, et al. Technetium-99m sestamibi myocardial perfusion imaging in the emergency room evaluation of chest pain. *J Am Coll Cardiol* 1994;23:1016–1022.
17. Iskander S, Iskandrian AE. Risk assessment using single-photon emission computed tomographic technetium-99m sestamibi imaging. *J Am Coll Cardiol* 1998;32:57–62.
18. Pamelia FX, Gibson RS, Watson DD, et al. Prognosis with chest pain and normal thallium-201 exercise scintigrams. *Am J Cardiol* 1985;55:920–926.
19. Brown KA. Prognostic value of cardiac imaging in patients with known or suspected coronary artery disease: comparison of myocardial perfusion imaging, stress echocardiography, and position emission tomography. *Am J Cardiol* 1995;75:35D–41D.
20. Pasquet A, Robert A, D'Hondt AM, et al. Prognostic value of myocardial ischemia and viability in patients with chronic left ventricular ischemic dysfunction. *Circulation* 1999;100:141–148.
21. Uren NG, Melin JA, De Bruyne B, et al. Relation between myocardial blood flow and the severity of coronary artery stenosis. *N Engl J Med* 1994;330:1782–1788.
22. Schwaiger M. Myocardial perfusion imaging with PET. *J Nucl Med* 1994;35:693–698.
23. Sabia PJ, Powers ER, Jayaweera AR, et al. Functional significance of collateral blood flow in patients with recent acute myocardial infarction. A study using myocardial contrast echocardiography. *Circulation* 1992;85:2080–2089.
24. Versaci F, Tomai F, Nudi F, et al. Differences of regional coronary flow reserve assessed by adenosine thallium-201 scintigra-

phy early and six months after successful percutaneous transluminal coronary angioplasty or stent implantation. *Am J Cardiol* 1996;78:1097–1102.

25. Kosa I, Blasini R, Schneider-Eicke J, et al. Early recovery of coronary flow reserve after stent implantation as assessed by positron emission tomography. *J Am Coll Cardiol* 1999;34:1036–1041.

26. Bax JJ, Cornel JH, Visser FC, et al. F18-fluorodeoxyglucose single-photon emission computed tomography predicts functional outcome of dyssynergic myocardium after surgical revascularization. *J Nucl Cardiol* 1997;4:302–308.

27. Rimoldi O, Burns SM, Rosen SD, et al. Measurement of myocardial blood flow with positron emission tomography before and after transmyocardial laser revascularization. *Circulation* 1999;100:II134–II138.

28. Iliceto S. Pharmacological agents for stress testing in the diagnosis of coronary artery disease. *Eur Heart J* 1995;16(Suppl M):1–2.

29. Bourdarias JP. Coronary reserve: concept and physiological variations. *Eur Heart J* 1995;16(Suppl I):2–6.

30. Goldstein RA, Kirkeeide RL, Demer LL, et al. Relation between geometric dimensions of coronary artery stenoses and myocardial perfusion reserve in man. *J Clin Invest* 1987;79:1473–1478.

31. Gould KL. Percent coronary stenosis: battered gold standard, pernicious relic or clinical practicality? *J Am Coll Cardiol* 1988;11:886–888.

32. White CW, Wright CB, Doty DB, et al. Does visual interpretation of the coronary arteriogram predict the physiologic importance of a coronary stenosis? *N Engl J Med* 1984;310:819–824.

33. Vassalli G, Hess OM. Measurement of coronary flow reserve and its role in patient care. *Basic Res Cardiol* 1998;93:339–353.

34. Hor G. Myocardial scintigraphy—25 years after start. *Eur J Nucl Med* 1988;13:619–636.

35. Keijer JT, Bax JJ, Van Rossum AC, et al. Myocardial perfusion imaging: clinical experience and recent progress in radionuclide scintigraphy and magnetic resonance imaging. *Int J Card Imaging* 1997;13:415–431.

36. Muzik O, Duvernoy C, Beanlands RS, et al. Assessment of diagnostic performance of quantitative flow measurements in normal subjects and patients with angiographically documented coronary artery disease by means of nitrogen-13 ammonia and positron emission tomography. *J Am Coll Cardiol* 1998;31:534–540.

37. Schwaiger M, Muzik O. Assessment of myocardial perfusion by positron emission tomography. *Am J Cardiol* 1991;67:35D–43D.

38. Schmermund A, Bell MR, Lerman LO, et al. Quantitative evaluation of regional myocardial perfusion using fast x-ray computed tomography. *Herz* 1997;22:29–39.

39. Georgiou D, Wolfkiel C, Brundage BH. Ultrafast computed tomography for the physiological evaluation of myocardial perfusion. *Am J Card Imaging* 1994;8:151–158.

40. Mulvagh SL. Myocardial perfusion by contrast echocardiography: diagnosis of coronary artery disease using contrast-enhanced stress echocardiography and assessment of coronary anatomy and flow reserve. *Coron Artery Dis* 2000;11:243–251.

41. Senior R, Kaul S, Soman P, et al. Power Doppler harmonic imaging: a feasibility study of a new technique for the assessment of myocardial perfusion. *Am Heart J* 2000;139:245–251.

42. Higgins CB, Sakuma H. Heart disease: functional evaluation with MR imaging. *Radiology* 1996;199:307–315.

43. Kramer CM. Integrated approach to ischemic heart disease. The one-stop shop. *Cardiol Clin* 1998;16:267–276.

44. Sensky PR, Jivan A, Hudson NM, et al. Coronary artery disease: combined stress MR imaging protocol—one-stop evaluation of myocardial perfusion and function. *Radiology* 2000;215:608–614.

45. Manning WJ, Atkinson DJ, Grossman W, et al. First-pass nuclear magnetic resonance imaging studies using gadolinium-DTPA in patients with coronary artery disease. *J Am Coll Cardiol* 1991;18:959–965.

46. Eichenberger AC, Schuiki E, Kochli VD, et al. Ischemic heart disease: assessment with gadolinium-enhanced ultrafast MR imaging and dipyridamole stress. *J Magn Reson Imaging* 1994;4:425–431.

47. Matheijssen NA, Louwerenburg HW, van Rugge FP, et al. Comparison of ultrafast dipyridamole magnetic resonance imaging with dipyridamole SestaMIBI SPECT for detection of perfusion abnormalities in patients with one-vessel coronary artery disease: assessment by quantitative model fitting. *Magn Reson Med* 1996;35:221–228.

48. Lauerma K, Virtanen KS, Sipila LM, et al. Multislice MRI in assessment of myocardial perfusion in patients with single-vessel proximal left anterior descending coronary artery disease before and after revascularization. *Circulation* 1997;96:2859–2867.

49. Fritz-Hansen T, Rostrup E, Sondergaard L, et al. Capillary transfer constant of Gd-DTPA in the myocardium at rest and during vasodilation assessed by MRI. *Magn Reson Med* 1998;40:922–929.

50. Wintersperger BJ, Penzkofer HV, Knez A, et al. Multislice MR perfusion imaging and regional myocardial function analysis: complimentary findings in chronic myocardial ischemia. *Int J Card Imaging* 1999;15:425–434.

51. Cullen JH, Horsfield MA, Reek CR, et al. A myocardial perfusion reserve index in humans using first-pass contrast-enhanced magnetic resonance imaging. *J Am Coll Cardiol* 1999;33:1386–1394.

52. Al-Saadi N, Nagel E, Gross M, et al. Noninvasive detection of myocardial ischemia from perfusion reserve based on cardiovascular magnetic resonance. *Circulation* 2000;101:1379–1383.

53. Gatehouse PD, Firmin DN. The cardiovascular magnetic resonance machine: hardware and software requirements. *Herz* 2000;25:317–330.

54. Lanzer P, Barta C, Botvinick EH, et al. ECG-synchronized cardiac MR imaging: method and evaluation. *Radiology* 1985;155:681–686.

55. Roth JL, Nugent M, Gray JE, et al. Patient monitoring during magnetic resonance imaging. *Anesthesiology* 1985;62:80–83.

56. Keijer JT, Van Rossum AC, Eenige MJ, et al. Magnetic resonance imaging of regional myocardial perfusion in patients with single-vessel coronary artery disease: quantitative comparison with 201-thallium-SPECT and coronary angiography. *J Magn Reson Imaging* 2000;11:607–615.

57. Keijer JT, Van Rossum AC, van Eenige MJ, et al. Semiquantitation of regional myocardial blood flow in normal human subjects by first-pass magnetic resonance imaging. *Am Heart J* 1995;130:893–901.

58. Hartnell G, Cerel A, Kamalesh M, et al. Detection of myocardial ischemia: value of combined myocardial perfusion and cine angiographic MR imaging. *AJR Am J Roentgenol* 1994;163:1061–1067.

59. Klein MA, Collier BD, Hellman RS, et al. Detection of chronic coronary artery disease: value of pharmacologically stressed, dynamically enhanced turbo-fast low-angle shot MR images. *AJR Am J Roentgenol* 1993;161:257–263.

60. Schaefer S, van Tyen R, Saloner D. Evaluation of myocardial perfusion abnormalities with gadolinium-enhanced snapshot MR imaging in humans. Work in progress. *Radiology* 1992;185:795–801.

61. Atkinson DJ, Burstein D, Edelman RR. First-pass cardiac perfusion: evaluation with ultrafast MR imaging. *Radiology* 1990;174:757–762.

62. Sensky PR, Horsfield MA, Samani NJ, et al. Is cardiac gating

beneficial for myocardial perfusion imaging? A non ECG-gated model and diagnostic performance evaluation in patients with coronary artery disease (CAD). *Proc Int Soc Magn Reson* 2001;9:1899.

63. Penzkofer H, Wintersperger BJ, Knez A, et al. Assessment of myocardial perfusion using multisection first-pass MRI and color-coded parameter maps: a comparison to 99mTc Sesta MIBI SPECT and systolic myocardial wall thickening analysis. *Magn Reson Imaging* 1999;17:161–170.

64. Stehling MK, Turner R, Mansfield P. Echo-planar imaging: magnetic resonance imaging in a fraction of a second. *Science* 1991;254:43–50.

65. Edelman RR, Li W. Contrast-enhanced echo-planar MR imaging of myocardial perfusion: preliminary study in humans. *Radiology* 1994;190:771–777.

66. Reeder SB, Atalar E, Faranesh AZ, et al. Multi-echo segmented k-space imaging: an optimized hybrid sequence for ultrafast cardiac imaging. *Magn Reson Med* 1999;41:375–385.

67. Iskandrian AS, Verani MS, Heo J. Pharmacologic stress testing: mechanism of action, hemodynamic responses, and results in detection of coronary artery disease. *J Nucl Cardiol* 1994;1:94–111.

68. Mathias WJ, Arruda A, Santos FC, et al. Safety of dobutamine-atropine stress echocardiography: a prospective experience of 4,033 consecutive studies. *J Am Soc Echocardiogr* 1999;12:785–791.

69. Pennell DJ, Underwood SR, Swanton RH, et al. Dobutamine thallium myocardial perfusion tomography. *J Am Coll Cardiol* 1991;18:1471–1479.

70. Al-Saadi N, Nagel E, Gross M, et al. Dobutamine magnetic resonance myocardial perfusion reserve: a step towards the one-stop shop. *J Cardiovasc Magn Reson Imaging* 1999;1:326.

71. Brasch RC. New directions in the development of MR imaging contrast media. *Radiology* 1992;183:1–11.

72. Tong CY, Prato FS, Wisenberg G, et al. Measurement of the extraction efficiency and distribution volume for Gd-DTPA in normal and diseased canine myocardium. *Magn Reson Med* 1993;30:337–346.

73. Diesbourg LD, Prato FS, Wisenberg G, et al. Quantification of myocardial blood flow and extracellular volumes using a bolus injection of Gd-DTPA: kinetic modeling in canine ischemic disease. *Magn Reson Med* 1992;23:239–253.

74. Higgins CB, Saeed M, Wendland M, et al. Contrast media for cardiothoracic MR imaging. *J Magn Reson Imaging* 1993;3:265–276.

75. Weinmann HJ, Brasch RC, Press WR, et al. Characteristics of gadolinium-DTPA complex: a potential NMR contrast agent. *AJR Am J Roentgenol* 1984;142:619–624.

76. Larsson HB, Stubgaard M, Sondergaard L, et al. In vivo quantification of the unidirectional influx constant for Gd-DTPA diffusion across the myocardial capillaries with MR imaging. *J Magn Reson Imaging* 1994;4:433–440.

77. Larsson HB, Fritz-Hansen T, Rostrup E, et al. Myocardial perfusion modeling using MRI. *Magn Reson Med* 1996;35:716–726.

78. Strich G, Hagan PL, Gerber KH, et al. Tissue distribution and magnetic resonance spin lattice relaxation effects of gadolinium-DTPA. *Radiology* 1985;154:723–726.

79. Weinmann HJ, Press WR, Gries H. Tolerance of extracellular contrast agents for magnetic resonance imaging. *Invest Radiol* 1990;25(Suppl 1):S49–S50.

80. Wilke N, Simm C, Zhang J, et al. Contrast-enhanced first pass myocardial perfusion imaging: correlation between myocardial blood flow in dogs at rest and during hyperemia. *Magn Reson Med* 1993;29:485–497.

81. Blomley MJ, Coulden R, Bufkin C, et al. Contrast bolus dynamic computed tomography for the measurement of solid organ perfusion. *Invest Radiol* 1993;28(Suppl 5):S72–S77.

82. Niendorf HP, Haustein J, Cornelius I, et al. Safety of gadolinium-DTPA: extended clinical experience. *Magn Reson Med* 1991;22:222–228.

83. Zierler KR. A simplified explanation of the theory of indicator-dilution for measurement of fluid flow and volume and other distributive phenomena. *Bull Johns Hopkins Hosp* 1958;103:1999.

84. Klocke FJ. Cognition in the era of technology: "seeing the shades of gray." *J Am Coll Cardiol* 1990;16:763–769.

85. Wilke N, Jerosch-Herold M, Stillman AE, et al. Concepts of myocardial perfusion imaging in magnetic resonance imaging. *Magn Reson Q* 1994;10:249–286.

86. Clough AV, al-Tinawi A, Linehan JH, et al. Regional transit time estimation from image residue curves. *Ann Biomed Eng* 1994;22:128–143.

87. Wilke N. MR measurement of myocardial perfusion. *MAGMA* 1998;6:147.

88. Jerosch-Herold M, Wilke N, Stillman AE. Magnetic resonance quantification of the myocardial perfusion reserve with a Fermi function model for constrained deconvolution. *Med Phys* 1998;25:73–84.

89. Vallee JP, Sostman HD, MacFall JR, et al. MRI quantitative myocardial perfusion with compartment analysis: a rest and stress study. *Magn Reson Med* 1997;38:981–989.

90. Jivan A, Horsfield MA, Moody AR, et al. Dynamic T1 measurement using snapshot-FLASH MRI. *J Magn Reson* 1997;127:65–72.

91. Vallee JP, Sostman HD, MacFall JR, et al. Quantification of myocardial perfusion by MRI after coronary occlusion. *Magn Reson Med* 1998;40:287–297.

92. Schwaiger M, Hutchins G. Quantification of regional myocardial perfusion by PET: rationale and first clinical results. *Eur Heart J* 1995;16(Suppl J):84–91.

93. Falsetti HL, Carroll RJ, Marcus ML. Temporal heterogeneity of myocardial blood flow in anesthetized dogs. *Circulation* 1975;52:848–853.

94. Austin REJ, Aldea GS, Coggins DL, et al. Profound spatial heterogeneity of coronary reserve. Discordance between patterns of resting and maximal myocardial blood flow. *Circ Res* 1990;67:319–331.

95. Bassingthwaighte JB, King RB, Roger SA. Fractal nature of regional myocardial blood flow heterogeneity. *Circ Res* 1989;65:578–590.

96. Canty JMJ. Methods of assessing coronary blood flow and flow reserve. *Am J Card Imaging* 1993;7:222–232.

97. Bremerich J, Buser P, Bongartz G, et al. Noninvasive stress testing of myocardial ischemia: comparison of GRE-MRI perfusion and wall motion analysis to 99m Tc-MIBI-SPECT, relation to coronary angiography. *Eur Radiol* 1997;7:990–995.

98. Sensky PR, Jivan A, Reek CR, et al. Magnetic resonance imaging in patients with coronary artery disease: a qualitative approach. *Proc Int Soc Magn Reson Med* 2000;8:1560.

99. Wolff SD, Day RA, Santiago L, et al. Assessment of first-pass myocardial perfusion imaging during rest and adenosine stress: comparison with cardiac catheterization. *Proc Int Soc Magn Reson Med* 1999;7:305.

100. McCrohon J, Rahman S, Lorenz CH, et al. Myocardial perfusion imaging with cardiac magnetic resonance in the assessment of patients with significant attenuation artifacts on stress scintigraphy. *J Cardiovasc Magn Reson* 2002;3(2):145.

101. Sensky PR, Samani NJ, Cherryman GR. Serial first pass contrast perfusion MRI following coronary artery angioplasty (PTCA) in patients with single vessel disease: qualitative and quantitative image analysis. *Proc Int Soc Magn Reson* 2001;9:1897.

102. Al-Saadi N, Nagel E, Gross M, et al. Myocardial perfusion re-

serve early after successful revascularisation: comparison of stent and balloon by cardiac MR. *Proc Soc Cardiovasc Magn Reson* 1999;1:324–325.

103. Eckstein FS, Scheule AM, Vogel U, et al. Transmyocardial laser revascularization in the acute ischaemic heart: no improvement of acute myocardial perfusion or prevention of myocardial infarction. *Eur J Cardiothorac Surg* 1999;15:702–708.

104. Pearlman JD, Laham RJ, Simons M. Coronary angiogenesis: detection *in vivo* with MR imaging sensitive to collateral neocirculation—preliminary study in pigs. *Radiology* 2000;214:801–807.

105. Laham RJ, Sellke FW, Edelman ER, et al. Local perivascular delivery of basic fibroblast growth factor in patients undergoing coronary bypass surgery: results of a phase I randomized, double-blind, placebo-controlled trial. *Circulation* 1999;100:1865–1871.

106. Higgins CB. Prediction of myocardial viability by MRI. *Circulation* 1999;99:727–729.

107. Nagel E, Lehmkuhl HB, Bocksch W, et al. Noninvasive diagnosis of ischemia-induced wall motion abnormalities with the use of high-dose dobutamine stress MRI: comparison with dobutamine stress echocardiography. *Circulation* 1999;99:763–770.

108. Niemi P, Poncelet BP, Kwong KK, et al. Myocardial intensity changes associated with flow stimulation in blood oxygenation sensitive magnetic resonance imaging. *Magn Reson Med* 1996;36:78–82.

109. Li D, Dhawale P, Rubin PJ, et al. Myocardial signal response to dipyridamole and dobutamine: demonstration of the BOLD effect using a double-echo gradient-echo sequence. *Magn Reson Med* 1996;36:16–20.

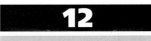

LEFT VENTRICULAR FUNCTION IN ISCHEMIC HEART DISEASE

EIKE NAGEL

Ischemic heart disease is one of the most common health problems of the Western world. A variety of tests are available in routine clinical practice for the noninvasive diagnosis of coronary artery disease, such as exercise electrocardiography (ECG), echocardiography, single photon emission computed tomography (SPECT), positron emission tomography (PET), and cardiovascular MR (CMR). The advantages and disadvantages of each technique are summarized in Table 12.1. Many noninvasive diagnostic tools are suboptimal, and both patients and physicians want a reliable diagnosis; as a consequence, 40% to 60% of all patients who undergo invasive cardiac catheterization procedures do not require a revascularization procedure, such as bypass surgery or angioplasty. Thus, a noninvasive test with a higher rate of diagnostic accuracy might reduce the number of overall cardiac catheterization procedures.

CMR has evolved into a new technique for the noninvasive detection of obstructive coronary artery disease. The ability of CMR to visualize global and regional wall motion and systolic thickening of the left ventricle (LV) with a high degree of spatial and temporal resolution makes it possible to detect abnormalities of wall motion. In addition, perfusion defects and reductions in coronary flow reserve can be assessed. Except for high-grade coronary artery stenosis, abnormalities can for the most part be identified only under stress conditions. These can be induced by physical exercise or by means of standardized stress protocols with infusions of pharmacologic agents such as dobutamine/atropine, dipyridamole, or adenosine. To date, the most reliable clinical data are based on the analysis of LV wall motion and thickening during pharmacologic stress. In this chapter, the results of recent studies and a detailed description of how to perform stress tests are presented.

PATHOPHYSIOLOGY

Ischemic heart disease can be caused by a variety of pathophysiologic conditions. Stenosis of the coronary arteries (coronary artery disease) is the most common of these, but LV hypertrophy, alterations of the microcirculation, and a reduction of energy uptake are other, less frequent causes. Patients with coronary artery disease usually have sufficient blood flow at rest; however, during stress, which induces a fourfold to fivefold increase in blood flow in healthy persons, the myocardium supplied by the stenotic coronary arteries does not receive enough blood because blood flow is impeded through the narrowed coronary artery lumen. Thus, except in very severe cases, in which the patients have ischemia at rest, stress testing is required to induce ischemia.

STRESS TESTING

Stress testing can be performed with either physical or pharmacologic stimulation. In general, to detect ischemic heart disease with a high level of sensitivity and reproducibility, a

E. Nagel: Department of Cardiology, German Heart Institute, Berlin, Germany.

TABLE 12.1. DIFFERENT TECHNIQUES FOR THE EVALUATION OF MYOCARDIAL ISCHEMIA

	Advantage	Disadvantage
Exercise ECG	Low cost Wide availability	Low diagnostic accuracy Many equivocal results Target heart rate not reached in many patients
Stress echocardiography	Low cost Wide availability	Nondiagnostic examinations in 10% to 15%
SPECT	Low cost	Radiation Low specificity Attenuation artifacts, especially in women
PET	Quantitative evaluation No attenuation artifacts	Limited availability High cost Radiation
EBT	High sensitivity	Low specificity
CMR	High diagnostic accuracy Combination of wall motion, perfusion, and anatomy No radiation	Limited availability High cost

ECG, electrocardiography; SPECT, single photon emission computed tomography; PET, positron emission tomography; EBT, electron beam computed tomography; CMR, cardiovascular MR.

defined end point (submaximal stress) must be reached. This end point is defined by the heart rate as follows:

$$\text{Target Heart Rate} = .85 \, (220 - \text{Age})$$

Ergometric Stress

Ergometric stress is the most physiologic stress test. Patients exercise on a bicycle or treadmill ergometer with incremental workloads. In general, this kind of stress has the disadvantages of relatively low reproducibility and the induction of motion artifacts. Because many patients with coronary artery disease also have other vessels that are stenotic (e.g., in their legs), they cannot be adequately stressed and frequently do not reach the required heart rate.

Ergometric stress in combination with CMR has additional limitations. Patients lie on their back within a relatively small-bore magnet, so that an optimal setup for ergometric stress is difficult to achieve. As a result, a large number of tests may be nondiagnostic because of an inadequate level of stress. In addition, CMR, which is sensitive to motion artifacts, is not compatible with exercise-induced stress testing. However, new techniques, such as real-time imaging, may overcome this problem.

Pharmacologic Stress

Pharmacologic stress is preferred by many clinicians because the results are highly reproducible and diagnostic in most patients. However, careful monitoring is required for patient safety (see below). Two different approaches are used:

Oxygen consumption can be increased by increasing the heart rate and contractility (dobutamine/arbutamine), or vasodilation can be induced (dipyridamole/adenosine). The different pharmacologic stress protocols are summarized in Table 12.2.

Dobutamine

Dobutamine is a sympathomimetic drug with β_1-, β_2-, and slight α_1-receptor–stimulating properties. Infusion of the drug increases the cardiac contractility and rate and decreases the systolic vascular resistance. Whereas during low-dose infusion (≤ 10 µg/kg per minute) increased contractility is the major effect, at higher doses the increased consumption of oxygen causes contraction abnormalities in myocardial segments supplied by stenotic coronary arteries.

A low dose of dobutamine is defined as an infusion of up to 10 µg/min per kilogram of body weight. Such a dose is sufficient to stimulate myocardium that does not contract at rest but may benefit from revascularization (viable or hibernating myocardium); however, this dose is insufficient to induce ischemia.

A high dose of dobutamine is defined as an infusion aimed at inducing ischemia. As explained above, it is essential that patients reach their target heart rate. To achieve this goal, atropine, which increases the heart rate by an anticholinergic mechanism, is commonly added. The stress protocol most widely used is described in the guidelines of the American Society of Echocardiography. Stress is induced by increasing doses of dobutamine, started at 10 µg/kg of body weight per minute for 3 minutes and increased in incre-

TABLE 12.2. STRESS PROTOCOLS

Stress Test	Patient Instructions	Protocol	Antidote
Dobutamine for the assessment of viability		5, 10 μg/kg BW per minute for >3 minutes	
Dobutamine/atropine for the detection of coronary artery disease (wall motion)	No β-blockers and nitrates 24 hours before the examination	(5), 10, 20, 30, 40 μg/kg BW per minute for 3 minutes each, up to 1 mg atropine (4 × 0.25 mg) until submaximal heart rate [(220 − age) × 0.85] is reached (half-life 2 minutes)	β-Blocker (esmolol) 0.5 mg mg/kg as slowly injected bolus, additional bolus of 0.2 mg/kg as needed, sublingual nitroglycerin
Dipyridamole (perfusion)	No caffeine (tea, coffee, chocolate, etc.) or medications such as aminophylline or nitrates 24 hours before the examination	0.56 mg/kg BW per minute for 4 minutes, maximal effect after approximately 3 to 4 minutes (half-life 30 minutes)	Aminophylline 250 mg i.v. slowly injected with ECG monitoring, sublingual nitroglycerin
Adenosine (perfusion)	Same as for dipyridamole	140 μg/kg BW per minute for 6 minutes (half-life 4 to 10 seconds)	Stop infusion (in occasional cases aminophylline 250 mg i.v. slowly injected with ECG monitoring)

BW, body weight; ECG, electrocardiogram.

ments of 10 μg/kg of body weight per minute every 3 minutes until a maximal dose of 40 μg/kg of body weight per minute is reached. (Some investigators use 50 μg/kg of body weight per minute as a maximum.) If the target heart rate is not reached, up to 1 mg of atropine is added in 0.25-mg fractions. The test must be stopped if certain criteria are fulfilled (Table 12.3).

Dipyridamole (Vasodilation)

Dipyridamole and its metabolic product and active component adenosine are vasodilators. They induce ischemia by a "steal effect," as follows: Coronary arteries with significant stenoses receive local stimuli (e.g., local adenosine produced by the endothelial cells) and are dilated to a maximum at rest. Thus, these vessels are not dilated any further if an external vasodilator is added. In contrast, healthy vessels react with significant vasodilation and increased blood flow after pharmacologic stimulation. This reaction can be measured as flow reserve in perfusion or flow measurements. Because of the increased flow in healthy areas, less blood is delivered

to the myocardial areas supplied by diseased coronary arteries (steal effect), so that ischemia develops in these myocardial regions. In clinical practice, a few centers use vasodilators to induce wall motion abnormalities, usually 140 μg of adenosine per minute for a maximum of 6 minutes. The sensitivity of wall motion testing with vasodilators is less than that with dobutamine/atropine, which is more frequently used. However, vasodilators are the preferred stressors for perfusion and flow measurements.

ACCURACY OF STRESS-INDUCED WALL MOTION ABNORMALITIES IN THE DIAGNOSIS OF ISCHEMIA

The echocardiographic detection of wall motion abnormalities during high-dose dobutamine or exercise stress has been shown to be an accurate diagnostic tool for screening patients with suspected coronary artery disease. Sensitivities of 54% to 96% and specificities of 60% to 100% have been reported (1), depending on the pretest likelihood of disease and the experience of the stress centers. However, the value of stress echocardiography is limited by a 10% to 15% rate of nondiagnostic results (1) and low specificities for the basal–lateral and basal–inferior segments of the LV (2).

CMR has yielded good results in the detection of wall motion abnormalities at intermediate doses of dobutamine (maximum of 20 μg/kg of body weight per minute intravenously) (3–5). However, echocardiographic studies have shown that high-dose dobutamine and additional atropine are required to ensure a high sensitivity. In a recent prospective study of 208 patients with suspected coronary artery dis-

TABLE 12.3. DOBUTAMINE TERMINATION CRITERIA

- Submaximal heart rate reached [(220 − age) × 0.85]
- Systolic pressure decrease >20 mm Hg below baseline systolic blood pressure or decrease >40 mm Hg from a previous level
- Blood pressure increase >240/120 mm Hg
- Intractable symptoms
- New or worsening wall motion abnormalities in at least 2 (of 16) adjacent left ventricular segments
- Complex cardiac arrhythmias

ease, stress with high-dose dobutamine/atropine (40 μg of dobutamine per kilogram of body weight per minute plus up to 1 mg of atropine intravenously) was used, and echocardiography and CMR were compared with angiography for the detection of significant coronary artery disease (stenosis of >50% the vessel diameter on angiography) (6). This study found significantly better values for the sensitivity (86% vs. 74%), specificity (86% vs. 70%), and diagnostic accuracy (86% vs. 73%) of CMR versus transthoracic echocardiography. These differences were most pronounced in the patients with moderate echocardiographic image quality (7) (Fig. 12.1). In a different study, by Hundley et al. (8), a similar protocol was used to assess patients with nondiagnostic echocardiographic image quality, and 94% of them could be adequately examined with CMR, for a sensitivity and specificity of 83% in those patients who also underwent coronary angiography.

Because high-dose dobutamine stress CMR is highly accurate and can be performed within less than 40 minutes, it has the potential to replace dobutamine stress echocardiography for the detection of coronary artery disease in patients with nondiagnostic or suboptimal echocardiographic image quality.

IMAGE ACQUISITION

For the assessment of wall motion, cine loops of the heart are acquired with gradient-echo or segmented k-space turbo gra-

dient-echo sequences. More rapid image acquisition is possible with echo-planar imaging, which allows either a reduced scan time or improved temporal resolution. The heart can be visualized with either contiguous short-axis slices or a combination of several short-axis (typically three to five) and long-axis (typically horizontal and vertical) views (Fig. 12.2).

Wall Motion Abnormalities (High-Dose Dobutamine)

For high-dose dobutamine stress tests, breath-hold cine imaging with turbo gradient-echo techniques, echo-planar imaging, or real-time imaging should ideally be used in preference to conventional non–breath-hold techniques. These fast techniques significantly reduce the scan time, improve image quality, and enable the rapid detection of wall motion abnormalities. The same imaging planes that are recommended for low-dose dobutamine studies should be acquired. Imaging starts immediately after the dobutamine dose is increased at each cardiac level. To achieve an adequate number of phases during tachycardia, the temporal resolution must be approximately 25 frames per second (<40 milliseconds). Studies published so far have used a spatial resolution of about 2×2 mm or better with a slice thickness of 6 to 10 mm. Images are acquired and reviewed at rest and during each stress level. The stress protocol, details of monitoring, contraindications, and termination criteria are summarized in Tables 12.2 through 12.5.

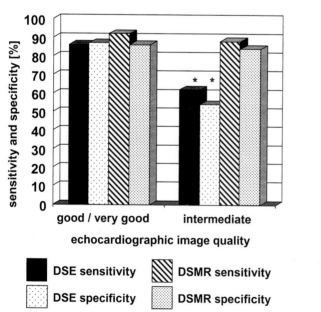

FIGURE 12.1. Sensitivity and specificity of dobutamine stress echocardiography (DSE) and dobutamine stress cardiovascular MR (DSMR). **Left columns:** Good or very good echocardiographic image quality. In these examinations, the diagnostic accuracy is similar for echocardiography and MRI. **Right columns:** Intermediate echocardiographic image quality. In these patients, the diagnostic accuracy of echocardiography is very low, and significantly better results are obtained with MRI. *$p < 0.05$ DSMR.

TABLE 12.4. CONTRAINDICATIONS TO MR STRESS TESTS

MR examination	Incompatible metallic implants (e.g., pacemakers, retroorbital metal, cerebral artery clips)
	Claustrophobia
Dobutamine	Severe arterial hypertension (≥220/120 mm Hg)
	Unstable angina pectoris
	Significant aortic stenosis (aortic valve gradient >50 mm Hg or aortic valve area <1 cm²)
	Complex cardiac arrhythmias
	Significant hypertrophic obstructive cardiomyopathy
	Myocarditis, endocarditis, pericarditis
	Other major disease
Dipyridamole/adenosine	Myocardial infarction <3 days
	Unstable angina pectoris
	Severe arterial hypertension
	Asthma or severe obstructive pulmonary disease
	Atrioventricular block >IIa

TABLE 12.5 MONITORING REQUIREMENTS FOR STRESS MRI

	Dobutamine + Atropine	Dipyridamole/ adenosine
Heart rate and rhythm (single-lead ECG)	Continuously	Continuously
Blood pressure	Every minute	Every minute
Pulse oximetry	Continuously	Continuously
Symptoms	Continuously	Continuously
Wall motion abnormalities	Every dose increment	At peak stress

Combination of Different Methods

In general, a combination of different imaging methods can be used within a CMR examination. The combined determination of wall motion and perfusion has been demonstrated in animals (9) and small numbers of patients (10,11). At the current time, it is not clear how much improvement in diagnostic accuracy can be achieved with such combinations. In addition, the optimal stress protocol (dobutamine, adenosine, or a combination of both) has not been defined. However, it seems reasonable to combine a test with high specificity (wall motion analysis) and a test with high sensitivity (perfusion) to increase overall diagnostic accuracy.

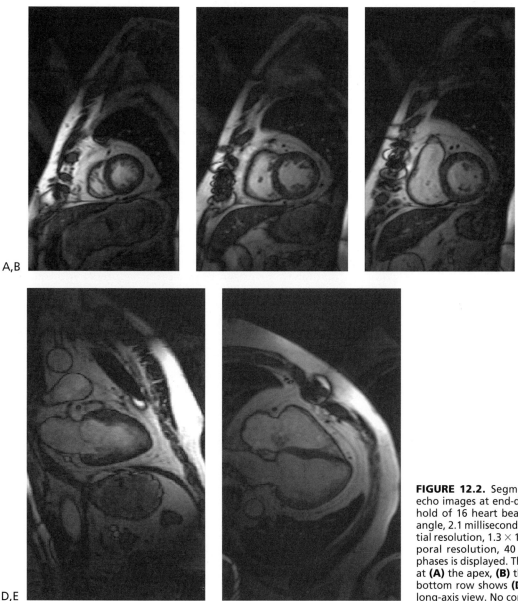

A,B

C

D,E

FIGURE 12.2. Segmented k-space spoiled gradient-echo images at end-diastole acquired during s breath-hold of 16 heart beats. Echo time/repetition time/flip angle, 2.1 milliseconds/5.9 milliseconds/25 degrees; spatial resolution, 1.3 × 1.3 mm; slice thickness, 8 mm; temporal resolution, 40 milliseconds. One of 18 cardiac phases is displayed. The top row shows short-axis views at **(A)** the apex, **(B)** the equator, and **(C)** the base, the bottom row shows **(D)** a vertical and **(E)** a horizontal long-axis view. No contrast agent was used.

IMAGE INTERPRETATION

Wall Motion Abnormalities in the Diagnosis of Ischemia

For image interpretation, a multiple cine loop display, which allows different stress levels to be assessed at the same time, is recommended. The ventricle is typically analyzed at 16 (or 17) LV segments per stress level according to the standards suggested by the American Society of Echocardiography (12) and the American Heart Association (Fig. 12.3). Each segment is assigned to a specific coronary artery; however, depending on the coronary artery anatomy or degree of collateralization, some segments may be supplied by different arteries. Thus, it is often not possible to define a stenotic coronary artery from a wall motion study. Image quality is graded as good, acceptable, or bad, and the number of diagnostic segments is reported. Segmental wall motion is classified as normokinetic, hypokinetic, akinetic, or dyskinetic and assigned one to four points. The sum of the points is divided by the number of analyzed segments to yield a wall motion score. Normal contraction results in a wall motion score of 1, and a higher score indicates wall motion abnormality. During stress with increasing doses of dobutamine, either a lack of increase in wall motion or systolic wall thickening or a reduction in wall motion or thickening is regarded as a pathologic finding (Figs. 12.4 and 12.5).

Quantitative Regional Wall Motion

The quantitative analysis of wall motion and systolic thickening is possible and has shown good results in small studies (13,14). Further improvements in diagnostic accuracy and reproducibility may be achieved with on-line or rapid off-line analysis or myocardial tagging (15), which allows the quantification of regional three-dimensional myocardial motion.

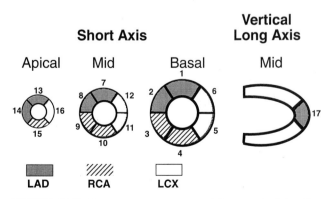

FIGURE 12.3. Seventeen-segment model suggested by the American Heart Association. The coronary artery territories are shown in the graph.

SAFETY

During stress examinations in which low or high doses of dobutamine, dipyridamole, or adenosine are administered, monitoring the patient within the magnet is mandatory. In general, monitoring during a CMR examination requires that the same precautions be taken and the same emergency equipment be available as in any other stress examination. A physician trained in cardiovascular emergencies and resuscitation must be at the scanner. Apart from specific contraindications to CMR, such as the presence of retroorbital metal, cerebral clips, or pacemakers, the contraindications are identical to those for stress echocardiography and are listed in Table 12.4.

Dobutamine

Although only minimal side effects are to be expected during low-dose dobutamine stress, high-dose dobutamine stress may cause severe complications in 0.25% of patients, including infarction (0.07%), ventricular fibrillation (0.07%), and sustained ventricular tachycardia (0.1%) (16,17). Thus, although adverse events are rare, the staff must be prepared to remove the patient from the magnet rapidly if necessary, and they must comply closely with the test termination criteria (Table 12.3). Whereas in most other modalities "eye-to-eye" contact between patient and examiner takes place, communication during CMR is usually via a microphone system and video cameras, although it can also be conducted personally. This does not hinder the safety process if the patient is carefully monitored for symptoms, blood pressure changes, and wall motion abnormalities and if pulse oximetry is performed (Table 12.2). Either standard equipment can be placed outside the scanner room and connected to the patient with special extensions through a waveguide in the radiofrequency cage, or special CMR-compatible equipment, currently available at many CMR sites, can be used. A defibrillator and all medications needed for emergency treatment must be available at the CMR site. A specific problem associated with monitoring within the magnet is that of assessing ST-segment changes from the ECG. Possible improvements may be achieved by the use of ECG tracings based on the spatial information of the vector cardiogram (18). However, because wall motion abnormalities precede ST changes (19,20) and because such abnormalities can be readily detected with fast CMR, monitoring is effective without a diagnostic ECG and can also be performed in patients with left bundle branch block, who are routinely evaluated with dobutamine stress echocardiography despite nondiagnostic ST segments. With conventional imaging, such wall motion abnormalities can be detected immediately after image reconstruction, which is completed 5 to 10 seconds after image acquisition. In addition, real-time imaging permits the immediate detection of wall motion

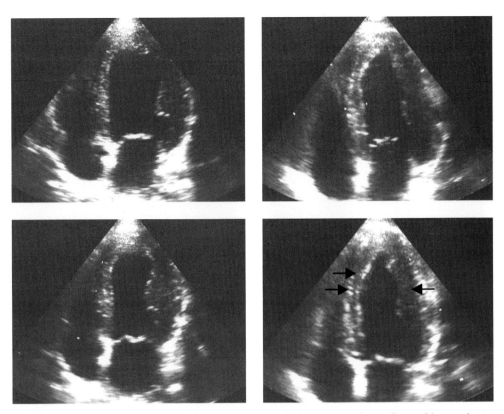

FIGURE 12.4. Horizontal long-axis views during dobutamine stress. Echocardiographic examination. **Left panel:** Rest. **Right panel:** Stress. **Top row:** End-diastole. **Bottom row:** End-systole. The *arrows* indicate wall motion abnormalities. (From Nagel E, Lehmkuhl HB, Bocksch W, et al. *Circulation* 1999;99:763–770, with permission.)

abnormalities and can be used for monitoring (21); however, it is not yet ready to be used for the diagnostic visualization of wall motion abnormalities.

Dipyridamole/Adenosine

The systemic vasodilator effects of adenosine or dipyridamole may lead to a mild or moderate reduction in systolic, diastolic, and mean arterial blood pressures of approximately 10 mm Hg. In addition, these agents have a depressant effect on the sinoatrial and atrioventricular nodes. Thus, for dipyridamole and adenosine stress tests, monitoring of the heart rate and rhythm, blood pressure, and symptoms is required, and patients with atrioventricular block grade IIa or higher must be excluded. Mild side effects such as hypotension or bradycardia are common (0.85%). Severe side effects are to be expected in only 0.07% of patients and include asystole, ventricular tachycardia, persistent angina pectoris, and myocardial infarction (22–24). Respiratory stimulation may lead to an increase in minute ventilation, a reduction in arterial carbon dioxide pressure, and respiratory alkalosis. Thus, this test is not suitable for patients with asthma or poor pulmonary function. Contraindications and monitoring requirements are listed in Tables 12.4 and 12.5.

FUTURE ASPECTS

A further reduction in acquisition time is possible with interactive or real-time CMR (25,26), which has been shown to provide similar or superior image quality in comparison with echocardiography (26). It also permits an accurate determination of the LV ejection fraction (27,28). Real-time imaging may also allow the application of physical rather than pharmacologic stress because the images are less sensitive to motion artifacts than are turbo gradient-echo images.

SUMMARY

CMR is a rapidly developing new modality that can be applied in clinical cardiology to detect and assess myocardial ischemia and viability. With currently available techniques, it is possible to detect ischemic myocardium during high-dose dobutamine stress MR examinations. These studies are safe and have a high rate of diagnostic accuracy, superior to that of dobutamine stress echocardiography. This technique should be used in patients with nondiagnostic or moderate echocardiographic image quality to detect stress-induced wall motion abnormalities. Although some further developments are pending, mainly in image postprocessing and dis-

myocardial tagging (19), which allows the accurate quantification of regional three-dimensional myocardial motion and therefore circumvents the inevitable inaccuracies of wall thickness measurements caused by systolic anterior movement of the apex.

Assessment of Viability from Contrast Enhancement

The distribution kinetics of contrast agents have been used to detect MI and define viable myocardium (20,21). In some patients after MI, a hypoenhanced zone in the core of a region of hyperenhancement appeared 1 to 2 minutes after injection in the equilibrium phase (21). This hypoenhanced core was explained by the presence of capillaries occluded by dying blood cells and debris (microvascular obstruction, or no-reflow region) and was a strong predictor of cardiac morbidity and mortality after MI. In experimental animals, various enhancement patterns correlated well with reversible and irreversible myocardial ischemia (22,23). In a study of 14 patients, various patterns of contrast agent kinetics after MI were assigned to different pathophysiologic situations, such as irreversible myocardial defect, predominantly viable myocardium, and mixture of viable and necrotic myocardium (24). The data seem thus far insufficient for broad clinical application, and the mechanisms underlying these

observations are not yet fully understood. Because the subject of this chapter is the measurement of regional LV function in the assessment of viable myocardium, perfusion studies are not discussed further here.

IMAGE ACQUISITION TECHNIQUES AND INTERPRETATION FOR MR VIABILITY STUDIES

Rest and Low-Dose Dobutamine Stress MRI

Because the time required for image acquisition is not critical in the assessment of viability, studies with low-dose dobutamine ($\leq$10 μg of dobutamine per kilogram of body weight per minute) can be performed with standard gradient-echo sequences. However, the examination time can be reduced with the use of segmented k-space turbo gradient-echo or echo-planar imaging techniques. The temporal resolution must be 20 frames per second or better, with a spatial resolution of less than 2 $\times$ 2 mm and a slice thickness of 6 to 10 mm, to allow the visual detection of small alterations in wall motion or the measurement of wall thickening in diastole and systole. Images are acquired at rest and during each stress level (usually 5 and 10 μg of dobutamine infused within a 5-minute time interval).

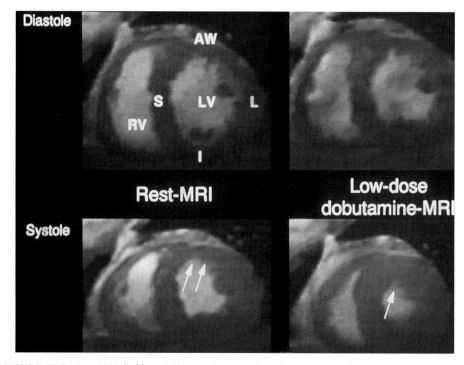

FIGURE 13.2. Rest MRI *(left)* and dobutamine MRI *(right)* short-axis tomogram at end-diastole *(top)* and systole *(bottom)*. The end-diastolic phase shows almost normal end-diastolic wall thickness in the anteroseptal region at rest *(upper left panel)* and lack of systolic wall thickening in the septum and anteroseptal portion of the anterior wall *(lower left panel, arrows)*. During dobutamine infusion *(lower right panel)*, significant wall thickening is present *(arrow)*. AW, anterior wall; I, inferior wall; L, lateral wall; LV, left ventricle; RV, right ventricle; S, septum.

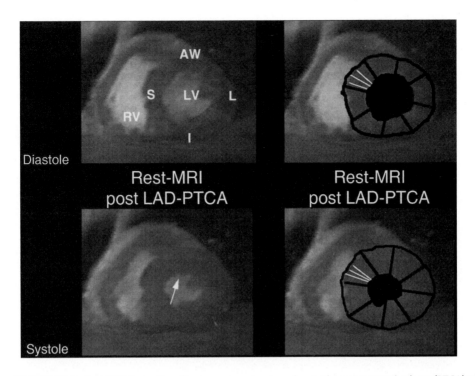

FIGURE 13.3. Rest MRI 6 months after percutaneous transluminal coronary angioplasty (PTCA) of the left anterior descending coronary artery *(left panel)* and illustration of quantitative analysis of wall thickening *(right panel)*. The end-diastolic still frame shows normal end-diastolic wall thickness, and the systolic still frame demonstrates a significant increase in systolic wall thickness in the anteroseptal region at rest *(lower right panel, arrow)*. In the left panel, systolic wall thickening is quantitatively evaluated by dividing the left ventricle into eight segments. For each segment, the mean diastolic wall thickness *(DWT, upper left panel)* and systolic wall thickness *(SWT, lower left panel)* are automatically calculated from serial measurements of the endocardial–epicardial distance (chords). Systolic wall thickening is derived from the difference between SWT and DWT. *AW,* anterior wall; *I,* inferior wall; *L,* lateral wall; *LV,* left ventricle; *RV,* right ventricle; *S,* septum.

Interpretation of MR Viability Studies

Viability studies can be analyzed qualitatively (visual analysis of wall motion at rest and during infusion of low-dose dobutamine (25) (Fig. 13.2), or preferably quantitatively by measuring wall thickness (Fig. 13.3) and wall thickening (9,10). A minimal end-diastolic wall thickness of more than 5 mm with resting thickening or resting akinesis and an improvement in systolic wall thickening of 2 mm or more during dobutamine stimulation are clinically robust diagnostic criteria for myocardial viability that have been used in the studies published so far (9,10,25,26).

STRESS MRI IN ACUTE MYOCARDIAL INFARCTION

Measurements of Wall Thickness and Wall Thickening

After an acute ischemic event, structural changes develop within the infarct zone, and infarct healing with scar forma-

tion is completed by approximately 3 to 4 months (27). Thinning of the infarct region may occur early, especially in large anterior myocardial infarcts. The consequence is an increase in the size of the infarcted segment, known as *infarct expansion* (28). However, infarct expansion is not usually seen in patients with open infarct-related arteries, which are encountered relatively often today because of the widespread use of thrombolysis and angioplasty of the infarct artery. Therefore, wall thickness may be the same in transmural necrosis and nontransmural necrosis early after MI. Both conditions may also be associated with a complete absence of resting function early after the acute event. Consequently, MRI studies of the anatomy and function of the LV at rest may not be helpful in detecting residual viability. However, even a small amount of wall thickening (e.g., severe hypokinesia) in a region-of-interest indicates the presence of residual contracting cells and hence viable myocardium.

Measurements of LV wall thickening by MRI are probably more accurate than echocardiographic measurements (29). However, as with all cross-sectional imaging tech-

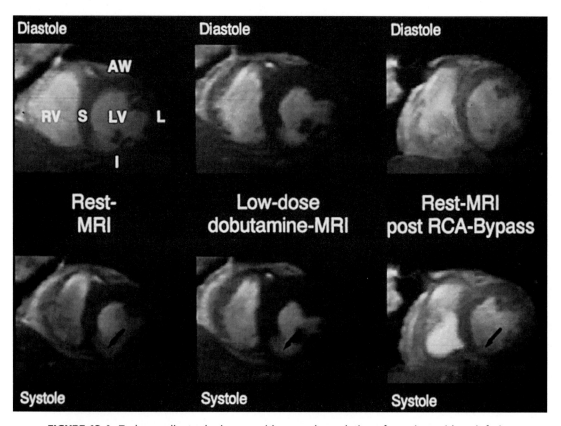

FIGURE 13.4. Turbo-gradient echo images with coronal angulation of a patient with an inferior myocardial infarct and multivessel coronary artery disease. The *left panel* demonstrates an end-diastolic and an end-systolic still frame at rest. Note the circumscript wall thinning (< 4 mm wall thickness and lack of wall thickening, *arrow*) of the inferior wall which is a typical morphologic parameter of a healed transmural infarct with persisting scar tissue. This is clearly in contrast to the anterior wall *(AW)* and the lateral wall *(LW)*, which show normal systolic wall thickening. The *middle panel* shows the identical slice at end-diastole and end-systole during dobutamine infusion (10 mcg/kg BW/min). The infarct region of the inferior wall remains thinned (< 4 mm, *arrow*) without a dobutamine inducible contraction reserve confirming the presence of scar tissue without significant remnants of viable myocardium. In contrast, the AW and LW demonstrate hyper-contractility during dobutamine infusion. The *right panel* shows the rest MRI study 6 months after coronary bypass grafting including the right coronary artery. The end-diastolic still frame shows permanent wall thinning of the inferior wall *(top)* and no sign of recovery of regional left ventricular function *(bottom)* confirming a transmural and therefore irreversible defect of the inferior wall.

niques, the complex motion of the heart in relation to the body axes makes it impossible to observe exactly the same portion of myocardium during systole and diastole in the same image. MR tagging techniques make it possible to trace the same portion of the myocardium, and wall thickening measurements by MRI based on this technique have been shown to be as accurate as the current gold standard, ultrasonic crystals sewn to the heart (30).

Inotropic Reserve

If no wall thickening is present or the degree of wall thickening is so small as to leave serious doubt about the potential for recovery of regional ventricular function, inotropic stimulation by dobutamine can be used with MRI to assess residual viability in patients with recent infarction (2,9). A

lack of contractile reserve shown by MRI was strongly associated with abnormalities of fatty acid metabolism demonstrated by β-methyl-iodophenyl-pentadecanoic acid (BMIPP) single photon emission tomography (31).

STRESS MRI IN CHRONIC MYOCARDIAL INFARCTS

As mentioned above, chronic myocardial infarcts are structurally different from acute myocardial infarcts. The most obvious difference is that chronic transmural infarcts are very thin (32). Consequently, this feature can be detected by MRI and can be used to distinguish between chronic transmural scar and residual viable myocardium in the infarct area (Fig. 13.4). However, when a small area of pronounced wall thinning is noted, one must be very cautious in assuming that the entire region perfused by an occluded coronary artery is completely scarred. Frequently, myocardial cells in the border zone survive, and ischemia of this border zone alone can cause substantial symptoms. Therefore, in a patient with single-vessel disease, previous MI, and anginal symptoms, restoring blood flow by reestablishing the patency of the occluded artery may be justified despite evidence of complete necrosis in the center of the infarct zone (33).

Myocardial Wall Thickness As a Feature of Viable Myocardium

The hypothesis that thinned and akinetic myocardium represents chronic scar has been tested by comparing MRI findings with those obtained by PET and SPECT in the same myocardial regions (9,33,34). The comparison of MR images with scintigraphic images is easily accomplished; because both techniques are three-dimensional, identical regions can be matched.

To define transmural scar by end-diastolic wall thickness, a cutoff value of 5.5 mm was selected. This value corresponded to the mean end-diastolic wall thickness in normal persons minus 2.5 standard deviations. It also corresponded well with the wall thickness of less than 6 mm found in a histopathologic study of transmural chronic scar (31). Regions that had a mean end-diastolic wall thickness of less than 5.5 mm showed a significantly reduced uptake of fluorodeoxyglucose (FDG) in comparison with regions that had an end-diastolic wall thickness of 5.5 mm or more (9). In 29 of 35 patients studied, the determination of viability based on FDG uptake was identical to the determination based on myocardial morphology as assessed by MRI. Importantly, relative FDG uptake did not differ between segments with systolic wall thickening at rest or akinesia at rest so long as wall thickness was preserved. These findings were applied to another group of patients, who underwent revascularization and control MRI at 3 months after revascularization (10). Of 125 segments with an end-diastolic wall thickness of less than 5.5 mm in 43 patients with chronic infarcts, only 12 segments recovered (corresponding to a negative predictive accuracy of 90% for the finding of end-diastolic wall thinning to predict transmural scar). In contrast, the positive predictive accuracy was only 62% for preserved end-diastolic wall thickness of 5.5 mm or more in predicting the presence of viable myocardium with the potential for recovery. The most likely explanation for this finding is that the amount of viable myocardium cannot be directly visualized on gradient-echo MR images. However, it is the amount of viable myocardium present in a particular region of the LV that determines whether the segment will recover function or not. Regions with preserved wall thickness may contain very small rims of epicardially located viable myocardium and yet not exhibit substantial wall thinning. However, such a small rim of viable myocardium may not be sufficient to result in improved wall

thickening after revascularization. Reduced end-diastolic wall thickness was also found to be a strong predictor of irreversibly damaged tissue in a study in which resting transthoracic echocardiography was used to assess patients with healed Q-wave anterior wall infarcts. This study, which defined myocardial viability as recovery of function after revascularization, found a predictive value of 87% for a pattern of increased acoustic reflectance combined with reduced end-diastolic wall thickness (35).

The relationship between end-diastolic wall thickness and viability has been disputed by other researchers (12), who found FDG uptake on PET images to be largely independent of regional end-diastolic wall thickness. However, this study included recent and chronic infarcts and used a suboptimal conventional spin-echo technique with a short echo time of 20 milliseconds to measure wall thickness. More recently, thallium 201 uptake was correlated with end-diastolic and end-systolic LV wall thickness as measured on cine MR images in patients with acute and healed myocardial infarcts (36). In this study, end-systolic wall thickness correlated better with normalized thallium activity than did end-diastolic wall thickness. Regions with normalized thallium activity of less than 50% showed wall thickening values of 12.3% ± 30.6%, and wall thickening was only slightly larger in regions with thallium activities between 50% and 60% (13.8% ± 27.0%). From a receiver-operating curve, an end-systolic wall thickness value of 9.8 mm had a sensitivity of 90% and a specificity of 94% for identifying regions with a normalized thallium uptake of less than 50%. In our opinion, this study does not really contradict our finding that end-diastolic wall thickness can distinguish between scarred and viable myocardium. The patient population of Lawson et al. (36) differed in one important aspect from ours; they included patients with hypokinesia in their study, whereas only patients with akinesia were included in ours. Obviously, any degree of wall thickening is related to the presence of contracting and hence viable cells in the region-of-interest. Nevertheless, it is undoubtedly true that end-systolic wall thickness indicates even larger differences between normal and viable myocardium if one includes zones of viability that are still contracting. However, viable zones in our studies did not contract (akinesia or dyskinesia), and systolic wall thickness was therefore not better than end-diastolic wall thickness for distinguishing between viable myocardium and scar.

Contractile Reserve during Low-Dose Dobutamine Infusion

Although severely reduced end-diastolic wall thickness is very helpful in identifying myocardium that is highly unlikely to recover after revascularization because it is completely scarred (10), the value of preserved end-diastolic wall thickness for predicting recovery of function following revascularization is disappointingly low. However, MRI offers the possibility to observe and measure wall thickening not only at rest but also during low-dose dobutamine infusion. Until recently, a protocol for the acquisition of cine MR images in multiple short-axis and two long-axis sections at rest and at 5 and 10 µg of dobutamine per kilogram per minute required an imaging time of more than 60 minutes. Because of the advent of fast MR sequences, the same protocol can now be completed within approximately 30 minutes. Image quality is often better with breath-hold cine MR images than with conventional MR images. Thus, it is not surprising that the sensitivity of dobutamine MRI for detecting viable myocardium as defined by a normalized FDG uptake on PET images was 81%, with a specificity of 95% (9). When recovery of wall thickening was considered to be the gold standard, the sensitivity of dobutamine MRI in predicting recovery of function after revascularization was 89%, with a specificity of 94%. The latter analysis was patient-related, which is clinically more meaningful than a segment-by-segment analysis (10). However, a study by Gunning et al. (11), performed in 30 patients with severe LV dysfunction (mean LV ejection fraction of 24%), showed a high specificity of 83% but a low sensitivity of only 45% for visually assessed dobutamine-induced wall thickening as a predictor of LV functional recovery after revascularization. The explanation for this difference is most likely patient selection. The higher mean LV ejection fraction (41%) in our study population (10), with possibly fewer profound ultrastructural changes and loss of contractile protein in areas of dysfunctional but viable myocardium, may have increased the likelihood of eliciting a dobutamine-stimulated contraction reserve. This explanation also fits with the observation that all patients (n = 3) with a false-negative result on dobutamine MRI had severely depressed LV function by left ventriculography (Table 13.1).

The Cologne MR Working Group also presented data on the relative values of dobutamine MRI and dobutamine transesophageal echocardiography (TEE) in the assessment of viable myocardium (25,26). Normalized FDG uptake on PET images was used as the standard against which both techniques were compared (26). The sensitivity and specificity of dobutamine TEE and dobutamine MRI for assessing FDG PET-defined myocardial viability were 77% versus 81% and 94% versus 100%, respectively. In a recently published study, the recovery of regional LV function after revascularization was chosen as the reference standard for the direct comparison of both imaging techniques on a qualitative visual basis (25). The positive and negative accuracy rates of dobutamine TEE and dobutamine MRI for the prediction of LV functional improvement were 85% versus 92% and 80% versus 85%, respectively. Thus, both imaging techniques provide similar accuracy rates in assessing viability in both quantitative (measurement of wall thickening) (26) and less time-consuming qualitative (evaluation of wall motion) (25) analysis. In the choice of an appropriate technique, patient acceptance becomes an important consideration. Although claustrophobia and electrocardiographic triggering may be problems in MRI, only a small number of patients are affected. In contrast, many patients do not like the experience of a TEE examination. On the other hand, TEE offers a clear economic advantage because the cost of an echo probe is only a fraction of that of an MR scanner.

FUTURE DEVELOPMENTS IN STRESS FUNCTIONAL MRI FOR THE ASSESSMENT OF MYOCARDIAL VIABILITY

In combination with low-dose dobutamine, which stimulates wall thickening without inducing ischemia, MRI has shown good results in detecting viable myocardium in comparison with PET and TEE (9). Moreover, it had a sensitiv-

TABLE 13.1. STRESS ECHOCARDIOGRAPHY AND LOW-DOSE DOBUTAMINE STRESS MRI FOR THE PREDICTION OF LEFT VENTRICULAR FUNCTIONAL RECOVERY AFTER SUCCESSFUL REVASCULARIZATION

Method of Viability Assessment	Reference Parameter	Sensitivity (%)	Specificity (%)	No. Patients Included	Study (Ref.)
Dobu-TTE	Wall motion recovery post revascularization	82	86	n = 25	Cigarroa et al., *Circulation* 1993 (7)
Dobu-TTE	Wall motion recovery post revascularization	86	90	n = 38	Smart et al., *Circulation* 1993 (8)
Dobu-TEE	Wall motion recovery post revascularization	92	88	n = 42	Baer et al., *JACC* 1996 (4)
Dobu-MRI	Wall motion recovery post revascularization	50	81	n = 23	Gunning et al., *Circulation* 1998 (11)
Dobu-MRI	Wall thickening improvement (>2 mm) post revascularization	89	94	n = 43	Baer et al., *JACC* 1998 (10)

Dobu, dobutamine; TTE, transthoracic echocardiography; TEE, transesophageal echocardiography; *JACC, Journal of the American College of Cardiology.*

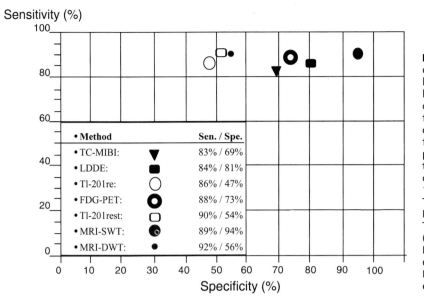

FIGURE 13.5. Diagnostic value of low-dose dobutamine stress-MRI in comparison to established imaging techniques for the prediction of left ventricular functional recovery following successful revascularization procedures. (Adapted from Bax JJ, Wijns W, Cornel JH, et al. Accuracy of currently available techniques for prediction of functional recovery after revascularization in patients with left ventricular dysfunction due to chronic coronary artery disease: comparison of pooled data. *J Am Coll Cardiol* 1997;30: 1451–1460.) Sen., sensitivity; Spe., specificity; TC-MIBI, technetium-methoxyisobutyl-isonitril; LDDE, low-dose dobutamine echocardiography; Tl-201re, thallium-201 reinjection scintigraphy (late); Tl-201rest, thallium-201 rest scintigraphy; MRI-SWT, magnetic resonance imaging assessed dobutamine induced systolic wall thickening; MRI-DWT, magnetic resonance imaging assessed end-diastolic wall thickness at rest.

ity of 89% and a specificity of 94% in predicting functional recovery after 4 to 6 months in 43 patients when an increase of systolic wall thickening of 2 mm or more was observed during stress MRI, values essentially identical to the sensitivity and specificity of PET (10).

Thus, low-dose dobutamine stress MRI has proved to be a valid and clinically robust tool for detecting viable myocardium and can compete with echocardiography and scintigraphic imaging techniques (Fig. 13.5). However, the current data have been obtained from only a few studies enrolling predominantly patients with chronic coronary artery disease. Therefore, multicenter studies of larger numbers of patients covering the entire spectrum of postischemic dysfunction (acute, subacute, and chronic infarction) are required to evaluate this technique fully.

With the now widespread availability of MR scanners that can assess perfusion and late enhancement and the development of infarct-specific contrast agents, it may in the future be possible to combine various MRI techniques within one examination to improve further the predictive accuracy of MRI in assessing and quantifying persisting viable myocardium within an infarct region (37,38,39).

REFERENCES

1. Gould KL. Myocardial viability. What does it mean and how to measure it? *Circulation* 1991;83:333–335.
2. Braunwald E, Rutherford J. Reversible ischemic left ventricular dysfunction: evidence of the "hibernating myocardium." *J Am Coll Cardiol* 1986;8:1467–1470.
3. Bax JJ, Wijns W, Cornel JH, et al. Accuracy of currently available techniques for prediction of functional recovery after revascularization in patients with left ventricular dysfunction due to chronic coronary artery disease: comparison of pooled data. *J Am Coll Cardiol* 1997;30:1451–1460.
4. Baer FM, Voth E, Deutsch H, et al. Predictive value of low-dose dobutamine transesophageal echocardiography and fluorine-18-fluorodeoxyglucose positron emission tomography for recovery of regional left ventricular function after successful revascularization. *J Am Coll Cardiol* 1996;28:60–69.
5. Lucignani G, Paolini G, Landoni C, et al. Presurgical identification of hibernating myocardium by combined use of technetium-99m hexakis 2-methoxyisobutylisonitrile single photon emission tomography and fluorine-18 fluoro-2-deoxy-D-glucose positron emission tomography in patients with coronary artery disease. *Eur J Nucl Med* 1992;19:874–881.
6. Bax JJ, Cornel JH, Visser FC, et al. Prediction of recovery of myocardial dysfunction following revascularization: comparison of F18-fluorodeoxyglucose/thallium-201 single photon computed emission tomography, thallium-201 stress-reinjection single photon emission tomography and dobutamine echocardiography. *J Am Coll Cardiol* 1996;28:558–564.
7. Cigarroa CG, deFilippi CR, Brickner ME, et al. Dobutamine stress echocardiography identifies hibernating myocardium and predicts recovery of left ventricular function after coronary revascularization. *Circulation* 1993;88:430–436.
8. Smart SC, Sawada S, Ryan T, et al. Low-dose dobutamine echocardiography detects reversible dysfunction after thrombolytic therapy of acute myocardial infarction. *Circulation* 1993;88:405–415.
9. Baer FM, Voth E, Schneider CA, et al. Dobutamine-gradient echo MRI: a functional and morphologic approach to the detection of residual myocardial viability. *Circulation* 1995;91:1006–1015.
10. Baer FM, Theissen P, Schneider CA, et al. Dobutamine magnetic resonance imaging predicts contractile recovery of chronically dysfunctional myocardium after successful revascularization. *J Am Coll Cardiol* 1998;31:1040–1048.
11. Gunning MG, Anagnostopoulos C, Knight CJ, et al. Comparison of 201-Tl, 99mTc-tetrofosmin, and dobutamine magnetic resonance imaging for identifying hibernating myocardium. *Circulation* 1998;98:1869–1874.
12. Perrone-Filardi P, Bacharach SL, Dilsizian V, et al. Metabolic evidence of viable myocardium in regions with reduced wall thickness and absent wall thickening in patients with chronic ischemic left ventricular dysfunction. *J Am Coll Cardiol* 1992;20:161–168.
13. Mallory GK, White PD, Salcedo-Galger J. The speed of healing

of myocardial infarction: a study of the pathologic anatomy in 72 cases. *Am Heart J* 1939;18:647–671.

14. Heusch G, Schulz R. Hibernating myocardium: a review. *J Mol Cell Cardiol* 1996;28:2359–2372.

15. Popio KA, Gorlin R, Bechtel D, et al. Postextrasystolic potentiation as a predictor of potential myocardial viability: preoperative analysis compared with studies after coronary bypass surgery. *Am J Cardiol* 1977;39:944–953.

16. Cigarroa CG, de Filippi CR, Brickner ME, et al. Dobutamine stress echocardiography identifies hibernating myocardium and predicts recovery of left ventricular function after coronary revascularization. *Circulation* 1993;88:430–436.

17. van Rugge FP, van der Wall EE, Spanjersberg SJ, et al. Magnetic resonance imaging during dobutamine stress for detection and localization of coronary artery disease. Quantitative wall motion analysis using a modification of the centerline method. *Circulation* 1994;90:127–138.

18. van der Geest RJ, Buller VGM, Jansen E, et al. Comparison between manual and semiautomated analysis of left ventricular volume parameters from short-axis MR images. *J Comp Assist Tomogr* 1997;21:756–765.

19. Power TP, Kramer CM, Shaffer AL, et al. Breath-hold dobutamine magnetic resonance myocardial tagging: normal left ventricular response. *Am J Cardiol* 1997;80:1203–1207.

20. Judd R, Lup-Olivieri C, Arai M, et al. Physiological basis of myocardial contrast enhancement in fast magnetic resonance images of 2-day-old reperfused canine infarcts. *Circulation* 1995;92:1902–1910.

21. Kim R, Fieno D, Parrish T, et al. Relationship of MRI delayed contrast enhancement to irreversible injury, infarct age and contractile function. *Circulation* 1999;100:1992–2002.

22. Wu KC, Zerhouni EA, Judd RM, et al. Prognostic significance of microvascular obstruction by magnetic resonance imaging in patients with acute myocardial infarction. *Circulation* 1998;97:765–772.

23. Kim RJ, Chen EL, Lima JA, et al. Myocardial Gd-DTPA kinetics determine MRI contrast enhancement and reflect the extent and severity of myocardial injury after acute reperfused infarction. *Circulation* 1996;94:3318–3326.

24. Rogers WJ, Kramer CM, Geskin G, et al. Early contrast-enhanced MRI predicts late functional recovery after reperfused myocardial infarction. *Circulation* 1999;99:744–750.

25. Baer FM, Theissen P, Crnac J, et al. Head-to-head comparison of dobutamine-transesophageal echocardiography and dobutamine-magnetic resonance imaging for the prediction of left ventricular functional recovery in patients with chronic coronary artery disease. *Eur Heart J* 2000;21:981–991.

26. Baer FM, Voth E, LaRosee K, et al. Comparison of dobutamine transesophageal echocardiography and dobutamine magnetic resonance imaging for detection of residual myocardial viability. *Am J Cardiol* 1996;78:415–419.

27. Mallory GK, White PD, Salcedo-Galger J. The speed of healing of myocardial infarction: a study of the pathologic anatomy in 72 cases. *Am Heart J* 1939;18: 647–671.

28. Pirolo JS, Hutchins GM, Moore GW. Infarct expansion: pathologic analysis of 204 patients with a single myocardial infarct. *J Am Coll Cardiol* 1986;7:349–354.

29. Sayad DE, Willett DL, Bridges WH, et al. Noninvasive quantitation of left ventricular wall thickening using cine magnetic resonance imaging with myocardial tagging. *Am J Cardiol* 1995;76: 985–989.

30. Lima JAC, Jeremy R, Guier W, et al. Accurate systolic wall thickening by nuclear magnetic resonance imaging with tissue tagging: correlation with sonomicrometers in normal and ischemic myocardium. *J Am Coll Cardiol* 1993;21:1741–1751.

31. Dendale P, Franken PR, van der Wall EE, et al. Wall thickening at rest and contractile reserve early after myocardial infarction: correlation with myocardial perfusion and metabolism. *Coron Artery Dis* 1997;8:259–264.

32. Dubnow MH, Burchell HB, Titus JL. Postinfarction left ventricular aneurysm. A clinicomorphologic and electrocardiographic study of 80 cases. *Am Heart J* 1965;70:753–760.

33. Braunwald E, Kloner RA. Myocardial reperfusion: a double-edged sword? *J Clin Invest* 1985;76:1713–1719.

34. Baer FM, Smolarz K, Jungehulsing M, et al. Chronic myocardial infarction: assessment of morphology, function, and perfusion by gradient-echo magnetic resonance imaging and ^{99m}Tc-methoxyisobutyl-isonitrile SPECT. *Am Heart J* 1992;123: 636–645.

35. Faletra F, Crivellaro W, Pirelli S, et al. Value of transthoracic two-dimensional echocardiography in predicting viability in patients with healed Q-wave anterior wall myocardial infarction. *Am J Cardiol* 1995;76:1002–1006.

36. Lawson MA, Johnson LL, Coghlan L, et al. Correlation of thallium uptake with left ventricular wall thickness by cine magnetic resonance imaging in patients with acute and healed myocardial infarcts. *Am J Cardiol* 1997;80:434–441.

37. Wendland MF, Saeed M, Arheden H, et al. Toward necrotic cell fraction measurement by contrast-enhanced MRI of reperfused ischemically injured myocardium. *Acad Radiol* 1998;1: 42–44.

38. Kim RJ, Wu E, Chen ARE, et al. The use of contrast-enhanced magnetic resonance imaging to identify reversible myocardial dysfunction. *N Engl J Med* 2000;343:1445–1453.

39. Klein C, Nekolla SG, Bengel FM, et al. Assessment of myocardial viability with contrast-enhanced magnetic resonance imaging: comparison with positron emission tomography. *Circulation* 2002;105:162–167.

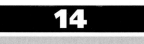

ASSESSMENT OF MYOCARDIAL VIABILITY BY CONTRAST ENHANCEMENT

RAYMOND J. KIM
KELLY M. CHOI
ROBERT M. JUDD

CLINICAL SIGNIFICANCE

In patients with ischemic heart disease, one of the most important determinants of long-term survival is the level of left ventricular (LV) dysfunction (1–3). It is important to recognize, however, that not all dysfunction of the LV is irreversible and represents previous infarction. In the setting of chronic coronary artery disease and LV dysfunction, it is well established that LV function can improve following revascularization procedures, such as percutaneous coronary angioplasty (PTCA) and coronary artery bypass grafting (CABG) (4–9). The mechanism for reversible myocardial dysfunction in this setting is not entirely clear, but terms such as *hibernating myocardium* (4,5) and *repetitive stunning* (10–12) have been used to describe the underlying pathophysiology. Regardless of the actual mechanism, several facts are known about this clinical syndrome. First, the prevalence is not inconsequential. Several studies have demonstrated that in up to one-third of patients with chronic coronary artery disease and LV dysfunction, LV

function improves after revascularization (13–16). Second, it is clear that diagnostic testing before revascularization can be useful in predicting functional improvement after revascularization (Fig. 14.1). Third, more recent studies have shown that patients with reversible dysfunction who undergo revascularization derive benefits beyond improved ventricular function, such as increased survival (17–20).

In the acute setting following an episode of myocardial ischemia and reperfusion, it is recognized that reversible myocardial dysfunction can also occur. In this setting, the underlying process is myocardial "stunning" (10,21,22), and the ventricular dysfunction should improve over time if the reperfusion therapy has been successful. It is important to distinguish between stunned and infarcted myocardium for several reasons. First, the prognosis is changed. Several studies have shown that patients with acute ventricular dysfunction primarily resulting from myocardial necrosis have a worse prognosis than patients with ventricular dysfunction that is primarily reversible (23,24). Second, patient management during the acute setting may be changed. Viable but injured myocardium, such as stunned myocardium, is potentially at risk for future infarction if the reperfusion therapy has not been complete and significant stenosis remains (24,25). Additionally, a determination of the extent of nonviable and viable myocardium across the ventricular wall in a dysfunctional region may be valuable in selecting

R. J. Kim and K. M. Choi: Duke Cardiovascular Magnetic Resonance Center, Duke University Medical Center, Durham, North Carolina.
R. M. Judd: Department of Medicine, Duke University Medical Center, Durham, North Carolina.

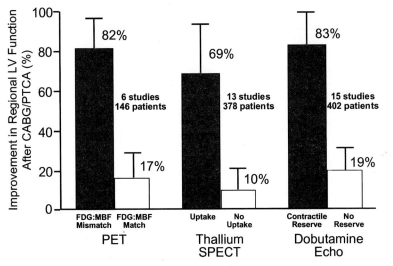

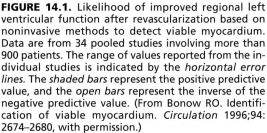

FIGURE 14.1. Likelihood of improved regional left ventricular function after revascularization based on noninvasive methods to detect viable myocardium. Data are from 34 pooled studies involving more than 900 patients. The range of values reported from the individual studies is indicated by the *horizontal error lines.* The *shaded bars* represent the positive predictive value, and the *open bars* represent the inverse of the negative predictive value. (From Bonow RO. Identification of viable myocardium. *Circulation* 1996;94: 2674–2680, with permission.)

patients most likely to benefit from therapy that can modulate ventricular remodeling after acute infarction, such as angiotensin-converting enzyme inhibitors (26). Third, infarct size determined accurately in the acute setting may prove to be an adequate surrogate end point for the assessment of new therapies (27,28). For example, the efficacy of current and experimental reperfusion therapies could be evaluated without the need for "mega" trials with large sample sizes that use mortality as an end point.

Thus, it is apparent that a diagnostic test capable of distinguishing between viable and nonviable myocardium independently of the level of contractile function in both acute and chronic settings is essential in the clinical assessment of patients with ischemic heart disease. In this chapter, we evaluate the ability of contrast MRI to fill this clinical role. We start, however, with the definition of myocardial viability. Although the definition may appear to be self-evident, discrepancies between the results of contrast MRI and various clinical indexes of viability may arise because of assumptions concerning the definition of viability.

DEFINITION OF MYOCARDIAL VIABILITY

The definition of myocardial viability is directly related to that of myocardial infarction (MI) because infarction is defined as the loss of viability. In the clinical setting, a number of techniques are available to determine whether or not infarction has occurred, and if so, how much of the injured territory is not yet infarcted and may be salvaged. In a review article, Kaul (29) summarized the clinical markers of infarct size and ranked them from least to most precise (Fig. 14.2). As previously discussed, the observation of a wall motion abnormality alone does not provide information regarding viability because both stunned and hibernating myocardium are dysfunctional. The electrocardiogram (ECG), although useful, is recognized as being insensitive to infarction be-

cause patients with smaller infarcts may demonstrate minimal ECG changes during the acute event and often do not have Q waves chronically. Serum markers such as creatine kinase (CK) and troponin I or T can be extremely useful, but even these are associated with several limitations. For example, CK and troponin levels may exhibit differing time courses depending on whether or not reperfusion has occurred (30), and neither can be used to localize the infarction to a specific coronary artery territory. Perhaps most importantly, serum levels of CK are not elevated beyond the first few days, and troponin levels are not elevated beyond the first 2 weeks following the ischemic event (31), so that they cannot be used to detect older infarcts.

Accordingly to Kaul (29), the most precise way to define infarction, and therefore the loss of viability, is to determine whether or not myocyte death has occurred. All ischemic events occurring before cell death are, at least in principle, reversible by the reestablishment of an adequate blood supply. The presence or absence of cell death can be established

Less Precise

- Wall motion abnormality
- Q waves
- Total enzyme leak
- No-reflow or low-reflow
- Change in tissue composition

More Precise

- Myocyte integrity

FIGURE 14.2. Clinical and physiologic markers to determine the size of infarction. (From Kaul S. Assessing the myocardium after attempted reperfusion: should we bother? *Circulation* 1998;98: 625–627, with permission.)

TABLE 14.1. DEFINITIONS OF MYOCARDIAL VIABILITY

Clinical
- Improvement in contraction after revascularization
- Improvement in contraction with low-dose dobutamine
- Absence of a fixed thallium defect
- Presence of glucose uptake
- Reduced perfusion
- Preserved wall thickness, wall thickening, or both

Histologic
- Presence of living myocytes

From Kim RJ, Hillenbrand HB, Judd RM. Evaluation of myocardial viability by MRI. *Herz* 2000; 25:417–430, with permission.

by light microscopy, electron microscopy, or histologic stains, such as triphenyltetrazolium chloride (TTC) (32).

Testing for myocardial viability by microscopy or histologic staining is obviously not practical in a clinical setting. Accordingly, a number of less precise definitions of viability have developed that are based on parameters more easily measured in patients (Table 14.1). It is important to recognize, however, that these clinical definitions are indirect and that only the presence of living myocytes can be considered to be the correct definition of viability. Moreover, the techniques that are used to measure these indexes can impose additional limitations. For example, the use of dobutamine echocardiography, positron emission tomography (PET), or single photon emission computed tomography (SPECT) usually leads to a binary determination of viability within a myocardial region because these tests cannot assess the transmural extent of viability across the ventricular wall. The discrepancy that can arise as a consequence of this limitation is demonstrated in Figure 14.3. In this particular ex-

ample, an assessment of the anterior wall by means of current clinical methods and definitions will be incorrect regardless of whether the anterior wall is determined to be viable or not viable because the correct assessment is that the subendocardial half of the wall is not viable and the epicardial half is viable.

SCOPE OF THE CHAPTER

This chapter focuses on the physiologic and clinical interpretation of myocardial delayed hyperenhancement, defined as regions of elevated image intensity on T1-weighted images acquired more than 5 minutes after the administration of a contrast agent. The phenomenon of delayed hyperenhancement was first described at least 15 years ago (33). Since that time, many reports of hyperenhancement in the setting of acute infarction have been published (34–44), although fewer studies have described delayed contrast enhancement patterns in chronic infarcts or reversibly injured myocardium (35,45–47). More recently, however, newer imaging pulse sequences have been developed that significantly improve the detection and sizing of regions of delayed hyperenhancement *in vivo* (48,49). Several excellent reviews of the literature concerning the interpretation of myocardial hyperenhancement before the development of the newer techniques have been published (50,51), and this literature is revisited here only briefly. Different interpretations of myocardial hyperenhancement may arise because of differences in image quality; accordingly, to provide a coherent view of contrast MRI, this chapter focuses on data acquired after the development of the newer imaging techniques.

IMAGING TECHNIQUE

History

The primary action of most MRI contrast agents currently approved for use in humans is to shorten the longitudinal relaxation time (T1). Accordingly, the goal of most MRI pulse sequences used for the purpose of examining contrast enhancement patterns is to make image intensities a strong function of T1 (T1-weighted images). Early approaches (about 1985) to acquiring T1-weighted images of the heart often used ECG-gated spin-echo images in which one k-space line was acquired during each cardiac cycle. Because the duration of the cardiac cycle (~800 milliseconds) is comparable with the myocardial T1, the resulting images were T1-weighted. Following the administration of a contrast agent, myocardial T1 was shortened and image intensities increased. Using this approach, a number of investigators reported that as image intensities increased throughout the heart, regions associated with acute MI became particularly bright (hyperenhanced) on a time scale of minutes to tens of minutes after contrast administration (34–39,42,44,

Ideal Imaging Method

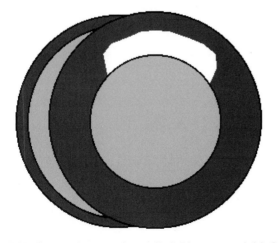

QUESTION: Is the anterior wall viable or not-viable?

FIGURE 14.3. Cartoon showing infarction of the subendocardial half of the anterior wall *(white area)*.

45,52). The use of ECG-gated spin-echo imaging, however, has several intrinsic limitations that adversely affect image quality. One such limitation is the need for relatively long acquisition times (minutes), which introduce artifacts caused by respiratory motion. Newer MRI techniques used for the purpose of examining myocardial contrast enhancement patterns have resulted in significant improvements in image quality.

New Technique

Since the early use of ECG-gated spin-echo imaging, a number of improvements have been made. One of the most important among these is the use of segmented k-space (53), in which multiple k-space lines are acquired during each cardiac cycle. As a result, imaging times are reduced to the point at which an entire image can be acquired during a single breath-hold (~8 seconds), so that image artifacts caused by respiration are eliminated. In addition, preparation of the magnetization before image acquisition with an inversion pulse

significantly increases the degree of T1 weighting in the images. In our laboratory, we recently compared a segmented inversion recovery pulse sequence with nine other MRI techniques in a dog model of MI (49). Table 14.2 summarizes the relative elevations in image intensities in infarcted and normal myocardial regions in humans and large-animal models *in vivo*. From 1986 to 1999, image intensities in "hyperenhanced" regions were generally 50% to 100% higher than in normal regions. The use of a segmented inversion recovery pulse sequence with the inversion time set to null signal from normal myocardium increased this differential approximately 10-fold, to 1,080% in animals and 485% in humans (labeled "current study" in Table 14.2).

The segmented inversion recovery sequence is shown in more detail in Figure 14.4. Following the R wave of the ECG, a delay period ("trigger delay") is used to ensure that the image is acquired during diastole to minimize cardiac motion. The magnetization of the heart is then prepared with a nonselective 180-degree inversion pulse to increase T1 weighting. The inversion delay time (TI) is then defined

TABLE 14.2. PERCENTAGE ELEVATIONS IN MR SIGNAL INTENSITY OF INFARCTED VERSUS NORMAL MYOCARDIUM AND VOXEL SIZES: PREVIOUSLY PUBLISHED AND CURRENT DATA

				Canine		Human	
Year	Reference	Technique[a]	Breath-Hold	ΔI/R (%)[b]	Voxel Size (mm³)	ΔI/R (%)[b]	Voxel Size (mm³)
1986	107	Spin echo	No	80	NS		
1986	108	Spin echo	No	70	NS		
1986	45	Spin echo	No			42[c]	29.3[d]
1988	109	Spin echo	No			60	29.3[d]
1989	110	Spin echo	No			36	29.3[d]
1990	111	Spin echo	No			32[c]	31.3[d]
1991	47	Spin echo	No			31[c]	27.5
1991	52	Spin echo	No			42	29.3[d]
1994	76	Spin echo	No			41[c]	29.3[d]
1995	40	MD-SPGR	Yes			103[c]	33.3
1995	41	MD-SPGR	Yes	123[e]	39.6		
1998	77	MD-SPGR	Yes			58[e]	30.8
1999	112	MD-SPGR	Yes	79[e]	14.7		
1999	56	Single-shot inversion-recovery FLASH	Yes			39	54.9[f]
Mean of previous studies				86	27.2	48	32.4
Current study				1,080	6.2	485	16.8

[a] All images were acquired *in vivo* at least 5 minutes after the administration of a United States Food and Drug Administration-approved MRI contrast agent.
[b] Percentage elevation in MR signal intensity of infarcted myocardium compared with signal intensity of normal myocardium.
[c] Published data were reported as precontrast versus postcontrast values; values in Table 14.2 were calculated as follows: (postcontrast value − precontrast value)/precontrast value.
[d] Assuming a field of view of 320 mm.
[e] Estimated from data reported in graphic format.
[f] Assuming a rectangular (6/8) field of view.
MD-SPGR, magnetization-driven spoiled gradient recalled; FLASH, fast low-angle shot; NS, not stated.
From Simonetti OP, Kim RJ, Fieno DS, et al. An improved MR imaging technique for the visualization of myocardial infarction. *Radiology* 2001; 218:215–223, with permission.

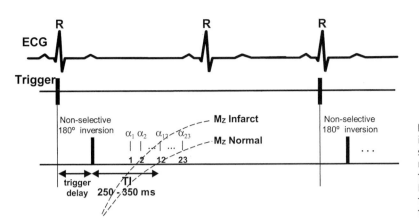

FIGURE 14.4. Timing diagram for the segmented inversion recovery turbo-FLASH (fast low-angle shot) sequence with inversion time set to null normal myocardium after the administration of contrast agent. See text for details. (From Simonetti OP, Kim RJ, Fieno DS, et al. An improved MR imaging technique for the visualization of myocardial infarction. *Radiology* 2001;218:215–233, with permission.)

as the time between this 180-degree pulse and the center of acquisition of the segmented k-space lines (lines 1 through 23 in Fig. 14.4). The TI is chosen such that the magnetization of normal myocardium is near its zero crossing, so that these regions appear as dark as possible. Infarcted myocardium, however, appears bright because of the lower T1 associated with infarcted myocardium following contrast administration.

MR images acquired with 10 different T1-weighted pulse sequences in the same imaging session are shown in Figure 14.5. The segmented inversion recovery sequence (SEG IR-TFL, large image in Fig. 14.5) produced the best delineation of the hyperenhanced region *(arrows)*. Table 14.3 compares the percentage elevation in image intensities in infarcted and normal myocardial regions obtained with the 10 different MRI pulse sequences in a series of animals. The segmented inversion recovery sequence produced the largest difference in regional myocardial image intensities of any sequence described to date. This sequence also produced the highest contrast-to-noise ratio.

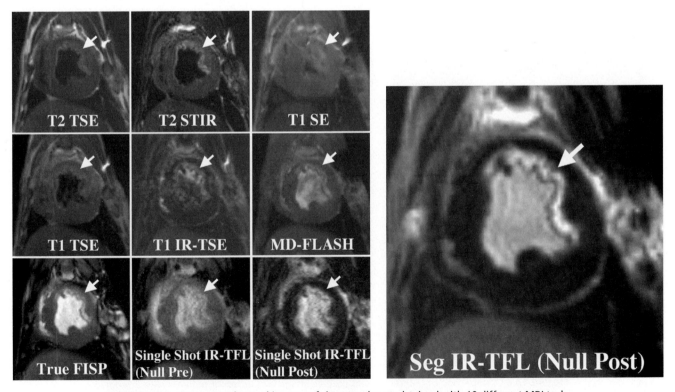

FIGURE 14.5. Contrast-enhanced images of the same heart obtained with 10 different MRI techniques. The segmented inversion recovery technique *(large image)* produced the clearest delineation of the hyperenhanced region *(arrows)*. (From Simonetti OP, Kim RJ, Fieno DS, et al. An improved MR imaging technique for the visualization of myocardial infarction. *Radiology* 2001;218:215–233, with permission.)

TABLE 14.3 SUMMARY OF RESULTS FROM 10 PULSE SEQUENCES TESTED IN A CANINE MODEL OF MYOCARDIAL INFARCTION

Sequence	Δ% INF/REM		CNR	
	Mean	SEM	Mean	SEM
T2-TSE	94.2	33.0	4.19	2.68
T2-STIR	120.1	62.2	3.16	1.94
T1-SE	67.2	26.0	2.95	1.63
T1-TSE	64.7	15.6	5.97	1.56
T1-IR-TSE	497.3	149.6	5.89	1.20
MD-FLASH	140.1	43.1	8.3	2.55
True FISP	148.1	31.9	14.44	4.23
IR-TFL (Null pre)	111.6	30.2	8.21	1.73
IR-SS-TFL (Null post)	510.4	181.4	10.14	2.54
SEG IR-TFL (Null post)	1,080.4	370.6	18.93	5.17

CNR, contrast-to-noise ratio; TSE, turbo spin-echo; IR, inversion recovery; MD-FLASH, magnetization-driven fast low-angle shot; FISP, fast imaging with steady-state free precession; TFL, turbo FLASH; SEG, segmented; SEM, standard error of the mean.
From Simoretti OP, Kim RJ, Fiero DS, et al. An improved MR imaging technique for the visualization of myocardial infarction. *Radiology* 2001;218:215–233, with permission.

Benefits of New Technique

Images acquired approximately 6 years ago are compared with those of today in Figure 14.6. The image in the left panel was published by our group in 1995 (40) and was acquired with the "magnetization-driven spoiled gradient recalled acquisition in the steady state" pulse sequence (MD-SPGR) (54). The image in the right panel was acquired more recently with the segmented inversion recovery pulse sequence shown in Figure 14.4 (49). As seen in Figure 14.6, the newer technique results in a sharper and better delineated region of hyperenhancement, and nontransmural involvement is clearly observed. This recent improvement in image quality underscores the need to understand fully the physiologic information portrayed by contrast-enhanced images of the heart.

ANIMAL STUDIES

The clinical utility of contrast MRI is determined both by the quality of the images and by their relationship to the underlying pathophysiology. Although clinical studies clearly help to define the information available, a direct comparison of the MR images with histologic tissue samples obtained from animals is a unique and important source of information. In principle, several species of animals can be used to study patterns of myocardial contrast enhancement. Large animals such as dogs, however, provide a practical advantage in that they can be studied in clinical scanners with the identical pulse sequences used for patients, so that the clinical relevance of the findings is ensured.

In humans, the type and age of an ischemic injury are complex and often only partially documented. Despite the clinical complexities, however, several well-defined states

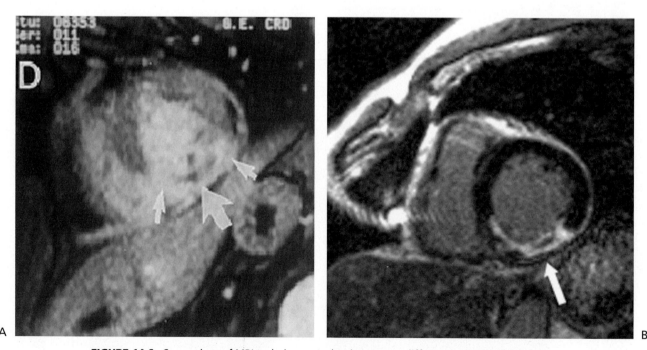

FIGURE 14.6. Comparison of MRI techniques used to image two different patients with inferior myocardial infarction in 1995 **(A)** and 2000 **(B).** The segmented inversion recovery sequence (B) better delineates the infarction and allows visualization of nontransmural involvement. (Panel A from Lima JA, Judd RM, Bazille A, et al. Regional heterogeneity of human myocardial infarcts demonstrated by contrast-enhanced MRI. Potential mechanisms. *Circulation* 1995;92:1117–1125, with permission.)

within the development of ischemic injury can be studied in a controlled setting in animals. These states include acute infarction, chronic infarction, and severe but reversible ischemic injury. In this section, we review the data concerning patterns of MRI contrast enhancement and their relationship to the underlying pathophysiology in the setting of these three pathologic circumstances.

Acute Myocardial Infarction

Patterns of contrast enhancement in the setting of acute infarction have been reported by a number of investigators both with and without reperfusion. Most if not all studies report that regions of acute infarction appear hyperenhanced on T1-weighted images acquired more than a few minutes after contrast administration (34–42,44,45,52,55–57). The exact relationship of the observed hyperenhanced regions to the underlying pathophysiology, however, has been a subject of debate and deserves some additional consideration. Understanding the issues requires some background regarding the development of ischemic myocardial injury.

In the traditional view of ischemic myocardial injury, an "area at risk" (58) is defined as a territory in which blood flow is reduced following occlusion of a coronary artery. Following occlusion, myocardial contractile function falls almost immediately throughout the "area at risk" (59). Little or no cellular necrosis, however, appears until about 15 minutes after occlusion (60,61). After 15 minutes, a "wavefront" of necrosis begins in the subendocardium and grows toward the epicardium during the next few hours (58,62). During this period, the size of the "area at risk" remains the same, but the size of the infarcted region within the "area at risk" increases. The interpretation of MRI hyperenhancement in the setting of acute infarction, therefore, requires a direct comparison of the MR images with the "area at risk" and the "area of infarction."

Both the "area at risk" and the "area of infarction" can be precisely defined only in histologic tissue sections. The "area at risk" can be identified experimentally with techniques involving microspheres (63) or blue dye (58), whereas the "area of infarction" can be defined by staining with TTC (32). Understanding the relationship of MRI contrast enhancement patterns to the underlying pathophysiology depends importantly, therefore, on registration of the *in vivo* MR images with the postmortem tissue samples.

In practice, the accurate registration of *in vivo* MR images with histologic tissue sections is difficult for several reasons. First, the three-dimensional shapes of both the "area at risk" and the "area of infarction" are very complex, and the details of their shapes are generally beyond the resolution of *in vivo* MRI. Second, after removal from the chest, the heart itself is easily deformed and almost impossible to cut along the exact same plane used for imaging. As a result, tissue slices aligned by eye and cut by hand almost certainly will not be registered precisely enough to allow slice-by-slice

comparisons of the detailed shapes of hyperenhanced regions observed *in vivo* by MRI with those defined histologically. In this setting, many investigators have avoided the image registration problem entirely by computing the percentage of the entire LV that is at risk or infarcted based on the sum of regions identified in a series of slices, usually short-axis slices from base to apex. This "one point per animal" approach, however, effectively discards the much larger amount of information that could be obtained by careful image registration.

To address this issue, we introduced in our laboratory the intermediate step of high-resolution *ex vivo* imaging. Immediately after the *in vivo* contrast-enhanced images were acquired, we removed the hearts, cooled them to 4°C, attached three MRI-visible registration markers, placed a balloon in the LV cavity (filled with deuterium to cause a proton signal void), and suspended the hearts in an extremity radiofrequency coil for high-resolution imaging. The absence of cardiac motion allowed us to acquire T1-weighted images with a spatial resolution of $500 \times 500 \times 500$ μm. After imaging, the hearts were further cooled and made partially stiff by repeated immersion in −80°C ethanol, and then sliced every 2 mm in a commercial rotating meat slicer along the same planes used for imaging (defined by the three MRI-visible markers). After this, each tissue slice was stained for myocyte necrosis with TTC (32) and compared with the MR images.

A comparison of MRI with histology in an animal with acute infarction made by means of this approach is shown in Figure 14.7. The "match" between TTC and MRI was extremely close, and even minute details, such as "fingers" of necrosis defined by TTC, were readily identified in the T1-weighted MR images. This "match" held in a series of animals with acute infarction that were studied both with and without reperfusion (Fig. 14.8). On the basis of these findings, we concluded that in the setting of acute infarction, the spatial extent of hyperenhancement by MRI is identical to the spatial extent of myocardial necrosis (48).

The mechanisms at the cellular level responsible for hyperenhancement have not been fully elucidated. Evidence suggests that concentrations of MRI contrast agents are elevated in regions of acute infarction (44,64), and this observation would explain the shortened T1 in these regions. One possible mechanism of hyperenhancement of acute infarcts is described in Figure 14.9. Whole body data strongly suggest that in normal myocardial regions, the MRI contrast agent is excluded from the myocyte intracellular space by intact sarcolemmal membranes (65,66). The hypothesis of Figure 14.9 is that in acutely infarcted regions, the myocyte membranes are ruptured, so that the MRI contrast agent can passively diffuse into the intracellular space. The result is an increased concentration of contrast agent at the tissue level and therefore hyperenhancement. Loss of sarcolemmal membrane integrity is thought to be very tightly related to cell death (59–61), and the idea that an event specific to cell death is related to hyperenhancement would explain the

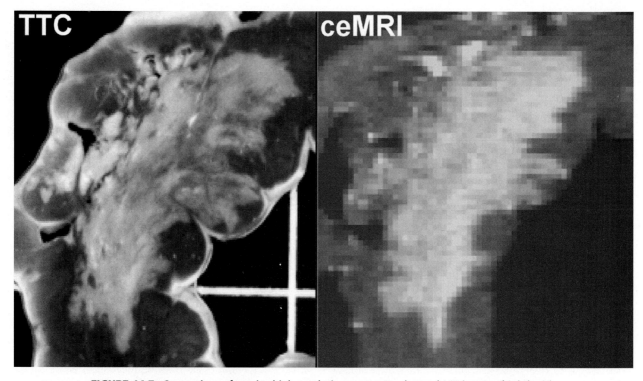

FIGURE 14.7. Comparison of *ex vivo* high-resolution contrast-enhanced MR images *(right)* with acute myocardial necrosis defined histologically by triphenyltetrazolium chloride staining *(left)*. See text for details. (From Kim RJ, Fieno DS, Parrish TB, et al. Relationship of MRI delayed contrast enhancement to irreversible injury, infarct age, and contractile function. *Circulation* 1999;100: 1992–2002, with permission.)

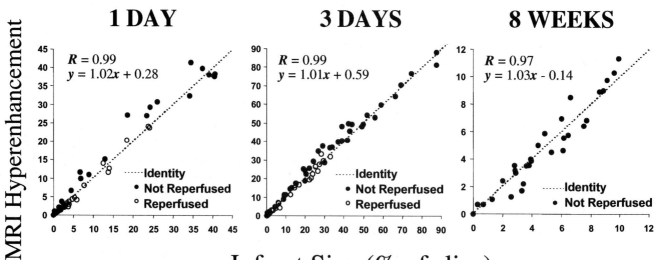

FIGURE 14.8. Comparison of hyperenhanced regions by MRI with infarct size measured by triphenyltetrazolium chloride at 1 day, 3 days, and 8 weeks with and without reperfusion. See text for details. (From Kim RJ, Fieno DS, Parrish TB, et al. Relationship of MRI delayed contrast enhancement to irreversible injury, infarct age, and contractile function. *Circulation* 1999;100:1992–2002, with permission.)

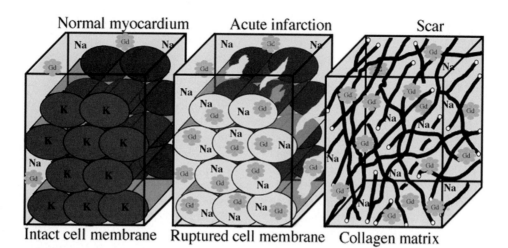

FIGURE 14.9. Potential mechanisms of hyperenhancement in acute and chronic myocardial infarcts. See text for details.

strong spatial relationship of MRI hyperenhancement to necrosis shown in Figure 14.7.

Chronic Myocardial Infarction

Unlike acute infarcts, which are characterized by necrotic myocytes, chronic infarcts are characterized by a dense collagenous scar. Because of these underlying structural differences, there is no reason a priori to believe that acute and chronic infarcts will appear similar in contrast-enhanced MR images. To address this issue, we scanned dogs 8 weeks after MI, when infarct healing had clearly progressed. The example of a dog with an 8-week-old infarct in which the hyperenhanced region observed *in vivo* is clearly associated with a dense collagenous scar defined histologically postmortem appears in Figure 14.10. When the same technique

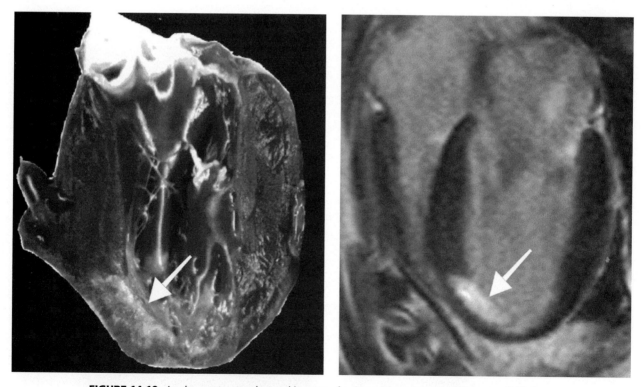

FIGURE 14.10. *In vivo* contrast-enhanced images of a dog with an 8-week-old myocardial infarction *(right)*. Despite replacement of necrotic myocytes with dense collagenous scar, hyperenhancement is still observed. (From Kim RJ, Fieno DS, Parrish TB, et al. Relationship of MRI delayed contrast enhancement to irreversible injury, infarct age, and contractile function. *Circulation* 1999;100:1992–2002, with permission.)

of high-resolution *ex vivo* imaging described above in the setting of acute infarcts was used, the regions of hyperenhancement observed in the setting of chronic infarcts also appeared to be identical to the infarcted regions defined histologically (48) (Fig. 14.8). These data indicate that chronic infarcts systematically hyperenhance.

The mechanism of hyperenhancement in chronic infarcts remains to be elucidated. One potential mechanism is proposed in Figure 14.9. Although myocardial scar is characterized by a dense collagenous matrix, at a cellular level, the interstitial space between collagen fibers may be significantly greater than the interstitial space between densely packed living myocytes that is characteristic of normal myocardium. In this case, the concentration of MRI contrast agent in scar would be greater than in normal myocardium because of the expanded volume of distribution of the contrast agent. Higher concentrations of the contrast agent would lower the T1, as in acute infarcts, and the regions of scar would appear hyperenhanced by MRI.

Reversible Ischemic Injury

Given that both acute and chronic myocardial infarcts exhibit hyperenhancement, the question of whether severe but reversible ischemic injury exhibits hyperenhancement takes on added importance. In our laboratory, we used two separate experimental approaches to examine this question. In the first approach, severe but reversible ischemic injury was induced in the magnet, and then contrast-enhanced images were acquired. In the second approach, high-resolution *ex vivo* images were compared with the "area at risk but not infarcted region" defined histologically.

Examples of the first approach appear in Figure 14.11 (48). Under sterile conditions, two coronary arteries were manipulated. The first coronary artery was permanently ligated to cause MI (left anterior descending diagonal of Fig. 14.11). The second coronary artery was instrumented with a reversible hydraulic occluder and a Doppler flowmeter. The animals were then allowed to recover and were studied 3 days later. While they were in the magnet, regional wall motion was examined with cine MRI. The reversible occluder was then inflated for 15 minutes. During the period of occlusion, cine MR images were again obtained to identify new regions of abnormal wall motion to ensure that the region distal to the reversible occluder was within the imaging plane. After 15 minutes, the occluder was released and flow was restored (verified by Doppler flow). The purpose of the 15-minute occlusion was to induce severe but reversible ischemic injury (60,61). A third set of cine MR images was then acquired. The gray scale bull's-eyes of Figure 14.11 correspond to wall thickening at this time (brighter indicates increased wall thickening). As can be seen in Figure 14.11, both the region associated with infarction *(filled arrows)* and the region associated with severe but reversible

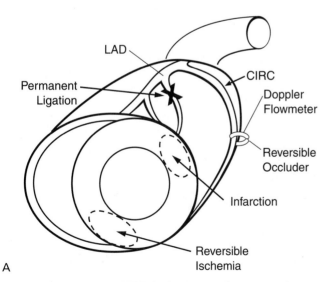

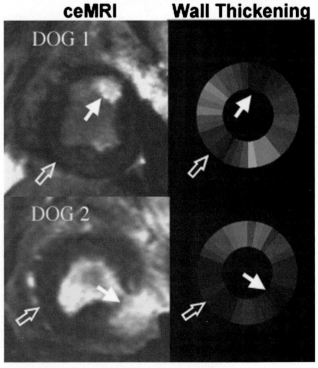

FIGURE 14.11. Hyperenhancement does not occur in regions of severe but reversible ischemic injury despite a persistent wall motion abnormality. See text for details. (From Kim RJ, Fieno DS, Parrish TB, et al. Relationship of MRI delayed contrast enhancement to irreversible injury, infarct age, and contractile function. *Circulation* 1999;100:1992–2002, with permission.)

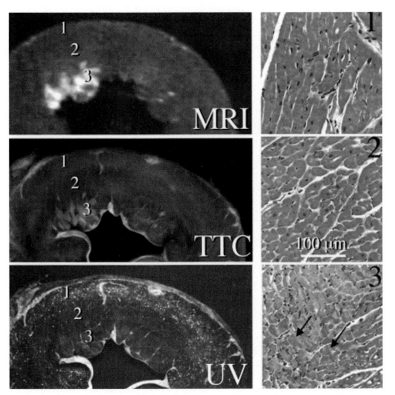

FIGURE 14.12. Hyperenhancement does not occur in regions "at risk but not infarcted." See text for details. (From Fieno DS, Kim RJ, Chen EL, et al. Contrast-enhanced magnetic resonance imaging of myocardium at risk: distinction between reversible and irreversible injury throughout infarct healing. *J Am Coll Cardiol* 2000;36:1985–1991, with permission.)

ischemic injury *(arrow outlines)* show abnormal wall thickening. The MRI contrast agent was then injected and the images inspected for hyperenhancement. As seen in Figure 14.11, the region of infarction exhibited hyperenhancement, but the region of severe but reversible ischemic injury did not. When these same animals were scanned 8 weeks later, wall thickening had returned to normal in the region of severe but reversible ischemic injury (48). Histologic examination (also at 8 weeks) revealed infarction in the territory subtended by the permanently occluded artery, but no evidence of infarction was found distal to the reversible occluder. These *in vivo* data support the view that severe but reversible ischemic injury does not result in hyperenhancement (48).

Another approach to this question is illustrated in Figure 14.12 (67). In these experiments, TTC was used to define the "area of infarction" *(middle left panel),* and fluorescent microparticles injected into the left atrium during occlusion were used to define the "area at risk" *(lower left panel).* In this way, we could identify the region that was "at risk but not infarcted," shown as zone 2 of Figure 14.12. As seen in Figure 14.12 *(upper panel),* the "at risk but not infarcted" region *(zone 2)* does not exhibit hyperenhancement as defined by carefully registered high-resolution *ex vivo* images. Light microscopy of this region revealed normal myocyte architecture *(middle right panel). Ex vivo* image intensities in the three zones defined in Figure 14.12—namely, "remote" *(zone 1),* "at risk but not infarcted" *(zone 2),* and "infarcted" *(zone 3)*—are summarized in Figure 14.13. No elevation of

image intensities was detected in "at risk but not infarcted" regions in comparison with normal myocardium. Consistent with the data of Figure 14.11, the data of Figures 14.12 and 14.13 strongly support the view that severe but reversible ischemic injury does not result in hyperenhancement (67).

The data of Figure 14.11 further underscore that a dissociation between wall thickening and contrast enhancement is possible, in which wall thickening is impaired but hyperenhancement is not observed. In the setting of acute ischemic injury, this condition is probably related to the phenomenon of myocardial "stunning" (10,21), in which cell death has not occurred but contractile dysfunction persists for days or even weeks after a severe ischemic event. The data of Figure 14.11 suggest that in the setting of an acute ischemic event, all regions exhibiting contractile dysfunction can be subdivided into irreversibly and reversibly injured regions, defined as those with and without hyperenhancement, respectively. This concept suggests that the presence or absence of hyperenhancement in regions of contractile dysfunction may be useful in detecting myocardial salvage early after acute infarction. If correct, this approach would represent a new technique to define myocardial salvage in patients following acute infarction.

To test the hypothesis that contrast enhancement can be used to index myocardial salvage, we initiated another study, in which animals were imaged 3 days, 10 days, and 4 weeks after transient coronary artery occlusion (68). The hypothesis was that recovery of contractile dysfunction at 4

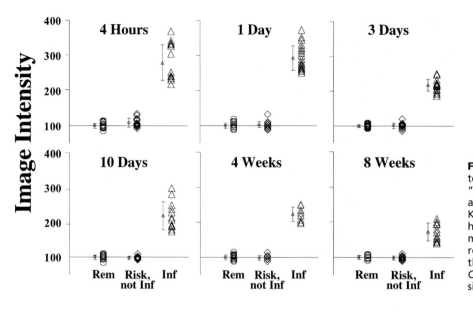

FIGURE 14.13. Summary of image intensities for all animals corresponding to "remote," "at risk but not infarcted," and "infarcted" regions. (From Fieno DS, Kim RJ, Chen EL, et al. Contrast-enhanced magnetic resonance imaging of myocardium at risk: distinction between reversible and irreversible injury throughout infarct healing. *J Am Coll Cardiol* 2000;36:1985–1991, with permission).

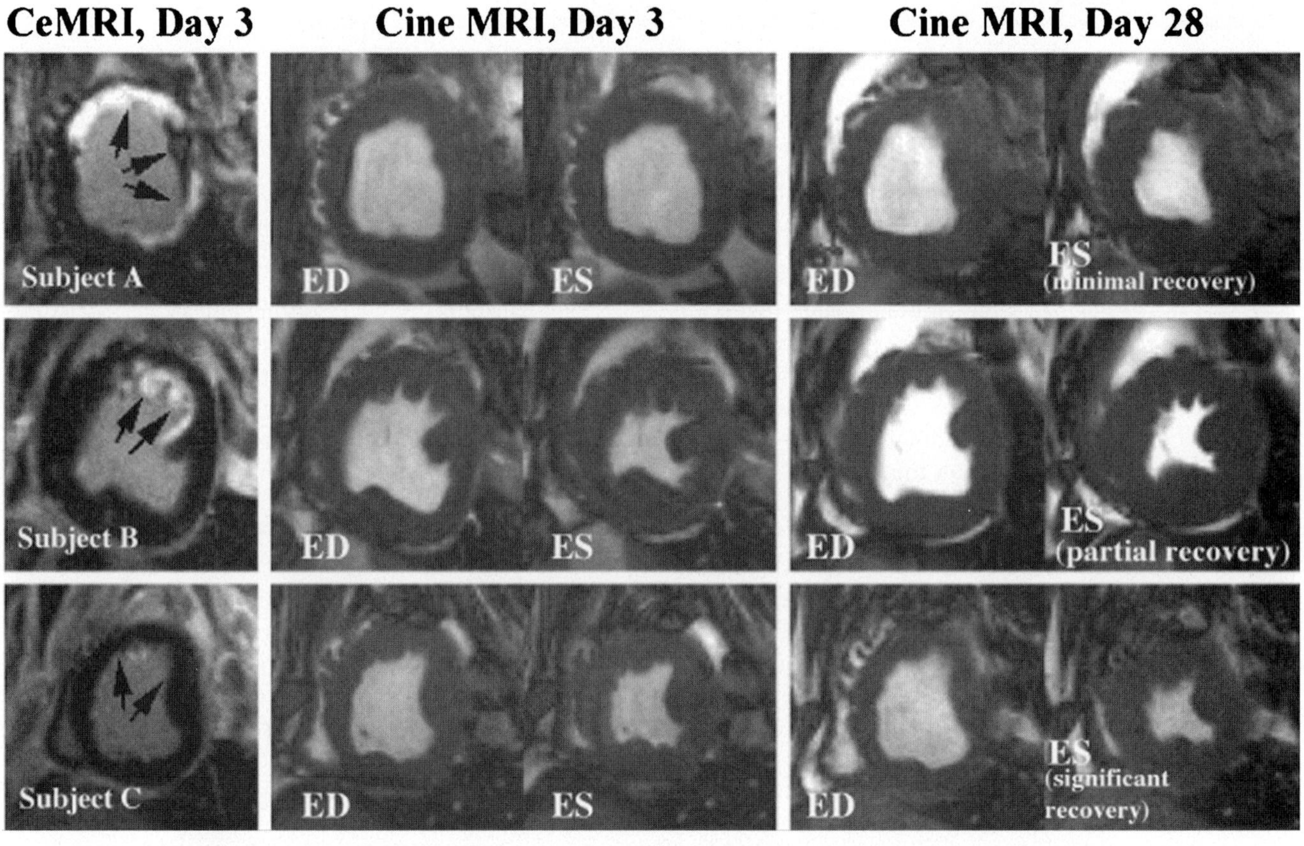

CeMRI, Day 3   Cine MRI, Day 3   Cine MRI, Day 28

Subject A | ED ES | ED ES (minimal recovery)

Subject B | ED ES | ED ES (partial recovery)

Subject C | ED ES | ED ES (significant recovery)

FIGURE 14.14. Contrast enhancement and wall thickening at 3 days *(columns 1–3)* compared with wall thickening at 28 days *(columns 4 and 5)* in three different animals *(rows)*. See text for details. (From Hillenbrand HB, Kim RJ, Parker MA, et al. Early assessment of myocardial salvage by contrast-enhanced magnetic resonance imaging. *Circulation* 2000;102:1678–1683, with permission. A full-motion version of this figure can be viewed on the Internet at *http://circ.ahajournals.org/cgi/content/full/102/14/1678/DC1/1.*)

weeks in comparison with that at 3 days could be predicted by contrast enhancement at 3 days. Specific examples from that study are shown in Figure 14.14, in which each row represents a different animal. The first three columns show MRI data acquired at 3 days, whereas the data in columns 4 and 5 were acquired at 4 weeks. At 3 days, all three animals showed contractile dysfunction in the territory of the left anterior descending artery by cine MRI *(columns 2 and 3)*. The first animal *(row 1)*, however, showed nearly transmural hyperenhancement, the second animal *(row 2)* about 50% transmural hyperenhancement, and the third animal *(row 3)* almost no hyperenhancement. Four weeks later, contractile function did not improve in the first animal, improved partially in the second animal, and completely recovered in the third animal. A summary of all data from this study appears in Figure 14.15. These data underscore that, as predicted by the results in Figures 14.11 through 14.13, contrast enhancement patterns observed early after MI can be used to index the extent of myocardial salvage (68). The full-motion version of Figure 14.14 can be viewed on the internet at the following address: *http://circ.ahajournals.org/cgi/content/full/102/14/1678/DC1/1.*

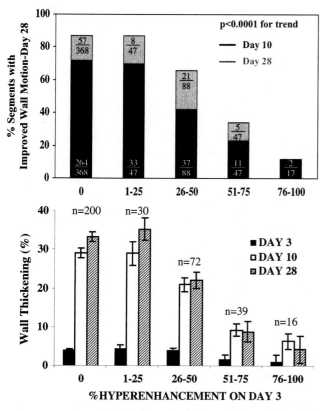

FIGURE 14.15. The likelihood of improvement in wall thickening *(upper panel)* and absolute wall thickening *(lower panel)* as a function of the transmural extent of hyperenhancement. *Black* and *gray bars* correspond to improvement by days 10 and 28 respectively. (From Hillenbrand HB, Kim RJ, Parker MA, et al. Early assessment of myocardial salvage by contrast-enhanced magnetic resonance imaging. *Circulation* 2000;102:1678–1683, with permission.)

The mechanism for the lack of hyperenhancement in regions of severe but reversible ischemic injury may be directly related to the mechanism for hyperenhancement in acute infarcts (i.e., it may be related to the integrity of the myocyte membrane). Although severe but reversible ischemic injury has many effects on the myocyte, the sarcolemmal membrane remains intact (60,61) and therefore presumably continues to exclude the MRI contrast agent from the intracellular space. In this setting, the volume of distribution of the contrast agent in regions of severe but reversible ischemic injury would be expected to remain similar to that in normal myocardium, and no hyperenhancement of these regions would be observed.

Potential Complexities

Several technical and physiologic issues can complicate the interpretation of the experimental data presented in the previous section. One such issue is that much of the evidence presented earlier was based on *ex vivo* images. Without additional evidence, the possibility exists that *in vivo* and *ex vivo* MR images show different findings. We examined this issue in a recent study in which we registered the three-dimensional *ex vivo* data set with 12 to 15 contiguous 5-mm thick *in vivo* images acquired in the same animals (67). As shown in Figure 14.16, the *in vivo* images were essentially identical to the *ex vivo* images, a result that supports the use of *ex vivo* data for the interpretation of *in vivo* contrast enhancement patterns.

Another technical issue concerning the comparison of *in vivo* and *ex vivo* images relates to the pulse sequence used to generate the T1-weighted images. For *in vivo* images, the segmented inversion recovery pulse sequence shown in Figure 14.4 was used. It is sometimes suggested that the spatial extent of hyperenhancement depends on the selected by the scanner operator, so that some laboratories may find a close correlation of hyperenhancement with infarction and others not. Certainly, if the TI is chosen incorrectly (i.e., is too short), the infarcted region can be made to appear *hypo*enhanced in comparison with normal myocardium. The definitive question, however, is whether infarcted regions but not reversibly injured regions have an increased concentration of contrast agent and therefore a shorter T1 than normal regions. In this context, it is important to note that all *ex vivo* imaging described in this chapter was performed with a standard gradient-echo sequence and a large flip angle to produce T1 weighting (i.e., no inversion pulse was used for the *ex vivo* images). The strong correlation between *ex vivo* MRI and histology (Fig. 14.8) underscores the existence of a fundamental relationship between nonviable myocardium and a shorter T1 after contrast (48,67).

A related issue concerns the suggestion that the spatial extent of hyperenhancement can change depending on how long after contrast administration imaging is performed. Clearly, issues may arise before 5 minutes that are related to

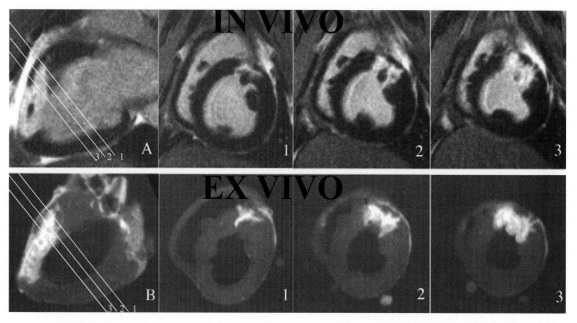

FIGURE 14.16. Hyperenhancement observed *in vivo* was similar to that observed *ex vivo*. (From Fieno DS, Kim RJ, Chen EL, et al. Contrast-enhanced magnetic resonance imaging of myocardium at risk: distinction between reversible and irreversible injury throughout infarct healing. *J Am Coll Cardiol* 2000;36:1985–1991, with permission.)

contrast agent delivery, and problems may develop after 30 to 40 minutes that are associated with contrast washout; however, in our laboratory, we have not observed significant changes in the spatial extent of hyperenhancement when imaging is performed between 5 to 30 minutes after contrast administration in patients. One caveat should be kept in mind. The longer one waits after contrast administration, the higher the TI should be set to obtain correct images. The basic premise is not that infarcted regions have a static T1 (which is obviously untrue *in vivo*), but that the T1 is always shorter than in normal regions in a relative sense. At all time points, the highest TI value should be selected in which normal myocardium is nulled to avoid mistakenly nulling regions with a shorter T1 than normal myocardium.

Other technical issues may play a role in the interpretation of *in vivo* MR images. The "partial volume" effect can play a role whenever the spatial resolution of the *in vivo* image is too poor to represent the complex three-dimensional nature of the pathophysiology adequately. An example of this is shown in Figure 14.17, in which an 8-mm-thick image *(panel B)* exhibits a "fuzzy" border, so that it is difficult to determined the exact edge of the hyperenhanced region (48). When this 8-mm-thick region is imaged at high resolution, however, the edges of the hyperenhanced region are clearly defined, and the "fuzzy" border is no longer present (Fig. 14.17, *lower 16 panels,* each with a thickness of 500 μm). Even with adequate spatial resolution, partial volume effects can occur with pulse sequences that require long acquisition times (minutes) as a consequence of respiratory and other subject motion. Figure 14.17 underscores how issues such as partial volume effects and, perhaps more importantly, even small errors related to misregistration of *in vivo* MR images with histologic sections can obscure the relationship of hyperenhancement to the underlying pathophysiology.

Another complexity related to both technical limitations and underlying physiology is the observation of regions of hypoenhancement at the core of large, acute infarcts. These dark regions are almost always completely surrounded by larger regions of hyperenhancement, and importantly, they slowly become hyperenhanced as repeated images are acquired at the same location. Figure 14.18 is an example of this phenomenon. The appearance of hypoenhanced regions on MR images has been related to the "no-reflow" phenomenon (41,69), which is a common feature of large, acute infarcts (70–73). Figure 14.19 shows the relationship of both hypoenhanced and hyperenhanced regions on contrast MR images to the traditional view of ischemic injury in more detail. The thin epicardial "rim" of dark myocardium in Figure 14.19 represents to viable myocytes salvaged by reperfusion, whereas the hyperenhanced region corresponds to necrotic myocytes with nearly normal perfusion. The dark region toward the endocardial core of the infarct corresponds to the "no-reflow" region, which is characterized by substantially reduced perfusion despite an open infarct-related artery. The reduced perfusion is thought to be caused by damage or obstruction at the microcirculatory level, which apparently impedes penetration of the MRI contrast agent into the core of the infarct. Because flow in these regions is low, but not absent, the regions appear dark initially, but as contrast accumulates, they slowly become hyperenhanced over time (Fig. 14.18). In practice, a "no-re-

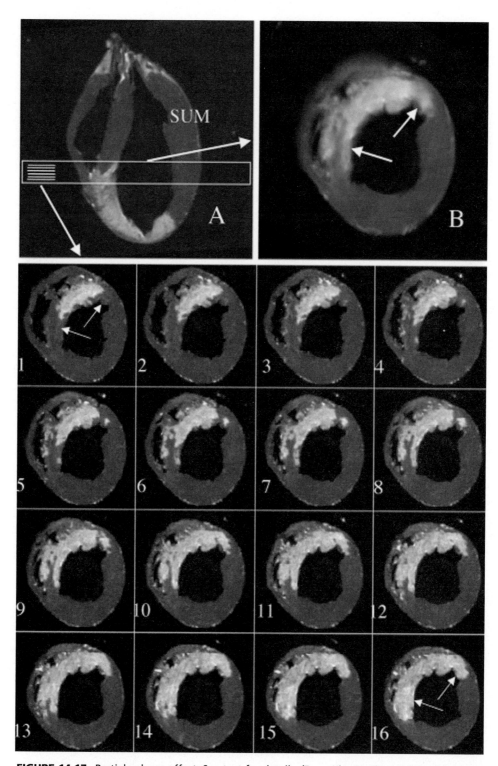

FIGURE 14.17. Partial volume effect. See text for details. (From Kim RJ, Fieno DS, Parrish TB, et al. Relationship of MRI delayed contrast enhancement to irreversible injury, infarct age, and contractile function. *Circulation* 1999;100:1992–2002, with permission.)

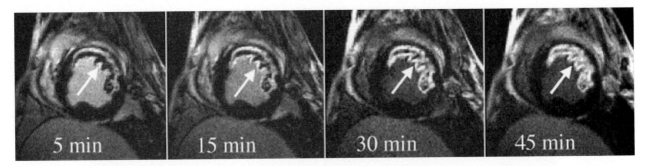

FIGURE 14.18. The "no-reflow" phenomenon revealed by contrast-enhanced MRI. Labels refer to time after the administration of contrast media. See text for details.

flow" region can be distinguished from viable myocardial regions, which are also not hyperenhanced, in several ways. First, because a "no-reflow" region is always surrounded (in three dimensions) by hyperenhanced regions, its nature is usually obvious on inspection of consecutive short-axis images. "No-reflow" regions are always located near the endocardium because ischemic injury is more severe in the endocardial layers of the heart wall (see explanation of the wavefront phenomenon in the section on acute MI under "Animal Studies"). It does not make sense physiologically, therefore, to interpret hypoenhancement near the subendocardium surrounded by hyperenhancement near the epicardium as an epicardial infarct surrounding viable endocardium. Second, the T1 in a "no-reflow" region is virtually unaffected by the administration of contrast agent and therefore is actually longer than in normal regions to which contrast agent has been delivered. Accordingly, repeated imaging with careful adjustment of the TI may help to distinguish a questionable "no-reflow" region from normal myocardium. When uncertainty remains, repeated imaging

over a longer period of time can be performed to test whether the region eventually becomes hyperenhanced (e.g., 30 to 45 minutes after contrast) (Fig. 14.18). It should be obvious from this discussion that when hypoenhanced regions are surrounded by hyperenhanced regions, the hypoenhanced region should be included in the measurement of infarct size.

Yet another complexity in the interpretation of MRI contrast enhancement patterns is the observation that regions with hyperenhancement sometimes exhibit an improvement in contractile function in the days and weeks that follow. The middle row of Figure 14.14 is an example of this phenomenon. Classically, myocardial viability is defined by an improvement in contractile function over time, and in the case of the middle row of Figure 14.14, it is clear that some improvement has occurred. Therefore, the observation of hyperenhancement at 3 days, as in the first column of Figure 14.14, might be interpreted as evidence that hyperenhancement can occur in viable myocardium. The problem with this interpretation is that myocardial viability

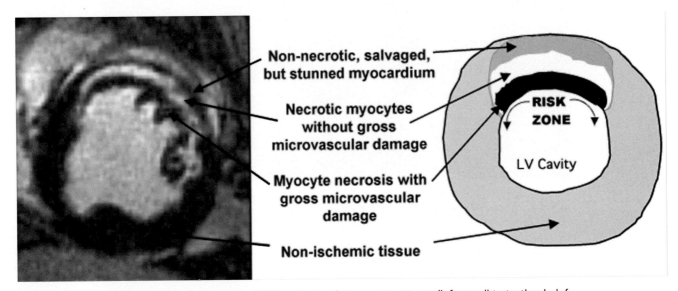

FIGURE 14.19. Relationship of MRI contrast enhancement patterns *(left panel)* to textbook definition of myocardial regions associated with ischemic injury *(right panel)*. (Right panel from Braunwald E, ed. *Heart disease: a textbook of cardiovascular medicine*, 5th ed. Philadelphia: W. B. Saunders, 1997:1178, with permission.)

is being intrinsically defined as an "all-or-none" phenomenon in which a transmural segment of myocardium must be either viable (improves) or not viable (does not improve). A more likely explanation, however, is that the entire thickness of the wall was within the "area at risk," and as the occlusion time increased, the "wavefront" of necrosis moved outward. Before the wavefront of necrosis reached the epicardium, however, the outer half of the heart wall was salvaged by reperfusion. In this case, the improvement in contractile function could be explained by "stunning" of the viable outer half of the heart at 3 days, which had recovered by 4 weeks. Because existing clinical imaging modalities that examine viability, such as dobutamine echocardiography and nuclear scintigraphy, cannot resolve nontransmural involvement, there has never been a compelling reason to consider viability as anything other than an "all-or-none" phenomenon. In this setting, the direct application of concepts derived from other imaging modalities may effectively ignore the new information (nontransmural involvement) portrayed by contrast MRI. This example also demonstrates the importance of image quality in contrast MRI. The precise transmural extent of hyperenhancement was often difficult to determine with earlier MRI techniques, so that the erroneous impression may have been acquired that contractile function sometimes improves in regions of "transmural" hyperenhancement.

A final complexity is the observation that the spatial extent of hyperenhancement appears to decrease during infarct healing. Figure 14.20 shows preliminary data from a study in which the spatial extent of hyperenhancement was serially examined in animals at 3 days, 10 days, 4 weeks, and 8 weeks after infarction. As can be seen in panel A, the size of the hyperenhanced region decreased approximately threefold from 3 days to 8 weeks. During this same period, the mass of non-hyperenhanced myocardium increased. One interpretation of these observations is that the hyperenhanced region was spatially larger than the infarcted territory at 3 days but became smaller by 8 weeks as reversibly injured regions healed and no longer exhibited hyperenhancement. This interpretation seems unlikely, however, in light of the strong correspondence between hyperenhancement and infarction defined histologically over multiple different time points (Fig. 14.8). An alternative interpretation of this finding is that infarcts shrink as the necrotic myocytes are replaced by collagenous scar. Direct evidence for infarct shrinkage can be found in the literature, and measurement of the degree of infarct shrinkage by techniques other than MRI also suggests a threefold to fourfold reduction in infarct volumes during healing. Panel B of Figure 14.20 shows an example of such data published in a review of myocardial ischemia by Reimer and Jennings (59). Although further study of these issues is clearly warranted, we have reason to believe that the changes in size of hyperenhanced and nonhyperenhanced regions during infarct healing represent a new perspective on the process of remodeling after infarction.

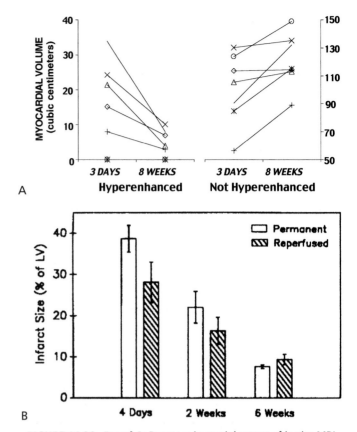

FIGURE 14.20. Panel A: Decrease in spatial extent of *in vivo* MRI hyperenhancement over time during infarct healing. Nonhyperenhanced regions increased in spatial extent over the same time period. (From Kim RJ, Fieno DS, Parrish TB, et al. Relationship of MRI delayed contrast enhancement to irreversible injury, infarct age, and contractile function. *Circulation* 1999;100:1992–2002, with permission.) **Panel B:** Infarct shrinkage determined by histopathology. (From Reimer KA, Jennings RB. Myocardial ischemia, hypoxia and infarction. In: Fozzard HA, et al., eds. *The heart and cardiovascular system*, 2nd ed. New York: Raven Press, 1992:1875–1973, with permission.)

HUMAN STUDIES

Few studies have been performed in humans with segmented inversion recovery turbo-FLASH (fast low-angle shot) imaging. In this section, the results of such studies are compared with the findings in the analogous animal models described in the previous section. Because histopathologic correlations are difficult to perform in human studies, particular attention should be paid to the "gold standard" used to define MI and determine the presence or absence of injured but viable myocardium.

MRI Protocol

All patient MRI data described in this section were acquired with the same imaging protocol. All images were acquired by using phased-array surface coils during repeated breathholds (about 8 seconds) and were gated to the ECG. Double-oblique long-axis scouts were taken to obtain true short-axis and long-axis references. Cine images were acquired in six to eight short-axis views and at least two long-axis views. Short-axis views were obtained every 1 cm throughout the whole LV starting at the mitral valve insertion plane. A clinically approved gadolinium-based contrast agent (e.g., 0.1 to 0.2 mmol of gadopentetate dimeglumine or gadoteridol per kilogram of body weight) was then administered intravenously by hand, and contrast-enhanced images were acquired 5 to 15 minutes later in the same views as the cine images. The contrast-enhanced images were acquired with the pulse sequence described earlier (Fig. 14.4), with typical inversion delays of 250 to 350 milliseconds and typical voxel sizes of $1.9 \times 1.4 \times 6.0$ mm. Figure 14.21 shows typical images of one patient acquired with this protocol. The total time required for MRI was approximately 30 minutes.

Acute Myocardial Infarction

We evaluated 18 consecutive patients referred for cardiac MRI who were known to have had a recent MI (49). Infarction was defined solely on the basis of an appropriate rise (more than twice the upper limit of normal) and fall in creatine kinase-myocardial band (CK-MB) isoenzyme levels. Patients underwent MRI 19 ± 7 days after documented en-

zyme elevations, and no patient was excluded for insufficient image quality or other reasons.

Representative images from three patients are shown in Figure 14.22. Starting at the left panel, infarction was caused by occlusion of the left anterior descending artery, left circumflex artery, and right coronary artery. Myocardial hyperenhancement is clearly visible in these patients in the appropriate infarct-related artery perfusion territory. Similar results were observed in the other 15 patients in the study. On average, the image intensities in hyperenhanced regions were 485% ± 43% higher than those in normal myocardial regions. As discussed previously, the degree of hyperenhancement was approximately 10-fold greater than that in previous reports (Table 14.2).

Ultimately, improved image quality is important only if it translates into improved diagnostic capability. Although prior studies showed that acute MI can be detected as hyperenhanced regions, the patients studied typically had large infarcts, and the transmural extent of infarction was not evaluated (37,39,40,74). Two relatively recent studies (57,75) distinguished between transmural and subendocardial hyperenhancement with the use of spin-echo techniques. Although nontransmural involvement was visualized in both studies, Dendale et al. (57) did not observe

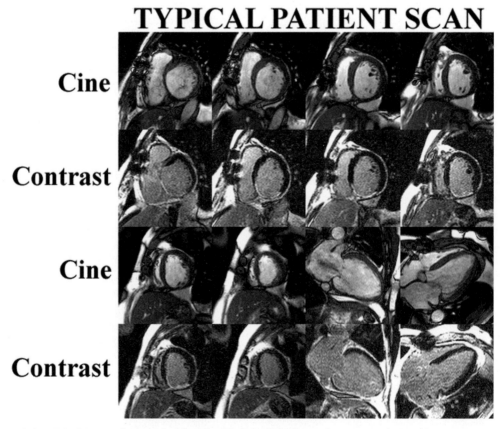

FIGURE 14.21. Imaging protocol for all patient studies. Cine and contrast-enhanced images were acquired at six to eight short and two long-axis locations during repeated breath-holds. This particular patient had a myocardial infarction caused by occlusion of the right coronary artery (determined at coronary angiography). Note hyperenhancement of the inferior wall.

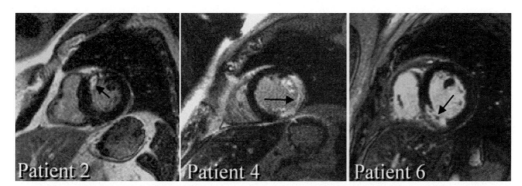

FIGURE 14.22. Short-axis images in three patients with acute myocardial infarction. The *arrows* point to the hyperenhanced region, which was in the appropriate infarct-related artery perfusion territory. (From Simonetti OP, Kim RJ, Fieno DS, et al. An improved MR imaging technique for the visualization of myocardial infarction. *Radiology* 2001;218:215–223, with permission.)

hyperenhancement in 15 (27%) of 56 infarct segments, and Yokota et al. (75) did not observe hyperenhancement in 6 (13%) of 44 patients with documented infarction. The infarcts that were missed were generally smaller infarcts with normal wall motion at rest (57) and lower peak CK levels (75). The inability to detect smaller infarcts may be a consequence of limitations in conventional spin-echo imaging, which requires image acquisition during several minutes of free-breathing. Partial volume effects caused by motional averaging over the respiratory cycle, image artifacts resulting from respiratory motion, and modest T1 weighting resulting from limited choices for repetition time may all decrease the conspicuity of hyperenhanced myocardium. Subendocardial infarction has been visualized with segmented inversion recovery turbo-FLASH techniques. This topic is discussed in the section entitled "Future Applications."

Chronic Myocardial Infarction

The studies of chronic infarction perhaps best demonstrate the importance of image quality in delayed contrast MRI. For example, Eichstaedt et al. (45), Nishimura et al. (46), and van Dijkman et al. (47) all observed gadolinium hyperenhancement in patients with acute MI but found no hyperenhancement in patients with chronic infarction. These reports formed the basis for the widespread conclusion that gadolinium does not accumulate in chronic infarcts (50,51). More recently, Fedele et al. (76) and Ramani et al. (77) suggested that this conclusion is erroneous. They described hyperenhancement in patients with chronic coronary artery disease and a high clinical likelihood of chronic infarction. Unfortunately, biochemical evidence for infarction was not provided, the age of infarction was unknown, and differences in image intensity were modest, with hyperenhanced regions having on average less than a 60% increase in image intensity in comparison with nonhyperenhanced regions.

Despite these conflicting results, we postulated in our laboratory that human chronic MI hyperenhances. This hypothesis was based on experimental animal data demon-

strating that collagenous scar hyperenhances in both *ex vivo* (Fig. 14.8) and *in vivo* imaging protocols (Fig. 14.10). To test this hypothesis, we enrolled patients at the time of acute infarction based on abnormal CK release and then performed MRI several months later after infarct healing (78). To assess the specificity of the findings, contrast MRI was also performed in patients with nonischemic cardiomyopathy and in healthy volunteers.

In the patients with chronic MI, we observed hyperenhancement in a variety of sizes, ranging from large, fully transmural hyperenhancement that extended over several short-axis slices to small, subendocardial hyperenhancement that was visible in only a single sector of a single view. Figure 14.23 shows typical short- and long-axis views of three patients with large transmural hyperenhancement in different coronary artery territories. The age of the infarct, the infarct-related artery, and the peak CK values are listed on the figure. In each of these patients, the hyperenhancement zone was in the appropriate infarct-related artery territory. Figure 14.24 demonstrates typical short- and long-axis views of three patients with minor CK-MB elevations and small regions of hyperenhancement in different coronary artery territories. Despite the small volume of hyperenhancement, the hyperenhancement zone was visually distinct, clearly nontransmural, and in the correct infarct-related artery territory in each patient. In all patients with hyperenhancement, the difference in image intensity between hyperenhanced and remote myocardium was more than six standard deviations of remote region intensity (mean difference, 17 standard deviations).

Twenty-nine (91%) of 32 patients with 3-month old infarcts and all 19 patients with 14-month old infarcts exhibited hyperenhancement. Among the patients with hyperenhancement in whom the infarct-related artery territory could be determined by coronary angiography, 24 of 25 patients with 3-month old infarcts (96%) and all 14 with 14-month old infarcts had hyperenhancement in the infarct-related artery territory. Regardless of the presence or absence of Q waves, the majority of patients with hyperenhance-

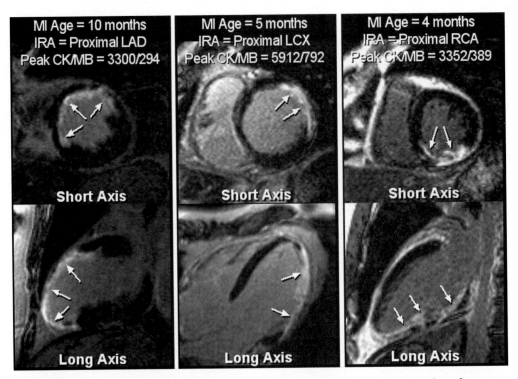

FIGURE 14.23. Typical short- and long-axis views of three patients with a large region of transmural hyperenhancement in different coronary artery territories. (From Wu E, Judd RM, Vargas JD, et al. Visualisation of presence, location, and transmural extent of healed Q-wave and non–Q-wave myocardial infarction. *Lancet* 2001;357:21–28, with permission.)

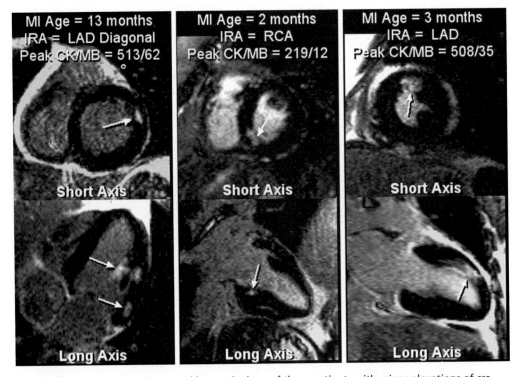

FIGURE 14.24. Typical short- and long-axis views of three patients with minor elevations of creatine kinase-myocardial band (CK-MB) isoenzyme and small regions of hyperenhancement in different coronary artery territories. (From Wu E, Judd RM, Vargas JD, et al. Visualisation of presence, location, and transmural extent of healed Q-wave and non–Q-wave myocardial infarction. *Lancet* 2001;357:21–28, with permission.)

TABLE 14.4. HYPERENHANCEMENT IN PATIENTS WITH HEALED INFARCTION

Hyperenhancement	Examined at 3 Months			Examined at 14 Months		
	Q-wave (n = 19)	Non–Q-wave (n = 13)	All (n = 32)	Q-wave (n = 11)	Non–Q-wave (n = 8)	All (n = 19)
Total	18	11	29	11	8	19
Transmural	8	1	9	4	2	6
Nontransmural	10	10	20	7	6	13
Infarct artery territory[a]	16/16	8/9	24/25	8/8	6/6	14/14

[a] Denominator given in each category.
From Wu E, Judd RM, Vargas JD, et al. Visualization of presence, location, and transmural extent of healed Q-wave and non–Q-wave myocardial infarction. *Lancet* 2001; 357:21–28, with permission.

ment had only nontransmural involvement (Table 14.4). None of the 20 patients with nonischemic dilated cardiomyopathy exhibited hyperenhancement despite significant LV systolic dysfunction. Likewise, none of the 11 normal volunteers exhibited hyperenhancement. The sensitivity of contrast MRI for the detection of healed infarction was 91% in the 3-month-old group and 100% in the 14-month old group. The specificity was 100% when patients with nonischemic dilated cardiomyopathy and normal volunteers were considered.

This study strongly suggests that contrast MRI can provide an accurate and permanent record of prior myocardial infarction. Nonetheless, routine clinical application will be improved by the further acquisition of data on the sensitivity and specificity of this technique in multiple different, clinically relevant patient populations.

Reversible Ischemic Injury

One obvious clinical application is in the patient cohort with known coronary artery disease and LV dysfunction. Given the animal and human data demonstrating that MI hyperenhances regardless of infarct age, and the animal data showing that viable myocardium does not hyperenhance despite contractile dysfunction, we hypothesized that contrast MRI could identify reversible myocardial dysfunction before coronary revascularization. To test this hypothesis, we performed cine and contrast MRI in 50 consecutive patients with LV dysfunction before they underwent surgical or percutaneous revascularization (79). Cine MRI was repeated approximately 11 weeks after revascularization to document changes, if any, in regional wall motion.

Representative cine and contrast images from two different patients in the study are shown in Figure 14.25. Re-

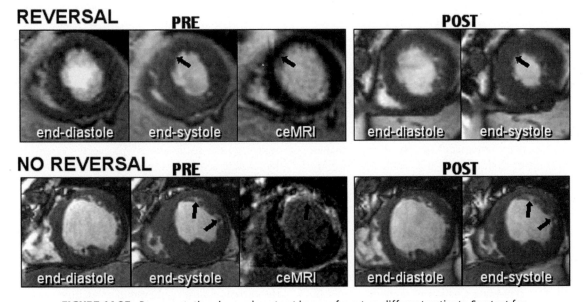

FIGURE 14.25. Representative cine and contrast images from two different patients. See text for details. (From Kim RJ, Wu E, Rafael A, et al. The use of contrast-enhanced magnetic resonance imaging to identify reversible myocardial dysfunction. *N Engl J Med* 2000;343:1445–1453, with permission.)

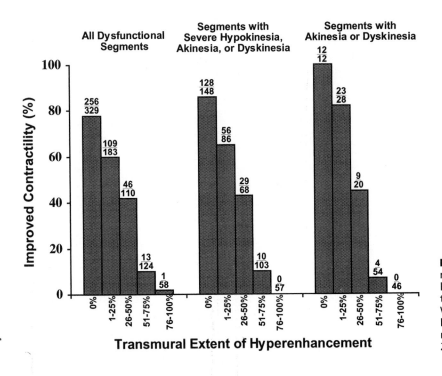

FIGURE 14.26. Relation between the transmural extent of hyperenhancement before revascularization and the likelihood of increased contractility after revascularization. (From Kim RJ, Wu E, Rafael A, et al. The use of contrast-enhanced magnetic resonance imaging to identify reversible myocardial dysfunction. *N Engl J Med* 2000;343:1445–1453, with permission.)

gional function recovered in the patient without hyperenhancement of the dysfunctional region, and did not recover in the patient with significant hyperenhancement of the dysfunctional region. The transmural extent of hyperenhancement was related significantly to improvement in wall thickening following revascularization (Fig. 14.26). When all dysfunctional segments before revascularization were considered, the proportion with contractile improvement decreased progressively as the transmural extent of hyperenhancement increased ($p <.001$). Thus, 256 (78%) of 329 segments with no hyperenhancement improved, whereas only 1 of 58 segments with more than 75% hyperenhancement improved. The same relation between the transmural extent of hyperenhancement and contractile improvement was found in segments with at least severe hypokinesia at baseline, and in segments with akinesia or dyskinesia at baseline ($p <.001$ for both). When the volume of dysfunctional but viable myocardium before revascularization was calculated on a patient-by-patient basis, we observed that an increasing extent of dysfunctional but viable myocardium correlated with greater improvements in both the mean wall motion score ($p <.001$) and the ejection fraction after revascularization ($p <.001$).

The relationship between the transmural extent of viability and the likelihood of functional improvement found in this study indicates that the use of a single cutoff value of hyperenhancement to predict functional improvement would not have a physiologic basis and therefore would be suboptimal. If a cutoff value of 25% hyperenhancement were chosen, the positive and negative predictive values for functional improvement would be 71% and 79%, respec-

tively, for all dysfunctional regions, and 88% and 89% for akinetic or dyskinetic regions. Although these predictive accuracy rates compare favorably with those reported previously for other imaging modalities (80), the full diagnostic information portrayed by contrast MRI is not utilized. For example, if regions with more than 75% hyperenhancement are considered, all 57 with at least severe hypokinesia at baseline did not improve, a negative predictive accuracy of 100%.

This example highlights the important advantage of contrast MRI over the other imaging modalities used to assess viability. Myocardial regions are not interpreted in a binary fashion as either viable or nonviable; rather, the transmural extent of viable myocardium is directly visualized. Knowledge of the transmural extent of viability can then be used to predict functional improvement more accurately, as in the example above, and can also be used to understand the underlying physiology of functional improvement. For instance, in the study above, the average extent of hyperenhancement across the ventricular wall was 10% ± 7% for all dysfunctional segments that improved and 41% ±14% for those that did not improve ($p <.001$). This result, which is consistent with those of previous studies that analyzed needle biopsy specimens taken during bypass surgery (81,82), indicates that significant degrees of myocardial viability can be present without eventual functional improvement. These data underscore the importance of differentiating between the current clinical "gold standard" definition of myocardial viability, which is improvement in wall motion after revascularization, and the actual definition, which is the presence of living myocytes (Table 14.1).

OVERVIEW OF IMAGE INTERPRETATION

The data presented under "Animal Studies" strongly support the following statements: In the setting of acute infarction, hyperenhancement is exclusively associated with myocyte necrosis. Regions within the "area at risk" but outside the "area of infarction" do not exhibit hyperenhancement. Large, acute infarcts often exhibit regions of hypoenhancement surrounded by larger hyperenhanced regions. These are associated with the "no-reflow" phenomenon. Regions subjected to severe but reversible ischemic injury do not hyperenhance, even in the presence of myocardial stunning. In the setting of chronic infarction, hyperenhancement is exclusively associated with myocardial scar.

The data presented under "Human Studies" strongly support the following statements: Both acute and chronic infarcts hyperenhance. In the setting of coronary artery disease and ventricular dysfunction, the transmural extent of hyperenhancement can predict those regions in which wall motion is most likely (minimal hyperenhancement) or least likely (large hyperenhancement) to improve. The extent of dysfunctional but nonhyperenhanced myocardium can predict on a case-by-case basis those patients whose LV ejection fraction is most likely to improve.

Taken together, these findings appear to be adequately summarized by the expression "bright is dead." This relationship is supported by a wealth of empiric data; nonetheless, it is difficult to understand how a "nonspecific" or "inert" contrast agent can distinguish between viable and nonviable myocardium, especially across the wide range of tissue environments that occur during infarct healing. An important physiologic fact, however, should be remembered, which is that the tissue volume in normal myocardium is predominantly intracellular (~75% of the water space) (83). Because extracellular contrast medium is excluded from this space, the volume of distribution of a contrast medium in normal myocardium is quite small (~25% of water space), and one can consider viable myocytes as actively excluding contrast media. The unifying mechanism for the hyperenhancement of nonviable myocardium may then be the *absence of viable myocytes* rather than any inherent properties that are specific for acutely necrotic tissue, collagenous scar, or other forms of nonviable tissue.

Combination of Cine and Contrast MRI

The combination of cine and contrast MRI in the imaging protocol (Fig. 14.21) facilitates comparisons of wall motion and contrast enhancement, with perfect registration of myocardial regions. The data from the previous sections show that although most regions with 76% to 100% transmural hyperenhancement are akinetic or dyskinetic, a diverse range of combinations of contrast enhancement and wall motion nonetheless exist. For example, in the study of pa-

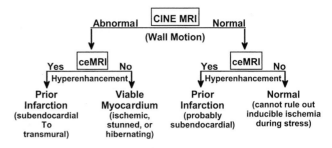

FIGURE 14.27. Combination of cine and contrast MRI to distinguish various forms of myocardial injury in patients with coronary artery disease.

tients with chronic infarction (see "Human Studies"), 71 (27%) of 259 segments with abnormal wall motion did not show hyperenhancement. Conversely, 62 (25%) of 250 segments that exhibited some hyperenhancement had normal wall motion. These data demonstrate that contrast enhancement patterns are frequently discordant with ventricular motion. They also underscore that contrast enhancement and wall motion index different physiologic parameters, and suggest that the combination of cine with contrast MRI might play an important clinical role in the evaluation of patients with ischemic heart disease. Specifically, the data suggest that combination MRI in the acute setting might be used to distinguish between myocardial infarction (hyperenhanced with or without contractile dysfunction), stunned myocardium (not hyperenhanced but with contractile dysfunction), and normal myocardium (not hyperenhanced with normal function). Likewise, in the chronic setting, combination MRI might be used to distinguish between myocardial scar, hibernating myocardium, and normal myocardium. Figure 14.27 summarizes how the different combination of contrast and cine MRI results might be used to identify different forms of myocardial injury.

FUTURE APPLICATIONS

The assessment of myocardial viability is generally thought to be synonymous with the detection of "hibernating" myocardium. We have already discussed the importance of detecting hibernating myocardium when coronary revascularization is being considered. However, the assessment of viability or, conversely, the detection of prior infarction may be important in many patients in whom coronary revascularization is not an issue. Viability assessment may not be considered in these patients because of assumptions derived from experience with other imaging modalities. We discuss three groups of patients in whom the role of viability assessment may not be readily evident at first glance. In each of these patient populations, the concept that the transmural extent of viable and nonviable myocardium can be distinguished is central in providing new information for the clinician. Given the abilities of contrast MRI, these examples in-

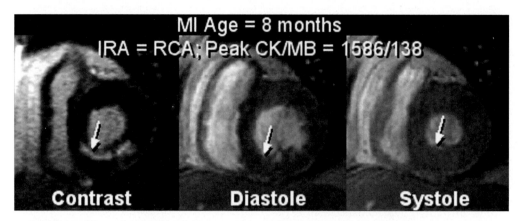

FIGURE 14.28. Typical MR images from a patient who had a myocardial infarction caused by occlusion of the right coronary artery. Although wall thickening is normal, the subendocardial infarction is demonstrated by the nontransmural hyperenhancement zone in the inferior wall. (From Wu E, Judd RM, Vargas JD, et al. Visualisation of presence, location, and transmural extent of healed Q-wave and non–Q-wave myocardial infarction. *Lancet* 2001;357:21–28, with permission.)

dicate that the clinical role of viability assessment should be reexamined.

Subendocardial Infarction

Lieberman et al. (84) studied a canine model of infarction and found an abrupt deterioration in systolic thickening in myocardial segments with more than 20% transmural infarction. Although the study considered only nonreperfused infarction evaluated during the acute phase (2 days) and did not account for the possibility of ongoing ischemia or myocardial stunning, it is often quoted as evidence that minor nontransmural infarction can lead to akinesia or dyskinesia. Such results, and others (85–87), have led to widespread agreement that measurement of the extent of wall motion abnormalities consistently leads to an overestimation of infarct size.

Few studies have focused on the possibility that measurements of regional wall motion can also *underestimate* infarct size. For example, in the study of patients with chronic infarction (see "Human Studies"), 10 patients had normal wall motion throughout the entire LV. Based on wall motion alone, these patients would not be suspected of having had a prior MI. Each of these patients showed evidence of subendocardial hyperenhancement in the infarct-related artery territory. Figure 14.28 shows typical MR images from one such patient, who had an inferior MI resulting from occlusion of the right coronary artery. The cine images demonstrate normal wall thickening in all regions, but the presence of hyperenhancement in the subendocardium of the inferior wall demonstrates the location of the prior infarction.

In this particular patient, one could argue that viability assessment was unnecessary because wall motion was normal at rest. However, if the studies had been performed, one can easily imagine that the inferior wall would have been called "viable" by dobutamine echocardiography, nuclear scintigraphy, or PET. Unfortunately, one can also imagine that the same tests would have failed to detect prior infarction in this patient because they interpret viability as an all-or-none phenomenon across the ventricular wall, and the majority of the inferior wall was indeed viable. Miller et al. (27) measured infarct size in patients by ^{99m}Tc sestamibi SPECT. Although cardiac enzyme levels were not reported, it is interesting to note that almost one-fourth of the patients with documented acute infarction had no detectable scintigraphic evidence of infarction. The median LV ejection fraction 6 weeks after hospital discharge was 50%; therefore, the distribution of infarct sizes in their study was likely biased toward smaller infarcts. Patients with subendocardial infarction and normal wall motion likely represent a particular cohort in whom current noninvasive imaging methods misdiagnose by failing to detect prior myocardial infarction.

The diagnosis of prior myocardial infarction is clinically important. Several studies have shown that survivors of MI have a mortality rate 3 to 14 times greater than that of the general population (88,89). The mortality rate is increased regardless of whether the index MI is classified electrocardiographically as Q-wave or non–Q-wave (90–93). The diagnosis of prior MI, however, can be difficult to confirm if infarction was not documented at the time of the acute event. The time window in which biochemical evidence of infarction is present is limited, and in many cases, the ECG is nondiagnostic because the majority of all acute MIs are not associated with the formation of Q waves (90). The identification of patients with prior MI is important not only for the determination of prognosis but also for the initiation of medical therapy because it is well established that cardiac morbidity and mortality can be reduced with appropriate therapy after infarction (94–97).

Unrecognized Myocardial Infarction

The patient in Figure 14.28 was given a diagnosis during the acute phase of infarction because he sought medical attention and appropriate blood tests were performed. It is known, however, that many patients with acute MI do not have significant symptoms and therefore do not seek medical attention within the time frame when elevated levels of cardiac enzymes can be documented. Population surveys, such as the Framingham Study, have surmised that up to 40% of all MIs are clinically "silent" or unrecognized (88,98–100). These conclusions are based on the appearance of new Q waves on annual 12-lead ECGs. Because non–Q-wave infarctions are not included, current estimates of the incidence of unrecognized infarction are likely underestimates. The risk associated with unrecognized MI has been demonstrated to be substantial, with long-term mortality comparable with that of recognized MI (88,98–100).

These data suggest that a large number of people have had prior MIs and are therefore at increased risk for future cardiac events and yet have not been identified for appropriate therapy. Necropsy studies have confirmed that undiagnosed healed MI is quite common, occurring in up to 50% of people who die suddenly outside the hospital (101) and in 16% of people in the general population (102). It may be difficult to identify this high-risk group with conventional imaging methods, however, because the infarcts are often quite small (102,103). A noninvasive method that can detect small infarcts long after the diagnostic window of cardiac enzyme assays has passed may be useful in patients who are at high-risk for coronary artery events but in whom viability assessment is not traditionally performed.

Subepicardial Viability

Increasing evidence suggests that the revascularization of viable myocardium may provide clinical benefit even in the absence of functional recovery. For instance, Lombardo et al. (104) reported that 22% of patients without substantial viability on dobutamine echocardiography manifested a reduction in symptoms of heart failure after revascularization although the LV ejection fraction remained unchanged. In the study of Samady et al. (105), postoperative survival and improvement in angina and heart failure scores were similar in patients with preoperative LV dysfunction whether or not the LV ejection fraction increased after coronary bypass surgery. These studies suggest that a certain degree of myocardial viability may influence outcome favorably after revascularization in terms of symptoms and survival without generating improvement in resting contractile function.

In the study of patients with reversible myocardial dysfunction (see "Human Studies"), 90% of regions with 51% to 75% transmural hyperenhancement did not show an improvement in contractility after revascularization. These regions would be considered nonviable according to criteria based on improvement in wall motion, even though a sizable epicardial "rim" of viable tissue was present (Fig. 14.29). These data underscore the important difference between using "recovery of wall motion following

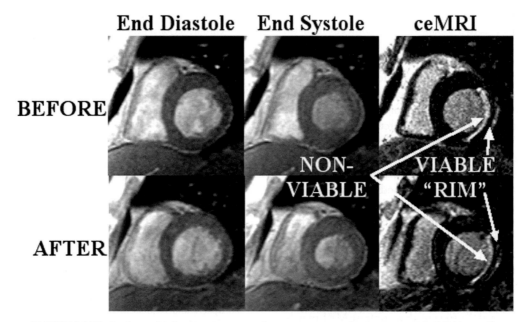

FIGURE 14.29. Patient with known three-vessel coronary artery disease scanned by MRI immediately before *(upper panels)* and 3 months after *(lower panels)* revascularization. Note that lateral wall hyperenhancement is not transmural. (From Kim RJ, Hillenbrand HB, Judd RM. Evaluation of myocardial viability by MRI. *Herz* 2000;25:417–430, with permission.)

poenhancement during the first pass without delayed enhancement (HYPO); (b) normal first-pass signal followed by hyperenhancement on delayed images (HYPER); and (c) hypoenhancement on first pass and delayed hyperenhancement (COMB). Regions characterized as HYPER exhibited significant improvement in function after 7 weeks, signifying viability, whereas HYPO regions did not improve and COMB regions showed borderline improvement (Table 15.2). In a subsequent study (62), these investigators confirmed their previous findings. Moreover, they demonstrated that contrast-enhanced MRI and stress MRI with tagging performed early after reperfusion impart similar information about the potential of functional recovery after several weeks. Dendale et al. (64), using conventional spin-echo imaging, also reported inotropic reserve in 83% and 41% of segments with subendocardial and transmural hyperenhancement, respectively, suggesting residual viability in these areas. Sandstede et al. (63) examined 12 patients with CHD, 10 of them with subacute infarction, before and after revascularization with contrast-enhanced MRI. Using a fast T1-weighted MR sequence, these investigators acquired both first-pass and delayed MR images. Three months after revascularization, 96% of hyperenhanced segments did not recover function, and it was therefore concluded that segments with delayed enhancement mainly comprise nonviable myocardium (Table 15.1). It should be noted that with one exception, all segments with delayed hyperenhancement exhibited hypoenhancement during the first pass. In the nomenclature of Rogers et al. (61,62), this pattern represents COMB, in which the investigators found at least some functional improvement. These discrepant findings may result from differences in the patient groups, such as age of the infarct and flow in the infarct-related artery, and in the assessment of functional recovery (qualitative or quantitative).

Few studies (65–70) have been performed in the nonacute setting. Most of them that used T1-weighted spin-echo imaging reported that no significant contrast enhancement could be observed in infarcts older than 3 to 4 weeks (65–68), but others did (69,70). With the use of rapid T1-weighted MRI sequences, a considerable increase in the signal intensity of infarcted myocardium made it possible to

demonstrate contrast enhancement, even in chronic infarcts. Ramani et al. (71) tested the feasibility of contrast-enhanced MRI to assess viability in patients with ischemic cardiomyopathy and compared their MR findings with rest–redistribution ^{201}Tl imaging. Their main conclusion was that hyperenhancement on delayed MR images is associated with nonviability by ^{201}Tl scintigraphy, particularly in regions exhibiting resting akinesis or dyskinesis.

Most recently, visualization of acute and chronic myocardial infarction after contrast administration has been further improved by the introduction of a segmented inversion recovery fast low-angle shot (FLASH) pulse sequence (72). Kim et al. (73,74) applied this technique and reported that the spatial extent of hyperenhancement in acute and chronic infarcts is identical to that of myocyte necrosis or scar in comparisons with *ex vivo* T1-weighted three-dimensional gradient-echo imaging and histochemical staining. Conversely, their previous studies (49,55) and studies of other groups (43,57–60) had suggested that hyperenhancement on delayed images occurs not only in regions of cellular necrosis but also in the border zone of injured but viable myocytes surrounding the acute infarct (periinfarction zone). Kim et al. (73,74) could not detect such a zone and stated that partial volume effects might have played a role in the overestimation of infarct size in some of these studies.

Using this new sequence (inversion recovery FLASH), Hillenbrand et al. (75) demonstrated that segments with a transmural extent of hyperenhancement greater than 75% early after infarction are unlikely to improve function 4 weeks later. Subsequently, Kim et al. (76) studied 50 patients with LV dysfunction caused by chronic coronary artery disease who underwent Gd-DTPA–enhanced MRI before coronary revascularization. Hyperenhancement on delayed MR images was present in 80% of all patients. The authors reported that the likelihood of improvement in regional contractility after successful revascularization decreases progressively as the transmural extent of hyperenhancement increases. Recently, Wu et al. (77) demonstrated the feasibility of this advanced contrast-enhanced MR technique to detect the presence, location, and transmural extent of healed transmural and nontransmural myocardial infarcts.

TABLE 15.2. ABNORMAL CONTRAST ENHANCEMENT PATTERNS IN INJURED AREAS AND THEIR FUNCTIONAL OUTCOME AFTER 7 WEEKS IN PATIENTS WITH ACUTE, REPERFUSED INFARCTS

Abnormal Pattern	First-pass Hypoenhancement	Delayed Hyperenhancement	Percentage Shortening Baseline (%)	Percentage Shortening Follow-up (%)	Functional Outcome After 7 Weeks
HYPO	+	−	5 ± 4	6 ± 3	No improvement (p = NS)
COMB	+	+	7 ± 6	11 ± 5	Borderline improvement (p = .06)
HYPER	−	+	9 ± 8	18 ± 5	Improvement (p < .001)

Based on Rogers WT Jr, Kramer CM, Geskin G, et al. Early contrast-enhanced MRI predicts late functional recovery after reperfused myocardial infarction. *Circulation* 1999;99:744–750.

Contrast-enhanced MRI allows visualization of the no-reflow zone and surrounding injured myocardium. Despite the restoration of epicardial blood flow, perfusion in the core of the infarct may be limited at the tissue level because of injury of the microvasculature and subsequent obstruction by erythrocytes, neutrophils, and debris, a phenomenon known as "no reflow" (78). Microvascular obstruction is characterized by hypoenhancement on either first-pass or delayed MR images and is associated with non-viability and greater regional dysfunction (49,52,54–56,61, 62,64). Moreover, it has been shown that the no-reflow phenomenon at the capillary level is a strong predictor of poor functional recovery, remodeling of the ventricle, and more frequent cardiovascular complications (54,56,79).

The interpretation of hyperenhancement on delayed MR images is less clear. In experimental models of acute MI (43,57–60,80), it has been demonstrated that hyperenhanced regions include the infarcted area per se in addition to a portion of the area at risk (periinfarction zone), so that the extent of necrosis is overestimated. Enhancement of the periinfarction zone is probably related to residual flow via collateral vessels and the presence of interstitial edema (68). During ischemia, blood vessels distal to the occlusion and collateral vessels dilate maximally in response to the release of several vasodilators, such as adenosine, bradykinins, lactic acid, and prostaglandins (81–83). Severe ischemia causes the extravasation of plasma proteins and the formation of edema, which may lead to further accumulation and slow washout of the contrast medium. In accordance with this observation, clinical studies (61,62) reported that viable myocardium can be found within hyperenhanced areas in acute, reperfused infarction. Conversely, the MR technique advanced by Kim et al. (73–75) could not detect the periinfarction zone. Their results indicated that the spatial extent of hyperenhancement is identical to the infarct size. It has been suspected that partial volume effects contribute to these discrepant findings, but the sensitivity of the applied pulse sequence to detect small T1 changes in the rim of the infarct should also be taken into account. Altogether, the following factors must be considered when the results of different studies defining myocardial viability from hyperenhanced regions are interpreted: (a) age of the infarct; (b) flow in the infarct-related artery; (c) type of imaging sequence and its sensitivity to T1 changes; (d) dose of the contrast medium and how long after contrast administration imaging is performed; (e) slice thickness and partial volume effects; and (f) the "reference standard" used to infer myocardial viability.

More importantly, with the introduction of fast contrast-enhanced MRI techniques, it has become feasible to detect contrast enhancement in the nonacute setting (Fig. 15.1). Several groups (63,70,71,73,74,76,77) reported similar findings in experimental animals and patients, suggesting that hyperenhancement in subacute or healed infarction

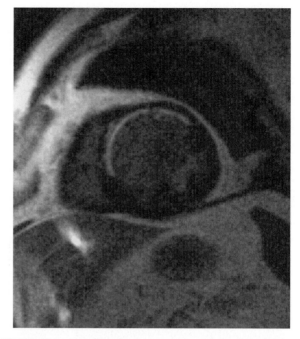

FIGURE 15.1. End-diastolic short-axis T1-weighted inversion recovery turbo-FLASH (fast low-angle shot) image (repetition time/inversion time/echo time 400/300/4 milliseconds) obtained 20 minutes after the administration of 0.1 mmol of Gd-DTPA (gadolinium diethylenetriamine pentaacetic acid) per kilogram in a patient with an old anterior myocardial infarction. Note the wall thinning and the hyperenhanced region in the anteroseptal wall.

represents nonviable tissue. However, the exact mechanism that leads to the enhancement of scar tissue is still unclear.

Nonspecific Extracellular MR Contrast Media to Detect the Breakdown of Cell Membranes

In this approach, the degree of myocardial injury is determined by estimating the breakdown of cellular membranes within the ischemic zone with the use of nonspecific extracellular contrast media. These agents can increase or decrease signal intensity, depending on the type and concentration of the contrast medium in the tissue and the MR sequence used. Relaxivity- or T1-enhancing contrast media, such as Gd-DTPA, usually increase the MR signal in tissue not excluded from blood supply on T1-weighted images, whereas susceptibility- or T2*-enhancing agents, such as dysprosium-DTPA (Dy-DTPA), cause a signal loss with T2-sensitive imaging sequences. Both these types of contrast media freely exit from the vascular space and are rapidly distributed in the extracellular space, but they are excluded from the intracellular compartment of cells with intact membranes.

After the administration of Dy-DTPA, the decrease in signal intensity is a function of magnetic susceptibility and distribution within the tissue, a greater effect being associated with a more heterogeneous distribution. In normal myocardium, cell membranes act as a barrier and limit the distribution of contrast agent to the extracellular space, causing a heterogeneous distribution in tissue with attenuation of signal. Because the loss of membrane selectivity is an indicator of cell death, it was hypothesized that alterations in the potency of susceptibility-dependent signal loss are related to the severity of myocardial injury. In a rat model of reperfused myocardial infarction, irreversibly injured regions, which appeared hyperintense on Gd-DTPA–enhanced T1-weighted spin-echo images, were also hyperintense on Dy-DTPA–enhanced T2-weighted spin-echo images (84). It was proposed that this effect is the result of a more homogeneous tissue distribution of dysprosium in the infarcted myocardium, signifying that the agent has entered the intracellular space. A subsequent study (85) in excised hearts corroborated this proposed mechanism. Geschwind et al. (85) administered Gd-DTPA and Dy-DTPA in tandem to rats subjected to irreversible myocardial injury followed by reperfusion and performed spin-echo and gradient-echo imaging. Gd-DPTA was used to document the presence of flow in the reperfused region and the delivery of contrast agents, whereas Dy-DTPA was used to assess myocardial viability. Although Gd-DTPA caused a greater increase in the signal of reperfused infarcted myocardium, Dy-DTPA-BMA (dysprosium diethylenetriamine pentaacetic acid-bis-methyamide) also delineated infarcted myocardium as a bright region. After imaging, the quantities of these agents present in reperfused infarcted and normal myocardium were measured by atomic absorption spectrometry. The tissue concentrations of both agents were found to be greatly increased in infarcted versus normal myocardium. Thus, the authors concluded that the loss of magnetic susceptibility effect exerted by Dy-DTPA is caused by the failure of myocardial cells to exclude the compound from the intracellular space rather than by a reduced tissue concentration.

In another experimental model of myocardial infarction, it was demonstrated that within the first 5 minutes after bolus injection, the tissue concentration of T1-enhancing extracellular MR contrast media such as Gd-DTPA is determined primarily by blood flow, and after about 10 minutes primarily by the agent's accessible space (fractional distribution volume, or fDV) (86). Moreover, it is well-known that Gd-DTPA produces considerably greater enhancement of irreversibly injured than of normal myocardium on MR images acquired several minutes after contrast injection (45,46). This observation also implies that a relatively larger quantity of contrast agent has been distributed into the injured region. With the loss of cellular membrane integrity, virtually no barrier is present between extracellular and intracellular compartments. Consequently, the fDV of gadolinium chelates is expanded from approximately 20% in normal myocardium to nearly 100% in complete myocardial necrosis. As the fDV increases, the bulk tissue con-

centration of extracellular contrast agents at the equilibrium phase also increases proportionally (86). Therefore, it was proposed that the calculation of the fDV in a region-of-interest encompassing a jeopardized myocardial region could provide a measure of the percentage of necrotic cells within this volume.

The concept of defining myocardial injury according to the distribution of MR contrast media into various myocardial compartments has been tested in several animal models (70,80,86–90). Using a constant infusion of Gd-DTPA, Pereira et al. (70,88) demonstrated that the partition coefficient (λ) of Gd-DTPA, which is proportional to the fDV, is maximal within the first week after infarction and progressively decreases thereafter, consistent with the time course of contrast enhancement in previous clinical studies (65–67). Measured values of the partition coefficient by MRI agreed well with values determined *ex vivo* by radioactive counting of ^{111}In-DTPA but were inversely correlated with ^{201}Tl uptake as a marker of residual viability (70,88). More importantly, MRI allowed monitoring of the partition coefficient during the initial minutes of reperfusion, and an observed increase from normal to maximal values during the first 2 hours suggested the ongoing rupture of myocardial cells (70).

Using an echo-planar MRI technique, Wendland et al. (90) measured the change in T1 relaxation rate ($\Delta R1$), which is proportional to the quantity of contrast medium within the tissue of interest, after bolus administration of gadolinium chelates. They found a constant proportionality between the $\Delta R1$ values of myocardium and blood during the first 30 minutes after contrast injection, and a failure of increased doses of the agent to alter this proportionality was considered indicative of an approximately equilibrated state of distribution. The authors proposed that direct measurement of the T1 changes in myocardium and blood at this steady state provides an estimate of the fDV of the contrast agent, which can be calculated by the following formula: $(\Delta R1_{myocardium}/\Delta R1_{blood}) \times (1 - \text{hematocrit})$. Subsequently, this hypothesis was tested in a rat model of reperfused myocardial infarction (80,87,89). Measured distribution volumes of gadolinium chelates were also compared with the results of ^{99m}Tc-DTPA autoradiography as an independent reference standard after sacrifice of the animals. Not surprisingly, a close agreement between both measurements was reported. In complete infarction, an fDV of approximately 90% suggests entrance of the indicators into nearly all myocardial cells. In animal models of graded myocardial injury, it was further shown that the fDV of extracellular contrast agents increases in relation to the duration of coronary occlusion (80,89) (Fig. 15.2). Additionally, it was found that cases subjected to 30 to 60 minutes of ischemia exhibit two regions of abnormally elevated count density on high-resolution ^{99m}Tc-DTPA autoradiography: a core of higher count density surrounded by a periphery of moderately increased count density (80,87). The fDV val-

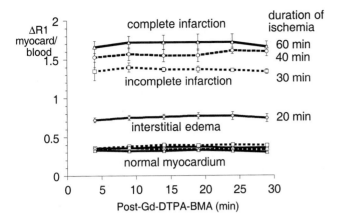

FIGURE 15.2. Plot of the effect of the duration of ischemia on ΔR1 ratio in rats subjected to 20, 30, 40, and 60 minutes of coronary occlusion followed by 1 hour of reperfusion. During repetitive measurements, the ΔR1 ratios for myocardium/blood remain constant during the initial 30 minutes after the injection of 0.2 mmol of Gd-DTPA-BMA (gadolinium diethylenetriamine pentaacetic acid-bis-methyamide) per kilogram, which suggests a state close to equilibrium. This means that the ΔR1 ratios represent partition coefficients (λ), which allow calculation of the fractional distribution volume. Note the increase in ΔR1 ratio as a function of the severity of injury. (From Arheden H, Saeed M, Higgins CB, et al. Reperfused rat myocardium subjected to various durations of ischemia: estimation of the distribution volume of contrast material with echo-planar MR imaging. *Radiology* 2000;215:520–528, with permission.)

ues of ^{99m}Tc-DTPA and its surrogate Gd-DTPA were approximately two times greater than those in normal myocardium in the periinfarction zone, but four times greater than those in normal myocardium in the infarcted core (Fig. 15.3). On electron microscopy, these regions contained moderately injured myocardium comprising largely viable cells (43,80). Consequently, it was inferred that this MRI approach has the potential to provide an estimate of the necrotic cell fraction and of potentially salvageable cells within the area at risk.

Thus, the concept of using nonspecific extracellular MR contrast media to detect the breakdown of cellular membranes after acute ischemic injury is now proven. It seems conceivable that quantifying the distribution volumes of extracellular MR contrast agents provides more information for determining the severity of myocardial injury than visually identifying regions of hyperenhancement. However, whether this approach is sufficiently practical and reliable to be applied clinically is another matter.

Necrosis-Specific MR Contrast Media to Determine the Necrotic Zone

The development of MR contrast agents with a high specific affinity for irreversibly damaged myocardium has been an elusive goal. Notable attempts have included binding an indicator to antibodies specific for intracellular compounds (91), and using phosphonate-modified gadolinium chelates

interactive with the calcium deposits that accumulate in necrotic tissue (92). All these efforts were discontinued because of concerns about agent toxicity.

Paramagnetic metalloporphyrins were originally developed as tumor-seeking contrast media because of their well-known tendency to accumulate in neoplastic tissue (93,94). However, the discovery that one such agent, gadolinium-mesoporphyrin (gadophrin-2), is necrosis-avid rather than tumor-selective opened up the field for new applications (95,96). Subsequently, gadolinium-mesoporphyrin was tested in several animal models to delineate areas of necrosis in both occlusive and reperfused infarcts (59,60,97–101). In all these reports, gadolinium-mesoporphyrin hyperenhancement of myocardial infarction resulted in a sharp demarcation on T1-weighted MR images and revealed details of necrotic tissue that matched those defined by TTC histochemical staining.

Pislaru et al. (100) induced coronary artery thrombosis in dogs and then administered thrombolytic therapy 90 minutes later to produce reperfused infarcts. Groups of animals were given gadolinium-mesoporphyrin on days 1, 2, and 6 after infarction, and MRI was performed *in vivo* and *in vitro* 24 hours later. In all groups, the infarct size demarcated by gadolinium-mesoporphyrin enhancement matched precisely the area of necrosis defined by TTC staining. Saeed et al. (59) induced reversible and irreversible myocardial injury in rats and administered a nonspecific T1-shortening agent, Gd-DTPA, in addition to the necrosis-specific compound

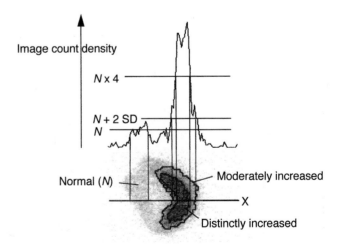

FIGURE 15.3. Profile of the image count density, through a section of an autoradiographic image, of a 20-μm-thick slice from a rat subjected to 60 minutes of coronary artery occlusion followed by reperfusion. Several levels of image count density are seen: low count density *(N)* corresponding to normal myocardium, moderately increased count density *(N + 2SD)* in the rim corresponding to ischemic injury, and high count density *(N × 4)* in the core, corresponding to severe ischemic injury. (From Arheden H, Saeed M, Higgins CB, et al. Measurement of the distribution volume of gadopentetate dimeglumine at echo-planar MR imaging to quantify myocardial infarction: comparison with ^{99m}Tc-DTPA autoradiography in rats. *Radiology* 1999;211:698–708, with permission.)

gadolinium-mesoporphyrin, at different time points after reperfusion. In animals with irreversibly injured myocardium, the size of the gadolinium- mesoporphyrin–enhanced regions closely matched the size of infarct defined by histochemical staining. Conversely, the zone delineated by Gd-DTPA overestimated the true infarction size but was more closely related to the area at risk (Figs. 15.4 and 15.5). In another study of Saeed et al. (60), the gadolinium-mesoporphyrin–enhanced region showed no wall thickening 24 hours after reperfusion, whereas the Gd-DTPA–enhanced area was characterized by moderately reduced function. It was concluded that the Gd-DTPA–enhanced zone encompasses viable and nonviable portions, and that the difference in size demarcated by the two compounds can be used to characterize the periinfarction zone.

Gadolinium-mesoporphyrin–enhanced MRI has not only the capability to distinguish between irreversibly and reversibly injured myocardium, but also the potential to visualize morphologic details, such nontransmural, subendo-

cardial, and scattered infarcts. Moreover, the enhancement of irreversibly damaged myocardium persists from 40 minutes to at least 48 hours (95,101), allowing more flexible timing between contrast administration and MRI. Although gadolinium-mesoporphyrin is not yet approved for human use, the discovery that metalloporphyrins can be used as necrosis-specific markers in MI should be considered a major breakthrough.

Ion Transport across Functional Cellular Membranes to Characterize Viable Myocardium

Manganese dipyridoxyl diphosphate (DPDP) is a hepatobiliary MR contrast agent approved for human use at a dose of 5 μmol/kg. Like Gd-DTPA, Mn-DPDP has a T1-shortening effect and nonspecific extracellular distribution properties. In animal models, the use of this agent to characterize MI was studied at high doses of up to 400 μmol/kg

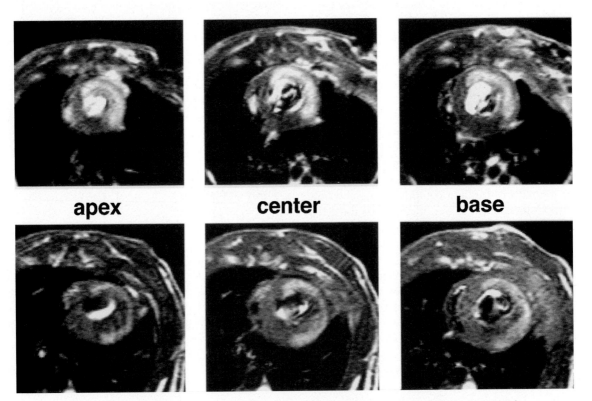

FIGURE 15.4. Multisection sets of short-axis T1-weighted spin-echo images (repetition time/echo time 300/12 milliseconds) at three levels (apex, center, and base) of the left ventricle in a rat heart subjected to reperfused irreversible myocardial injury. Images were obtained after the administration of Gd-DTPA (gadolinium diethylenetriamine pentaacetic acid) 1 hour after reperfusion *(top row)*, and after the administration of gadolinium-mesoporphyrin at 24 hours following reperfusion *(bottom row)*. Both MR contrast media can delineate irreversibly injured myocardium as a hyperenhanced zone in comparison with normal myocardium. Note the smaller size of the hyperenhanced zone on the gadolinium-mesoporphyrin–enhanced images than on the images obtained after administration of Gd-DTPA. The difference in size of the hyperenhanced regions produced by the two compounds may represent salvageable periinfarcted myocardium. (From Saeed M, Bremerich J, Wendland MF, et al. Reperfused myocardial infarction as seen with use of necrosis-specific versus standard extracellular MR contrast media in rats. *Radiology* 1999;213:247–257, with permission.)

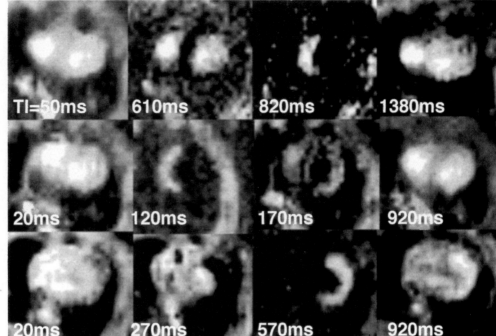

FIGURE 15.5. Axial inversion recovery echo-planar MR images (repetition time/echo time 7000/10 milliseconds) obtained in a heart subjected to reperfused irreversible myocardial injury. The images were obtained before the administration of contrast medium, after the administration of 0.3 mmol of Gd-DTPA (gadolinium diethylenetriamine pentaacetic acid) per kilogram, and after the administration of 0.05 mmol of gadolinium-mesoporphyrin (gadophrin-2) per kilogram. The images in these sets demonstrate that different regions-of-interest pass the null point of longitudinal magnetization recovery at different inversion time (TI) settings. On Gd-DTPA–enhanced images, reperfused irreversibly injured myocardium passes through the null point first at a TI of 120 milliseconds because it has the highest Gd-DTPA content and largest distribution volume. This is followed by left ventricular chamber blood at a TI of 170 milliseconds, which contains less Gd-DTPA than infarcted myocardium but more than normal myocardium, and finally by normal myocardium. The reperfused irreversibly injured myocardium passes through the null point at a TI of 270 milliseconds because it has the highest gadolinium-mesoporphyrin content, followed by left ventricular chamber blood and normal myocardium at a TI of 570 milliseconds. The difference in TI effect between the two contrast media is related to the injected dose, distribution volume, and binding of the two agents, and the time of imaging after injection.

(102–104). Studies have shown that the manganese cation (Mn^{2+}) is slowly released from the ligand (105), quickly taken up via voltage-operated calcium channels, and retained in viable myocardial cells (106–108). Because intact Mn-DPDP and dissociated Mn^{2+} have distinct distributional and kinetic properties, it was proposed that it might be possible to obtain MR images after Mn-DPDP administration in which the contrast is primarily provided by the uptake of Mn^{2+} released from the chelate and accumulated in viable myocytes. This was attempted in a study by Bremerich et al. (109), in which three groups of rats were prepared with reperfused infarctions and given either 25, 50, or 100 μmol of Mn-DPDP per kilogram. With inversion recovery echoplanar imaging, ΔR1 was measured successively for 60 minutes after contrast administration to monitor the accumulation of manganese in myocardial cells. The ΔR1 values in normal myocardium increased linearly, whereas the values in infarcted myocardium and blood decreased with time, indi-

cating clearance from these regions. The enhancement provided by the accumulation of manganese in normal myocardium was also apparent on high-resolution inversion recovery spin-echo images (Fig. 15.6). Because only viable cells can retain manganese, it was suggested that Mn-DPDP might be useful to assess myocardial viability with MRI.

Normally functioning cells maintain a membrane potential and control of electrochemical gradients. In normal myocardium, the intracellular sodium concentration is usually less than that in the extracellular space because of active transport across cell membranes. During ischemia, the intracellular sodium concentration rises and remains elevated in irreversible myocardial injury (110). Cannon et al. (111), using sodium (^{23}Na) MRI in an animal model, showed that regions of irreversibly damaged myocardium are clearly visible as areas of increased signal. Similar findings reported by Kim et al. (112) suggest that this MRI technique has the potential to distinguish between viable and nonviable my-

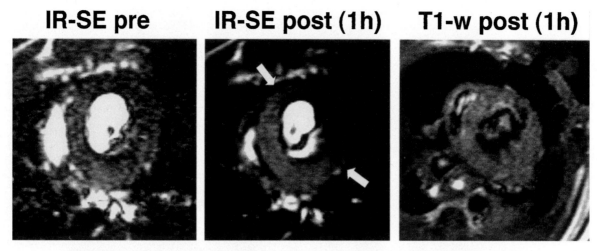

IR-SE pre   **IR-SE post (1h)**   **T1-w post (1h)**

FIGURE 15.6. Short-axis inversion recovery spin-echo (repetition time/inversion time/echo time 1,000/500/12 milliseconds) and conventional T1-weighted spin-echo (repetition time/echo time 300/12 milliseconds) images acquired before *(left panel)* and after contrast injection of 100 μmol of Mn-DPDP per kilogram *(middle and right panels)* at the midventricular level. Note the dark appearance of the infarcted zone *(arrows)* 1 hour after injection on inversion recovery spin-echo imaging, whereas normal myocardium appears bright because of the uptake of paramagnetic Mn^{2+} ions. The nonviable zone is not visualized on unenhanced inversion recovery spin-echo images and enhanced conventional T1-weighted spin-echo images.

ocardium by using sodium ions as endogenous markers. Moreover, the feasibility of performing sodium MRI has been demonstrated in healthy volunteers (113), and studies in patients can be expected in the near future.

FUTURE APPLICATIONS

The versatility of the approaches used to characterize myocardial injury is intriguing, and MRI shows substantial promise in providing an unambiguous determination of myocardial viability. Improvements in MR hardware, software, and imaging speed in conjunction with the development of MR contrast media targeted to highlight hallmarks of viable or nonviable cells have led to increased interest and further research in recent years. Even though MRI has the capability to provide information regarding coronary anatomy, blood flow, and microvascular integrity in one single examination, it is still applied in ischemic heart disease less frequently than echocardiography and radionuclide imaging, which are familiar and ubiquitous. In this regard, the development of a robust and uncomplicated methodology for MRI coronary angiography must be considered the ultimate breakthrough. However, the general strengths of MRI, such as noninvasiveness and excellent spatial resolution and tissue contrast, in conjunction with the latest advances in the field may increase its use in the assessment of myocardial viability in the near future. Prospective, randomized trials are warranted to determine the value and cost-effectiveness of MRI in detecting reversible myocardial dysfunction as a means of guiding therapeutic interventions in patients with CHD and impaired ventricular function.

SUMMARY

MRI is a highly accurate method of characterizing reversible and irreversible myocardial injury and obtaining information on residual myocardial viability. The various approaches used to achieve these important goals have been described. Preserved wall thickness and contractile reserve can be assessed by cine MRI qualitatively and quantitatively. Contrast-enhanced MRI provides information on tissue perfusion and cellular membrane function. A thorough assessment of all accepted parameters used to characterize myocardial viability, such as structure, function, perfusion, and cellular integrity, can be readily performed with MRI. In this regard, MRI has the potential to replace or complement other commonly used techniques in the diagnostic armamentarium of physicians caring for patients with ischemic heart disease.

REFERENCES

1. Higgins CB, Saeed M, Wendland M. MRI in ischemic heart disease: expansion of the current capabilities with MR contrast. *Am J Card Imaging* 1991;5:38–50.
2. van der Wall EE, Vliegen HW, de Roos A, et al. Magnetic resonance imaging in coronary artery disease. *Circulation* 1995;92: 2723–2739.
3. Kramer CM. Integrated approach to ischemic heart disease. The one-stop shop. *Cardiol Clin* 1998;16:267–276.
4. van der Wall EE, Vliegen HW, de Roos A, et al. Magnetic resonance techniques for assessment of myocardial viability. *J Cardiovasc Pharmacol* 1996;28(Suppl 1):S37–S44.
5. Higgins CB. Prediction of myocardial viability by MRI. *Circulation* 1999;99:727–729.

6. Bax JJ, de Roos A, van Der Wall EE. Assessment of myocardial viability by MRI. *J Magn Reson Imaging* 1999;10:418–422.
7. Stillman AE, Wilke N, Jerosch-Herold M. Myocardial viability. *Radiol Clin North Am* 1999;37:361–378.
8. Herman MV, Gorlin R. Implications of left ventricular asynergy. *Am J Cardiol* 1969;23:538–547.
9. Lewis SJ, Sawada SG, Ryan T, et al. Segmental wall motion abnormalities in the absence of clinically documented myocardial infarction: clinical significance and evidence of hibernating myocardium. *Am Heart J* 1991;121:1088–1094.
10. Birnbaum Y, Kloner RA. Myocardial viability. *West J Med* 1996;165:364–371.
11. Bax JJ, van Eck-Smit BL, van der Wall EE. Assessment of tissue viability: clinical demand and problems. *Eur Heart J* 1998;19:847–858.
12. Hendel RC, Chaudhry FA, Bonow RO. Myocardial viability. *Curr Probl Cardiol* 1996;21:145–221.
13. Rahimtoola SH. The hibernating myocardium. *Am Heart J* 1989;117:211–221.
14. Braunwald E, Rutherford JD. Reversible ischemic left ventricular dysfunction: evidence for the "hibernating myocardium." *J Am Coll Cardiol* 1986;8:1467–1470.
15. Tillisch J, Brunken R, Marshall R, et al. Reversibility of cardiac wall-motion abnormalities predicted by positron tomography. *N Engl J Med* 1986;314:884–888.
16. Di Carli MF. Predicting improved function after myocardial revascularization. *Curr Opin Cardiol* 1998;13:415–424.
17. Mickleborough LL, Maruyama H, Takagi Y, et al. Results of revascularization in patients with severe left ventricular dysfunction. *Circulation* 1995;92:II73–II79.
18. Haas F, Haehnel CJ, Picker W, et al. Preoperative positron emission tomographic viability assessment and perioperative and postoperative risk in patients with advanced ischemic heart disease. *J Am Coll Cardiol* 1997;30:1693–1700.
19. Braunwald E, Kloner RA. The stunned myocardium: prolonged, postischemic ventricular dysfunction. *Circulation* 1982;66:1146–1149.
20. Bolli R, Zhu WX, Thornby JI, et al. Time course and determinants of recovery of function after reversible ischemia in conscious dogs. *Am J Physiol* 1988;254:H102–H114.
21. Berman DS. Use of 201Tl for risk stratification after myocardial infarction and thrombolysis. *Circulation* 1997;96:2758–2761.
22. Gropler RJ, Bergmann SR. Myocardial viability—what is the definition? *J Nucl Med* 1991;32:10–12.
23. Bax JJ, Wijns W, Cornel JH, et al. Accuracy of currently available techniques for prediction of functional recovery after revascularization in patients with left ventricular dysfunction due to chronic coronary artery disease: comparison of pooled data. *J Am Coll Cardiol* 1997;30:1451–1460.
24. Saeed M, Wendland MF, Higgins CB. Contrast media for MR imaging of the heart. *J Magn Reson Imaging* 1994;4:269–279.
25. Saeed M, Wendland MF, Watzinger N, et al. MR contrast media for myocardial viability, microvascular integrity and perfusion. *Eur J Radiol* 2000;34:179–195.
26. Atkinson DJ, Edelman RR. Cineangiography of the heart in a single breath hold with a segmented turboFLASH sequence. *Radiology* 1991;178:357–360.
27. van Rugge FP, van der Wall EE, Spanjersberg SJ, et al. Magnetic resonance imaging during dobutamine stress for detection and localization of coronary artery disease. Quantitative wall motion analysis using a modification of the centerline method. *Circulation* 1994;90:127–138.
28. Baer FM, Smolarz K, Jungehülsing M, et al. Chronic myocardial infarction: assessment of morphology, function, and perfusion by gradient echo magnetic resonance imaging and 99mTc-methoxy-isobutyl-isonitrile SPECT. *Am Heart J* 1992;123:636–645.
29. Perrone-Filardi P, Bacharach SL, Dilsizian V, et al. Regional left ventricular wall thickening. Relation to regional uptake of 18fluorodeoxyglucose and 201Tl in patients with chronic coronary artery disease and left ventricular dysfunction. *Circulation* 1992;86:1125–1137.
30. Lawson MA, Johnson LL, Coghlan L, et al. Correlation of thallium uptake with left ventricular wall thickness by cine magnetic resonance imaging in patients with acute and healed myocardial infarcts. *Am J Cardiol* 1997;80:434–441.
31. Pennell DJ, Underwood SR. Stress cardiac magnetic resonance imaging. *Am J Card Imaging* 1991;5:139–149.
32. Pennell DJ, Underwood SR, Manzara CC, et al. Magnetic resonance imaging during dobutamine stress in coronary artery disease. *Am J Cardiol* 1992;70:34–40.
33. Nagel E, Lehmkuhl HB, Bocksch W, et al. Noninvasive diagnosis of ischemia-induced wall motion abnormalities with the use of high-dose dobutamine stress MRI: comparison with dobutamine stress echocardiography. *Circulation* 1999;99:763–770.
34. Hundley WG, Hamilton CA, Thomas MS, et al. Utility of fast cine magnetic resonance imaging and display for the detection of myocardial ischemia in patients not well suited for second harmonic stress echocardiography. *Circulation* 1999;100:1697–1702.
35. Dendale PA, Franken PR, Waldman GJ, et al. Low-dosage dobutamine magnetic resonance imaging as an alternative to echocardiography in the detection of viable myocardium after acute infarction. *Am Heart J* 1995;130:134–140.
36. Sechtem U, Baer FM, Voth E, et al. Stress functional MRI: detection of ischemic heart disease and myocardial viability. *J Magn Reson Imaging* 1999;10:667–675.
37. Sayad DE, Willett DL, Hundley WG, et al. Dobutamine magnetic resonance imaging with myocardial tagging quantitatively predicts improvement in regional function after revascularization. *Am J Cardiol* 1998;82:1149–1151, A10.
38. Baer FM, Voth E, Schneider CA, et al. Comparison of low-dose dobutamine gradient-echo magnetic resonance imaging and positron emission tomography with [18F]fluorodeoxyglucose in patients with chronic coronary artery disease. A functional and morphological approach to the detection of residual myocardial viability. *Circulation* 1995;91:1006–1015.
39. Baer FM, Theissen P, Schneider CA, et al. Dobutamine magnetic resonance imaging predicts contractile recovery of chronically dysfunctional myocardium after successful revascularization. *J Am Coll Cardiol* 1998;31:1040–1048.
40. Bouchard A, Reeves RC, Cranney G, et al. Assessment of myocardial infarct size by means of T2-weighted 1H nuclear magnetic resonance imaging. *Am Heart J* 1989;117:281–289.
41. Dulce MC, Duerinckx AJ, Hartiala J, et al. MR imaging of the myocardium using nonionic contrast medium: signal-intensity changes in patients with subacute myocardial infarction. *AJR Am J Roentgenol* 1993;160:963–970.
42. Ryan T, Tarver RD, Duerk JL, et al. Distinguishing viable from infarcted myocardium after experimental ischemia and reperfusion by using nuclear magnetic resonance imaging. *J Am Coll Cardiol* 1990;15:1355–1364.
43. Choi SI, Jiang CZ, Lim KH, et al. Application of breath-hold T2-weighted, first-pass perfusion and gadolinium-enhanced T1-weighted MR imaging for assessment of myocardial viability in a pig model. *J Magn Reson Imaging* 2000;11:476–480.
44. Wisenberg G, Prato FS, Carroll SE, et al. Serial nuclear magnetic resonance imaging of acute myocardial infarction with and without reperfusion. *Am Heart J* 1988;115:510–518.
45. Masui T, Saeed M, Wendland MF, et al. Occlusive and reperfused myocardial infarcts: MR imaging differentiation with nonionic Gd-DTPA-BMA. *Radiology* 1991;181:77–83.

46. Saeed M, Wendland MF, Takehara Y, et al. Reperfusion and irreversible myocardial injury: identification with a nonionic MR imaging contrast medium. *Radiology* 1992;182:675–683.

47. Atkinson DJ, Burstein D, Edelman RR. First-pass cardiac perfusion: evaluation with ultrafast MR imaging. *Radiology* 1990; 174:757–762.

48. Manning WJ, Atkinson DJ, Grossman W, et al. First-pass nuclear magnetic resonance imaging studies using gadolinium-DTPA in patients with coronary artery disease. *J Am Coll Cardiol* 1991;18:959–965.

49. Judd RM, Lugo-Olivieri CH, Arai M, et al. Physiological basis of myocardial contrast enhancement in fast magnetic resonance images of 2-day-old reperfused canine infarcts. *Circulation* 1995;92:1902–1910.

50. Kim RJ, Chen EL, Lima JA, et al. Myocardial Gd-DTPA kinetics determine MRI contrast enhancement and reflect the extent and severity of myocardial injury after acute reperfused infarction. *Circulation* 1996;94:3318–3326.

51. Saeed M, Wendland MF, Yu KK, et al. Identification of myocardial reperfusion with echo planar magnetic resonance imaging. Discrimination between occlusive and reperfused infarctions. *Circulation* 1994;90:1492–1501.

52. Lima JA, Judd RM, Bazille A, et al. Regional heterogeneity of human myocardial infarcts demonstrated by contrast-enhanced MRI. Potential mechanisms. *Circulation* 1995;92:1117–1125.

53. Judd RM, Reeder SB, Atalar E, et al. A magnetization-driven gradient echo pulse sequence for the study of myocardial perfusion. *Magn Reson Med* 1995;34:276–282.

54. Wu KC, Zerhouni EA, Judd RM, et al. Prognostic significance of microvascular obstruction by magnetic resonance imaging in patients with acute myocardial infarction. *Circulation* 1998;97:765–772.

55. Rochitte CE, Lima JA, Bluemke DA, et al. Magnitude and time course of microvascular obstruction and tissue injury after acute myocardial infarction. *Circulation* 1998;98:1006–1014.

56. Gerber BL, Rochitte CE, Melin JA, et al. Microvascular obstruction and left ventricular remodeling early after acute myocardial infarction. *Circulation* 2000;101:2734–2741.

57. Nishimura T, Yamada Y, Hayashi M, et al. Determination of infarct size of acute myocardial infarction in dogs by magnetic resonance imaging and gadolinium-DTPA: comparison with indium-111 antimyosin imaging. *Am J Physiol Imaging* 1989;4:83–88.

58. Schaefer S, Malloy CR, Katz J, et al. Gadolinium-DTPA–enhanced nuclear magnetic resonance imaging of reperfused myocardium: identification of the myocardial bed at risk. *J Am Coll Cardiol* 1988;12:1064–1072.

59. Saeed M, Bremerich J, Wendland MF, et al. Reperfused myocardial infarction as seen with use of necrosis-specific versus standard extracellular MR contrast media in rats. *Radiology* 1999;213:247–257.

60. Saeed M, Lund G, Wendland MF, et al. Magnetic resonance characterization of the peri-infarction zone of reperfused myocardial infarction with necrosis-specific and extracellular nonspecific contrast media. *Circulation* 2001;103:871–876.

61. Rogers WJ Jr, Kramer CM, Geskin G, et al. Early contrast-enhanced MRI predicts late functional recovery after reperfused myocardial infarction. *Circulation* 1999;99:744–750.

62. Kramer CM, Rogers WJ, Mankad S, et al. Contractile reserve and contrast uptake pattern by magnetic resonance imaging and functional recovery after reperfused myocardial infarction. *J Am Coll Cardiol* 2000;36:1834–1840.

63. Sandstede JJ, Lipke C, Beer M, et al. Analysis of first-pass and delayed contrast-enhancement patterns of dysfunctional myocardium on MR imaging: use in the prediction of myocardial viability. *AJR Am J Roentgenol* 2000;174:1737–1740.

64. Dendale P, Franken PR, Block P, et al. Contrast enhanced and functional magnetic resonance imaging for the detection of viable myocardium after infarction. *Am Heart J* 1998;135:875–880.

65. Eichstaedt HW, Felix R, Dougherty FC, et al. Magnetic resonance imaging (MRI) in different stages of myocardial infarction using the contrast agent gadolinium-DTPA. *Clin Cardiol* 1986;9:527–535.

66. Nishimura T, Kobayashi H, Ohara Y, et al. Serial assessment of myocardial infarction by using gated MR imaging and Gd-DTPA. *AJR Am J Roentgenol* 1989;153:715–720.

67. van Dijkman PR, van der Wall EE, de Roos A, et al. Acute, subacute, and chronic myocardial infarction: quantitative analysis of gadolinium-enhanced MR images. *Radiology* 1991;180:147–151.

68. Saeed M, Wendland MF, Masui T, et al. Myocardial infarction: assessment with an intravascular MR contrast medium. Work in progress. *Radiology* 1991;180:153–160.

69. Fedele F, Montesano T, Ferro-Luzzi M, et al. Identification of viable myocardium in patients with chronic coronary artery disease and left ventricular dysfunction: role of magnetic resonance imaging. *Am Heart J* 1994;128:484–489.

70. Pereira RS, Prato FS, Sykes J, et al. Assessment of myocardial viability using MRI during a constant infusion of Gd-DTPA: further studies at early and late periods of reperfusion. *Magn Reson Med* 1999;42:60–68.

71. Ramani K, Judd RM, Holly TA, et al. Contrast magnetic resonance imaging in the assessment of myocardial viability in patients with stable coronary artery disease and left ventricular dysfunction. *Circulation* 1998;98:2687–2694.

72. Simonetti O, Kim RJ, Fieno DS, et al. An improved MR imaging technique for the visualization of myocardial infarction. *Radiology* 2001;218:215–223.

73. Kim RJ, Fieno DS, Parrish TB, et al. Relationship of MRI delayed contrast enhancement to irreversible injury, infarct age, and contractile function. *Circulation* 1999;100:1992–2002.

74. Fieno DS, Kim RJ, Chen EL, et al. Contrast-enhanced magnetic resonance imaging of myocardium at risk: distinction between reversible and irreversible injury throughout infarct healing. *J Am Coll Cardiol* 2000;36:1985–1991.

75. Hillenbrand HB, Kim RJ, Parker MA, et al. Early assessment of myocardial salvage by contrast-enhanced magnetic resonance imaging. *Circulation* 2000;102:1678–1683.

76. Kim RJ, Wu E, Rafael A, et al. The use of contrast-enhanced magnetic resonance imaging to identify reversible myocardial dysfunction. *N Engl J Med* 2000;343:1445–1453.

77. Wu E, Judd RM, Vargas JD, et al. Visualization of presence, location, and transmural extent of healed Q-wave and non–Q-wave myocardial infarction. *Lancet* 2001;357:21–28.

78. Kloner RA, Ganote CE, Jennings RB. The "no-reflow" phenomenon after temporary coronary occlusion in the dog. *J Clin Invest* 1974;54:1496–1508.

79. Ito H, Tomooka T, Sakai N, et al. Lack of myocardial perfusion immediately after successful thrombolysis. A predictor of poor recovery of left ventricular function in anterior myocardial infarction. *Circulation* 1992;85:1699–1705.

80. Arheden H, Saeed M, Higgins CB, et al. Reperfused rat myocardium subjected to various durations of ischemia: estimation of the distribution volume of contrast material with echo-planar MR imaging. *Radiology* 2000;215:520–528.

81. Cobb FR, Bache RJ, Rivas F, et al. Local effects of acute cellular injury on regional myocardial blood flow. *J Clin Invest* 1976;57:1359–1368.

82. Berne RM, Rubio R. Acute coronary occlusion: early changes that induce coronary dilatation and the development of collateral circulation. *Am J Cardiol* 1969;24:776–781.

83. Factor SM, Okun EM, Kirk ES. The histological lateral border of acute canine myocardial infarction. A function of microcirculation. *Circ Res* 1981;48:640–649.

84. Saeed M, Wendland MF, Masui T, et al. Reperfused myocardial infarctions on T1- and susceptibility-enhanced MRI: evidence for loss of compartmentalization of contrast media. *Magn Reson Med* 1994;31:31–39.

85. Geschwind JF, Wendland MF, Saeed M, et al. AUR Memorial Award. Identification of myocardial cell death in reperfused myocardial injury using dual mechanisms of contrast-enhanced magnetic resonance imaging. *Acad Radiol* 1994;1:319–325.

86. Diesbourg LD, Prato FS, Wisenberg G, et al. Quantification of myocardial blood flow and extracellular volumes using a bolus injection of Gd-DTPA: kinetic modeling in canine ischemic disease. *Magn Reson Med* 1992;23:239–253.

87. Arheden H, Saeed M, Higgins CB, et al. Measurement of the distribution volume of gadopentetate dimeglumine at echo-planar MR imaging to quantify myocardial infarction: comparison with ^{99m}Tc-DTPA autoradiography in rats. *Radiology* 1999;211:698–708.

88. Pereira RS, Prato FS, Wisenberg G, et al. The determination of myocardial viability using Gd-DTPA in a canine model of acute myocardial ischemia and reperfusion. *Magn Reson Med* 1996;36:684–693.

89. Wendland MF, Saeed M, Arheden H, et al. Toward necrotic cell fraction measurement by contrast-enhanced MRI of reperfused ischemically injured myocardium. *Acad Radiol* 1998;5(Suppl 1):S42–S46.

90. Wendland MF, Saeed M, Lauerma K, et al. Alterations in T1 of normal and reperfused infarcted myocardium after Gd-BOPTA versus GD-DTPA on inversion recovery EPI. *Magn Reson Med* 1997;37:448–456.

91. Weissleder R, Lee AS, Khaw BA, et al. Antimyosin-labeled monocrystalline iron oxide allows detection of myocardial infarct: MR antibody imaging. *Radiology* 1992;182:381–385.

92. Adzamli IK, Blau M, Pfeffer MA, et al. Phosphonate-modified Gd-DTPA complexes. III: The detection of myocardial infarction by MRI. *Magn Reson Med* 1993;29:505–511.

93. Hindre F, Le Plouzennec M, de Certaines JD, et al. Tetra-*p*-aminophenylporphyrin conjugated with Gd-DTPA: tumor-specific contrast agent for MR imaging. *J Magn Reson Imaging* 1993;3:59–65.

94. Nelson JA, Schmiedl U, Shankland EG. Metalloporphyrins as tumor-seeking MRI contrast media and as potential selective treatment sensitizers. *Invest Radiol* 1990;25(Suppl 1):S71–S73.

95. Ni Y, Marchal G, Yu J, et al. Localization of metalloporphyrin-induced "specific" enhancement in experimental liver tumors: comparison of magnetic resonance imaging, microangiographic, and histologic findings. *Acad Radiol* 1995;2:687–699.

96. Ni Y, Petre C, Miao Y, et al. Magnetic resonance imaging-histomorphologic correlation studies on paramagnetic metalloporphyrins in rat models of necrosis. *Invest Radiol* 1997;32:770–779.

97. Marchal G, Ni Y, Herijgers P, et al. Paramagnetic metalloporphyrins: infarct avid contrast agents for diagnosis of acute myocardial infarction by MRI. *Eur Radiol* 1996;6:2–8.

98. Ni Y, Marchal G, Herijgers P, et al. Paramagnetic metalloporphyrins: from enhancers of malignant tumors to markers of myocardial infarcts. *Acad Radiol* 1996;3(Suppl 2):S395–S397.

99. Herijgers P, Laycock SK, Ni Y, et al. Localization and determination of infarct size by Gd-mesoporphyrin–enhanced MRI in dogs. *Int J Card Imaging* 1997;13:499–507.

100. Pislaru SV, Ni Y, Pislaru C, et al. Noninvasive measurements of infarct size after thrombolysis with a necrosis-avid MRI contrast agent. *Circulation* 1999;99:690–696.

101. Choi SI, Choi SH, Kim ST, et al. Irreversibly damaged myocardium at MR imaging with a necrotic tissue-specific contrast agent in a cat model. *Radiology* 2000;215:863–868.

102. Saeed M, Wagner S, Wendland MF, et al. Occlusive and reperfused myocardial infarcts: differentiation with Mn-DPDP–enhanced MR imaging. *Radiology* 1989;172:59–64.

103. Pomeroy OH, Wendland M, Wagner S, et al. Magnetic resonance imaging of acute myocardial ischemia using a manganese chelate, Mn-DPDP. *Invest Radiol* 1989;24:531–536.

104. Saeed M, Wendland MF, Takehara Y, et al. Reversible and irreversible injury in the reperfused myocardium: differentiation with contrast material-enhanced MR imaging. *Radiology* 1990;175:633–637.

105. Gallez B, Bacic G, Swartz HM. Evidence for the dissociation of the hepatobiliary MRI contrast agent Mn-DPDP. *Magn Reson Med* 1996;35:14–19.

106. Chauncey DM Jr, Schelbert HR, Halpern SE, et al. Tissue distribution studies with radioactive manganese: a potential agent for myocardial imaging. *J Nucl Med* 1977;18:933–936.

107. Hunter DR, Haworth RA, Berkoff HA. Cellular manganese uptake by the isolated perfused rat heart: a probe for the sarcolemma calcium channel. *J Mol Cell Cardiol* 1981;13:823–832.

108. Brurok H, Schjott J, Berg K, et al. Effects of MnDPDP, DPDP^{--}, and MnCl$_2$ on cardiac energy metabolism and manganese accumulation. An experimental study in the isolated perfused rat heart. *Invest Radiol* 1997;32:205–211.

109. Bremerich J, Saeed M, Arheden H, et al. Normal and infarcted myocardium: differentiation with cellular uptake of manganese at MR imaging in a rat model. *Radiology* 2000;216:524–530.

110. Pike MM, Kitakaze M, Marban E. ^{23}Na-NMR measurements of intracellular sodium in intact perfused ferret hearts during ischemia and reperfusion. *Am J Physiol* 1990;259:H1767–H1773.

111. Cannon PJ, Maudsley AA, Hilal SK, et al. Sodium nuclear magnetic resonance imaging of myocardial tissue of dogs after coronary artery occlusion and reperfusion. *J Am Coll Cardiol* 1986;7:573–579.

112. Kim RJ, Lima JA, Chen EL, et al. Fast ^{23}Na magnetic resonance imaging of acute reperfused myocardial infarction. Potential to assess myocardial viability. *Circulation* 1997;95:1877–1885.

113. Parrish TB, Fieno DS, Fitzgerald SW, et al. Theoretical basis for sodium and potassium MRI of the human heart at 1.5 T. *Magn Reson Med* 1997;38:653–661.

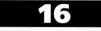

CORONARY MRA—TECHNICAL APPROACHES

MATTHIAS STUBER
RENÉ M. BOTNAR
KRAIG V. KISSINGER
WARREN J. MANNING

Coronary artery disease is one of the major causes of morbidity and mortality in the Western world. The current gold standard for the diagnosis of coronary disease is x-ray coronary angiography. In the United States (1) and Europe, more than 1,000,000 of these diagnostic procedures are performed each year. Roentgenographic (x-ray) coronary angiography is used to define coronary anatomy and guide patient therapy. However, x-ray coronary angiography is expensive and invasive, exposes both patient and operator to potentially harmful ionizing radiation, and carries a small risk for serious complications. Furthermore, a significant minority of patients undergoing x-ray angiography are found not to have significant disease (2) but remain exposed to the costs and morbidity of this invasive procedure. Thus, a more cost-effective, noninvasive approach for defining luminographic disease is urgently needed.

Coronary MRA combines several advantages and great potential. It is noninvasive and can survey the heart in any image plane, and it does not involve the use of possibly harmful ionizing radiation or iodinated contrast media. In addition to providing a high degree of spatial resolution, MR is not associated with any known short- or long-term side effects.

The utility of MRA for visualizing the coronary anatomy has been investigated since the late 1980s (3,4). Although no coronary stenoses were identified in these early studies, demonstrations of the potential of MRI to assess the anatomy of the coronary vessels triggered intense interest in the field.

Successful coronary MRA data acquisition is technically demanding because of the small caliber and tortuosity of the coronary arteries and the presence of signal from surrounding epicardial fat and myocardium. In addition, cardiac motion results from the natural periodic contractions of the heart and the movements of breathing. Both of these motion components exceed the coronary artery dimensions by a multiple, so that efficient strategies to suppress motion must be applied. Furthermore, enhancement of the contrast between the coronary vessel lumen and the surrounding tissue (myocardium, epicardial fat) is mandatory for a successful visualization of the coronary anatomy.

The general approaches described in this chapter are available on current state-of-the-art cardiac MR units from all vendor platforms, but some nuances may be vendor-specific (e.g., navigator implementation). Established and advanced coronary MRA methods are reviewed. Specific strategies for motion suppression and contrast enhancement are discussed, and representative image material is displayed.

TECHNICAL CONSIDERATIONS

The bulk of research studies and methods development in coronary MRA has been conducted on 1.5-tesla (T) whole body systems. However, high-quality coronary MRA data have also been obtained at a lower field strength on 0.5-T systems (5–7).

M. Stuber: Cardiovascular Division, Harvard Medical School, Boston, Massachusetts.

R. M. Botnar: Cardiovascular Division, Beth Israel Deaconess Medical Center and Harvard Medical School, Boston, Massachusetts.

K. V. Kissinger: Beth Israel Deaconess Medical Center, Cardiac MR Center, Boston, Massachusetts.

W. J. Manning: Departments of Medicine (Cardiovascular Division) and Radiology, Beth Israel Deaconess Medical Center and Harvard Medical School, Boston, Massachusetts.

Suppression of Motion Artifacts

The heart is subject to intrinsic and extrinsic motion. Intrinsic myocardial motion is the occurrence of natural contraction and relaxation during the R-R interval. Extrinsic myocardial motion is bulk motion of the heart induced by breathing. Both extrinsic and intrinsic myocardial motion may greatly exceed the coronary artery diameter and so cause blurring and ghosting of the coronary vessels on images. Therefore, strategies that minimize the adverse effects of both motion components are needed.

Suppression of Intrinsic Myocardial Motion

For submillimeter coronary MRA, the image data cannot be collected during one R-R interval. Therefore, the coronary MRA data acquisition must be synchronized with the cardiac cycle, and k-space segmentation must be applied (Fig. 16.1). For segmented k-space techniques, an accurate electrocardiographic (ECG) synchronization is mandatory. Less robust peripheral pulse detection methods yield inferior results. Even though ECG triggering is superior to peripheral pulse detection, reliable R-wave detection in the presence of a strong static magnetic field (hydrodynamic effect) and

switching magnetic field gradients is technically challenging. However, by using a vector ECG approach, a more robust ECG triggering can be obtained (8).

To minimize motion artifacts in the images further, the coronary MRA data should be acquired during a short acquisition window (<100 milliseconds) and during a period of minimal myocardial motion. The coronary arteries are relatively quiescent during isovolumic relaxation (approximately 350 to 400 milliseconds after the R wave) and at mid-diastole (9). Because bright blood (gradient-echo) coronary MRA depends on the inflow of unsaturated spins, mid-diastole is generally preferred for image acquisition because it also represents a period of rapid coronary blood flow. However, recent studies suggest that the onset of the mid-diastolic diastasis is patient-specific and cannot be predicted from heart rate data (10,11). Therefore, subject-specific trigger delays may have to be defined by using a visual inspection of cine images or more advanced automated approaches (11).

Suppression of Extrinsic Myocardial Motion

Breath-Hold Techniques

Among the major limitations of coronary MRA are the artifacts resulting from the bulk cardiac motion associated with

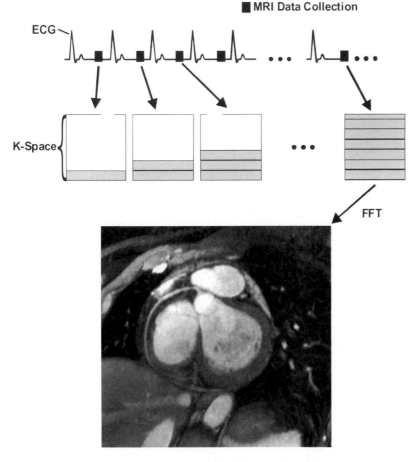

Coronary MRA

FIGURE 16.1. Principle of electrocardiogram triggering, k-space segmentation, and diastolic data acquisition for coronary MRA. After the completion of data collection in k-space, images are generated by means of a fast Fourier transform.

respiration. These motion artifacts cause ghosting, blurring, and image degradation, which compromise the visualization of the coronary arteries and the assessment of focal stenoses. To compensate for respiratory motion, breath-holding was implemented early to suppress respiratory motion (12). Two-dimensional (2D) breath-hold coronary MRA relied on the acquisition of contiguous parallel images, with the goal of surveying the proximal segments of the coronary arteries during serial breath-holds (13). More recently, three-dimensional (3D) breath-hold techniques for coronary MRA have also been implemented (14–16) and are currently under investigation (17). Breath-hold approaches offer the advantage of rapid imaging and are technically easy to implement in compliant healthy volunteers and subjects with coronary artery disease. For coronary MRA techniques that utilize first-pass contrast enhancement of intravenously injected extracellular contrast agents, breath-holding is a requirement at the present time.

However, breath-hold strategies have several practical limitations. Major patient and operator involvement is required for serial breath-holds. Patients with cardiac or pulmonary disease frequently have difficulty sustaining adequate breath-holds, particularly when the duration exceeds 5 to 10 seconds. For a sufficient anatomic coverage, serial (30 to 40) breath-holds are often needed. Alternative breath-holding techniques, including serial brief breath-holds (18) and coached breath-holding with visual or audible feedback (19–21), have been used to minimize respiratory motion artifacts and patient inconvenience, but these are practical only for highly motivated subjects. Even with cooperative patients, breath-holding may be problematic. With a sustained breath-hold, cranial diaphragmatic drift, which is often substantial (~1 cm), may occur (12,22–25). During serial breath-holds, the diaphragmatic and cardiac positions frequently vary by up to 1 cm, so that image registration errors result (25). Misregistration causes apparent gaps between the segments of the visualized coronary arteries, which can be misinterpreted as signal voids from coronary stenoses. Finally, the use of signal enhancement techniques, such as 3D imaging, signal averaging, and fold-over suppression, is not practical within a breath-hold of reasonable duration (15 seconds).

Signal Averaging and Respiratory Bellows

Initial free-breathing coronary MRA approaches utilized multiple signal averaging to minimize motion artifacts (26,27). This averaging approach is reasonable for relatively low (>1 to 2 mm) spatial resolutions but inadequate for accurate stenosis detection. Another early free-breathing approach utilized a thoracic respiratory bellows to gate to the end-expiratory position (24,27) and showed promise in comparison with breath-holding. Respiratory bellows have been used to monitor chest wall expansion and thereby gate image acquisition to the end-expiratory position. Enhancements included respiratory feedback monitoring (21). However, respiratory bellows gating is often not reliable, and a relative phase shift between chest wall expansion and diaphragmatic motion may occur and introduce motion artifacts into the images. Subsequently, more accurate and flexible MR navigators have replaced bellows gating.

Free-Breathing Navigator Approaches

The use of free breathing with respiratory navigators, first proposed by Ehman and Felmlee (28), serves to overcome the time constraints and cooperation imposed by breath-hold approaches. Free-breathing navigator methods are particularly well suited for prolonged 3D coronary MRA approaches, combining the postprocessing benefits of thin, adjacent slices with the submillimeter spatial resolution afforded by an improved signal-to-noise ratio (SNR). They further enable the flexibility to use signal enhancement techniques, such as signal averaging and fold-over suppression. The use of navigator gating has received considerable attention, and implementations vary from "simple" to "complex" (Table 16.1). In principle, the MR navigator "monitors" the motion of an interface. Data are accepted only when the selected interface falls within a user-defined window (usually 3 to 5 mm) positioned around the end-expiratory level of the interface (Figs. 16.2 and 16.3). Although the need for patient cooperation and operator involvement is reduced

TABLE 16.1. NAVIGATOR GATING

Breath-holding	Free Breathing
• Sustained end-expiratory	• Multiple averages
• Sustained end-inspiratory	• Bellows gating
• Multiple breath-holds (coached)	• Navigators
• Visual/auditory feedback	• Intersecting planes
• Hyperventilation	• 2D selective pencil beam
• Supplemental oxygen	• Retrospective gating
	• Prospective gating
	• Real-time motion correction ("tracking")
	• Motion-adaptive gating
	• Real-time adaptive averaging
	• Multiple navigators

Increasing complexity ↓ (applies to Navigators sub-list)

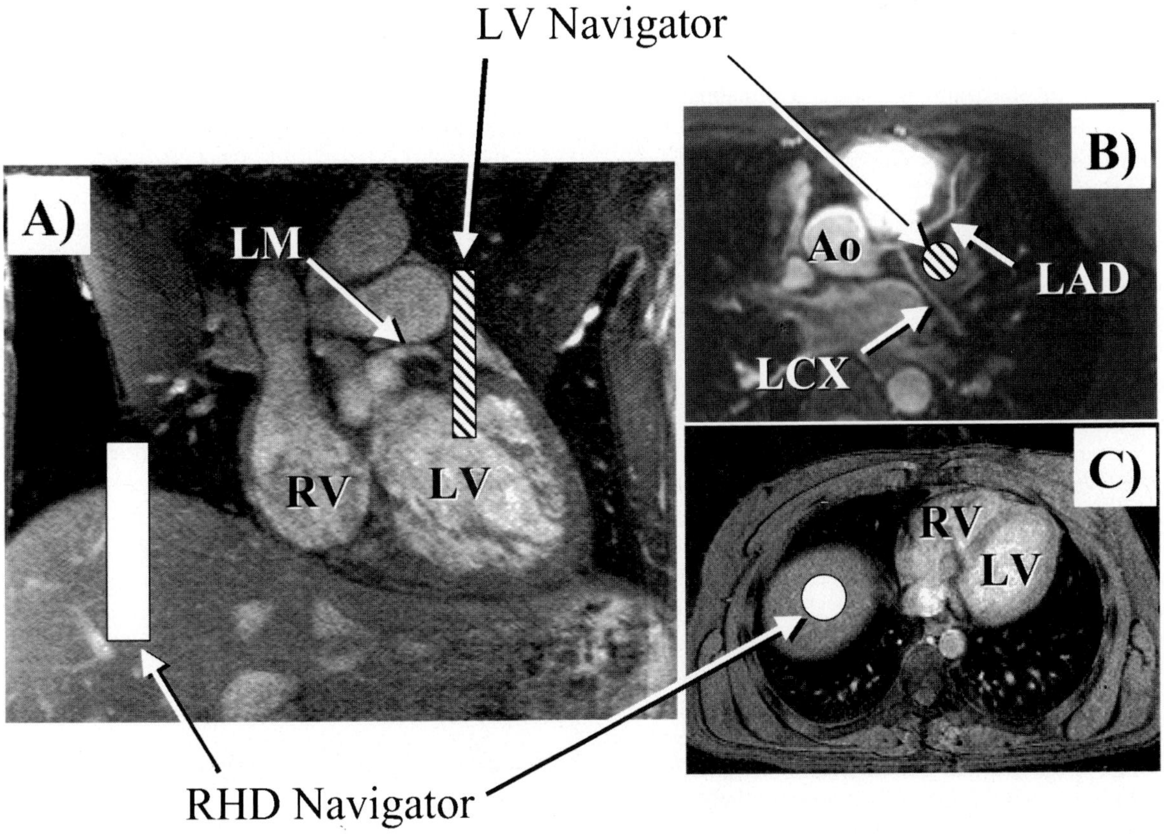

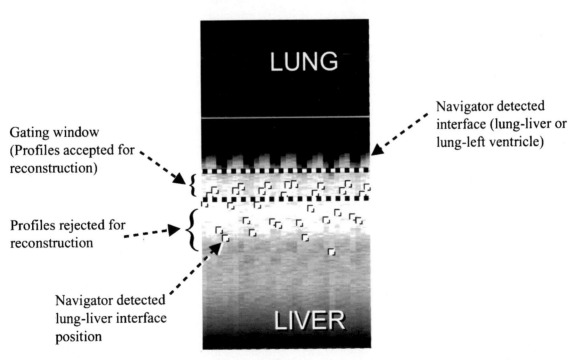

FIGURE 16.2. Planning the position of the navigator at the dome of the right hemidiaphragm *(RHD Navigator)* **(A,C)** and at the free wall of the left ventricle *(LV Navigator)* **(A,B)** as depicted in the coronal (A) and transverse (B,C) views obtained in the scout scans. *LV,* left ventricle; *RV,* right ventricle; *LM,* left main coronary artery; *Ao,* ascending aorta; *LAD,* left anterior descending coronary artery; *LCX,* left circumflex coronary artery.

FIGURE 16.3. Free-breathing navigator display as visualized in run time on the system console. Time is on the x-axis, and the lung–liver interface is displayed on the y-axis. If a navigator-detected lung–liver or lung–left ventricle position *(white squares)* falls into a certain window *(dotted lines, gating window),* the subsequently acquired k-space profiles are accepted for reconstruction. Otherwise, they are rejected for reconstruction and are remeasured in the next R-R interval.

with navigator/free-breathing methods, diaphragmatic drift and patient motion remain relevant issues (24,29). Chest wall motion during free breathing may result in motion artifacts overlaid to the image. By using an anterior local saturation band and fat saturation, signal originating from the anterior chest wall may be minimized, with a resultant suppression of chest wall artifacts (30). Although less comfortable, as an alternative, prone imaging also reduces these problems and serves to suppress chest wall motion (not accounted for by the diaphragmatic navigator) while improving navigator efficiency (31).

Navigator Localization and Geometry. Navigators can be positioned at any interface that accurately reflects respiratory motion, including the dome of the right hemidiaphragm (20,27,32) (Fig. 16.2), the left hemidiaphragm, and the anterior chest wall, or directly through the anterior free wall of the left ventricle (24,33) (Fig. 16.2). Navigators have been implemented as two intersecting planes (34,35) and as 2D selective pencil beam excitations (36). Although the intersecting planes are easier to implement, they may compromise magnetization (leading to local signal voids), and intersecting plane navigator positioning directly at the heart is therefore not recommended. In contrast, 2D selective pencil beam excitations can be implemented with the use of shallow radiofrequency (RF) excitation angles, so that they only minimally affect the magnetization in the region-of-interest. Therefore, 2D selective pencil beam excitations can be directly localized at the left ventricle, and no interference with the imaged slices has been reported (24,33). Nevertheless, studies suggest that the bulk of cardiac motion related to breathing is in the superior–inferior axis (37) and that most single-navigator locations yield similar image quality (24,33). Thus, the right hemidiaphragm is now preferred because of the relative ease of identifying the interface from a series of coronal, sagittal, and transverse scout images.

Navigator Gating. The gating process can be either prospective (i.e., determined before coronary data acquisition and offering the opportunity to correct for slice position) (27,38) or retrospective (i.e., following data acquisition but before image reconstruction) (35,39,40). Collected image data are accepted for reconstruction only if the navigator-detected interface falls into a certain range or window (the gating window) (Fig. 16.3). With navigator gating (without tracking), a 3-mm end-expiratory diaphragmatic window is used, and data are collected on average from one-third of R-R intervals (33% navigator efficiency) (24).

Navigator Gating and Tracking. From MR studies of cardiac borders, Wang et al. (37) noted that the dominant impact of respiration on cardiac position is in the superior–inferior direction. At the end-expiratory position, the relationship between diaphragmatic and cardiac motion is about 0.6 for the right coronary artery and about 0.7 for the left coronary artery. Advances in computer processing and knowledge of this relatively fixed relationship offer the opportunity for prospective navigator gating with real-time tracking of the imaged volume position (32,41). This facilitates the use of wider gating windows and shortens scan time through increased navigator efficiency. Navigator tracking is often also referred to as *prospective adaptive motion correction.* The correction of the imaged volume position is obtained by a prospective run-time adaptation of the frequency of the slice-selective RF excitation and of the demodulator phase and frequency (dependent on the navigator-detected interface position). With real-time tracking implementations, a 5-mm diaphragmatic gating window is often used with a navigator efficiency close to 50% (41), versus about 33% with a 3-mm window and navigator gating alone. Coronary MRA with real-time navigator tracking has been shown to minimize registration errors (in comparison with breath-holding), and image quality is maintained or improved in both 2D and 3D approaches (24,33).

Navigator Tracking Alone. Limitations of breath-hold techniques include diaphragmatic drift and inconsistencies of the end-expiratory position between serial breath-holds. To overcome these limitations, breath-held coronary MRA has been combined with navigator tracking (42,43). With the use of these techniques, coronary MRA data can be acquired in serial breath-holds, and adverse effects of diaphragmatic drift during or between serial breath holds can be minimized.

Reordering of k-Space. Sophisticated navigator algorithms have also been implemented to collect important k-space profiles more efficiently based on the navigator-detected interface position. Implementations of such k-space–reordered techniques include the following: motion adaptive gating (MAG) (44), the diminishing variant algorithm (DVA) (45), phase ordering with automated window selection (PAWS) (46), and the zonal motion adaptive reordering technique (ZMART), which includes a prospective adaptive RF excitation angle adjustment (47).

Adaptive Averaging. Recently, preliminary data for a novel respiratory suppressive approach that does not utilize ECG gating, breath-holds, or navigator gating have suggested that it may prove useful, particularly for patients with an irregular heart rhythm or irregular breathing pattern. With real-time imaging and adaptive averaging (48), cross-correlation is used to identify automatically those real-time imaging frames in which a coronary vessel is present and to determine the location of the vessel within each frame. This information is then used for selective averaging of frames to increase the SNR and improve vessel visualization. The robustness of this technique in patients with coronary disease remains to be defined.

Navigators, Prepulses, and Imaging Sequences. Most of the navigator concepts described above can be freely combined with prepulses and 2D or 3D imaging sequences (Fig. 16.4). Because the navigator data are intended to reflect the position of the heart during the subsequent acquisition period, positioning of the navigator *immediately* before the data acquisition block and rapid navigator analysis are crucial (49). However, prepulses preceding the navigator excitation may adversely affect navigator detection of the interface position. This factor must be considered in the sequence design. In the presence of nonselective prepulses, such as inversion or dual-inversion prepulses, the magnetization for subsequent navigator interface detection may be compromised. Therefore, countermeasures such as the Nav-Restore prepulse (which locally reinverts the magnetization after the inversion or dual-inversion prepulses) have been developed and successfully applied (50).

Contrast Enhancement

The native epicardial coronary arteries are surrounded by both epicardial fat and myocardium. For successful visualization of the coronary arteries, a high level of contrast between the coronary lumen and the surrounding tissue is desirable. The contrast between the coronary blood pool and the surrounding tissue can be manipulated by using the inflow effect (unsaturated protons entering the imaging field between successive RF pulses), by the application of MR prepulses (endogenous contrast enhancement), or by the administration of contrast agents (exogenous contrast enhancement) with or without preparatory pulses. Preparatory pulses such as fat saturation (51), magnetization transfer contrast (26), T2 preparation (52,53) (Fig. 16.5), local saturation bands (REST), and inversion (54,55) and dual-inversion (56) prepulses have all been shown to enhance contrast in coronary MRA.

Endogenous Contrast Enhancement

Fat Saturation in Bright Blood Coronary MRA
In most subjects, the coronary arteries are surrounded by epicardial fat. Fat has a relatively short T1 (250 milliseconds at 1.5 T), and the resultant MR signal intensity similar to that of flowing blood. Fat saturation prepulses are used to suppress signal from surrounding fat selectively to allow visualization of the underlying coronary arteries. This is often accomplished with a frequency-selective prepulse that minimizes the

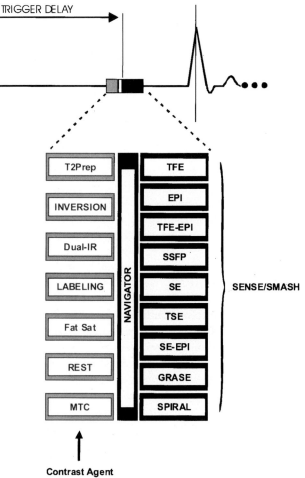

FIGURE 16.4. Conceptualized building blocks of a coronary MRA sequence. Electrocardiogram triggering is used to suppress intrinsic myocardial motion. Extrinsic motion caused by respiration can be suppressed by means of a navigator preceding the imaging sequence, breath-hold, respiratory bellows gating, or signal averaging. Contrast enhancement is obtained by means of prepulses *(gray boxes)* with or without the application of a contrast agent. *T2Prep,* T2 preparation; *inversion,* inversion prepulse; *dual-IR,* dual-inversion prepulse; *labeling,* spin labeling or arterial spin tagging prepulse; *FatSat,* fat saturation prepulse; *REST,* saturation band for local signal suppression; *MTC,* magnetization transfer contrast prepulses. Prepulses typically precede the imaging part of the sequence and can be used individually or combined (e.g., T2Prep and FatSat) if necessary. Candidate imaging sequences *(black boxes)* include segmented k-space gradient-echo sequences *(TFE),* echo-planar imaging sequences *(EPI),* segmented hybrid EPI techniques *(TFE-EPI),* steady-state free-precession imaging *(SSFP),* spin-echo *(SE),* turbo spin-echo *(TSE),* spin-echo in conjunction with echo-planar readouts *(SE-EPI),* turbo spin-echo combined with echo-planar readouts *(GRASE),* and spiral k-space acquisition *(SPIRAL).* All the imaging sequences may theoretically be combined with parallel imaging, such as simultaneous acquisition of spatial harmonics *(SMASH)* or sensitivity encoding *(SENSE).* Only a few of the multiple potential combinations of prepulses, motion suppression strategies, and imaging sequences documented in this figure have been explored.

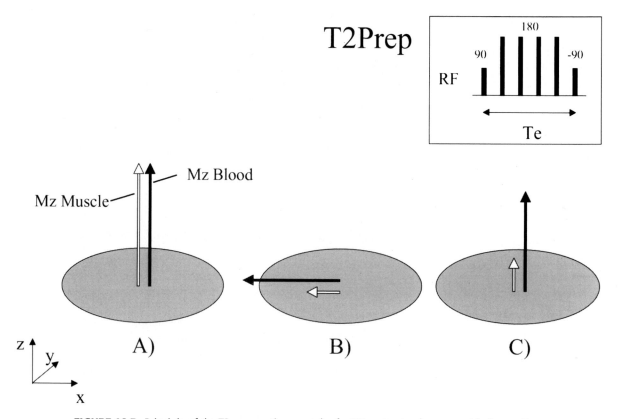

FIGURE 16.5. Principle of the T2 preparation prepulse for T2 contrast enhancement between the coronary blood pool and the myocardium (52). The blood T2 (250 milliseconds) is prolonged in comparison with that of muscle (50 milliseconds). Starting at the same equilibrium magnetization, the Mz-magnetization of blood *(black arrow)* and that of myocardium *(white arrow)* are rotated into the transverse plane by means of a non–slice-selective 90-degree radiofrequency (RF) pulse **(A)**. During a train of repetitive nonselective 180-degree refocusing pulses, both the transverse blood magnetization and the transverse muscle magnetization experience a T2 decay during an "echo time" (TE). This T2 decay is enhanced for the myocardium with the shorter T2 value **(B)**. After a final nonselective 90-degree tip-up RF excitation, the transverse blood magnetization and transverse muscle magnetization are rotated back into z-direction **(C)**. The configuration in C represents the Mz-magnetization of blood and myocardium before imaging. Because of the increased relative Mz-magnetization of the blood (in comparison with that of the myocardium), a signal-enhanced blood pool and a signal-attenuated myocardium are obtained in the images.

fat signal and thereby allows visualization of the coronary vessels. In the case of spiral imaging, a spectral spatial RF excitation pulse may be used, which selectively excites water (57).

Signal from the Myocardium in Bright Blood Coronary MRA

In addition to epicardial fat, the coronary arteries run in close proximity to the epimyocardium. The relatively similar T1 relaxation values of myocardium and coronary blood (850 and 1,200 milliseconds, respectively, at 1.5 T) complicate the differentiation of the coronary arteries for 3D coronary MRA as blood exchange (inflow effect) is reduced between successive RF excitations. Different methods can be used to enhance the contrast between the coronary arteries and myocardium. The most promising are prepulses such as T2 preparation (52,53) and magnetization transfer contrast (26). Because the T2 relaxation times of coronary arterial blood (250 milliseconds) and myocardium (50 milliseconds) are substantially

different, the application of a T2 preparation prepulse serves to suppress myocardial signal, with relative preservation of the signal from coronary arterial blood (Fig. 16.5). As an added benefit, the signal of deoxygenated blood in the cardiac veins, which has a T2 of 35 milliseconds, is also suppressed when T2 preparation is used (53). This suppression is particularly helpful if minimal epicardial fat is present or the great cardiac vein runs in close proximity to the left anterior descending and left circumflex coronary arteries. Thus, with the use of fat saturation and T2 preparation (or magnetization transfer contrast) prepulses, the coronary lumen appears bright, and the signal intensity of the surrounding tissue (including fat and myocardium) is reduced.

Signal from the Myocardium and Epicardial Fat in Black Blood Coronary MRA

In black blood coronary MRA, a signal-enhanced myocardium and a signal-attenuated coronary lumen are desirable. For this purpose, a dual-inversion prepulse consisting of a nonselective inversion followed by a slice-selective inversion is used to reestablishing the initial magnetization of the myocardium at the level of interest (58). For black blood coronary MRA, a high signal from the myocardium and epicardial fat is necessary to maximize the contrast between the signal-attenuated coronary blood pool and the surrounding myocardium. Therefore, no fat saturation is used in this approach (56).

Exogenous Contrast Enhancement

Bright blood, time-of-flight (TOF) coronary MRA methods depend heavily on the inflow of unsaturated protons/blood into the imaging plane. If, however, flow is slow, saturation effects will cause a loss of signal. Furthermore, vessel wall, plaque, and thrombus can have signal intensities similar to that of coronary blood (59). In contrast-enhanced MRA, enhancement of the blood signal is based primarily on the intravascular T1 relaxation rate and therefore may allow for "true" lumen imaging. With the use of MR contrast agents, the T1 relaxation of blood can be markedly shortened to increase the contrast-to-noise ratio (CNR) for coronary MRA (54,55,60–62). For this purpose, the U.S. Food and Drug Administration has approved extracellular agents, such as gadopentetate dimeglumine (Magnevist; Berlex Laboratories, Wayne, New Jersey), gadodiamide (Omniscan; Nycomed Amersham, Buckinghamshire, United Kingdom), and gadoteridol (ProHance; Bracco Diagnostics, Princeton, New Jersey), and intravascular agents, such as iron oxide (AMI 227; Advanced Magnetics, Cambridge, Massachusetts), MS-325 (Epix Medical, Cambridge, Massachusetts), and NC100150 (Clariscan; Nycomed Amersham). Because *extracellular* agents quickly extravasate into the extravascular space, their use requires rapid first-pass imaging and therefore breath-hold techniques (14). However, first-pass coronary MRA with extravascular contrast agents is limited by the need for repeated injections of contrast when more than one slab is imaged. With each subsequent injection, the CNR becomes lower as the signal from the extracellular space continuously increases (because of a progressively decreasing T1) following initial contrast administration. The use of intravascular agents has the inherent advantage of allowing image acquisition for longer periods of time. Thus, non–breath-hold schemes can be used, and repeated scans have similar CNRs without the need for repeated injections (55). When intravascular contrast agents are used in conjunction with navigator technology, free-breathing, high-resolution coronary MRA data acquisition is enabled, and signal enhancement strategies such as 3D imaging, signal averaging, and fold-over suppression can be applied.

Spatial Resolution

The spatial resolution requirements for coronary MRA depend on whether the goal is simply to identify the ostial takeoff and proximal course of the coronary artery (as in suspected cases of congenital anomalous coronary arteries), or to identify focal stenoses. Figure 16.6 displays an x-ray coronary angiogram displayed at spatial resolutions of 300, 500, 1,000, and 2,000 μm. At resolutions of 500 and 1,000 μm, the focal coronary stenoses *(arrows)* are readily detectable, whereas at in-plane resolutions above 1,000 μm, only the coronary artery is visible, potentially allowing the identification of anomalous coronary vasculature but not focal

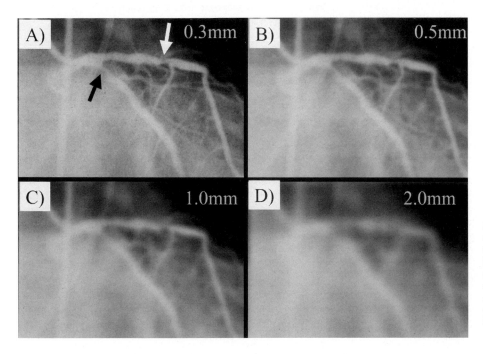

FIGURE 16.6. Conventional x-ray coronary angiogram acquired with a spatial resolution of 300 μm is shown in **(A)**. Focal lesions in the proximal left anterior descending *(LAD, white arrow)* and proximal left circumflex *(LCX, black arrow)* coronary arteries are documented. The images display simulated spatial resolutions of 500 **(B)**, 1,000 **(C)**, and 2,000 μm **(D)**.

stenoses. Thus, it appears that submillimeter spatial resolution is necessary for the visual identification of focal stenoses.

Although submillimeter in-plane spatial resolution appears important, the use of relatively thick (1.5- to 3-mm) slices for coronary MRA results in anisotropic voxels. This anisotropic voxel size may lead to vessel blurring with oblique and multiplanar reconstructions. The use of isotropic voxel sizes has been shown to be advantageous for coronary MRA, with resultant improved vessel sharpness (63), but at the "cost" of a reduced SNR.

Dedicated Coils

In-plane spatial resolution requirements for coronary MRA mandate maximizing the SNR with the use of appropriate cardiac receiver coils. Because the SNR decreases sharply with the distance of the organ-of-interest from the receiver coil, cardiac-specific coils have been optimized for the size of the heart and the distance of the heart from the chest wall. Fortunately, the right, left main, and left anterior descending coronary arteries are relatively anterior structures. Nearly all vendors offer cardiac-specific phased-array coils. The use of these coils allows flexibility (a single or multiple anterior coils can be combined with posterior elements) and enhances the SNR in comparison with use of the body coil as the receiver. The use of cardiac-specific coils should be the standard for all coronary MRA examinations.

Scout Scanning and Volume-Targeted Acquisition

The shape, geometry, and orientation of the heart and the coronary arteries are highly variable among individuals. As a consequence, the orientation of the imaged plane in parallel to the major axes of the left and right coronary systems must be adjusted for each individual (5,15). Because of the tortuosity of the coronary arteries, it must be ascertained that the imaged volume encompasses the vessel-of-interest. For this purpose, a survey scan with reduced resolution that is capable of visualizing the gross anatomy of the coronary arteries is required. We have found it extremely valuable to have the timing and method of respiratory suppression for all scout images (Scout Scan) (Fig. 16.7) be coherent with the higher-resolution coronary imaging sequences (HR-Scan) (30) (Fig. 16.7). If the high-resolution coronary MRA data are acquired during a breath-hold, a preceding breath-hold localizer is advised. Similarly, if the coronary MRA data are acquired in mid-diastole, the localizer scan must be acquired at the same point in time within the cardiac cycle. For free-breathing navigator coronary MRA, a preceding low-resolution localizer scan acquired during free breathing is mandatory. For our first scout, we use an ECG-triggered, free-breathing, multislice, 2D, segmented gradient-echo thoracic acquisition with nine transverse, nine coronal, and nine sagittal interleaved acquisitions. From this data set, the navigator position at the dome of the right hemidiaphragm and its location of the base of the heart can be readily identified (Fig. 16.2). A second ECG-triggered 3D fast gradient-echo echo-planar imaging scout is then acquired with navigator gating about a volume that includes the coronary arteries. From this second scout, the location of the ostial takeoff of the left main and right coronaries can be delineated.

Volume targeting along the major axes of the left and right coronary systems is facilitated with a three-point plan-scan tool (Fig. 16.8). With this software, the user identifies three points with an interactive mouse click along the vessel-of-interest on the second scout scan. Plane offset and orientation are then automatically calculated for the subsequent high-resolution coronary MRA scan (30).

Two-Dimensional versus Three-Dimensional Data Acquisition

With the rapid acquisition of multiple phase-encoding steps during each heart beat, the acquisition of one 2D image during fewer than 20 heart beats is possible, so that breath-

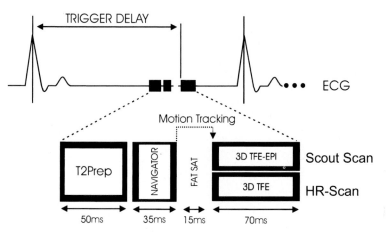

FIGURE 16.7. Schematic of pulse sequences for three-dimensional (3D) scout scanning *(Scout Scan)* and high-resolution 3D MR angiography *(HR-Scan)* based on prospective navigator gating and real-time motion tracking. The elements of the sequence—T2 preparation prepulse, saturation prepulse *(REST)*, navigator, fat saturation prepulse *(FatSat)*, and the 3D imaging sequence—are shown in temporal relationship to the electrocardiogram and trigger delay. Note the parallel structure for the scout and the high-resolution coronary MRA scans. (From Stuber M, Botnar RM, Danias PG, et al. Double-oblique free-breathing high-resolution 3D coronary MRA. *J Am Coll Cardiol* 1999;34:524–531, with permission.)

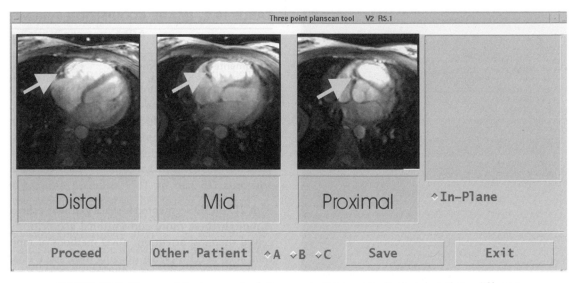

FIGURE 16.8. Three-point planscan tool. Transverse images are displayed at three different anatomic levels acquired with a free-breathing navigator-gated three-dimensional turbo-field echo–echo-planar imaging (TFE-EPI) scout sequence. On all three levels, the user manually identifies the right coronary artery *(arrows)* with a three-point planscan tool. The double-oblique imaging plane through all three points is automatically determined. (From Stuber M, Botnar RM, Danias PG, et al. Double-oblique free-breathing high-resolution 3D coronary MRA. *J Am Coll Cardiol* 1999;34:524–531, with permission.)

holds can be used for respiratory compensation. This technique, first described in humans by Edelman and colleagues (12), takes full advantage of the inflow-related contrast between coronary blood and surrounding stationary tissues. Still, 2D approaches are limited by the tortuous nature of the coronary vessels; focal signal loss related to the deviation of the coronary artery out of the image plane may be misinterpreted as a focal stenosis. SNR constraints, registration errors related to inconsistency between serial breath-holds, and diaphragmatic drift during sustained respiration are additional impediments to 2D breath-hold coronary MRA. With the development of advanced gradient systems and improvements in scanner software, respiration-compensated 3D coronary MRA approaches have become widely available (35,53). Three-dimensional coronary MRA overcomes several of the limitations of 2D techniques (5,26) and offers significant advantages, including enhanced SNR, improved slice registration, and less operator interaction with the patient. The improved SNR is particularly valuable because it can be "traded" for improved spatial resolution. Additionally, thinner adjacent slices can be obtained, and the volumetric image data can be postprocessed in any orientation. However, 3D approaches for coronary MRA often offer a lower CNR because of the attenuated blood inflow effect. Thus, the use of contrast agents in 3D coronary MRA techniques may have greater potential than in 2D approaches. With recent 3D acquisition schemes, such as spiral imaging (64,65) and free-breathing real-time navigator approaches, submillimeter spatial resolution has been achieved (33) (Figs. 16.9 and 16.10).

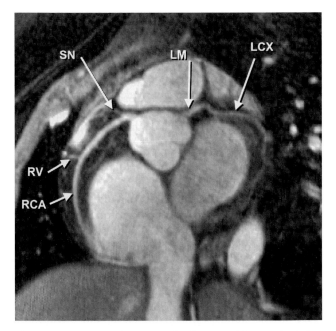

FIGURE 16.9. Three-dimensional reformatted image depicting the right coronary artery *(RCA)*, left main coronary artery *(LM)*, and left circumflex coronary artery *(LCX)*. The in-plane spatial resolution is 0.7 × 1.0 mm. The sinus node branch *(SN)* and an acute marginal branch *(RV)* are also seen. The image was acquired with a double-oblique T2 preparation navigator-gated and -corrected three-dimensional segmented k-space gradient-echo imaging sequence. (From Stuber M, Botnar RM, Danias PG, et al. Double-oblique free-breathing high-resolution 3D coronary MRA. *J Am Coll Cardiol* 1999;34:524–531, with permission.)

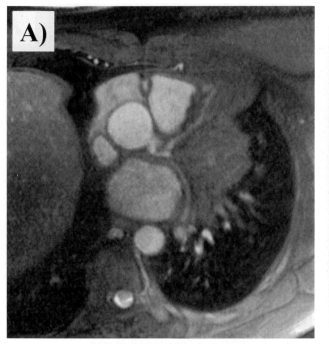
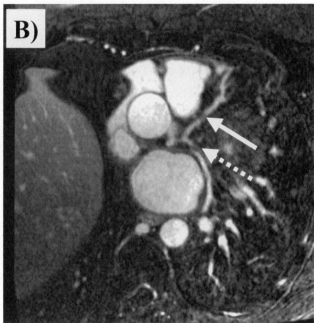

Endogenous Contrast Enhancement (T2Prep)

Exogenous Contrast Enhancement (MS-325/AngioMARK + Inversion)

FIGURE 16.15. Coronary MRA of a left coronary system acquired in a patient with x-ray–defined left anterior descending *(solid arrow)* and proximal left coronary circumflex *(dotted arrow)* disease. The image in **(A)** was acquired by means of a free-breathing three-dimensional (3D) T2 preparation navigator-gated and -corrected segmented k-space gradient-echo sequence. After administration of an intravascular T1-lowering contrast agent (MS-325), the image in **(B)** was acquired during free breathing with use of an inversion prepulse, a right hemidiaphragmatic navigator for gating and motion correction, and a 3D segmented k-space gradient-echo imaging sequence. (From Stuber M, Botnar RM, Danias PG, et al. Contrast agent-enhanced, free-breathing, three-dimensional coronary magnetic resonance angiography. *J Magn Reson Imaging* 1999;10: 790–799, with permission.)

sionally successful in identifying coronary ostia, this approach was not reliable for assessing anomalous vessels or disease. In one of the earliest studies, Lieberman et al. (3) used an ECG-gated spin-echo technique and were able to visualize portions of the native coronary arteries in only 7 (30%) of 23 subjects. Subsequently, Paulin et al. (4) used a similar methodology in six patients who had undergone x-ray coronary angiography. Even though the data were acquired during ventricular systole, respiratory motion was not suppressed, and the data were acquired over several minutes, the origin of the left main coronary artery was seen in all six subjects and the ostium of the right coronary artery in four of six subjects. No stenoses were visualized in either report. Subsequently, bright blood gradient-echo techniques came into greater use and made it possible to visualize proximal to middle portions of the coronary arteries in healthy and diseased states.

Two-Dimensional and Three-Dimensional Fast Spin-Echo Black Blood Coronary MRA

Although it has been used successfully, it is difficult to delineate luminal stenosis accurately with bright blood TOF coronary MRA because focal turbulent flow may result in artifactual "darkening" (83). The vessel luminal diameter may therefore be underestimated, and results appear biased in comparison with those of conventional x-ray angiography. In addition, the signal intensity of thrombus, vessel wall, and various components of plaque may appear high on bright blood coronary MRA (59), so that focal stenosis is obscured. Methods based on spin-echo imaging also have the potential for enhancing CNR in comparison with gradient-echo approaches. Thus, a "black blood" spin-echo–based coronary MRA technique that exclusively displays the coronary blood pool may offer advantages in coronary MRA.

Submillimeter black blood coronary MRA images have been acquired successfully with the use of ECG-triggered navigator-gated free-breathing dual-inversion 2D fast spin-echo MRA (56) (Figs. 16.17 and 16.18). Black blood methods appear to be particularly advantageous for patients with metallic implants, such as vascular clips, markers, and sternal wires. These metallic objects are a source of local magnetic field inhomogeneities. The size of the artifacts is increased with gradient-echo bright blood coronary MRA but

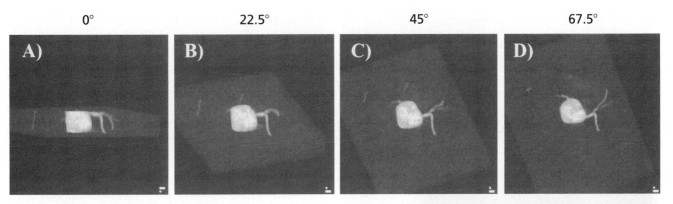

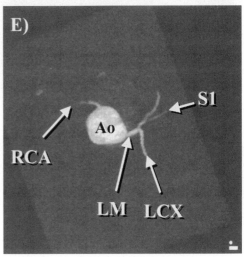

FIGURE 16.16. Coronary MRA data of a left coronary system acquired by means of aortic spin tagging (spin labeling) in conjunction with a free-breathing three-dimensional (3D) interleaved navigator-gated and -corrected spiral imaging sequence. For signal labeling in parallel to the ascending aorta, a 2D selective "pencil beam" inversion of the magnetization was applied. **A–E:** The images display maximum intensity projections of the same data at incremental viewing angles about the left–right axis. On these images, the ascending aorta *(Ao)*, left main *(LM)* coronary artery, left anterior descending *(LAD)* coronary artery, and a septal branch *(S1)* can be seen. A situation acquired 200 milliseconds after spin tagging is displayed.

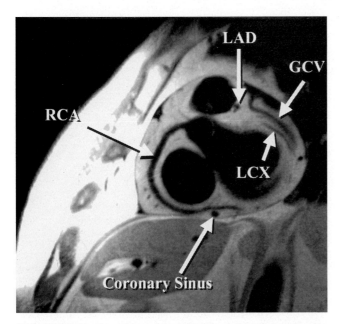

FIGURE 16.17. Two-dimensional dual-inversion fast spin-echo black blood coronary MRA of a right coronary system *(RCA)* acquired during free breathing with the use of navigator gating and motion correction. The image also shows a perpendicular cut through the left anterior descending *(LAD)* coronary artery and the coronary sinus, a proximal segment of the left circumflex *(LCX)* coronary artery, and a portion of the great cardiac vein *(GCV)*. (From Stuber M, Botnar RM, Danias PG, et al. Free-breathing black blood coronary magnetic resonance angiography: initial results. *Radiology* 2001;219:278–283, with permission.)

minimized with black blood approaches (Fig. 16.18). The high CNR between the coronary blood pool and the surrounding tissue on 2D fast spin-echo dual-inversion coronary MRA also suggested that an extension with a 3D fast spin-echo imaging sequence might further enhance the CNR and that CNR enhancement could be traded for an enhanced spatial resolution. Therefore, a 3D implementation with a "technical" in-plane spatial resolution of 500 μm has been proposed (50) (Fig. 16.19).

CORONARY MRA—FUTURE OUTLOOK

Current research in coronary MRA is focused on the clinical assessment of many of the advanced methods described in this chapter. The goal is to provide a novel noninvasive test that makes it possible to screen for major disease of the proximal and middle coronary arteries. Despite many advances during the past decade, the SNR and speed of data acquisition still must be improved for high-resolution coronary MRA. To overcome these hurdles, several groups are working on novel approaches, including spiral acquisition, MR contrast agents, tagging of blood in the aortic root, black blood coronary MRA, and rapid acquisition schemes, such as SMASH and SENSE. Although beyond the scope of

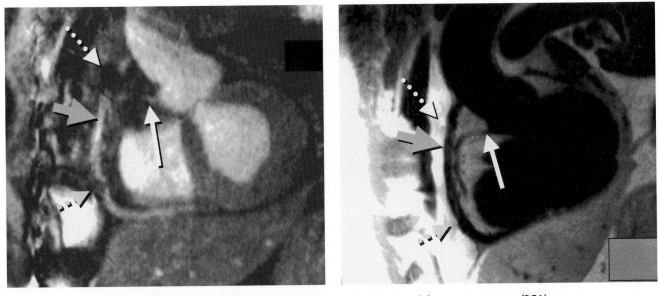

A

B

FIGURE 16.18. A 65-year-old man with a 100% proximal native right coronary artery *(RCA)* occlusion *(solid white arrow)* and RCA bypass graft *(bold gray arrow)*. A conventional bright blood coronary MRA **(A)** is compared with a black blood coronary MRA **(B)**. Both images were acquired in the same double-oblique view in parallel to the RCA bypass graft. Local artifacts induced by a vascular clip *(dotted white arrow)* and a sternal wire *(dashed gray arrow)* obscure the bright blood coronary MRA. These artifacts are minimized on the black blood coronary MRA, in which a long, continuous segment of the RCA bypass graft is visualized. (From Stuber M, Botnar RM, Danias PG, et al. Free-breathing black blood coronary magnetic resonance angiography: initial results. *Radiology* 2001;219:278–283, with permission.)

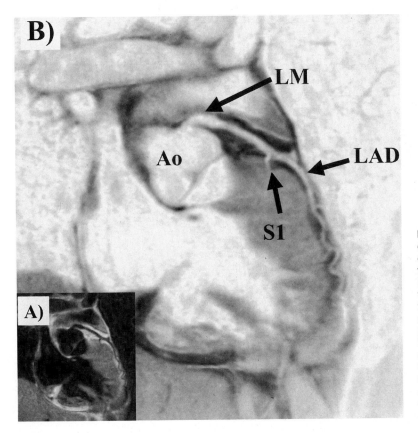

FIGURE 16.19. Three-dimensional black blood dual-inversion fast spin-echo coronary MRA of a left coronary system acquired with an in-plane resolution of 500 μm. The data were acquired during free breathing with the use of navigator gating and motion correction. A continuous 11.4-cm segment of the combined left main *(LM)* and left anterior descending *(LAD)* coronary arteries is displayed together with a portion of a septal branch *(S1)*. In the image in **(A)**, the multiplanar reformatted original data are displayed, and in the image in **(B)**, a zoomed video-inverted version of the same data is shown. (From Stuber M, Botnar RM, Spuentrup E, et al. Three-dimensional high-resolution fast spin-echo coronary magnetic resonance angiography. *Magn Reson Med* 2001;45:206–211, with permission.)

this chapter, cardiac MR also has the potential to image the coronary vessel wall noninvasively and detect subclinical atherosclerotic plaque, so that new insights may be acquired into the development and progress of subclinical atherosclerosis.

Parallel Imaging Techniques

Parallel imaging techniques such as SMASH (70) and SENSE (71) offer a novel method of markedly abbreviating the time required for image acquisition. Both SMASH and SENSE require minimal hardware modifications. Traditionally, the imaging speed depended on gradient performance. In contrast, these parallel imaging methods take advantage of the sensitivity maps of multiple coil arrays, so that image reconstruction is possible following the acquisition of a fraction of k-space. The remaining data are then reconstructed by using the sensitivity information of the individual coil elements. The "cost" is an expected loss of SNR, with a "benefit" of imaging speed. In principle, these two novel parallel imaging techniques can be combined with any of the above-described imaging sequences, and promising results have already been obtained in combinations with a free-breathing, navigator-gated and -corrected, T2 preparation coronary MRA technique (84) (Fig. 16.20).

Stents

The number of cardiac patients who undergo percutaneous revascularization with intracoronary stents is increasing. Stents are metallic implants that locally distort the magnetic field, and they may appear as signal voids on MR images. As a consequence, the direct assessment of stent patency with MR is not practical. In comparison with gradient-echo approaches, techniques based on fast spin-echo imaging may minimize such artifacts; however, no large patient studies have been reported. The stent geometry, material, and orientation with respect to the main magnetic field are variables that cannot be controlled and that substantially influence the appearance of artifacts (85–87). Therefore, MR-compatible stents may have to be developed, and the use of MR techniques (e.g., spin tagging) to assess stent patency remains to be studied in more detail.

Interventional Coronary MRA

Recently developed receiver coil designs, MR-compatible catheters, interactive real-time user interfaces, and short-bore systems may be combined in interventional coronary MRA (88). Even though presently at a very early developmental stage, catheter tracking, contrast injection, coronary stent placement, and coronary angioplasty under real-time MR surveillance are currently under active investigation. However, the fundamental noninvasive advantage of MRI would be sacrificed, and the specific benefit of interventional coronary MRA would have to be defined in comparison with that of conventional x-ray coronary angiography.

High-Field-Strength Coronary MRA

A growing number of research centers are investigating the potential role of high-field-strength (>1.5 T) whole body

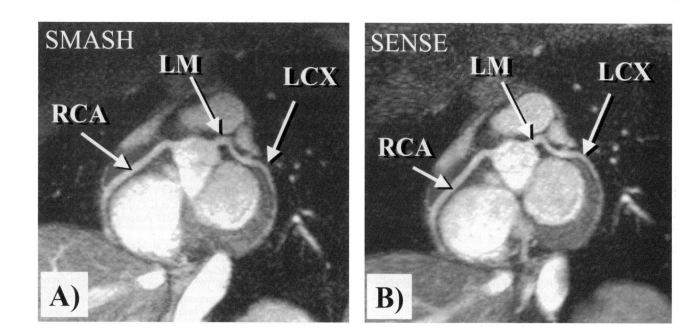

FIGURE 16.20. Right coronary artery *(RCA)* and left main *(LM)* and left circumflex *(LCX)* coronary arteries acquired by means of simultaneous acquisition of spatial harmonics (SMASH) **(A)** (84) and sensitivity encoding (SENSE) **(B)** with an acceleration factor of 2 for both techniques. (Images courtesy of D. K. Sodickson.)

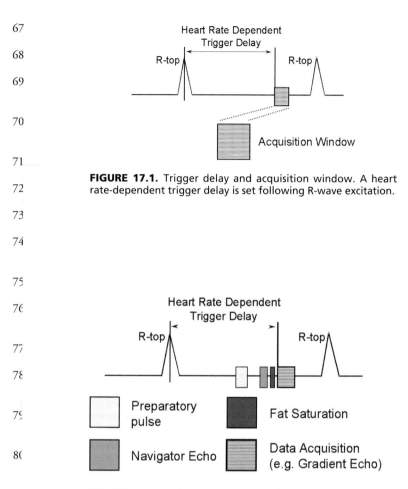

FIGURE 17.1. Trigger delay and acquisition window. A heart rate-dependent trigger delay is set following R-wave excitation.

FIGURE 17.2. Navigator sequence. Before the acquisition window, a navigator echo detects a diaphragm level that includes or excludes acquisition data. Usually, a preparation pulse for contrast enhancement and a fat saturation pulse are applied (see Chapter 16).

expiratory period of the respiratory cycle. This is achieved by applying a navigator echo that tracks diaphragm motion during coronary MRA (Figs. 17.2 and 17.3). Within the end-expiratory period, the imaging scanplane translates parallel according to the remaining diaphragm motion. This technique is called *slice tracking* and minimizes the respiratory motion artifacts. The navigator sequence usually is an ultrafast three-dimensional (3D) gradient-echo sequence that is preceded by the navigator echo. The navigator technique is very robust and reliable, but it prolongs the scan time and is not yet widely available clinically (2–5). The alternative technique is the breath-hold approach. Respiratory motion artifacts are reduced when patients hold their breath. A variant, called *volume coronary angiography with targeted scans* (VCATS), is a breath-hold technique wherein the coronary artery tree is covered in one or multiple breath-holds (6) (Fig. 17.4). The breath-hold sequence usually is an ultrafast ECG-triggered 3D gradient-echo or echo-planar sequence. The breath-hold approach has the advantage of limiting the duration of acquisition, but patients must be able to cooperate and be physically able to hold their breath. Coronary MRA techniques are discussed in further detail in Chapter 16.

ANOMALOUS CORONARY ARTERIES

Background

The most generally accepted clinical application of coronary MRA today is the evaluation of anomalous coronary arteries. Coronary anomalies represent a potentially lethal disorder in a number of cases.

Major coronary anomalies are found in 0.3% to 0.8% of the population (7). Of all adults referred to x-ray angiography for chest pain, approximately 0.85% are found to have at least one anomalous coronary artery. Particularly in children and young adults, this condition is among the main

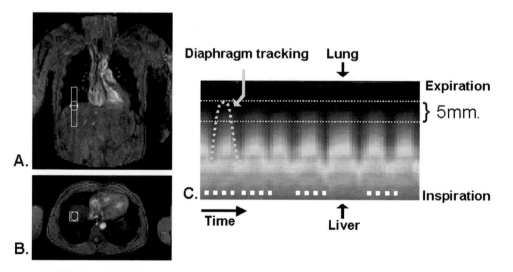

FIGURE 17.3. Planning the navigator beam. During data acquisition, the navigator beam *(white rectangular area)* scans the diaphragm. Coronal **(A)** and transverse **(B)** views. **C:** The motion of the diaphragm in time. Data are accepted only during expiration over a small, 5-mm trajectory.

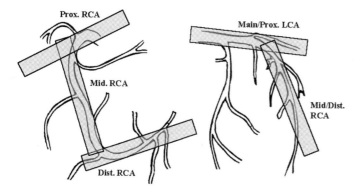

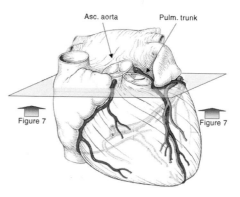

FIGURE 17.4. Example breath-hold planning according to volume coronary angiography with targeted scans (2).

causes of sudden cardiac death (8). In a 20-year prospective study of young athletes, an anomalous coronary artery was identified as the cause of death in 12% of all athletes who died suddenly (9). The prevalence of anomalous coronary arteries is higher in patients with congenital anomalies; anomalies may be detected in 3% to 36% of all cases of congenital heart disease. Because patients with congenital heart disease often undergo operative procedures and detailed information regarding the coronary anatomy is required to avoid damage to the arteries, it is essential that anomalies be identified correctly. In particular, in patients with tetralogy of Fallot, an anomalous artery or large conus branch may pass over the right ventricular outflow tract; if not correctly identified, this is likely to be severed during ventriculotomy (2).

Coronary anomalies:

- High incidence in congenital heart disease
- Associated with sudden death
- High-risk when interarterial course

Diagnostic x-ray angiography is generally accepted as the method of first choice for detecting coronary anomalies. Recent advances in high-resolution coronary MRA, however, have shown coronary MRA to be a very reliable tool for evaluating coronary anomalies. It may be difficult to identify anomalous coronary arteries with conventional x-ray angiography because it does not provide 3D information that relates the course of the anomalous coronary artery to that of the great vessels. However, 3D visualization is an unsurpassed feature of coronary MRA, which therefore is now generally proposed as the new gold standard for detecting coronary anomalies (Fig. 17.5).

Anatomy and Pathology

In the normal anatomic situation, the right coronary artery (RCA) originates from the right coronary sinus and travels in the right atrioventricular groove. The left coronary artery (LCA) originates from the left coronary sinus and after 10 mm bifurcates to form the left main (LM) and left circumflex coronary arteries (LCx). The LM artery travels in the interventricular groove, whereas the LCx artery runs in the left atrioventricular groove (Fig. 17.6).

In anomalous situations, the origin of the anomalous coronary artery is often at the wrong, opposite side of the aorta, whereas the distal part is in situ. In other words, the anomalous artery runs from its anomalous origin to its

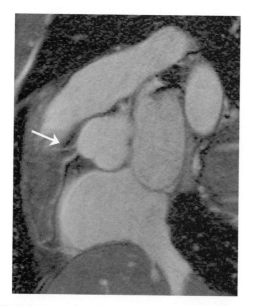

FIGURE 17.5. Example of coronary MRA revealing separate origins of a nondominant right coronary artery and conus artery (*white arrow*).

FIGURE 17.6. Normal anatomy. Coronary arteries in relation to the origin of the great vessels. A cross-sectional plane is applied. A schematic projection of this cross-sectional plane is shown in Figure 17.7, which illustrates the anatomical variants of coronary anomalies.

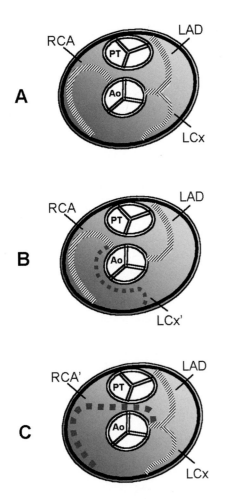

FIGURE 17.7. Examples of aberrant coronary arteries. **A:** Normal anatomy. **B:** Common anomaly of the left circumflex artery originating in the right sinus. **C:** Malignant interarterial anomaly of the right coronary artery originating in the left sinus. *PT,* pulmonary trunk; *Ao,* ascending aorta.

blood-supplying area at the opposite site of the aorta. This "detour" may be posterior to the aorta (retroaortic), between the ascending aorta and pulmonary trunk/right ventricular outflow tract (interarterial), or anterior to the pulmonary trunk (Fig. 17.7). The most common adult form of coro-

nary anomaly is an aberrant origin of the LCx from the right sinus of Valsalva (Fig. 17.7B). The second most common anomaly is an aberrant origin of the RCA from the left sinus of Valsalva (8) (Fig. 17.7C). In the latter, the course of the anomalous artery may be interarterial, running between aorta and main pulmonary artery, a pattern that is associated with a high risk for sudden cardiac death. Fig. 17.8 shows an MR example of a malignant anomalous coronary artery.

Most coronary anomalies are not of hemodynamic significance, except for the interarterial variant. An anomalous coronary artery with an interarterial course is associated with exercise-induced ischemia, myocardial infarction, and sudden cardiac death in young patients. This type of anomaly is therefore said to be "malignant." Several hypotheses for the malignant association have been proposed: (a) impingement on the anomalous coronary artery by the aorta and pulmonary artery, particularly during exercise, when aortic and pulmonary dilation occur in response to increased cardiac output, in combination with increased coronary flow; (b) limitation of flow caused by a sharp turn or bend at the aberrant origin of the coronary vessel; (c) ostial stenosis of the aberrant origin. These factors may individually or together contribute to the malignant properties. An anomaly in which the LM coronary artery originates from the right sinus of Valsalva and follows an interarterial course is considered to be associated with the highest risk for ischemia and sudden cardiac death (8).

Clinical Applications

Coronary MRA has proved to be a relatively easy-to-use and noninvasive diagnostic tool for detecting coronary anomalies in combination with respiratory navigator and breath-hold techniques. Several studies have been performed to evaluate the accuracy of anomaly identification with coronary MRA. Sensitivities of 88% to 100% and specificities of 100% for detecting a proximal anomalous course have been reported repeatedly (2,7). The accuracy of x-ray angiography, the current gold standard, in detecting anomalies has previously been discussed (10,11). The lack of anatomic 3D

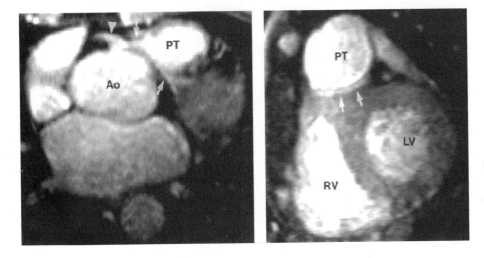

FIGURE 17.8. Coronary MRA of a malignant coronary anomaly. The left main coronary artery originates from the right aortic sinus and crosses to the left, following an interarterial course between the aorta and pulmonary trunk. (Courtesy of J. C. Post.)

visualization relating the course of the coronary artery to other thoracic structures is a major shortcoming of x-ray angiography. MRI may prove very useful in filling this gap.

In conclusion, MRI is an accurate tool for evaluating anomalous coronary arteries. In clinical practice, coronary MRA may serve as a final diagnostic procedure whenever the results of x-ray angiography are inconclusive (2,12). On the other hand, because of the excellent MR image quality and 3D anatomic visualization it provides, coronary MRA may be considered the first-choice diagnostic method for detecting anomalies.

CORONARY ARTERY STENOSIS

Background

Coronary artery disease remains the leading cause of death in Western society (13). In clinical practice today, patients with suspected coronary disease are routinely scheduled for conventional x-ray angiography to confirm or exclude stenotic lesions, and x-ray angiography is the gold standard for quantifying stenosis. Despite its indisputable efficacy in detecting coronary stenosis, x-ray angiography is an invasive technique associated with a definite risk for severe complications: ventricular tachycardia or fibrillation (0.2% to 0.3%), myocardial infarction (<0.1%), and death (0.1%) (14–16). In response, several less invasive imaging modalities for evaluating coronary pathology have been investigated that entail less risk and provide safer and less costly alternatives for patient screening and follow-up; these include computed tomography, echocardiography, and coronary MRA. Coronary MRA is one of the most promising techniques.

Technical Coronary MRA requirements for stenosis detection:

- High spatial resolution (submillimeter)
- Contrast to background
- Cardiac motion compensation
- Respiratory motion compensation

Imaging techniques:

- 2D breath hold
- 3D breath hold
- 3D navigator gating

MRI Technique

Coronary MRA for detecting and quantifying coronary artery stenosis is still at an experimental stage but is rapidly evolving. Evaluation of the carotid arteries, aorta, intracerebral arteries, and other peripheral arteries with MRA is an established method in many centers. Accurate and reliable MRA of the coronary arteries, however, is technically more challenging. Obstacles are the relatively small size of the vessels, their tortuous anatomic course, and the persistent spatial shift caused by cardiac and respiratory motion (1,17,18). Therefore, an accurate quantification of coronary stenosis with coronary MRA depends on several technical factors. First, a reasonable spatial resolution relative to vessel diameter should be achieved. The vessel diameter should exceed voxel size several times to allow for accurate quantification. In comparison with the spatial resolution of invasive x-ray angiography, which is 0.3 mm, that of coronary MRA currently ranges from 0.7 to below 0.4 mm in experimental studies (5,19). Voxel size (spatial resolution) is related to hardware capabilities, applied scan sequences, and slab volume. Second, the contrast between vessel and background should be optimally enhanced to depict and delineate the coronary vessels. Contrast may be enhanced with any of the following: (a) flow phenomena; (b) the physiologic relaxation difference between blood and myocardium (T2 preparation); (c) new imaging techniques, such as steady-state free precession [balanced FFE (fast-field echo), true FISP (fast imaging with steady-state free precession)] and spiral k-space acquisition; (d) contrast agents. Third, compensation for cardiac and respiratory movement should be applied, as previously described in the section on coronary MRA techniques.

Clinical Applications

Numerous studies have been performed in which breath-hold and navigator techniques were used to evaluate the capabilities and diagnostic value of coronary MRA. The first clinical attempts at visualizing the coronary arteries were possible only after the introduction of segmented k-space strategies, in which multiple phase-encoding steps are acquired during one heartbeat. Therefore, a single 2D image can be covered in 16 heartbeats, so that breath-hold coronary MRA can be applied clinically. This 2D approach is fully dependent on in-flow phenomena for signal and contrast properties.

Two-Dimensional Breath-Hold Approach

The first study of a series of patients in which a 2D breath-hold approach was used to detect stenosis was published by Manning and Edelman in 1993 (20). This study reported a sensitivity of 90% and a specificity of 92% for the correct identification of stenoses of 50% or more; x-ray angiography was used as a reference. Since then, several other studies in which 2D breath-hold acquisitions were used have been performed with varying outcomes; overall sensitivities between 36% and 90% and specificities between 82% and 95% were observed (21,22). The reported ranges vary according to the specific segments of the coronary tree imaged. For example, Post et al. (23) reported a sensitivity of 0% (n = 30) for the LCx artery, 53% (n = 30) for the left anterior descending (LAD) artery, 71% (n = 31) for the RCA, and 100% (n = 34) for the LM artery in the detection of significant coronary artery stenosis. Sensitivities in the study of Manning and

Edelman (20) were 71% (n = 7) for the LCx artery, 87% (n = 23) for the LAD artery, 100% (n = 2) for the LM artery, and 100% (n = 20) for the RCA. Three years later, Pennell et al. (24) reported a sensitivity of 75% for the LCx artery, 75% to 100% for the RCA, 88% for the LAD artery, and 100% for the LM artery, resulting in an overall sensitivity of 85% (47 of 55) in the detection of stenosis. Several factors that may influence study outcome hinder 2D breath-hold techniques. Considerable operator skill is required since multiple slices are needed to image the tortuous coronary arteries. The acquisition of multiple slices may result in slice misregistration due to inconsistent diaphragm levels during breath-holding. Additional impediments are the relatively long duration of the acquisition and the suboptimal signal of vessels that are not close to the receiver coil. The latter particularly affects the LCx artery. This problem can be overcome by applying combined coils, called *phased-array coils.* The long time required for planning the scan and performing multiple breath-holds may be overcome in part as operator skills are perfected.

Consequently, 3D volume acquisitions were developed (Fig. 17.9). The advantages of 3D coronary MRA in comparison with the 2D approach are the following: improved signal-to-noise ratio, improved slice registration, less operator dependency, and increased possibilities for image post-processing. However, in 3D acquisitions, the contrast-to-noise ratio may be hampered because in-flow effects are reduced. In addition, spatial resolution may not be as high as in the equivalent 2D acquisitions because a whole volume must be covered in one breath-hold instead of a single 2D slice. The latter problem does not arise in the navigator approach, which is not restricted by the time required for the breath-hold. Breath-hold or navigator respiratory approaches may be combined with 3D acquisitions.

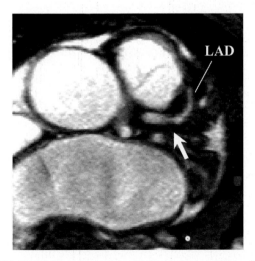

FIGURE 17.9. Stenotic lesion. High-resolution three-dimensional navigator acquisition of the left anterior descending artery (one slice of a 20-slice slab, in-plane resolution 0.7 × 1.1 mm). The *white arrow* indicates an angiographically confirmed stenotic lesion.

Three-Dimensional Breath-Hold Approach

Few clinical trials of the 3D breath-hold approach have been performed with an adequate patient cohort. Similar to 2D imaging, the sensitivity and specificity for stenosis detection vary for the individual segments. For example, Van Geuns et al. (25) reported sensitivities of 0 (n = 4) for the LCx artery, 64% for the RCA (n = 14), and 77% (n = 13) for the LM and LAD arteries, for an overall sensitivity of 68% in the detection of significant stenosis with a VCATS technique (25).

Three-Dimensional Navigator Approach

When navigator respiratory correction is used, the duration of the acquisition is not restricted to the physical breath-holding capacity of the subject. Therefore, a high spatial resolution in large slabs can be achieved, even at the submillimeter level in routinely used acquisitions. The use of navigator in combination with T2 preparation has been proposed to improve the contrast between the coronary vessels and surrounding myocardial tissue and epicardial fat (5). Huber et al. (26) reported sensitivities of 71% for the proximal and middle segments of the LAD artery, 80% for the proximal and middle segments of the LCx artery, and 89% for the proximal and middle segments of the RCA. A sensitivity of 100% was reported for the proximal LCx artery.

The clinical utility of 3D navigator coronary MRA was recently evaluated in a multicenter trial performed by Kim and colleagues (27). In this trial, the sensitivities for coronary MRA to correctly identify significant stenosis (≥50%) were 67% for the left main, 88% for the LAD, 53% for the LCx, and 93% for the RCA. The specificities were 90%, 52%, 70%, and 72%, respectively. The identification of left main or three-vessel disease could be performed with 100% sensitivity and 85% specificity. This study shows that 3D coronary MRA allows for accurate detection of coronary arery disease in multiple cardiovascular research centers.

In conclusion, currently feasible 3D breath-hold and navigator techniques can provide excellent high-resolution images. Several studies have shown that coronary MRA may accurately detect proximal coronary artery stenosis. Current technical developments such as parallel image acquisition, spiral imaging, steady state free precession, and the introduction of blood pool contrast agents may result in improved visualization of the middle and distal coronary artery segments. This may allow coronary MRA to be clinically applied for diagnosis of coronary artery stenosis.

QUANTIFICATION OF CORONARY FLOW AND FLOW RESERVE

Background

As part of the examination of coronary artery disease, it is important to assess the hemodynamic significance of a coronary artery lesion because the extent of ischemia is a strong predictor of the development of cardiac disease (28). The hemodynamic significance of coronary stenosis can be quantified by measuring coronary flow and flow reserve. Conventionally, coronary flow is quantified with an intravascular Doppler flowmeter during cardiac catheterization. Alternative and less invasive measures include single photon emission computed tomography (SPECT), transthoracic echocardiography, and transesophageal echocardiography. In addition, MRI has the potential to measure coronary flow noninvasively with a high rate of accuracy.

MRI Technique

Coronary flow is usually measured with phase-shift velocity mapping. This technique is based on the observation that as spins move with a velocity along a magnetic field gradient, they acquire a phase shift. The accumulation of flow-induced shift is proportional to the velocity and is directly correlated with signal intensity. The flow acquisition data are calculated to an image called a *phase velocity map*. In this image, velocity differences in moving spins can be depicted and calculated to flow. If phase-shift velocity mapping is combined with a fast segmented k-space acquisition and cine imaging, multiphase coronary flow can be acquired within a single breath-hold (14,29).

Measurements of flow reserve express functional properties of diseased and healthy coronary arteries. Coronary flow reserve is calculated as the ratio of flow at stress to baseline flow. In the normal situation, coronary vessels dilate in response to physical stress to allow for an increase in coronary flow. In a diseased coronary system, the stenotic vessels do not respond to stress and so prevent coronary flow from increasing in response to stress. Therefore, the coronary flow reserve is a measure of coronary stenotic disease. Flow reserve can be measured by acquiring MR images before and after the application of stress. Stress can be clinically induced either by exercise (treadmill) or pharmacologically (e.g., adenosine or dobutamine).

Coronary flow reserve (CFR)

Stress induction:

- Pharmacologic
- Exercise

Imaging:

- Cine gradient echo
- Echo planar imaging

Flow reserve calculation:

$$CFR = \frac{\text{Coronary flow}_{stress}}{\text{Coronary flow}_{baseline}}$$

In MR flow measurements, several types of error may affect accuracy: (a) With a low spatial resolution relative to vessel diameter, an overestimation of coronary blood flow may be caused by intravoxel averaging of the signal of flowing blood and the signal of static tissue at the vessel edge. (b) With insufficient temporal resolution, image blurring and subsequent inaccurate flow measurements may be caused by a long acquisition window (29). It has been calculated that for reliable coronary flow measurements, the acquisition window should be less than 25 milliseconds for the RCA and less than 120 milliseconds for the LAD artery (30).

Clinical Applications

Several studies have successfully measured coronary flow with MRI acquisitions. Hundley et al. (31) measured coronary flow and coronary flow reserve with phase-contrast MRI and adenosine stress and compared the results with measurements obtained with an intravascular flowmeter. Excellent correlation with the invasive Doppler flowmeter measurements ($r = .89$ for both coronary flow and coronary flow reserve) suggested accurate MR flow measurements. Sakuma et al. (32) demonstrated a correlation of MR measurements of coronary flow reserve with positron emission tomography (PET) measurements ($r = .79$). Schwitter et al. (33) assessed coronary sinus flow and showed MR flow measurement to be highly accurate in comparison with PET flow measurement (mean difference of 2.2% between MRI and PET). A clinical application of the MRI measurement of coronary flow reserve may be the use of serial measurements of flow reserve to detect restenosis after balloon angioplasty (29). In a recent study of Hundley and colleagues (34), MR coronary flow reserve measurement was highly sensitive and specific for coronary stenosis with x-ray angiography used as the standard of reference. A coronary flow reserve of 2.0 or less was 100% sensitive and 89% specific for detecting luminal narrowing of 70% or more, and 82% sensitive and 100% specific for detecting luminal narrowing of 50% or more.

In conclusion, MRI coronary flow measurements as part of an evaluation for coronary disease may be highly effective in the follow-up of patients who have undergone coronary angioplasty. MR flow measurement has the potential to be a cost-effective, noninvasive, and accurate tool for detecting asymptomatic coronary artery disease.

CONTRAST-ENHANCED CORONARY MRA

MR contrast agents act by altering the T1 or T2 of blood and thereby inducing a change in blood signal that is independent of flow. A variety of contrast agents are currently available for clinical use. These include short-acting agents (extravascular) and long-acting blood pool contrast agents (intravascular).

Contrast Agents

The active substance of a contrast agent may be iron or gadolinium. Ferrous agents consist of ultrasmall particles of iron oxide (USPIOs). USPIO agents are super-paramagnetic macromolecular compounds with a low r1/r2 relaxivity ratio and increase the signal intensity of blood only at low concentrations. USPIOs are not well suited for coronary artery imaging because of the rapid occurrence of T2* effects (signal loss caused by local field inhomogeneities) and a moderate T1-lowering capacity.

Gadolinium, one of the lanthanide elements, is chelated to a core to eliminate its toxic properties. The molecular structure of the core accounts for the pharmacokinetic properties of the compound and its effects on relaxation time. Currently, the gadolinium compounds are the first-choice agents for coronary MRA.

Gadolinium compounds are categorized as extravascular or intravascular contrast agents. Extravascular gadolinium agents have a small molecular weight that allows them to diffuse freely through the capillary endothelium (Fig. 17.10). Extravascular gadolinium agents, such as gadoterate meglumine (DOTAREM, Guerbet, Aulnay sous Bois, France) and Magnevist (gadopentetate dimeglumine; Berlex Laboratories, Wayne, New Jersey), are widely used for imaging the carotid, renal, and peripheral arteries. Extravascular agents, however, are of limited value in coronary MRA because they diffuse rapidly to interstitium and myocardial tissue. As a result, coronary background tissue is enhanced and image contrast decreased. Particularly during acquisitions with long imaging times, such as VCATS and respiratory navigator, extravasation significantly affects image quality. Recently, however, extravascular contrast agents have been shown to be useful in delayed enhancement techniques. These relatively simple imaging techniques exploit the diffusion of small contrast agent molecules into ischemic myocardial areas. Once injected, the contrast agent spreads over the myocardium, including the ischemic regions. Because of local flow disturbances and diminished local tissue metabolism in ischemic areas, the contrast agent is eliminated from ischemic areas more slowly than from healthy, perfused areas. The imaging technique may be a spin-echo sequence or a gradient-echo sequence with inversion prepulse following a time delay after injection (35). Extravascular agents can also be used for myocardial perfusion imaging. However, once injected, no additional coronary MRA examination can be performed because rapid extravasation distorts image contrast.

To solve extravasation-related problems, new contrast agents have been developed. These agents, commonly referred to as *blood pool contrast agents* (BPCAs), are currently undergoing clinical evaluation. Advantages of BPCAs include the following: (a) They have a high R1 relaxivity time, up to 10-fold that of conventional agents. This enhances the coronary signal and increases the contrast-to-noise ratio. (b) Their intravascular properties prevent extravasation to the background tissue. Blood pool confinement and therefore prolonged T1 shortening enable acquisitions that require a longer scan time or multiple sequential images. Examples of long acquisitions are multiple breath-holds and respiratory navigator acquisitions. Currently, the most promising BPCAs are gadolinium chelates. A subgroup of the BPCAs are the rapid clearance BPCAs, which combine intravascular confinement with rapid (e.g., 5 minutes) renal clearance. These features enable multiple injection schemes. When rapid clearance BPCAs are used, rest-stress perfusion imaging can be combined with coronary MRA.

T1 and Blood Pool Properties

The T1-lowering capacity of a contrast medium depends on the R1 relaxivity time because T1 and R1 are inversely related. The R1 depends on the gadolinium compound and its molecular structure. BPCAs have specific properties that limit transcapillary diffusion. The intravascular properties of a specific agent depend on several factors: absorption, distribution, metabolism, and elimination. Absorption is 100% when injection is intravenous. Distribution accounts almost entirely for the blood pool properties. A small distribution volume reflects slow extravasation. Extravasation may be limited by (a) linking the contrast agent to an intravascular carrier protein, such as serum albumin, or (b) incorporating the active substance into a macromolecule to make it larger than capillary fenestrations (Fig. 17.10). Metabolism depends on drug substance and solubility. In practice, metabolism is limited by the rapid excretion of the contrast agent. Elimination is renal or hepatic.

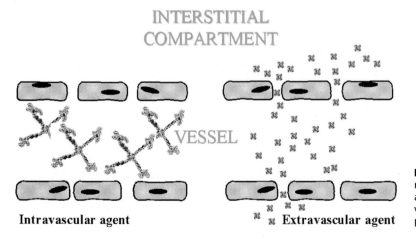

INTERSTITIAL COMPARTMENT

VESSEL

Intravascular agent

Extravascular agent

FIGURE 17.10. Intravascular mechanism. **Left:** The macromolecular structure of the blood pool contrast agent prevents transcapillary diffusion. **Right:** Conventional small-molecule contrast agent can freely pass the capillary endothelium.

T1 and R1 have an inverse relation:

$$T1 = \frac{1}{R1}$$

R1 depends on:

- Gadolinium compound
- Molecule structure

Blood pool properties depend on pharmacokinetics:

- Absorption
- Distribution
- Metabolism
- Elimination

Clinical Applications

The most promising applications of BPCAs in coronary MRA include contrast-enhanced detection of stenosis, contrast-enhanced bypass imaging, and contrast-enhanced diagnosis of coronary anomalies. Furthermore, rapid clearance BPCAs may prove useful in delayed enhancement strategies and perfusion imaging. The main advantage of rapid clearance BPCAs is that multiple injections can be administered because after each injection, the agent is rapidly excreted without extravasation (Fig. 17.11). Rapid clearance BPCAs may therefore contribute to the "one-stop shop" concept, wherein multiple MR examinations are performed within a single imaging session; for example, detection of stenosis is combined with quantification of coronary flow reserve and myocardial perfusion imaging.

Several studies have evaluated the use of contrast agents in coronary MRA. Regenfus et al. (36) performed an angiographically controlled study of 50 patients with suspected coronary artery disease in which they used a 3D sin-gle breath-hold method and an extravascular gadolinium agent. In this study, on a patient basis, coronary artery stenosis could be identified with a sensitivity of 94% and a specificity of 57%. Vrachliotis et al. (37) used angiographically controlled coronary MRA to study the patency of coronary artery bypass grafts. Breath-hold imaging was performed after administration of an extravascular contrast agent. A close agreement with conventional angiography was found, expressed by a sensitivity of 93% and a specificity of 97% (37).

Experimental studies have been performed in which BPCAs were used. It was shown that the application of a BPCA results in an increased contrast-to-noise ratio in comparison with noncontrast enhancement or the application of extravascular agents (38–42). In an animal experiment, Li and colleagues (39) demonstrated a substantial improvement in the contrast-to-noise ratio with the use of an intravascular contrast agent in comparison with an extravascular agent. Both breath-hold and navigator approaches benefited from the intravascular agent. Stuber and colleagues (38) demonstrated an improvement in the contrast-to-noise ratio after the application of a carrier-linked BPCA in six patients.

In conclusion, contrast agents, particularly BPCAs, may prove extremely useful in coronary MRA; however, large clinical trials must still be performed.

STENTS AND PACEMAKERS IN MRI: SAFETY CONSIDERATIONS

Coronary stents and cardiac pacemakers are implanted daily in the practice of cardiovascular medicine. The placement of coronary stents has become the major method of treating obstructive cardiovascular disease. Patients with coronary stents or implanted cardiac pacemakers may have to undergo MRI for a medical indication. In addition, MRI may be used to evaluate stent patency. Questions have arisen about the safety of stents and cardiac pacemakers in the

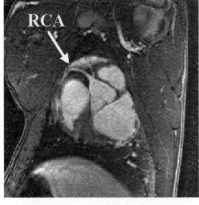

BPCA combined with
saturation background
suppression

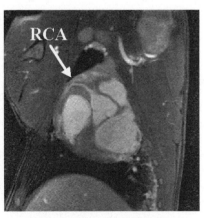

No contrast agent,
no saturation background
suppression

FIGURE 17.11. Example of a blood pool contrast agent (BPCA) application. **Left:** BPCA application is combined with active background suppression (saturation prepulse). Therefore, the surrounding tissue (myocardium and epicardial fat) is very well suppressed to facilitate vessel depiction. **Right:** No contrast agent was applied, so that a saturation prepulse for background suppression was not applied. (Data from an animal experiment.)

presence of the continuously increasing field strengths of modern MR systems, and the use of MRI to evaluate stent patency has been investigated.

Coronary Stents in MRI

Coronary stents typically consist of tantalum or stainless steel. After a stent is placed with a guidewire under x-ray control, it undergoes endothelialization and becomes part of the vessel wall. It has been shown that patients with implanted stents are not necessarily excluded from MR examination. However, with the strong static and gradient magnetic fields currently in use, the safety of patients with coronary stents has again been questioned. On the other hand, the demand for a noninvasive method to assess stent patency is increasing. MRI may play a significant role in the noninvasive assessment of stent patency with MRA and flow measurements.

It is generally recommended that patients with a coronary stent wait for several weeks after stent placement before undergoing an MR examination. Metallic stents made of weakly ferromagnetic materials are considered to be safe for patients in the MRI environment after 6 to 8 weeks (43). Exposing a stent to a strong magnetic field may cause displacement or heating. A recent study by Hug and colleagues (44) evaluated the translational forces and heating effects to which stents are subjected in strong magnetic fields. Even with fast gradients, no migration or heating of the investigated stents was noted. The risk for the displacement and heating of a metallic implant depends on several factors (44): (a) the static and gradient magnetic field strength (stent heating is most likely to occur in the presence of rapidly switching gradient fields, as in fast cardiac MRI schemes such as gradient-echo and echo-planar imaging); (b) the degree of ferromagnetism of the implanted device (tantalum and stainless steel are weakly ferromagnetic, so that they are less likely to become displaced or hot); (c) the geometry of the implanted device; and (d) the location and orientation of the implant in situ during MRI. These factors should always be carefully considered in MRI, particularly when the implanted device is located in a potentially dangerous area of the body, such as near a vascular structure, where possible migration or heating could cause severe injury.

Cardiac Pacemakers and Related Risks

Cardiac pacemakers and implantable cardioverter defibrillators (also called *implantable pulse generators*) constitute a potential hazard in strong magnetic fields such as those of MR systems. These implantable devices are subjected to several risks in strong magnetic fields (45): (a) Depending on the composition of the material, a static magnetic field may exert translational and torsional forces on a pacemaker, electrode wires, and connectors. This force theoretically may be strong enough to cause displacement of a pacemaker or disconnection of the wires and electrodes. The rapid change of field gradients and radiofrequency pulses can damage pacemaker electronics or alter pacemaker programs. (b) Currents induced by a magnetic field in pacemaker wires can cause alterations in sensing and triggering that may result in rapid or runaway pacing or even pacing arrest. (c) Reed switches (magnetic contact switches that are commonly used in pacemaker devices) may prematurely close or be damaged. (d) Heating of metallic parts with thermal damage to body tissues theoretically may occur.

The Medical Devices Agency and Food and Drug Administration guidelines strongly emphasize that pacemakers should not be exposed to magnetic fields that reach or exceed 0.5 millitesla (mT) [5 gauss (G)] because of the above-mentioned hazards. Exceptions may be made if the clinical need and risk-to-benefit ratio warrant exposure of an implanted pacemaker to an MR system (45). However, in such cases, a cardiac emergency team should always be on site. *In vitro* and *in vivo* experiments have been performed to evaluate the effects of MR examination on cardiac pacemakers. In a clinical study published by Sommer and colleagues (46), the authors state that MRI of patients with specific types of pacemakers can be performed safely with a 0.5-T system (46). Various other studies have concluded that the safety of exposing implanted pacemakers to magnetic fields strongly depends on the type of pacemaker device. For further information, see the Medical Devices Agency guidelines and the U.S. Food and Drug Administration guidelines (www.fda.gov), or consult your local center/authority.

In conclusion, depending on their anatomic location, stents are not a contraindication to MR investigation. MRI provides opportunities to assess stent patency. Precautions must be taken if a pacemaker is exposed to a strong magnetic field.

ACKNOWLEDGMENTS

We thank Albert de Roos and Joost Doornbos (of the Department of Radiology, Leiden University Medical Center, Leiden, The Netherlands) for advice and revision.

REFERENCES

1. Wang Y, Vidan E, Bergman GW. Cardiac motion of coronary arteries: variability in the rest period and implications for coronary MR angiography. *Radiology* 1999;213:751–758.
2. Taylor AM, Thorne SA, Rubens MB, et al. Coronary artery imaging in grown-up congenital heart disease: complementary role of magnetic resonance and x-ray coronary angiography. *Circulation* 2000;101:1670–1678.
3. Stuber M, Botnar RM, Danias PG, et al. Submillimeter three-dimensional coronary MR angiography with real-time navigator correction: comparison of navigator locations. *Radiology* 1999; 212:579–587.
4. Sardanelli F, Molinari G, Zandrino F, et al. Three-dimensional, navigator-echo MR coronary angiography in detecting stenoses of the major epicardial vessels, with conventional coronary angiography as the standard of reference. *Radiology* 2000;214:808–814.
5. Botnar RM, Stuber M, Danias PG, et al. Improved coronary artery definition with T2-weighted, free-breathing, three-dimensional coronary MRA. *Circulation* 1999;99:3139–3148.
6. Wielopolski PA, van Geuns RJ, de Feyter PJ, et al. Breath-hold coronary MR angiography with volume-targeted imaging. *Radiology* 1998;209:209–219.

7. Post JC, van Rossum AC, Bronzwaer JG, et al. Magnetic resonance angiography of anomalous coronary arteries. A new gold standard for delineating the proximal course? *Circulation* 1995; 92:3163–3171.

8. McConnell MV, Stuber M, Manning WJ. Clinical role of coronary magnetic resonance angiography in the diagnosis of anomalous coronary arteries. *J Cardiovasc Magn Reson* 2000;2:217–224.

9. Corrado D, Basso C, Schiavon M, et al. Screening for hypertrophic cardiomyopathy in young athletes. *N Engl J Med* 1998;339:364–369.

10. Ishikawa T, Brandt PW. Anomalous origin of the left main coronary artery from the right anterior aortic sinus: angiographic definition of anomalous course. *Am J Cardiol* 1985;55:770–776.

11. Serota H, Barth CW, Seuc CA, et al. Rapid identification of the course of anomalous coronary arteries in adults: the "dot and eye" method. *Am J Cardiol* 1990;65:891–898.

12. Vliegen HW, Doornbos J, de Roos A, et al. Value of fast gradient-echo magnetic resonance angiography as an adjunct to coronary arteriography in detecting and confirming the course of clinically significant coronary artery anomalies. *Am J Cardiol* 1997; 79:773–776.

13. American Heart Association. *2001 Heart and stroke statistical update.* Dallas, TX: American Heart Association, 2000.

14. American Heart Association. *1993 Heart and stroke facts and statistics.* Dallas, TX: American Heart Association, 1993:8.

15. Johnson LW, Krone R. Cardiac catheterization 1991: a report of the Registry of the Society for Cardiac Angiography and Interventions (SCA&I). *Cathet Cardiovasc Diagn* 1993;28:219–220.

16. Krone RJ, Johnson L, Noto T. Five-year trends in cardiac catheterization: a report from the Registry of the Society for Cardiac Angiography and Interventions. *Cathet Cardiovasc Diagn* 1996;39:31–35.

17. Hofman MB, Wickline SA, Lorenz CH. Quantification of in-plane motion of the coronary arteries during the cardiac cycle: implications for acquisition window duration for MR flow quantification. *J Magn Reson Imaging* 1998;8:568–576.

18. Holland AE, Goldfarb JW, Edelman RR. Diaphragmatic and cardiac motion during suspended breathing: preliminary experience and implications for breath-hold MR imaging. *Radiology* 1998;209:483–489.

19. Stuber M, Botnar RM, Spuentrup E, et al. Three-dimensional high-resolution fast spin-echo coronary magnetic resonance angiography. *Magn Reson Med* 2001;45:206–211.

20. Manning WJ, Li W, Edelman RR. A preliminary report comparing magnetic resonance coronary angiography with conventional angiography. *N Engl J Med* 1993;328:828–832.

21. Duerinckx AJ. Imaging of coronary artery disease—MR. *J Thorac Imaging* 2001;16:25–34.

22. Nitatori T, Yoshino H, Yokoyama K, et al. Coronary MR angiography—a clinical experience in Japan. *J Magn Reson Imaging* 1999;10:709–712.

23. Post JC, van Rossum AC, Hofman MB, et al. Clinical utility of two-dimensional magnetic resonance angiography in detecting coronary artery disease. *Eur Heart J* 1997;18:426–433.

24. Pennell DJ, Bogren HG, Keegan J, et al. Assessment of coronary artery stenosis by magnetic resonance imaging. *Heart* 1996;75: 127–133.

25. van Geuns RJ, Wielopolski PA, de Bruin HG, et al. MR coronary angiography with breath-hold targeted volumes: preliminary clinical results. *Radiology* 2000;217:270–277.

26. Huber A, Nikolaou K, Gonschior P, et al. Navigator echo-based respiratory gating for three-dimensional MR coronary angiography: results from healthy volunteers and patients with proximal coronary artery stenoses. *AJR Am J Roentgenol* 1999;173:95–101.

27. Kim WY, Danias PG, Stuber M, et al. Coronary magnetic resonance angiography for the detection of coronary stenoses. *N Engl J Med* 2001;345:1863–1869.

28. Ladenheim ML, Pollock BH, Rozanski A, et al. Extent and severity of myocardial hypoperfusion as predictors of prognosis in patients with suspected coronary artery disease. *J Am Coll Cardiol* 1986;7:464–471.

29. Sakuma H, Kawada N, Takeda K, et al. MR measurement of coronary blood flow. *J Magn Reson Imaging* 1999;10:728–733.

30. Keegan J, Gatehouse P, Yang GZ, et al. Interleaved spiral cine coronary artery velocity mapping. *Magn Reson Med* 2000;43: 787–792.

31. Hundley WG, Lange RA, Clarke GD, et al. Assessment of coronary arterial flow and flow reserve in humans with magnetic resonance imaging. *Circulation* 1996;93:1502–1508.

32. Sakuma H, Koskenvuo JW, Niemi P, et al. Assessment of coronary flow reserve using fast velocity-encoded cine MR imaging: validation study using positron emission tomography. *AJR Am J Roentgenol* 2000;175:1029–1033.

33. Schwitter J, DeMarco T, Kneifel S, et al. Magnetic resonance-based assessment of global coronary flow and flow reserve and its relation to left ventricular functional parameters: a comparison with positron emission tomography. *Circulation* 2000;101: 2696–2702.

34. Hundley WG, Hillis LD, Hamilton CA, et al. Assessment of coronary arterial restenosis with phase-contrast magnetic resonance imaging measurements of coronary flow reserve. *Circulation* 2000;101:2375–2381.

35. Kim RJ, Wu E, Rafael A, et al. The use of contrast-enhanced magnetic resonance imaging to identify reversible myocardial dysfunction. *N Engl J Med* 2000;343:1445–1453.

36. Regenfus M, Ropers D, Achenbach S, et al. Noninvasive detection of coronary artery stenosis using contrast-enhanced three-dimensional breath-hold magnetic resonance coronary angiography. *J Am Coll Cardiol* 2000;36:44–50.

37. Vrachliotis TG, Bis KG, Aliabadi D, et al. Contrast-enhanced breath-hold MR angiography for evaluating patency of coronary artery bypass grafts. *AJR Am J Roentgenol* 1997;168:1073–1080.

38. Stuber M, Botnar RM, Danias PG, et al. Contrast agent-enhanced, free-breathing, three-dimensional coronary magnetic resonance angiography. *J Magn Reson Imaging* 1999;10:790–799.

39. Li D, Zheng J, Weinmann HJ. Contrast-enhanced MR imaging of coronary arteries: comparison of intra- and extravascular contrast agents in swine. *Radiology* 2001;218:670–678.

40. Hofman MB, Henson RE, Kovacs SJ, et al. Blood pool agent strongly improves 3D magnetic resonance coronary angiography using an inversion pre-pulse. *Magn Reson Med* 1999;41:360–367.

41. Dirksen MS, Lamb HJ, Kunz P, et al. Improved coronary MRA using a new blood pool contrast agent (P-792) and respiratory navigator gating. Presented at the International Society for Magnetic Resonance in Medicine and European Society for Magnetic Resonance in Medicine and Biology Joint Annual Meeting, 2001:1854(abst).

42. Li D, Dolan RP, Walovitch RC, et al. Three-dimensional MRI of coronary arteries using an intravascular contrast agent. *Magn Reson Med* 1998;39:1014–1018.

43. Shellock FG, Shellock VJ. Metallic stents: evaluation of MR imaging safety. *AJR Am J Roentgenol* 1999;173:543–547.

44. Hug J, Nagel E, Bornstedt A, et al. Coronary arterial stents: safety and artifacts during MR imaging. *Radiology* 2000;216:781–787.

45. Bhachu DS, Kanal E. Implantable pulse generators (pacemakers) and electrodes: safety in the magnetic resonance imaging scanner environment. *J Magn Reson Imaging* 2000;12:201–204.

46. Sommer T, Vahlhaus C, Lauck G, et al. MR imaging and cardiac pacemakers: *in vitro* evaluation and *in vivo* studies in 51 patients at 0.5 T. *Radiology* 2000;215:869–879.

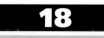

CORONARY BLOOD FLOW MEASUREMENT

HAJIME SAKUMA
CHARLES B. HIGGINS

Selective coronary angiography has been used to evaluate coronary artery disease. However, an assessment of the anatomic severity of a coronary stenosis does not adequately determine the functional significance of the lesion (1,2). Quantitative coronary angiography, which was designed to minimize variability in interpretation, cannot reliably predict the physiologic significance of a stenosis of intermediate severity (3). An assessment of the functional significance of a stenosis is particularly important in lesions of intermediate severity because the interpretation of such lesions significantly influences therapeutic decisions in patients with coronary artery disease. The functional significance of a coronary arterial stenosis can be evaluated by measuring the coronary flow reserve, which is the ratio of maximal hyperemic coronary flow to the baseline coronary flow (4,5). In the presence of a normal epicardial coronary artery and myocardial microcirculation, the administration of a vasodilator (e.g., dipyridamole and adenosine) induces more than a threefold to fourfold increase in coronary blood flow. In patients with significant coronary arterial stenosis, however, compensatory dilation takes place in the downstream microcirculation to maintain myocardial blood flow. Thus, the ability to augment coronary blood flow during pharmacologic stress is attenuated in patients with significant coronary arterial stenosis.

The evaluation of blood flow velocity and flow velocity reserve with an intracoronary Doppler guidewire is well established and allows a functional assessment of the severity of a stenosis. A study in which an intracoronary Doppler

guidewire was used showed that the sensitivity, specificity, and overall predictive accuracy of the coronary flow velocity reserve were 94%, 95%, and 94%, respectively, when stress thallium 201 single photon emission computed tomography (^{201}Tl-SPECT) was used as a gold standard (6). Another study demonstrated that a coronary flow velocity reserve below 2.0 by the Doppler technique had a sensitivity of 92% and a specificity of 82% for predicting the presence of a significant stenosis in the coronary artery on selective coronary angiography (7). However, intracoronary flow velocity measurement with the Doppler guidewire is invasive and available only during cardiac catheterization.

Fast phase-contrast cine MRI is an emerging application of MRI that can provide noninvasive assessments of blood flow and flow reserve in human coronary arteries. Several studies have demonstrated the usefulness of this technique in detecting coronary arterial restenosis after percutaneous revascularization procedures and in assessing patency and stenosis in coronary artery bypass conduits. In addition, MR measurement of the coronary sinus blood flow allows the noninvasive assessment of global myocardial blood flow. This chapter reviews the current status and potential clinical applications of MR measurements of blood flow and flow reserve in the coronary artery, coronary artery bypass graft (CABG), and coronary sinus.

MRI TECHNIQUES FOR MEASURING CORONARY BLOOD FLOW

Phase-contrast cine MRI can provide noninvasive flow measurements at multiple temporal phases in the cardiac cycle.

H. Sakuma: Department of Radiology, Mie University Hospital, Tsu, Mie, Japan.
C. B. Higgins: Department of Radiology, University of California San Francisco, San Francisco, California.

The MR measurement of blood flow in large vessels, such as the aorta, pulmonary artery, and carotid artery, is well established and validated (8). However, MR blood flow quantification in the coronary artery has been very challenging because the coronary artery is small (<3 to 4 mm) and subject to both cardiac and respiratory motion. Several different approaches have been proposed in the past for quantifying blood flow in the coronary arteries with MRI, including a time-of-flight method (9), MR bolus tagging (10), and a phase-contrast method (11). A phase-contrast cine MR technique has been most commonly used to measure blood flow in the human coronary vessels in recent studies.

MR flow measurement in the coronary artery can be achieved with either a breath-hold acquisition or a respiration-triggered acquisition. In 1993, Edelman et al. (11) demonstrated the feasibility of breath-hold measurement of blood flow velocity in the coronary artery at a single diastolic phase with the use of a segmented k-space phase-contrast MR acquisition. Keegan et al. (12) then measured coronary blood flow at multiple phases in the cardiac cycle within a single breath-hold time by using segmented k-space phase-contrast cine MRI. We measured diastolic peak velocities in the left anterior descending artery in the basal state and after intravenous administration of dipyridamole by means of this technique (13). The average coronary flow velocity reserve in eight normal subjects was 3.14 ± 0.59 (Fig. 18.1). Volumetric blood flow in the coronary arteries can be calculated in theory by integrating the product of the mean velocity and area of the vessel over the cardiac cycle (14–17). The normal coronary flow reserve with volumetric MR flow measurement was 4.2 ± 1.8 according to Grist et al. (16) and 5.0 ± 2.6 according to Davis et al. (17).

Errors from several sources affect blood flow quantification with phase-contrast MR sequences (18–20). Currently,

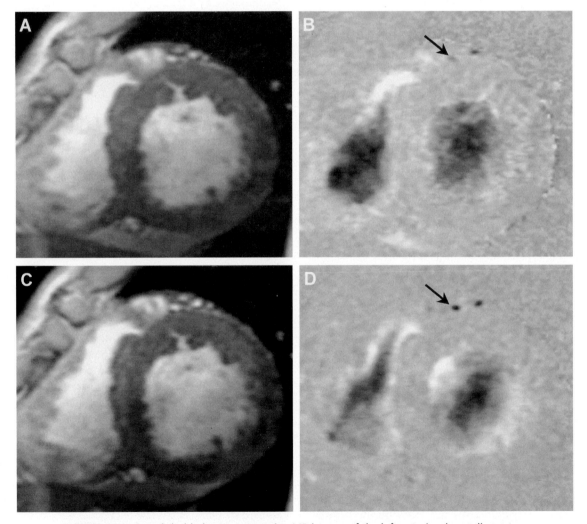

FIGURE 18.1. Breath-hold phase-contrast cine MR images of the left anterior descending artery *(arrows)* in a subject without significant stenosis in that vessel. Magnitude image **(A)** and phase-difference image **(B)** at rest and magnitude image **(C)** and phase-difference image **(D)** after intravenous administration of dipyridamole. The increase in the coronary blood flow velocity after pharmacologic stress is observed as a darkening of the signal on the phase-difference image.

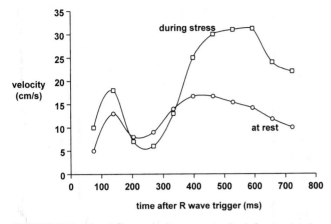

FIGURE 18.2. Blood flow velocity curves in the left anterior descending artery at rest and after intravenous administration of dipyridamole in a patient with significant stenosis. The coronary flow velocity reserve can be calculated from the flow velocity curves of the coronary artery before and during pharmacologic stress. The coronary flow velocity reserve in this patient (1.9) was reduced by stenosis in the left anterior descending artery.

the major limitations of breath-hold MR measurement of coronary blood flow are suboptimal spatial and temporal resolution. If the spatial resolution of MRI is compromised relative to the vessel size, partial volume averaging of bright signal from flowing blood and attenuated signal from static tissue around the vessel lumen results in an overestimation of blood flow volume on phase-difference images. In addition, the peak flow velocity in the coronary artery measured by phase-contrast MRI is substantially lower than the peak velocity by intracoronary Doppler guidewire because the highest velocity at the center and lower velocities at the peripheral areas of the vessel lumen are averaged within an MRI voxel (21). Insufficient temporal resolution of the cardiac cycle is another source of error. If the data acquisition window in the cardiac cycle is not sufficient, blurring of the vessel by in-plane motion results in inaccurate measurements of blood flow velocity and flow volume. Hofman et al. (22) reported that the duration of the acquisition window for an accurate MR flow volume quantification should be less than 25 milliseconds for the right coronary artery and 120 milliseconds for the left coronary artery; these figures indicate that further improvement is necessary to obtain accurate flow volume quantification in the right coronary artery. It should be noted that blood flow measured during breath-hold MR acquisition may be different from physiologic blood flow during regular breathing because breath-holding at inspiration causes an increase in intrathoracic pressure, which then reduces systemic venous return to the heart. Our recent study showed that MR measurements of cardiac output are significantly depressed during breath-holding at deep inspiration (23). No significant difference was observed between breath-hold measurement at shallow inspiration and non–breath-hold measurement, a finding that indicates the importance of using shallow inspiration to

obtain physiologic blood flow measurement in breath-hold MR sequences.

Phase-contrast cine MR sequences with respiration-triggered acquisition permit the non–breath-hold assessment of coronary blood flow. Navigator techniques are based on one-dimensional image acquisitions; these are used to monitor the position of the diaphragm and accept image data only if the position of the diaphragm is within a certain range. Because image data can be acquired for a prolonged scan time during regular breathing, navigator techniques make it possible to acquire phase-contrast cine MR images with better spatial and temporal resolution. Nagel et al. (24) reported that a higher degree of temporal resolution and shorter acquisition window in the cardiac cycle with navigator-corrected non–breath-hold MRI increased the accuracy of measurements of coronary blood flow velocity, especially in the right coronary arteries.

The use of a stronger gradient system and newer, fast scan techniques can improve the accuracy of breath-hold MR flow quantification in the coronary vessels (25). In comparison with respiration-triggered acquisition, the breath-hold method requires less scan time; this feature is critically important in studies in which pharmacologic stress is used and may make it possible to assess blood flow and flow reserve in multiple coronary arteries within a short scan time. Langerak et al. (26) used turbo-field echo-planar MRI to measure blood flow in CABGs. In this approach, breath-hold flow mapping with spatial and temporal resolutions of 0.8 mm^2 and 23 milliseconds, respectively, can be achieved. These investigators showed that breath-hold turbo-field echo-planar MRI provides fast and accurate flow measurements and allows motion-compensated flow quantification in multiple CABGs during a short infusion of adenosine

MR MEASUREMENT OF CORONARY FLOW RESERVE IN PATIENTS WITH CORONARY ARTERIAL STENOSIS

Measurements of coronary flow reserve obtained with phase-contrast cine MRI can be used to evaluate the functional significance of stenoses in the left main and left anterior descending coronary arteries in patients (Fig. 18.2). To validate this approach, Shibata et al. (21) compared coronary flow velocity reserve measurements obtained by breath-hold phase-contrast cine MRI with measurements obtained by intracoronary Doppler guidewire in 19 patients with varying degrees of stenosis in the left anterior descending artery. Although the mean MR flow velocity in the coronary artery in the baseline state was significantly lower than that assessed by Doppler guidewire (12.5 ± 4.9 cm/s vs. 32.4 ± 12.1 cm/s, $p < 0.001$), a significant linear correlation was observed between MR and Doppler measurements of the coronary flow velocity reserve, with a correlation coefficient of .91. In a recent study (27), breath-hold MR measurement of the coronary flow velocity reserve in the proximal left anterior descending artery correlated well with myocardial perfusion reserve in the anterior wall of the left ventricle (LV) measured by positron emission tomography (PET) and water labeled with oxygen 15 (^{15}O).

The noninvasive MR measurement of coronary flow reserve has been shown to be useful in identifying the functional significance of stenoses in the left anterior descending artery in patients with coronary artery disease. Hundley et al. (28) demonstrated a statistically significant correlation between MR assessments of coronary flow reserve and the severity of coronary arterial stenosis by quantitative coronary angiography. The sensitivity and specificity of MR coronary flow velocity reserve for identifying stenosis of 70% or greater in the left main or left anterior descending artery were 100% and 83%, respectively.

Restenosis of the coronary artery is a major clinical problem in patients who undergo coronary interventions. MR assessment of coronary flow reserve can be performed in outpatients repeatedly and allows the noninvasive detection of restenosis after coronary interventions. Saito et al. (29) showed that restenosis after coronary balloon angioplasty and stent placement can be detected noninvasively by monitoring serial changes of the coronary flow velocity reserve with breath-hold phase-contrast MRI. Coronary flow velocity reserve in segments distal to angioplasty and stent placement was repeatedly evaluated by MRI after interventional procedures. A metallic stent in the coronary artery was useful as a marker for determining the slice location of MR blood flow measurement. In patients without restenosis at follow-up x-ray angiography after 6 months, the flow velocity reserve was 1.97 ± 0.37 at 1 month and 2.29 ± 0.31 at 6 months. In contrast, the coronary flow velocity reserve showed a gradual decrease in patients with restenosis at follow-up x-ray angiography. The coronary flow velocity reserve was 2.27 ± 0.49 at 1 month and 1.52 ± 0.15 at 6 months (Fig. 18.3). A recent study by Hundley et al. (30) also indicated that phase-contrast cine MRI can be used to detect restenosis noninvasively in patients with recurrent chest pain after percutaneous revascularization. A coronary flow reserve value of 2.0 or less was 100% sensitive and 89% specific for detecting a luminal diameter narrowing of 70% or greater, and it was 82% sensitive and 100% specific for detecting a luminal diameter narrowing of 50% or greater.

MR FLOW MEASUREMENT IN CORONARY ARTERY BYPASS GRAFTS

In many circumstances, a CABG must be assessed postoperatively for patency or stenosis. Selective x-ray angiography is the routine procedure and gold standard for assessing bypass grafts, but this technique is invasive and entails some risks. MRI techniques such as electrocardiogram (ECG)-gated spin-echo MRI (31,32), cine MRI (33,34) and three-dimensional contrast-enhanced MR angiography (35,36) have been shown to be useful for predicting graft patency. However, in most of these previous studies, imaging was confined to the proximal and middle segments of the grafts, and direct visualization of the distal anastomosis to the native coronary artery requires a higher degree of spatial and temporal resolution. Therefore, these MRI methods of morphologic assessment do not differentiate between nonoccluded stenotic grafts and normal grafts (37). MR flow measurement is an effective method of functionally assessing a CABG, and it noninvasively detects stenosis and occlusion in a graft.

MR blood flow quantification in saphenous vein grafts was initially reported by Hoogendoorn et al. (38), who used non–breath-hold MRI. They reported that the average blood flow volume in normal saphenous vein grafts was 71 ± 17 mL/min, whereas the average blood flow volume in stenotic/occluded grafts was significantly reduced to 9 ± 8 mL/min ($p < 0.001$). In the study of Galjee et al. (39), adequate MR flow velocity profiles were obtained in 85% of angiographically patent grafts with non–breath-hold phase-contrast cine MRI. Graft flow was characterized by a biphasic pattern, with one peak during systole and a second peak

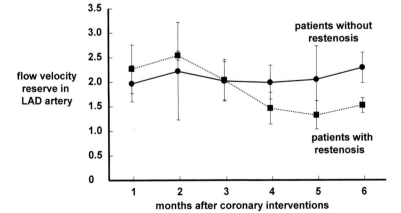

FIGURE 18.3. Serial changes in the coronary flow velocity reserve after percutaneous balloon angioplasty and stent placement in the left anterior descending artery in patients without restenosis and in patients with significant stenosis at follow-up selective coronary angiography. The coronary flow velocity reserve gradually decreased after several months in the patients who demonstrated restenosis in the coronary artery.

during diastole. The feasibility of MR blood flow measurements in internal mammary artery grafts was demonstrated with the use of non–breath-hold phase-contrast cine MRI (40) and breath-hold phase-contrast cine MRI (41). Ishida et al. (42) measured blood flow in internal mammary artery bypass grafts in 26 patients with a breath-hold phase-contrast cine MR sequence (Figs. 18.4 and 18.5). Titanium clips were used to avoid metal artifacts on the MR images in this study protocol. The ratio of diastolic to systolic peak velocity in patients with stenotic grafts (>70% diameter) on selective angiography was 0.61 ± 0.44, which was significantly lower than that in patients without graft stenosis (1.88 ± 0.96,

p <0.01). In addition, the average blood flow volume in stenotic grafts (16.9 ± 5.5 mL/min) was significantly lower than that in normal grafts (79.8 ± 38.2 mL/min, p <0.01) (Fig. 18.6). The sensitivity and specificity of MR blood flow measurement in predicting significant stenosis were 85.7% and 94.1%, respectively. These results indicate that MR blood flow measurement is useful in predicting significant stenosis in internal mammary arterial grafts.

It has been suggested that determining the flow reserve ratio in a CABG may be useful for identifying graft stenosis. Langerak et al. (26) used a turbo-field echo-planar sequence to measure blood flow in 20 normal grafts (18 venous and 2

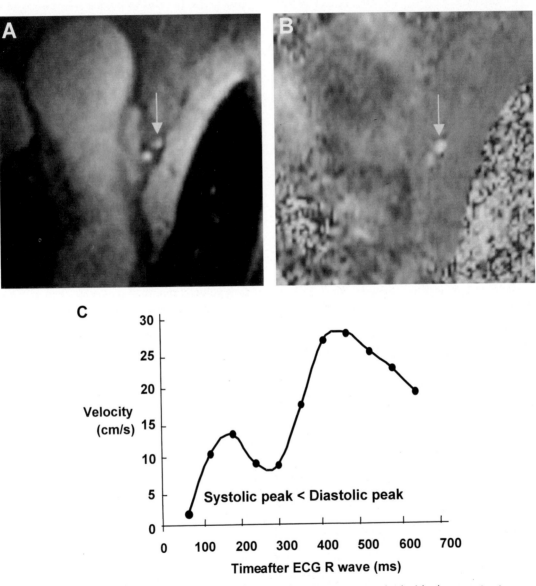

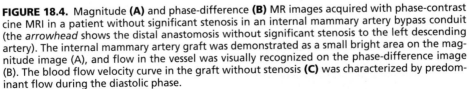

FIGURE 18.4. Magnitude **(A)** and phase-difference **(B)** MR images acquired with phase-contrast cine MRI in a patient without significant stenosis in an internal mammary artery bypass conduit (the *arrowhead* shows the distal anastomosis without significant stenosis to the left descending artery). The internal mammary artery graft was demonstrated as a small bright area on the magnitude image **(A)**, and flow in the vessel was visually recognized on the phase-difference image **(B)**. The blood flow velocity curve in the graft without stenosis **(C)** was characterized by predominant flow during the diastolic phase.

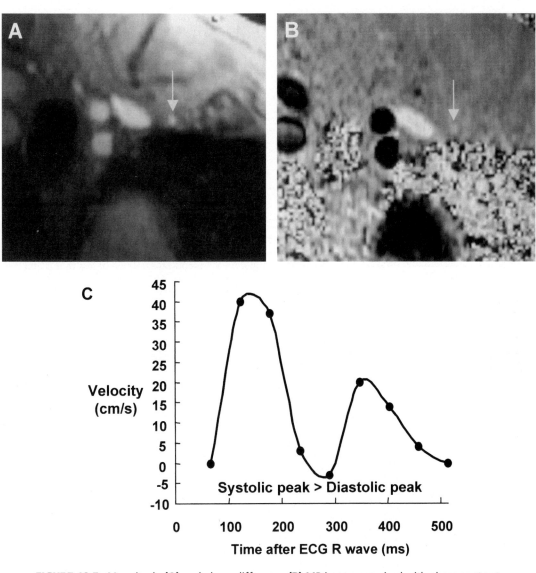

FIGURE 18.5. Magnitude **(A)** and phase-difference **(B)** MR images acquired with phase-contrast cine MRI in a patient with significant stenosis in an internal mammary artery bypass conduit (the *arrowhead* shows the distal anastomosis with significant stenosis to the left descending artery). The blood flow velocity curve in the graft with stenosis **(C)** showed predominant flow during the systolic phase.

arterial) before and during adenosine stress. The mean bypass graft flow increased from 30.8 ± 13.5 mL/min to 76.7 ± 36.5 mL/min ($p < 0.05$) to yield a flow reserve of 2.7. When Ishida et al. (42) evaluated pharmacologic flow reserve in internal mammary artery grafts with dipyridamole, the mean flow velocity reserve ratio in grafts with significant stenosis (1.39 ± 1.46) was reduced in comparison with that in normal grafts (2.0 ± 1.43, $p < 0.01$). However, this study indicated that MR measurement of the vasodilator flow reserve does not further increase the detection of graft stenosis in patients early after operation because blood flow volume and the ratio of diastolic to systolic velocity measured at rest can effectively discriminate between normal and stenotic grafts. The limited diagnostic value of flow reserve

measurements for detecting stenosis in internal mammary arterial grafts early after operation was mainly a consequence of the small diameter and limited flow reserve ratios of the normal grafts. Akasaka et al. (43) measured flow velocity in internal mammary artery grafts by Doppler guidewire and showed that internal mammary artery grafts early after operation are characterized by a higher peak velocity at baseline to compensate for their small diameter. The early postoperative flow reserve (1.8 ± 0.3) is significantly lower than that in older grafts (2.6 ± 0.3) because of the high baseline flow velocity. Further studies are required to determine the diagnostic value of MR measurement of pharmacologic flow reserve in the noninvasive detection of stenosis in internal mammary artery grafts and saphenous venous grafts.

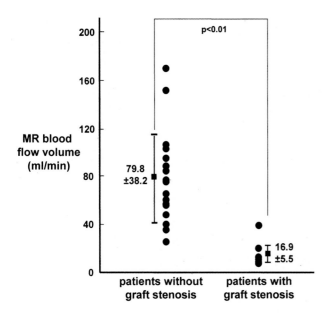

FIGURE 18.6. Blood flow volume in internal mammary artery grafts in patients with and without significant stenosis on selective angiography. An MR blood flow volume of less than 35 mL/min predicts significant graft stenosis (stenosis of more than 70% of the luminal diameter) with a sensitivity of 85.7% and a specificity of 94.1%.

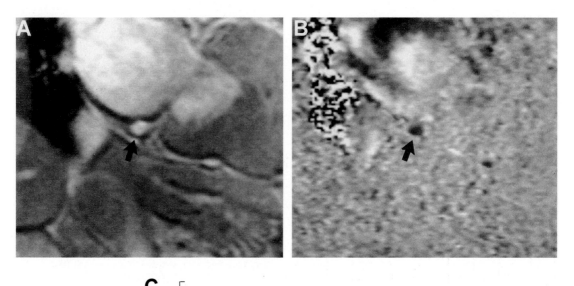

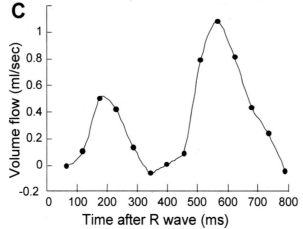

FIGURE 18.7. MR measurement of blood flow volume through the coronary sinus. Magnitude **(A)** and phase-difference **(B)** images were acquired on the imaging plane that is perpendicular to the coronary sinus with a phase-contrast cine MR sequence. The volume flow curve **(C)** can be generated by integrating the product of the blood flow velocity and vessel area over the cardiac cycle.

MR BLOOD FLOW QUANTIFICATION IN THE CORONARY SINUS

Blood flow in the coronary sinus reflects the global myocardial blood flow because it represents approximately 96% of the total myocardial blood flow of the LV (44). If blood flow in the coronary sinus is measured with phase-contrast cine MRI and LV myocardial mass is measured with cine MRI, both the total myocardial blood flow and the average coronary blood flow per gram of myocardial mass can be quantified (Fig. 18.7). To validate this approach, several investigators compared MR measurements of coronary sinus blood flow with values determined by reference methods. Lund et al. (45) compared blood flow in the coronary sinus measured by MRI with that assessed by an ultrasonic volumetric flowmeter in dogs. Coronary sinus flow measured by phase-contrast cine MRI and total coronary blood flow measured by flowmeter showed a good correlation ($r = 0.98$, $p < 0.001$); the mean difference between total coronary blood flow by flowmeter and coronary sinus flow by MRI was 3.1 ± 8.5 mL/min. Mean blood flow per gram of myocardial mass was 0.40 ± 0.09 mL/min per gram by MRI and 0.44 ± 0.08 mL/min per gram by flowmeter ($p = $ NS). Schwitter et al. (46) measured coronary sinus blood flow by phase-contrast cine MRI and myocardial blood flow by PET and [^{13}N]ammonia in healthy volunteers. Coronary sinus flow divided by LV mass correlated highly with the ^{13}N-PET flow data (0.77 ± 0.19 mL/min per gram by MRI and 0.73 ± 0.15 mL/min per gram by PET, $r = 0.95$). Koskenvuo et al. (47) compared breath-hold MR measurements of coronary blood flow per gram of myocardial mass with myocardial blood flow determined by PET and ^{15}O-labeled water, which is regarded as the most accurate approach for measuring myocardial blood flow. Coronary sinus blood flow divided by myocardial mass was 0.65 ± 0.20 mL/min per gram with breath-hold MRI, which showed a good agreement with the PET measurement of myocardial blood flow of 0.65 ± 0.20 mL/min per gram.

This integrated MR approach for measuring global myocardial blood under resting and hyperemic conditions has been shown to be useful in evaluating diffuse myocardial diseases, such as hypertrophic cardiomyopathy, and cardiac transplants. In a study in 29 patients with hypertrophic cardiomyopathy, the baseline myocardial blood flow was 0.74 ± 0.23 mL/min per gram in normal subjects and 0.62 ± 0.27 mL/min per gram in patients with hypertrophic cardiomyopathy ($p = $ NS) (48). After the administration of dipyridamole, the myocardial blood flow in patients with hypertrophic cardiomyopathy increased to a level significantly lower than that healthy subjects (1.03 ± 0.40 mL/min per gram vs. 2.14 ± 0.51 mL/min per gram, $p < 0.01$), so that the patients with hypertrophic cardiomyopathy had a severely decreased flow reserve ratio ($1.72 \pm$ 0.49 vs. 3.01 ± 0.75, $p < 0.01$). A significant inverse relationship was found between the coronary flow reserve ratio and LV mass ($r = -0.46$, $p < 0.05$). Schwitter et al. (46) evaluated myocardial blood flow and flow reserve in recipients of orthotopic heart transplants with phase-contrast MRI. The coronary flow reserve was reduced in the patients with transplanted hearts (2.0 ± 0.4) in comparison with that in control subjects (3.9 ± 1.4, $p < 0.005$). A moderate but significant negative correlation was noted between myocardial blood flow after pharmacologic stress and LV mass index ($r = -0.56$, $p < 0.005$).

SUMMARY

Recent advances in fast MRI sequences have considerably extended the capabilities of cardiac MRI in the functional assessment of coronary blood flow and flow reserve. The MR measurement of coronary flow reserve can be used to identify restenosis of the left main and left anterior descending coronary arteries after percutaneous interventions in clinical patients. Further refinements in MR pulse sequences, including the use of phase-contrast echo-planar or spiral MR methods, may make it possible to quantify blood flow volume and flow reserve more accurately in all major branches of the coronary arteries.

The MR measurement of blood flow in CABGs permits a functional evaluation of the graft and is useful in the noninvasive detection of graft stenosis. In most clinical patients with coronary bypass conduits, however, it is necessary to know the status of the native coronary arteries or detect the presence of myocardial ischemia. Although the MR measurement of flow in bypass grafts cannot by itself replace invasive coronary angiography, comprehensive assessments of myocardial perfusion and blood flow in coronary artery bypass conduits during stress and at rest within a single MR examination will be highly useful after bypass graft surgery and may reduce the need for invasive catheterization.

The MR measurement of blood flow through the coronary sinus allows a noninvasive assessment of global coronary hemodynamics. Because the coronary sinus is larger than the native coronary arteries, the errors in blood flow quantification associated with the limited spatial and temporal resolution of current phase-contrast MR sequences are substantially smaller. The MR quantification of total coronary blood flow and coronary blood flow per gram of myocardium during stress and at rest seems to be an ideal method for evaluating coronary hemodynamics in diffuse myocardial diseases of the heart (49), such as hypertensive heart diseases and cardiomyopathies, and may be useful in evaluating endothelial dysfunction of the coronary circulation, which develops in the earliest stages of atherosclerotic disease and may precede obstruction of the epicardial coronary arteries.

REFERENCES

1. White CW, Wright CB, Doty DB, et al. Does visual interpretation of the coronary angiogram predict the physiological importance of a coronary stenosis? *N Engl J Med* 1984;310:819–824.
2. Marcus ML, Skorton DJ, Johnson MR, et al. Visual estimates of percent diameter coronary stenosis: a battered gold standard. *J Am Coll Cardiol* 1988;11:882–885.
3. Vogel RA. Assessing stenosis significance by coronary angiography. Are the best variables good enough? *J Am Coll Cardiol* 1988;12:692–693.
4. Gould KL, Lipscomb K, Hamilton GW. Physiologic basis for assessing critical coronary stenosis: instantaneous flow response and regional distribution during coronary hyperemia as measures of coronary flow reserve. *Am J Cardiol* 1974;33:87–94.
5. White CW. Clinical applications of Doppler coronary flow reserve measurements. *Am J Cardiol* 1993;71:10D–16D.
6. Joye JD, Schulman DS, Lasorda D, et al. Intracoronary Doppler guide wire versus stress single-photon emission computed tomographic thallium-201 imaging in assessment of intermediate coronary stenoses. *J Am Coll Cardiol* 1994;24:940–947.
7. Redberg RF, Sobol Y, Chou TM, et al. Adenosine-induced coronary vasodilatation during transesophageal Doppler echocardiography: rapid and safe measurement of coronary flow reserve ratio can predict significant left anterior descending coronary stenosis. *Circulation* 1995;92:190–196.
8. Szolar DH, Sakuma H, Higgins CB. Cardiovascular application of magnetic resonance flow and velocity measurements. *J Magn Reson Imaging* 1996;6:78–89.
9. Poncelet BP, Weisskoff RM, Wedeen WJ, et al. Time of flight quantification of coronary flow with echo-planar MRI. *Magn Reson Med* 1993;30:447–457.
10. Chao H, Burstein D. Multibolus-stimulated echo imaging of coronary artery flow. *J Magn Reson Imaging* 1997;7:603–605.
11. Edelman RR, Manning WJ, Gervino E, et al. Flow velocity quantification in human coronary arteries with fast breath-hold MR angiography. *J Magn Reson Imaging* 1993;3:699–703.
12. Keegan J, Firmin D, Gatehouse P, et al. The application of breath-hold phase velocity mapping techniques to the measurement of coronary artery blood flow velocity: phantom data and initial *in vivo* results. *Magn Reson Med* 1994;31:526–536.
13. Sakuma H, Blake LM, Amidon TM, et al. Noninvasive measurement of coronary flow reserve in humans using breath-hold velocity encoded cine MR imaging. *Radiology* 1996;198:745–750.
14. Clarke GD, Eckels R, Chaney C, et al. Measurement of absolute epicardial coronary artery flow and flow reserve with breath-hold cine phase-contrast magnetic resonance imaging. *Circulation* 1995;91:2627–2634.
15. Hundley WG, Lange RA, Clarke GD, et al. Assessment of coronary arterial flow and flow reserve in humans with magnetic resonance imaging. *Circulation* 1996;93:1502–1508.
16. Grist TM, Polzin JA, Bianco JA, et al. Measurement of coronary blood flow and flow reserve using magnetic resonance imaging. *Cardiology* 1997;88:80–89.
17. Davis CP, Liu P, Hauser M, et al. Coronary flow and coronary flow reserve measurements in humans with breath-hold magnetic resonance phase contrast velocity mapping. *Magn Reson Med* 1997;37:537–544.
18. Polzin JA, Korosec FR, Wedding KL, et al. Effect of through-plane myocardial motion on phase-difference and complex-difference measurements of absolute coronary artery flow. *J Magn Reson Imaging* 1996;6:113–123.
19. Frayne R, Polzin JA, Mazaheri Y, et al. Effect of and correction for in-plane myocardial motion on estimates of coronary volume flow rates. *J Magn Reson Imaging* 1997;7:815–828.
20. Hofman MBM, van Rossum AC, Sprenger M, et al. Assessment of flow in the right human coronary artery by magnetic resonance phase contrast velocity measurement: effects of cardiac and respiratory motion. *Magn Reson Med* 1996;35:521–531.
21. Shibata M, Sakuma H, Isaka N, et al. Assessment of coronary flow reserve with fast cine phase contrast magnetic resonance imaging: comparison with the measurement by Doppler guide wire. *J Magn Reson Imaging* 1999;10:563–568.
22. Hofman MB, Wickline SA, Lorenz CH. Quantification of in-plane motion of the coronary arteries during the cardiac cycle: implication for acquisition window duration for MR flow quantification. *J Magn Reson Imaging* 1998;8:568–576.
23. Sakuma H, Kawada N, Kubo H, et al. Effect of breath holding on blood flow measurement using fast velocity encoded cine MRI. *Magn Reson Med* 2001;45:346–348.
24. Nagel E, Bornstedt A, Hug J, et al. Noninvasive determination of coronary blood flow velocity with magnetic resonance imaging: comparison of breath-hold and navigator techniques with intravascular ultrasound. *Magn Reson Med* 1999;41:544–549.
25. Sakuma H, Saeed M, Takeda K, et al. Quantification of coronary arterial volume flow rate using fast velocity encoded cine MR imaging. *AJR Am J Roentgenol* 1997;168:1363–1367.
26. Langerak SE, Kunz P, Vliegen HW, et al. Improved MR flow mapping in coronary artery bypass grafts during adenosine-induced stress. *Radiology* 2001;218:540–547.
27. Sakuma H, Koskenvuo JW, Niemi P, et al. Assessment of coronary flow reserve using fast velocity-encoded cine MR imaging: validation study using positron emission tomography. *AJR Am J Roentgenol* 2000;175:1029–1033.
28. Hundley WG, Hamilton CA, Clarke GD, et al. Visualization and functional assessment of proximal and middle left anterior descending coronary stenoses in humans with magnetic resonance imaging. *Circulation* 1999;99:3248–3254.
29. Saito Y, Sakuma H, Shibata et al. Assessment of coronary flow reserve using cine phase contrast MRI for noninvasive detection of restenosis after angioplasty and stenting. *J Cardiovasc Magn Reson* 2001;3:209–214.
30. Hundley WG, Hillis LD, Hamilton CA, et al. Assessment of coronary arterial restenosis with phase-contrast magnetic resonance imaging measurements of coronary flow reserve. *Circulation* 2000;101:2375–2381.
31. White RD, Caputo GR, Mark AS, et al. Coronary artery bypass graft patency: noninvasive evaluation with MR imaging. *Radiology* 1987;164:681–686.
32. Rubinstein RI, Askenase AD, Thickman D, et al. Magnetic resonance imaging to evaluate patency of aortocoronary bypass grafts. *Circulation* 1987 76:786–791.
33. White RD, Pflugfelder PW, Lipton MJ, et al. Coronary artery bypass grafts: evaluation of patency with cine MR imaging. *AJR Am J Roentgenol* 1988;150:1271–1274.
34. Aurigemma GP, Reichek N, Axel L, et al. Noninvasive determination of coronary artery bypass graft patency by cine magnetic resonance imaging. *Circulation* 1989;80:1595–1602.
35. Vrachliotis TG, Bis KG, Aliabadi D, et al. Contrast-enhanced breath-hold MR angiography for evaluating patency of coronary artery bypass grafts. *AJR Am J Roentgenol* 1997;168:1073–1080.
36. Wintersperger BJ, Engelmann MG, von Smekal A, et al. Patency of coronary bypass grafts: assessment with breath-hold contrast-enhanced MR angiography—value of a non-electrocardiographically triggered technique. *Radiology* 1998;208:345–351.
37. van Rossum AC, Bedaux WL, Hofman MB. Morphologic and functional evaluation of coronary artery bypass conduits. *J Magn Reson Imaging* 1999;10:734–740.

38. Hoogendoorn LI, Pattynama PMT, Buis B, et al. Noninvasive evaluation of aortocoronary bypass grafts with magnetic resonance flow mapping. *Am J Cardiol* 1995;75:845–848.

39. Galjee MA, van Rossum AC, Doesburg T, et al. Value of magnetic resonance imaging in assessing patency and function of coronary artery bypass grafts: an angiographically controlled study. *Circulation* 1996;93:660–666.

40. Debatin JF, Strong JA, Sostman HD, et al. MR characterization of blood flow in native and grafted internal mammary arteries. *J Magn Reson Imaging* 1993;3:443–450.

41. Sakuma H, Globits S, O'Sullivan M, et al. Breath-hold MR measurements of blood flow velocity in internal mammary arteries and coronary artery bypass grafts. *J Magn Reson Imaging* 1996;6:219–222.

42. Ishida N, Sakuma H, Cruz BP, et al. MR flow measurement in the internal mammary artery-to-coronary artery bypass graft: comparison with graft stenosis at radiographic angiography. *Radiology* 2001;220:441–447.

43. Akasaka T, Yoshikawa J, Yoshida K, et al. Flow capacity of internal mammary artery grafts: early restriction and later improvement assessed by Doppler guide wire; comparison with saphenous vein grafts. *J Am Coll Cardiol* 1995;25:640–647.

44. van Rossum AC, Visser FC, Hofman MBM, et al. Global left ventricular perfusion: noninvasive measurement with cine MR imaging and phase velocity mapping of coronary venous outflow. *Radiology* 1992;182:685–691.

45. Lund GK, Wendland MF, Schimawaka A, et al. Coronary sinus flow measurement by means of velocity-encoded cine MR imaging: validation by using flow probes in dogs. *Radiology* 2000;217:487–493.

46. Schwitter J, De Marco T, Kneifel S, et al. Magnetic resonance-based assessment of global coronary flow and flow reserve and its relation to left ventricular function parameters: a comparison with positron emission tomography. *Circulation* 2000;101:2696–2702.

47. Koskenvuo JW, Sakuma H, Niemi P, et al. Global myocardial blood flow and global flow reserve measurements by MRI and PET are comparable. *J Magn Reson Imaging* 2001;13:361–366.

48. Kawada N, Sakuma H, Yamakado T, et al. Hypertrophic cardiomyopathy: MR measurement of coronary blood flow and vasodilator flow reserve in patients and healthy subjects. *Radiology* 1999;211:129–135.

49. von Schulthess GK, Schwitter J. Cardiac MR imaging: facts and fiction. *Radiology* 2001;218:326–328.

19

CORONARY ARTERY BYPASS GRAFTS

JOHANNES C. POST
WILLEMIJN L. F. BEDAUX
ALBERT C. VAN ROSSUM

Introduced in 1968 by Favoloro (1), coronary artery bypass graft (CABG) surgery has become a common revascularization procedure for patients with coronary artery disease, especially those with multiple-vessel disease. In the United States, approximately 1 in every 1,000 persons undergoes coronary artery surgery each year, for an annual case load of 300,000 operations (2). Different types of autologous vessel grafts may be used to bypass a severely stenosed coronary artery segment and provide the myocardium with a blood supply sufficient to avoid ischemia. Saphenous vein grafts are extensively used. Often, they serve as bypass grafts to distal branches of the right and circumflex coronary arteries. Proximally, they are anastomosed to the ascending aorta, and distally, either one end-to-side anastomosis ("single" graft) or one to several side-to-side and a final end-to-side anastomosis ("sequential" or "jump" grafts) are created. Because of their superior long-term patency, left internal mammary artery grafts are preferred for revascularizing the important left anterior descending artery and its diagonal branches. Other potential arterial conduits include the right internal mammary artery and the right gastroepiploic artery, which usually are anastomosed to the right coronary artery.

The clinical outcome of CABG surgery depends largely on the maintenance of graft patency (3). The operation provides excellent early symptomatic benefit. However, 25% of saphenous vein grafts become occluded within the first year, and of these, about half become occluded in the first 2 weeks following surgery. During the next 5 years, the annual occlusion rate is 2%, increasing to about 5% in subsequent years. Thus, 10 years after surgery, 50% to 60% of venous grafts are occluded, and many more are severely narrowed (4). The mechanisms involved in occlusion are thought to be thrombosis in the first weeks after surgery, followed by intimal proliferation and progressive atherosclerosis. Internal mammary artery (IMA) grafts become occluded less frequently, but significant stenosis develops in some of these grafts at the distal anastomosis at an early stage (5,6). Finally, stenoses may develop in the recipient coronary artery distal to the graft anastomosis, or progressive atherosclerosis may affect a nongrafted coronary artery. Unfortunately, then, recurrent chest pain after bypass surgery is not uncommon. Only a few patients require early repeated surgery or angioplasty, but after 12 years, 31% have undergone a second or third revascularization procedure (7).

Because atherosclerosis is a progressive disease and grafts may become occluded or severely diseased, diagnostic techniques are needed that make it possible to visualize bypass grafts together with the native coronary anatomy. In many patients, such assessments may be necessary several times.

IMAGING TECHNIQUES TO ASSESS BYPASS GRAFTS

Selective x-ray contrast angiography is the technique usually used to assess the patency of aortocoronary bypass grafts. Although it normally provides excellent visualization of bypass grafts, the procedure has some important disadvantages. It is invasive, and the use of contrast material and ionizing radiation is associated with a small but definite risk for complications. If a catheter fails to fit with an aortic graft anasto-

J. C. Post, W. L. F. Bedaux, and A. C. van Rossum: Department of Cardiology, Vrije Universiteit Medical Center, Amsterdam, The Netherlands.

mosis, doubt may persist regarding whether the graft has become occluded or has merely not been engaged. The technique can be extended to obtain functional information by measuring flow velocity with a Doppler wire, but doing so increases invasiveness, expense, and risk (8).

Several noninvasive techniques have been used to assess bypass grafts. Echocardiography has been used to assess grafts anastomosed to the left anterior descending artery, but its utility is limited (9–11). Computed tomography, in particular electron beam computed tomography, is a more promising technique for visualizing graft anatomy, but it entails the use of a contrast agent and relatively high doses of ionizing radiation (12–16). MRI has the advantage of being noninvasive and does not require the application of ionizing radiation, and it does not necessarily depend on the use of potentially nephrotoxic contrast agents. The technique offers the unique possibility of gathering not only anatomic data but also functional data on blood flow at the same time. Therefore, MRI is a very promising diagnostic technique for the combined noninvasive imaging and functional assessment of aortocoronary bypass grafts (17,18).

MRI OF BYPASS GRAFTS

Several MR techniques have been introduced to assess the patency of bypass grafts (Table 19.1). In general, the techniques that are useful in imaging the coronary arteries serve also for imaging bypass grafts, although the reverse is not necessarily true. In many studies, assessment has been limited to the proximal segment of the graft. For several reasons, the proximal segments of grafts are more easily studied than the distal segments; they are less subject to cardiac mo-

tion, and no confounding native coronary arteries and veins are nearby. Furthermore, the great majority of studies have included only venous grafts. This may be because venous grafts are larger in diameter than arterial grafts, and because metallic hemostatic clips are frequently used in the preparation of IMA grafts, which create ferromagnetic artifacts on MRI.

Conventional Spin-Echo and Gradient-Echo Imaging

The assessment of saphenous vein aortocoronary bypass graft anatomy has been a relatively early indication for cardiac MR studies. Several groups reported the feasibility of using conventional spin-echo techniques to determine the patency of bypass grafts (19–22). Patent grafts appear as conduits with a signal void because of rapid laminar blood flow, whereas occluded grafts or stenotic grafts with slow flow have an intermediate signal intensity. In comparative studies with conventional x-ray angiography as the reference, sensitivities in predicting graft patency ranged from 90% to 98% and specificities from 72% to 90%.

Conventional nonsegmented gradient-echo techniques with a relatively long echo time (TE) and repetition time (TR) have also been used at an early stage. Sensitivities were in the same range (88% to 98%), whereas specificities were slightly higher (86% to 100%) (23–25). With gradient-echo techniques, blood flow in patent grafts appears as a bright signal. The specificity of gradient-echo techniques in detecting graft patency is supposedly higher because the false-positive results that may appear with spin-echo techniques, when signal voiding is caused by metallic hemostatic clips, stents, calcifications, and thickened pericardium, are avoided.

TABLE 19.1. DETECTION OF BYPASS GRAFT PATENCY ACCORDING TO VARIOUS MR TECHNIQUES

Reference	Technique	No. Grafts	Sensitivity (%)	Specificity (%)	Accuracy (%)
White et al. (19)	SE	65	91	72	86
Rubinstein et al. (20)	SE	44	92	85	89
Jenkins et al. (21)	SE	60	90	90	90
Frija et al. (22)	SE	52	98	78	94
White et al. (23)	Cine	28	93	86	89
Aurigemma et al. (24)	Cine	45	88	100	91
Galjee et al. (25)	SE	98	98	85	96
	Cine		98	88	96
	Combined		98	76	94
Kalden et al. (29)	HASTE	59	95	93	95
	3D CE (ECG-trigg)	93	93	93	93
Kessler et al. (32)	3D navigator	19	87	100	89
Molinari et al. (33)	3D navigator	51	91	97	96
Wintersperger et al. (35)	3D CE (non–ECG-trigg)	76	95	81	92
Vrachliotis et al. (36)	3D CE (ECG-trigg)	44	93	97	95

HASTE, half-Fourier acquisition single-shot turbo spin echo; 3D, three-dimensional; CE, contrast-enhanced; ECG-trigg, electrocardiogram-triggered; SE, spin-echo.

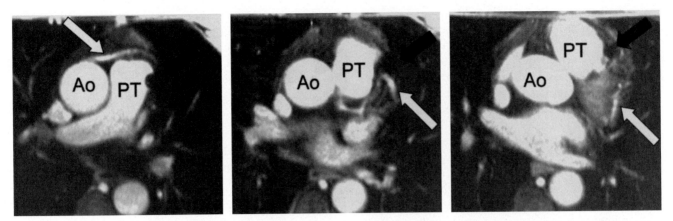

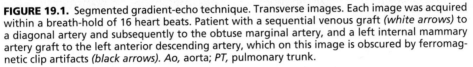

FIGURE 19.1. Segmented gradient-echo technique. Transverse images. Each image was acquired within a breath-hold of 16 heart beats. Patient with a sequential venous graft *(white arrows)* to a diagonal artery and subsequently to the obtuse marginal artery, and a left internal mammary artery graft to the left anterior descending artery, which on this image is obscured by ferromagnetic clip artifacts *(black arrows)*. *Ao,* aorta; *PT,* pulmonary trunk.

Two-Dimensional Breath-Hold MRA

Two-dimensional (2D) breath-hold techniques that have been extensively tested in coronary artery imaging can also be applied successfully to visualize bypass grafts (26,27) (Fig. 19.1). Within a breath-hold of 16 to 20 heart beats, a segmented gradient-echo image is acquired, typically with a 4- or 5-mm slice thickness and an in-plane resolution of about 1.0×1.4 mm. A surface coil is used. To cover the entire course of a bypass graft, repetitive breath-holds are necessary, so that the technique depends greatly on the ability of the patient to cooperate. It is also time-consuming, especially when multiple grafts are to be evaluated. A high degree of susceptibility to metallic materials introduced during CABG surgery has been reported (Fig. 19.1). The feasibility of evaluating separate segments of sequential "jump" grafts has been demonstrated (28).

In another 2D breath-hold approach, a multislice half-Fourier acquisition single-shot turbo spin-echo (HASTE) sequence is used. Within a breath-hold of approximately 14 seconds, seven T2-weighted images are acquired with a 1.3×1.4-mm in-plane resolution and a 5-mm slice thickness (Figs. 19.2 and 19.3). A sensitivity of 95% and a specificity of 93% in detecting graft patency have been reported (29). Furthermore, the percentage of distal anastomoses delineated is high (93%). The sequence is less susceptible to metallic implant artifacts than are gradient-echo techniques. This may be why a high rate of accuracy has been reported in detecting the patency of arterial grafts, whereas visualization with gradient-echo techniques in many patients is hampered by the presence of metallic hemostatic clips; a sensitivity as high as 90% and a specificity of 100% have been reported. However, the low pretest likelihood of detecting an occluded arterial graft is undoubtedly related to the low false-positive rate. In our personal experience, HASTE sequences have been very useful for visualizing bypass grafts, but the detection of graft disease is rather poor.

Three-Dimensional Respiratory-Gated MRA

A 3D data set of truly contiguous slices may be obtained with respiratory-gated 3D gradient-echo techniques. Gating to the respiratory cycle is achieved with navigators that monitor the position of the diaphragm (30). MR data ac-

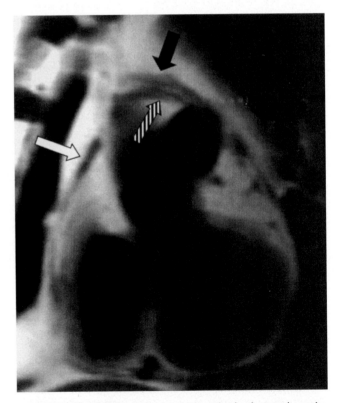

FIGURE 19.2. Half-Fourier acquisition single-shot turbo spin-echo (HASTE) technique. Coronal image. Patient with three single venous grafts: to the right coronary artery *(white arrow)*, to a diagonal artery *(striped arrow)*, and to the obtuse marginal artery *(black arrow)*.

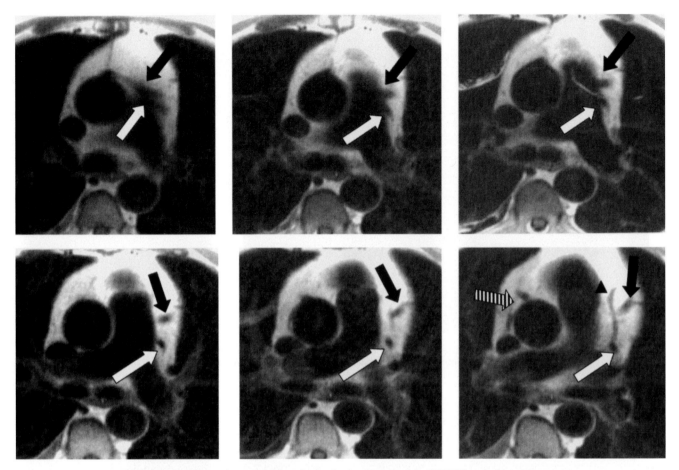

FIGURE 19.3. Half-Fourier acquisition single-shot turbo spin-echo (HASTE) technique. Transverse images. Patient with three single venous grafts: to the right coronary artery *(striped arrow)*, to a diagonal artery *(black arrows)*, and to the obtuse marginal artery *(white arrows)*. The native left anterior descending artery is indicated by an *arrowhead.*

quired with a preset acceptance window of respiration-induced diaphragm excursion are used for image reconstruction. The patient is allowed to breathe freely without the need for repetitive breath-holding, at the expense of an increase in imaging time. Several refinements of this gating procedure have been developed for imaging the coronary arteries (31). In the assessment of bypass graft patency, sensitivities of 87% to 91% have been reported, with specificities of 97% to 100% (32,33).

Three-Dimensional Contrast-Enhanced Breath-Hold MRA

Breath-hold contrast-enhanced MRA is a relatively new technique that was first applied in imaging the aorta (34). The T1-shortening effect of the contrast agent on blood makes it possible to obtain a high degree of vascular contrast with the use of short-TR/TE gradient-echo sequences. After an interstitial contrast agent has been injected intravenously, preferably with an MR-compatible power injector, a 3D gradient-echo sequence with a short TR/TE (4.4/1.4 milliseconds or even shorter) is applied. Within a

breath-hold of approximately 30 seconds, a 3D volume slab with a typical thickness of 6 to 9 cm is imaged that consists of 24 to 32 contiguous slice partitions. Before the 3D slab is acquired, a single-slice 2D turbo gradient-echo sequence is used to time the arrival in the aorta of a test bolus of the contrast agent. To maximize the contrast-enhancing effect, the acquisition of the central k-space lines of the 3D data is set to coincide with the peak arrival of contrast. This is achieved by introducing a time delay between the contrast injection and the start of the imaging sequence (delay equals arrival time minus one-half or one-third the acquisition time). With newly introduced rapid scan techniques, real-time tracking of the contrast bolus is possible, so that the calculations for an optimized contrast arrival are not needed. The spatial resolution is typically 1 × 1.5 mm in-plane and the section thickness 2 to 3 mm, depending on the field of view, matrix size, number of partitions, and slab thickness. Each partition of the 3D acquisition yields a source image. Studies may be evaluated by reading the source images and by postprocessing techniques such as maximum intensity projection and planar or curved reformatting (Figs. 19.4, 19.5, and 19.6).

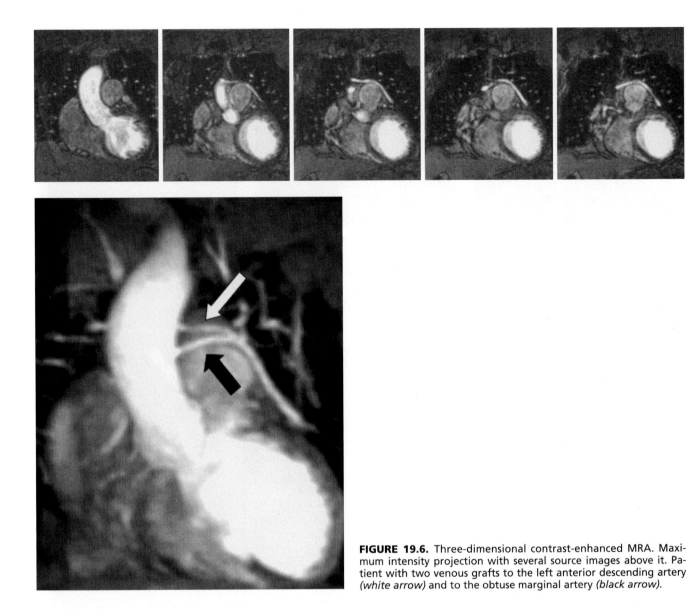

FIGURE 19.6. Three-dimensional contrast-enhanced MRA. Maximum intensity projection with several source images above it. Patient with two venous grafts to the left anterior descending artery *(white arrow)* and to the obtuse marginal artery *(black arrow)*.

used because of their better long-term patency, but they have been excluded from most MR studies because of metallic clip artifacts. Flow reserve measurements proximal to the clip artifacts may be of diagnostic help. The use of alternative methods to obtain hemostasis without such clips would improve imaging results.

So far, the application of MRI in CABGs has been limited to demonstrating patency versus total occlusion. The documentation of nonocclusive graft disease has not been convincing with the techniques available to date. The MR measurements of blood flow at rest and after pharmacologic stress to calculate functional flow parameters may prove helpful, in addition to anatomic imaging, in determining the functional status of diseased bypass grafts and their recipient coronary arteries.

However, even a clear demonstration of graft segment patency or narrowing is often insufficient for clinical deci-

sion making. In most cases, information about the status of the native coronary arteries is also needed. A recipient coronary artery may have narrowed beyond the anastomosis of a patent graft segment, and a progression of disease in other coronary arteries must be excluded. Thus, MRI currently is not expected to eliminate the need for conventional x-ray coronary angiography when coronary reinterventions are under consideration.

INDICATIONS

Nonetheless, in some cases, MRI of bypass grafts may be clinically indicated even when a knowledge of the status of the native coronary arteries is not immediately needed. For example, a patient may have chest pain shortly after CABG surgery. Also, later after CABG surgery, knowing that a graft

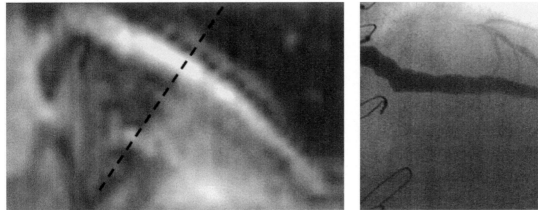

A   B

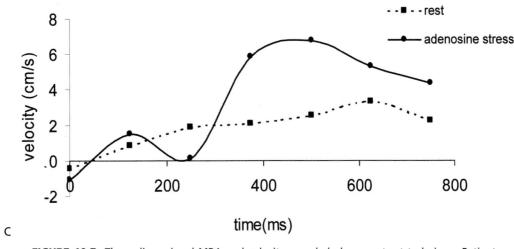

C

FIGURE 19.7. Three-dimensional MRA and velocity-encoded phase-contrast technique. Patient with single venous graft to the left anterior descending (LAD) artery and venous sequential graft to posterior descending and posterolateral branches of the right coronary artery. **A:** Curved planar reformatted image of single LAD graft. *Dashed line* indicates plane orientation used for flow measurement. **B:** Coronary x-ray angiography of single LAD graft. **C:** Cross-sectional averaged velocity measured at multiple phases throughout the cardiac cycle. Calculated volume flow was 38 mL/min at rest and 68 mL/min during adenosine stress, yielding a flow reserve of 1.8.

is patent and functioning well may be helpful in deciding whether coronary angiography can be postponed in a patient with ambiguous thoracic pain or only mild angina pectoris. Noninvasive monitoring of flow parameters might then be useful in detecting a gradual increase of graft stenosis and deciding whether to proceed to x-ray angiography and possibly angioplasty with stent placement before the onset of a total occlusion.

Furthermore, MRI can be used as a screening procedure before x-ray angiography to indicate the number of grafts to be visualized and thereby shorten the angiographic procedure considerably. Another useful indication appears to be in assessing the patency of grafts that are not visualized at conventional angiography. Although such an assessment will often indicate proximal occlusion of the graft, failure of the catheter to fit with the aortic graft anastomosis may result in a false diagnosis of graft occlusion. In case of doubt, MRA can rapidly confirm or discard the diagnosis. Finally, when

angiography has demonstrated graft narrowing, MR assessment may be helpful in further management by assessing functional flow parameters when Doppler wires are not available.

Notwithstanding these indications, most patients at present still require conventional x-ray angiography to assess the status of their native coronary arteries and bypass grafts. Unless MRI can also provide more detailed information regarding the status of the native coronary arteries, a wide application is unlikely to occur. Further improvements in MRI of the coronary arteries and bypass grafts may be expected based on new developments in hardware, including more powerful gradient systems, new and sophisticated pulse sequence designs, and the increased use of contrast agents. Whether MRI will ever develop into a diagnostic tool that can obviate the need for repeated invasive diagnostic procedures in postsurgical patients is presently unknown.

REFERENCES

1. Favaloro RG. Saphenous vein autograft replacement of severe segmental coronary artery occlusion. Operative technique. *Ann Thorac Surg* 1968;5:334–339.

2. Gersh BJ, Braunwald E, Rutherford JD. Chronic coronary artery disease: coronary artery bypass graft surgery. In: Braunwald E, ed. *Heart disease, a textbook of cardiovascular medicine,* 5th ed. Philadelphia: WB Saunders, 1997:1316.

3. Chesebro JH, Clements IP, Fuster V, et al. A platelet-inhibitor-drug trial in coronary artery bypass operations. Benefit of perioperative dipyridamole and aspirin therapy on early post-operative vein-graft patency. *N Engl J Med* 1982;307:73–78.

4. Henderson WG, Goldman S, Copeland JG, et al. Antiplatelet or anticoagulant therapy after coronary artery bypass surgery. A meta-analysis of clinical trials. *Ann Intern Med* 1989;111:743–750.

5. van der Meer J, Hillege HL, van Gilst WH, et al. A comparison of internal mammary artery and saphenous vein grafts after coronary artery bypass surgery: no difference in 1-year occlusion rates and clinical outcome. *Circulation* 1994;90:2367–2374.

6. Cameron A, Davis KB, Green G, et al. Coronary bypass surgery with internal-thoracic-artery grafts: effects on survival over a 15-year period. *N Engl J Med* 1996;334:216–219.

7. Weintraub WS, Jones EL, Craver JM, et al. Frequency of repeat coronary bypass or coronary angioplasty after coronary artery bypass surgery using saphenous venous grafts. *Am J Cardiol* 1994;73:103–112.

8. Bach R, Kern M, Donohue T, et al. Comparison of phasic flow velocity characteristics of arterial and venous coronary artery bypass conduits. *Circulation* 1993;88:133–140.

9. Fusejima K, Takahara Y, Sudo Y, et al. Comparison of coronary hemodynamics in patients with internal mammary artery and saphenous vein coronary artery bypass grafts: a noninvasive approach using combined two-dimensional and Doppler echocardiography. *J Am Coll Cardiol* 1990;15:131–139.

10. Takagi T, Yoshikawa J, Yoshida K, et al. Noninvasive assessment of left internal mammary artery graft patency using duplex Doppler echocardiography from supraclavicular fossa. *J Am Coll Cardiol* 1993;22:1647–1652.

11. Voudris V, Athanassopoulos G, Vassilikos V, et al. Usefulness of flow reserve in the left internal mammary artery to determine graft patency to the left anterior descending coronary artery. *Am J Cardiol* 1999;83:1157–1163.

12. Stanford W, Galvin JR, Skorton DJ, et al. The evaluation of coronary bypass graft patency: direct and indirect techniques other than coronary arteriography. *AJR Am J Roentgenol* 1991;156:15–22.

13. Stanford W, Brundage BH, MacMillan R, et al. Sensitivity and specificity of assessing coronary bypass graft patency with ultrafast computed tomography: results of a multicenter study. *J Am Coll Cardiol* 1988;12:1–7.

14. Tello R, Costello P, Ecker C, et al. Spiral CT evaluation of coronary artery bypass graft patency. *J Comput Assist Tomogr* 1993;17:253–259.

15. Engelmann MG, Von Smekal A, Knez A, et al. Accuracy of spiral computed tomography for identifying arterial and venous coronary graft patency. *Am J Cardiol* 1997;80:569–574.

16. Achenbach S, Moshage W, Ropers D, et al. Noninvasive, three-dimensional visualization of coronary artery bypass grafts by electron beam tomography. *Am J Cardiol* 1997;79:856–861.

17. van Rossum AC, Galjee MA, Doesburg T, et al. The role of magnetic resonance in the evaluation of functional results after CABG/PTCA. *Int J Card Imaging* 1993;9:59–69.

18. Galjee MA, van Rossum AC, Doesburg T, et al. Quantification of coronary artery bypass graft flow by magnetic resonance phase velocity mapping. *Magn Reson Imaging* 1996;14:485–493.

19. White RD, Caputo GR, Mark AS, et al. Coronary artery bypass graft patency: noninvasive evaluation with MR imaging. *Radiology* 1987;164:681–686.

20. Rubinstein RI, Askenase AD, Thickman D, et al. Magnetic resonance imaging to evaluate patency of aortocoronary bypass grafts. *Circulation* 1987;76:786–791.

21. Jenkins JPR, Love HG, Foster CJ, et al. Detection of coronary artery bypass graft patency as assessed by magnetic resonance imaging. *Br J Radiol* 1988;61:2–4.

22. Frija G, Schouman-Claeys E, Lacombe P, et al. A study of coronary artery bypass graft patency using MR imaging. *J Comput Assist Tomogr* 1989;13:226–232.

23. White RD, Pflugfelder PW, Lipton MJ, et al. Coronary artery bypass grafts: evaluation of patency with cine MR imaging. *AJR Am J Roentgenol* 1988;150:1271–1274.

24. Aurigemma GP, Reichek N, Axel L, et al. Noninvasive determination of coronary artery bypass graft patency by cine magnetic resonance imaging. *Circulation* 1989;80:1595–1602.

25. Galjee MA, van Rossum AC, Doesburg T, et al. Value of magnetic resonance imaging in assessing patency and function of coronary artery bypass grafts: an angiographically controlled study. *Circulation* 1996;93:660–666.

26. Manning WJ, Li W, Boyle NG, et al. Fat-suppressed breath-hold magnetic resonance coronary angiography. *Circulation* 1993;87:94–104.

27. Hartnell GG, Cohen MC, Charlamb M, et al. Segmented k-space magnetic resonance angiography for the detection of coronary artery bypass graft patency. Book of abstracts of the 4th annual meeting of the International Society for Magnetic Resonance in Medicine, New York, 1996;1:178(abst).

28. Post JC, van Rossum AC, Bronzwaer JGF, et al. Magnetic resonance angiography of sequential aortocoronary bypass grafts. *Circulation* 1997;96(Suppl):I-133.

29. Kalden P, Kreitner KF, Wittlinger T, et al. Assessment of coronary artery bypass grafts: value of different breath-hold MR imaging techniques. *AJR Am J Roentgenol* 1999;172:1359–1364.

30. Hofman MBM, Paschal CB, Li D, et al. MRI of coronary arteries: 2D breath-hold versus 3D respiratory-gated acquisition. *J Comput Assist Tomogr* 1995;19:56–62.

31. Danias PG, McConnell MV, Khasgiwala VC, et al. Prospective navigator correction of image position for coronary MR angiography. *Radiology* 1997;203:733–736.

32. Kessler W, Achenbach S, Moshage W, et al. Usefulness of respiratory gated magnetic resonance coronary angiography in assessing narrowings ≥50% in diameter in native coronary arteries and in aortocoronary bypass conduits. *Am J Cardiol* 1997;80:989–993.

33. Molinari G, Sardanelli F, Zandrino F, et al. Value of navigator echo magnetic resonance angiography in detecting occlusion/patency of arterial and venous, single and sequential coronary bypass grafts. *Int J Card Imaging* 2000;16:149–160.

34. Prince MR, Narasimham DL, Stanley JC, et al. Breath-hold gadolinium-enhanced MR angiography of the abdominal aorta and its major branches. *Radiology* 1995;197:785–792.

35. Wintersperger BJ, Engelmann MG, von Smekal A, et al. Patency of coronary artery bypass grafts: assessment with breath-hold contrast-enhanced MR angiography—value of a non-electrocardiographically triggered technique. *Radiology* 1998;208:345–351.

36. Vrachliotis TG, Bis KG, Aliabadi D, et al. Contrast-enhanced breath-hold MR angiography for evaluating patency of coronary artery bypass grafts. *AJR Am J Roentgenol* 1997;168:1073–1080.

37. Goldfarb JW, Edelman RR. Coronary arteries: breath-hold, gadolinium-enhanced, three-dimensional MR angiography. *Radiology* 1998;206:830–834.

38. Voigtländer T, Kreitner KF, Wittlinger T, et al. MR measurement of flow reserve in coronary grafts. Book of abstracts of the 2nd annual meeting of the Society for Cardiovascular Magnetic Resonance, 1999:53(abst).

39. Debatin JF, Strong JA, Sostman HD, et al. MR characterization of blood flow in native and grafted internal mammary arteries. *J Magn Reson Imaging* 1993;3:443–450.

40. Sakuma H, Globits S, O'Sullivan M, et al. Breath-hold MR measurements of blood flow velocity in internal mammary arteries and coronary artery bypass grafts. *J Magn Reson Imaging* 1996;6:219–222.

41. Kawada N, Sakuma H, Cruz BC, et al. Noninvasive detection of significant stenosis in the coronary artery bypass grafts using fast velocity-encoded cine MRI. Book of abstracts of the 2nd annual meeting of the Society for Cardiovascular Magnetic Resonance, 1999:82(abst).

42. Langerak, SE, Kunz P, Vliegen HW, et al. Improved MR flow mapping in coronary artery bypass grafts during adenosine-induced stress. *Radiology* 2001;218:540–547.

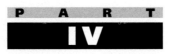

PART

IV

CONGENITAL HEART DISEASE

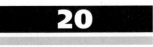

20

CONGENITAL HEART DISEASE: MORPHOLOGY AND FUNCTION

PHILIP A. ARAOZ
GAUTHAM P. REDDY
CHARLES B. HIGGINS

The primary objectives of imaging in congenital heart disease (CHD) are the precise delineation of cardiovascular anatomy and the quantitative assessment of function. The evaluation of CHD was one of the first applications of cardiac MRI and continues to be one of its most important indications. MRI has significant advantages over other modalities, including echocardiography and angiography, for the definitive assessment of congenital cardiovascular anomalies. MRI does not require the use of a contrast agent or ionizing radiation. The absence of ionizing radiation is a major advantage of MRI in children, who in the past have been exposed to large doses of radiation during cine angiography for initial diagnosis and postoperative monitoring.

The role of MRI has been greatly influenced by the perceived success of echocardiography as the primary noninvasive imaging technique in CHD. The major applications have been for lesions incompletely evaluated by echocardiography, most notably coarctation of the aorta, branch stenosis of pulmonary arteries, and the depiction of three-dimensional (3D) relationships in very complex CHD. However, substantial technologic improvements, especially fast imaging, now make MRI competitive with echocardiography in all areas of CHD, both for the evaluation of morphology and for the quantification of function and flow. MRI may now be readily used to appraise collateral circulation in coarctation of the aorta, quantify shunts, measure flow in the left and right pulmonary arteries, and quantify valvular regurgitation.

TECHNIQUES

Morphologic information is obtained primarily with electrocardiogram (ECG)-gated multislice spin-echo images through the heart, usually with a slice thickness of 5 mm and a gap between slices of 1 mm, and with thinner (3 mm) slices at increased numbers-of-excitations through areas of interest. Respiratory compensation is used to minimize artifacts caused by respiratory motion. Gadolinium-enhanced MRA provides an increased spatial resolution of the great vessels and their branches and lends itself to 3D reconstruction. In older children, adults, and patients on mechanical ventilation, MRA is performed while respiration is suspended. Functional information can be derived from a variety of techniques. Two of the most commonly used are fast gradient-echo sequences gated to the cardiac cycle, played in

P. A. Araoz, G. P. Reddy, and C. B. Higgins: Department of Radiology, University of California San Francisco, San Francisco, California.

cine mode to quantify ventricular volumes and masses, and velocity-encoded cine MRI (VEC MRI), a phase-contrast technique. VEC MRI provides velocity measurements from which blood flow can be calculated. These techniques are described further below.

MAJOR CLINICAL INDICATIONS

The applications of MRI in CHD are influenced by the greater experience and availability of echocardiography. Echocardiography is particularly useful in infants and young children because the acoustic window usually allows clear visualization of the heart and great vessels. MRI is an alternative imaging technique in older children and adults, in whom echocardiography is less effective. In addition, MRI can provide complementary information, especially in the evaluation of complex anomalies and supracardiac structures.

The major clinical indications of MRI are the following:

1. Assessment of thoracic aortic anomalies
2. Determination of the presence and size of the pulmonary arteries in tetralogy of Fallot and pulmonary atresia
3. Delineation of the anatomy of complex ventricular anomalies
4. Definition of pulmonary venous anomalies, including anomalous pulmonary venous connections
5. Follow-up after surgery
6. Assessment of situs abnormalities
7. Definition of systemic venous abnormalities
8. Differential measurement of blood flow in the right and left pulmonary arteries
9. Quantification of shunts
10. Measurement of collateral circulation in coarctation of the aorta
11. Measurement of the pressure gradient across coarctation and surgical conduits
12. Quantification of ventricular masses and volumes
13. Measurement of pulmonary regurgitant fraction after repair of tetralogy of Fallot

SEGMENTAL APPROACH TO CARDIAC ANATOMY

The analysis of complex CHD requires a systematic approach. The approach most widely used today is the segmental one, in which the heart is thought of as comprising three main segments (atria, ventricles, and great vessels) and the connections between them (venous, atrioventricular, and ventriculoarterial connections) (1). Cardiac anatomists have different opinions about which part of the segmental approach should be emphasized and about how some abnormalities should be classified, especially complex ventricular abnormalities (1–3). Because the intent of this chapter is not to create a definitive, robust categorization system but rather to present a helpful scan pattern, abnormalities have been

organized according to where they would be encountered during the evaluation of an MRI examination of the heart.

Axial sections from the aortic arch to the upper abdomen demonstrate the segmental cardiovascular anatomy. The relationships and relative sizes of the great arteries are delineated at the base of the heart. Normally, the aorta is to the right of and posterior to the pulmonary artery, and the two vessels are nearly equal in size.

The reliability of MRI for delineating the segmental cardiac anatomy was reported in 74 patients suspected of having CHD (4). In all subjects in whom images encompassed a sufficient portion of the heart, MRI defined the relationships among the great vessels, the situs, and the type of ventricular loop. The findings on MRI were validated by other imaging studies in all cases.

ATRIA

The embryology, functions, and structures of the right and left atria are different. Therefore, the chamber called the *right atrium* (RA) is not defined by its position on the right side of the heart, but by its structure. If the chamber that is structurally an RA is found on the left side of the heart, it is called a *morphologic RA* to emphasize that its name describes its internal architecture, not its location (3).

The most definitive distinguishing feature of the atria are the atrial appendages. On an axial MR image, the RA appendage appears as a triangular structure with a broad-based opening into the RA. This is in distinction to the left atrial (LA) appendage, which is a long, narrow, finger-like projection with a narrow orifice (5) (Fig. 20.1). The atrial

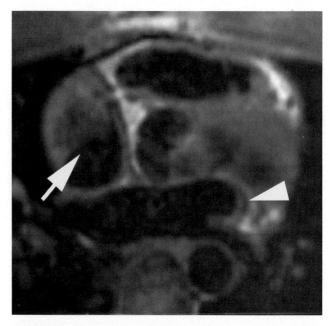

FIGURE 20.1. Normal atrial appendages. Axial T1-weighted spin-echo images. The right atrial appendage has a characteristic wide attachment to the right atrium *(arrow)*. The opening of the left atrial appendage is narrow *(arrowhead)*.

appendages are the most constant part of the atria, even in the face of complex abnormalities. Therefore, if the atrial appendages can be identified, the atria can be categorized as morphologically right or left (3). In cases in which the atrial appendages are difficult to identify, the next most reliable structure is the drainage of the inferior vena cava (IVC). Superior vena caval and pulmonary venous drainage are variable and are not used to identify atrial morphology (6).

Situs Abnormalities

Atrial morphology develops primarily as a result of the RA absorbing a confluence of veins that collect systemic venous return in the embryo (5). Thus, many of the defining features of the RA are intimately related to its development as the atrium that receives the systemic venous return from the

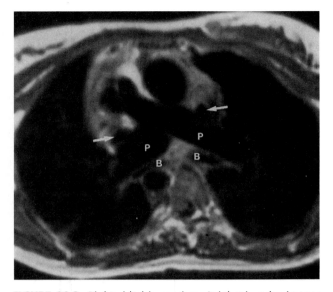

FIGURE 20.3. Right-sided isomerism. Axial spin-echo images show both pulmonary arteries *(P)* running anterior to the bronchi *(B)*. Note the bilateral superior venae cavae *(arrows)*. (From Higgins CB. Congenital heart disease. In: Higgins CB, Hricak H, Helms CA, eds. *Magnetic resonance imaging of the body,* 3rd ed. Philadelphia: Lippincott–Raven Publishers, 1997:470, with permission.)

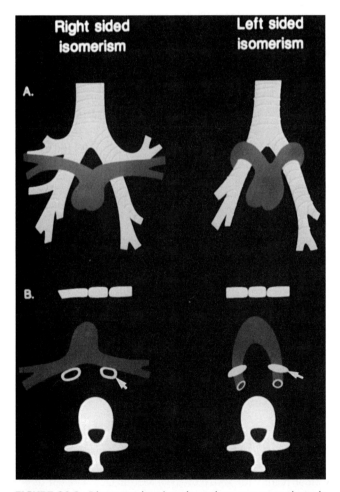

FIGURE 20.2. Diagrams showing the pulmonary artery branching in right-sided isomerism *(right)* and left-sided isomerism *(left)* in the coronal **(A)** and axial **(B)** planes. In right-sided isomerism, the course of the pulmonary arteries is anterior to the bronchi. In left-sided isomerism, the course of the pulmonary arteries is superior and then posterior to the bronchi. (From Higgins CB. Congenital heart disease. In: Higgins CB, Hricak H, Helms CA, eds. *Magnetic resonance imaging of the body,* 3rd ed. Philadelphia: Lippincott–Raven Publishers, 1997:466, with permission.)

body. The atria and the venous return from the body form at the same time, and the formation of the atria in part depends on the formation of venous return from the body, so that abnormalities of atrial position are usually associated with abnormalities in the situs of organs in the rest of the body (7). Abnormalities of atrial location develop early in fetal life and are usually associated with serious and widespread anomalies. MRI is a very attractive modality for evaluating abnormalities of the heart, abdomen, and lungs in a single examination.

The right-sided abdominal and thoracic structures are usually on the same side as the morphologic RA. Likewise, the left-sided organs are usually on the same side as the morphologic LA. In a developmental anomaly in which both atria have morphologic features of an RA *(RA isomerism)*, the visceral and thoracic structures tend to be right-sided. Likewise, bilateral left atria *(LA isomerism)* are associated with bilateral left-sided visceral and thoracic structures (7).

The bronchi and pulmonary arteries have a characteristic relationship (Fig. 20.2). In RA isomerism, both lungs usually have three lobes, and both bronchi have the pattern of a right bronchus—that is, the pulmonary artery runs in front of and beneath the main bronchus (a type of bronchus known as an *eparterial bronchus*) (Fig. 20.3). Right-sided isomerism is often associated with asplenia syndrome. The liver is large and crosses the midline, and the spleen is often absent.

In LA isomerism, both lungs have two lobes, and both the right and left pulmonary arteries pass over their respective bronchi. This type of bronchial pattern is known as

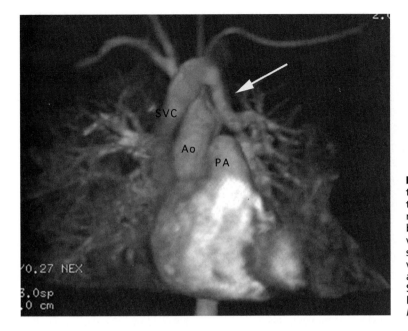

FIGURE 20.6. Partial anomalous pulmonary venous return. Three-dimensional volume-rendered image obtained from a breath-hold gadolinium MRA. An abnormal vessel, a left-sided vertical vein *(arrow)*, drains blood from the left upper lobe into the brachiocephalic vein. Note that the left vertical vein is derived from the same embryologic remnant as the left-sided superior vena cava *(SVC)*, and they have a similar appearance on axial images through the upper thorax. The left-sided SVC and the vertical vein can be distinguished by following the vessels on consecutive images. *Ao,* aorta; *PA,* pulmonary artery.

PVC, the anomalous veins can drain into supracardiac (SVC, left vertical vein), cardiac (RA), or infracardiac (IVC) sites (9). In all cases of CHD, it is important to identify the connections of all four pulmonary veins, a function for which spin-echo MRI has been shown to be accurate (11). Accuracy should be even better with the use of gadolinium-enhanced MRA (12) (Fig. 20.6).

PAPVC is a left-to-right shunt because oxygenated pulmonary venous blood flows into the right side of the heart. Therefore, ancillary findings of left-to-right shunting may be identified, including RA and possibly RV enlargement, depending on the magnitude of the shunt. The shunt can be quantified, as discussed later in the section on intracardiac defects. PAPVC is associated with atrial septal defect (ASD) and occurs in almost all patients with a sinus venosus ASD. Axial or coronal MR images can clearly depict the connections of the pulmonary veins. These connections also can be demonstrated with gadolinium-enhanced MRA. MRI shows the right upper pulmonary vein connecting to the SVC, which is the most frequent type of PAPVC. On axial MR images, dilation of the coronary sinus raises the possibility of anomalous drainage into this vessel. MR tomograms and gadolinium-enhanced MRA can depict the common right pulmonary artery entering the IVC in patients with scimitar syndrome.

VENTRICLES AND ATRIOVENTRICULAR CONNECTIONS

Abnormalities of the atrioventricular connections consist primarily of discordant connections (e.g., congenitally corrected transposition of the great arteries) or of atrioventric-

ular stenosis or atresia (e.g., tricuspid atresia, double-inlet ventricle, straddling atrioventricular valve) (2,3,13). The first step in analyzing atrioventricular connections is to identify the ventricles and determine their morphology.

Axial and coronal MR images through the ventricles can be used to identify these chambers as morphologically right or left. In early embryonic development, the heart is a straight tube with the two ventricles connected in series. The tube then folds over, so that the distal ventricle (the primitive RV) is placed beside and to the right of the primitive LV (5,14,15). Because the outflow of the primitive heart arises from the primitive RV, the morphologic RV has a muscular infundibulum. This muscular infundibulum and well-defined outflow region separate the RV atrioventricular valve (the tricuspid valve) from the semilunar valve (5) (Fig. 20.7). These findings are readily identified on axial MRI, in which several axial slices usually separate the tricuspid valve and pulmonic valve. On the other hand, in the morphologic LV, the atrioventricular valve and semilunar valve are in fibrous continuity (5) and are seen on adjacent images in the axial plane (Fig. 20.8). The atrioventricular valve of the morphologic RV (the tricuspid valve) is slightly more apical in location than the atrioventricular valve of the morphologic LV (the mitral valve). As a result, in the normal heart, a small septum, called the *atrioventricular septum,* divides the LV from the RA (3,5) (Fig. 20.9).

The morphologic RV has more trabeculations than the morphologic LV. The ventricular septum at the apex is heavily trabeculated in the RV but smooth in the LV. A muscular band (moderator band) connecting the RV free wall and septum is depicted on axial images (5) (Fig. 20.10).

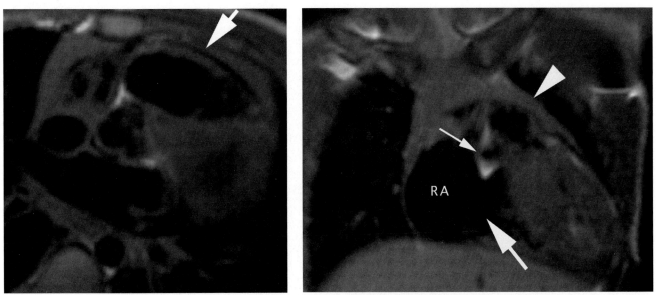

FIGURE 20.7. Normal right ventricle. **A:** Axial T1-weighted spin-echo images show the muscular infundibulum of the right ventricle *(arrow)*. **B:** Coronal image in the same patient shows that the pulmonary valve *(arrowhead)* is not continuous with the tricuspid valve *(large arrow)*. The proximal right coronary artery *(small arrow)* is seen in cross section as it runs through the right atrioventricular groove. *RA,* right atrium.

Abnormalities of Ventricular Location/Position

The normal rightward bending of the primitive cardiac tube places the morphologic right ventricle on the right side of the heart. This rightward bending is called *D-looping* (*D* for the Latin *dextro,* "right"). If the primitive heart tube bends to the left, the result is called *L-looping* (*L* for *levo,* "left"), in which the morphologic RV is placed on the left side of the heart. The normal heart has a D-ventricular loop. Any heart in which the morphologic RV is on the left side may be said to have an L-ventricular loop (13).

Atrioventricular connections can be concordant or discordant. In normal, concordant atrioventricular connections, the RA is connected to the RV, and the LA to the LV.

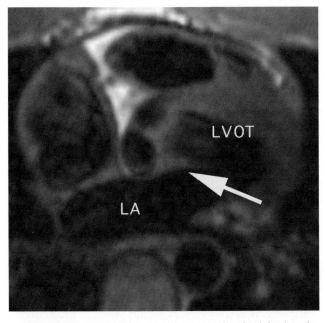

FIGURE 20.8. Normal left ventricle. T1-weighted axial spin-echo images show normal fibrous continuity *(arrow)* of the aortic valve and mitral valve. *LA,* left atrium; *LVOT,* left ventricular outflow tract.

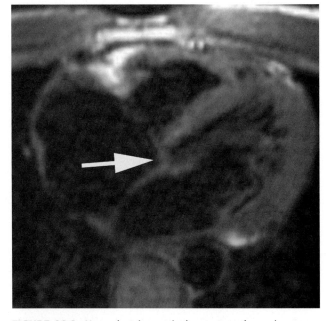

FIGURE 20.9. Normal atrioventricular septum *(arrow)* seen on axial T1-weighted spin-echo images.

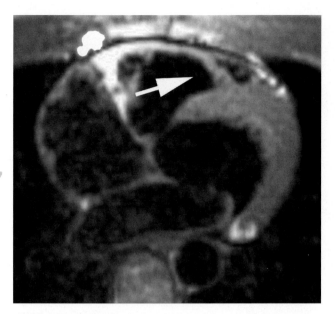

FIGURE 20.10. Moderator band. Axial T1-weighted spin-echo image shows a prominent moderator band *(arrow)*, a characteristic feature of the normal right ventricle.

The atrioventricular valves remain with their respective ventricles, regardless of the type of ventricular loop. The mitral valve resides with the LV, and the tricuspid valve is part of the RV, except in patients with double-inlet ventricle. Although MRI cannot directly distinguish the atrioventricular valves, the identification of ventricular morphology indicates the type of atrioventricular valve within the ventricle.

RA-LV and LA-RV connections are discordant atrioventricular connections. Congenitally corrected transposition of the great arteries is an example of an anomaly with atrioventricular discordance.

Congenitally Corrected Transposition of the Great Arteries (Atrioventricular and Ventriculoarterial Discordance)

A pattern in which the morphologic ventricles are on the wrong side of the heart (L-loop) but the atria are in the appropriate location (normal atrial situs) and the great vessels come off the appropriate side of the heart (and therefore the inappropriate morphologic ventricles) is most commonly called *congenitally corrected transposition of the great arteries* (Fig. 20.11). Authors who use classification systems that emphasize connections use the term *atrioventricular and ventriculoarterial discordance* (1,3).

Corrected transposition can be understood as a ventricular inversion anomaly—the morphologic ventricles are transposed. The remaining structures (atria and great vessels) may be displaced to accommodate the abnormally located ventricles but are otherwise normal. As a result, blood flows to the appropriate location. On the right side, deoxygenated blood flows from the body into the RA, passes into

a ventricle with fibrous continuity between its atrioventricular and ventriculoarterial valves (i.e., a morphologic LV), and ultimately into the pulmonary arteries and lungs. Oxygenated blood then returns to the LA, flows into a ventricle with a muscular outflow tract (i.e., a morphologic RV), and eventually into the aorta and systemic circulation (16,17).

In almost all cases of atrioventricular discordance and ventriculoarterial discordance, the aorta is anterior to and to the left of the pulmonary artery—a spatial relationship known as *L-transposition*. As a result, the position of the great vessels was often formerly used to predict the position of the ventricles before the advent of cross-sectional imaging (17). However, the position of the great vessels is not always predictive of the ventricular morphology (17); moreover, with MRI, ventricular morphology can be determined directly (18). Therefore, abnormalities of ventricular location should be defined by the position of the ventricles, and the position of the great vessels should be described separately.

In corrected transposition, blood flows in the appropriate direction, and if no other abnormalities are present, patients are asymptomatic. However, the morphologic RV is not designed to pump against systemic pressures for the long term, and failure of the morphologic RV (clinically left-sided heart failure) or arrhythmias may develop when patients reach their 40s or 50s (19). In 99% of patients with congenitally corrected transposition, other abnormalities dominate the clinical picture. The diagnosis is usually made in childhood. One associated anomaly is Ebstein malformation (described below) of the morphologic RV. Because Ebstein anomaly is an abnormality of the tricuspid valve, and the tricuspid valve is a part of the morphologic RV, Ebstein anomaly with corrected transposition is associated with obstruction of blood flow or regurgitation into the LA. Ventricular septal defect (VSD) or pulmonic stenosis may also be present (16,17).

Inadequate Ventricular Size/Decreased Flow through a Ventricle

For the cardiac chambers to grow to normal size and function properly, adequate blood must flow through them during embryonic life. If the atrioventricular or ventriculoarterial valves are stenotic, or if blood is preferentially shunted away from a ventricle, then the ventricle fails to develop normally. Depending on the severity of the underlying problem, the lesser ventricle may be simply small, or it may be rudimentary with no visible lumen. Many clinicians and authors refer to such hearts as functionally *univentricular*—a term that has created controversy among anatomists, who have debated the strict definition of a ventricle (20). Nevertheless, the concept of "univentricular" is helpful in thinking about surgical correction for this group of problems. In most cases, the surgeon's goal is to use the larger, more functional ventricle to pump blood to the systemic circulation. Usually, the smaller ventricle is bypassed by connecting the

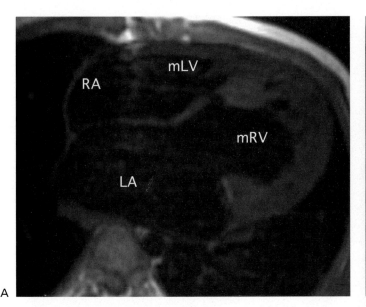

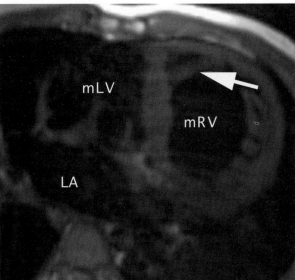

FIGURE 20.11. Corrected transposition of the great vessels. Axial T1-weighted spin-echo images. **A:** The most inferior image shows the right atrium *(RA)* and left atrium *(LA)* in their normal position. The LA connects to the morphologic right ventricle *(mRV)*, which is on the left side of the heart. The RA connects to the morphologic left ventricle *(mLV)*, which is on the right side of the heart. **B:** A more superior image from the same examination shows the moderator band *(arrow)*, a characteristic feature of the mRV. **C:** A more superior image shows that the aorta *(Ao)* is anterior to and to the left of the pulmonary artery *(PA)*. This spatial orientation is called *L-transposition* (L indicates the leftward position of the aorta). This orientation is usually present in corrected transposition, but rare exceptions occur. Note the muscular outflow around the aorta, also a feature of the morphologic right ventricle.

systemic venous return directly into the pulmonary arteries (21).

Tricuspid Atresia

In tricuspid atresia, a direct communication between the RA and RV is lacking. The tricuspid valve may be imperforate, in which case a fibrous band is seen on MR images. More commonly, the atrioventricular connection is absent, in which case transverse MR images demonstrate a solid bar of fat and muscle interposed between the atrium and ventricle (22,23).

If any blood is to reach the RV, an ASD must be present to shunt blood from the RA to the LA, and a VSD to shunt blood from the LV to the RV (Fig. 20.12). If both of these shunts are large and no pulmonic stenosis is present, the RV may be close to normal size. On the other hand, if the ASD,

VSD, or pulmonary outflow is small, the RV may be small and rudimentary. Thus, in tricuspid atresia, the hemodynamics and therefore the chamber sizes are variable (24). A restrictive VSD is one in which the maximal diameter is less than the diameter of the pulmonary annulus in a person with normally related great arteries, or less than the diameter of the aortic annulus in a person with transposition of the great arteries. Differentiation of tricuspid atresia with a large VSD from a single ventricle requires demonstration of the atretic valve. In tricuspid atresia, MRI depicts the size of the VSD in addition to hypoplasia or absence of the RV inflow region. For accurate measurement of the defect, the imaging plane must be nearly perpendicular to the VSD.

The incidence of abnormalities of ventriculoarterial connection is high in tricuspid atresia. Transposition of the great vessels (described below) occurs in 25% to 40% of these patients, in which the aorta arises from the diminutive

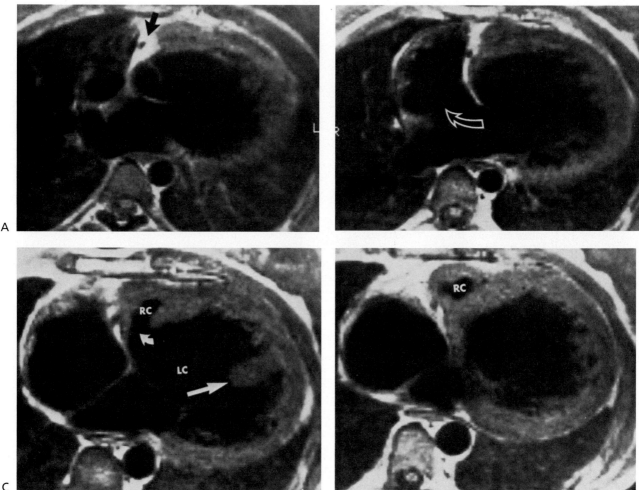

FIGURE 20.12. Tricuspid atresia. Axial T1-weighted spin-echo image at the level of the left ventricular outflow tract **(A)** show that fat from the atrioventricular groove is interposed between the right ventricle and right atrium *(arrow)*. **B:** A more inferior image shows that a large atrial septal defect *(open arrow)* allows blood to flow from the right atrium to the left atrium. **C,D:** More inferiorly, the right ventricle is seen as a hypoplastic chamber *(RC)* with hypertrophied walls. This communicates with the left ventricular chamber *(LC)* via a large ventricular septal defect *(curved arrow)*. Note the thickened papillary muscle *(straight arrow in C)* in the left ventricle. (From Higgins CB. Congenital heart disease. In: Higgins CB, Hricak H, Helms CA, eds. *Magnetic resonance imaging of the body,* 3rd ed. Philadelphia: Lippincott–Raven Publishers, 1997:488, with permission.)

RV and the pulmonary artery arises from the larger, more functional LV (24).

Most infants with tricuspid atresia undergo palliative correction, usually one or more of several types of systemic-to-pulmonary artery shunts. At 1 year of age, which many authors consider the minimal age for definitive correction (25), a Fontan procedure is performed. In this operation, all systemic venous blood is surgically rerouted to the pulmonary circulation, so that the right side of the heart is bypassed entirely. In its classic form, the Fontan procedure rerouted blood from the RA to the pulmonary artery; however, many adaptations have since been made (26). Preoperatively, important selection criteria for the Fontan procedure are a low mean pulmonary arterial pressure and

pulmonary vascular resistance (25), which are measured by catheter angiography. Other selection criteria are an adequate LV ejection fraction and mass, which are most accurately determined with MRI, especially in patients with abnormal ventricular geometry (27). Postoperatively, MRI can be used to assess the Fontan shunt and any complications (28).

Hypoplastic Left Heart Syndrome

The term *hypoplastic left heart syndrome* refers to several different anomalies, all of which lead to underdevelopment of the LV. It is usually caused by aortic stenosis/atresia, mitral stenosis/atresia, or both. As in tricuspid atresia, the degree of ventricular hypoplasia varies, depending on the location and severity of the obstruction (29). For example, in mitral atresia without a large ASD and VSD, the LV may be a small mass of muscle with no visible lumen (Fig. 20.13). On the other hand, if the mitral valve is patent and the problem is primarily one of aortic valvular hypoplasia, the LV may be normal in size and hypertrophic (Fig. 20.14A). In all cases, the RA tends to be enlarged, and the RV to be dilated and hypertrophic (29). Axial MRI can readily depict the chamber enlargement and ventricular hypertrophy.

In most cases of hypoplastic left heart syndrome, little blood flows through the ascending aorta. Blood tends to flow from the pulmonary artery through the ductus arteriosus into the aorta, then in retrograde fashion to the aortic root to supply the coronary arteries. As a result, the ascending aorta is usually very small, and the main pulmonary artery, which receives most of the cardiac output, is very large (Fig. 14B). The diameters of the great arteries are clearly defined on axial MR images.

The prognosis for hypoplastic left heart syndrome was very poor until the development of the Norwood procedure, in which the large RV is made to pump blood to the systemic circulation. This is accomplished by severing the main pulmonary artery from the RV and anastomosing the proximal pulmonary stump to the ascending aorta. The pulmonary circulation is reestablished by routing systemic blood into the pulmonary circulation, initially with a systemic-to-pulmonary shunt and later with a Fontan procedure (30) (Fig. 20.14C). An important role for MRI in hypoplastic left heart syndrome has been the evaluation of the morphology and function of the various stages of the Norwood procedure (31,32).

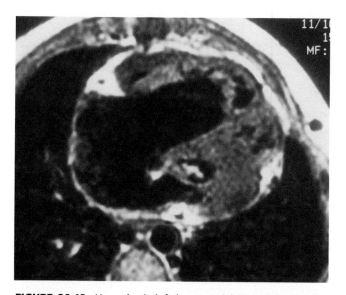

FIGURE 20.13. Hypoplastic left heart. Axial T1-weighted spin-echo image shows a small left ventricle with hypertrophied walls and a very small lumen.

Ebstein Malformation

Ebstein malformation is a primary abnormality of the tricuspid valve in which the septal and anterior leaflets of the valve adhere to the RV wall. The leaflets become free at a variable distance, at a location more apical than usual, so that the tricuspid valve orifice is displaced toward the apex. The right atrioventricular ring still defines the border of the anatomic RV; however, because the valve orifice is more apical than usual, the functional part of the RV becomes smaller. The portion of the RV that is basal to the valve orifice becomes "atrialized," meaning that it functions as part of the atrium rather than as part of the RV. The atrialized portion of the RV becomes progressively thin-walled and smooth-walled, and it may become markedly enlarged (33). Ebstein anomaly is frequently associated with an ASD (34). MRI can readily delineate the pathologic anatomy (Fig. 20.15), and cine MRI can be used to quantify chamber size and ejection fraction of the functional RV (27,35).

Atrioventricular Septal Defect/Atrioventricular Canal (Endocardial Cushion Defect)

These terms denote a spectrum of abnormalities that have in common an abnormal septation between the atria and ventricles. Some authors prefer the term *endocardial cushion defects* because the defects are all presumed to result from abnormalities of the embryologic endocardial cushions, which grow together in the center of the heart and divide the atria from the ventricles. The structures that are derived from the endocardial cushions and that are abnormal in this group of defects are the apical portion of the interatrial septum, the basal portion of the interventricular septum, the septal leaflet of the tricuspid valve, and the septal leaflet of the mitral valve. Other authors question some of the proposed embryology underlying the term "endocardial cushion defects" and instead call this group of abnormalities *atrioventricular septal defects* because they can be unified by a deficiency of the atrioventricular septum (36).

In the normal heart, the atrioventricular septum separates the RA from the LV. The atrioventricular septum is created by the normal apical displacement of the tricuspid valve relative to the mitral valve (5) (Fig. 20.9). In all cases of atrioventricular septal defect, the tricuspid and mitral valves originate at the same level, and the atrioventricular septum is absent (36). This abnormal relationship is depicted on axial MRI (Fig. 20.16). In the mildest form of atrioventricular septal defect, the only additional abnormality is a cleft septal leaflet of the mitral valve, which is usually not detectable on MRI. In more severe cases, the atrial septum adjacent to the atrioventricular valve orifice may be absent. This condition is known as *ostium primum ASD*. Some patients may have an inlet VSD, usually located in the same axial image as the atrioventricular valve(s). In still more se-

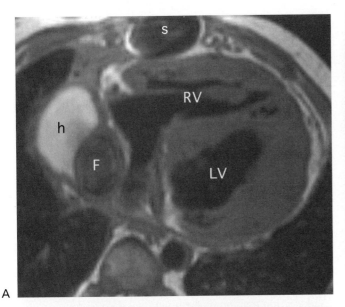

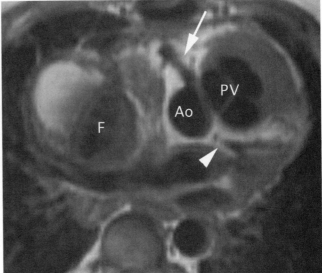

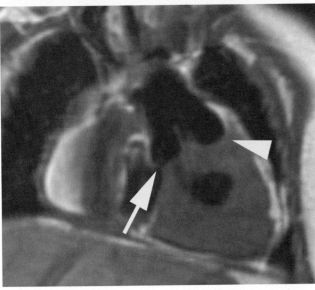

FIGURE 20.14. Hypoplastic left heart after a Norwood procedure. **A:** Axial T1-weighted spin-echo images show a Fontan shunt *(F)*. On other images (not included), this could be seen to run from the inferior vena cava to the right pulmonary artery. The circumscribed area of increased T1 signal around the Fontan is a postoperative hematoma *(h)*. The left ventricle *(LV)* is hypertrophied but not atretic because this patient had good-sized atrial septal and ventricular septal defects (not shown) and relatively mild aortic stenosis, which allowed flow through the left ventricle. *RV*, right ventricle; *s*, artifact from prior sternotomy. **B:** In the same patient, more superior images at the level of the pulmonary valve *(PV)* show that the aorta *(Ao)* is smaller than the pulmonary artery. The right coronary artery *(arrow)* and left main coronary artery *(arrowhead)* are seen originating from the aorta. **C:** Coronal T1-weighted spin-echo images in the same patient show the anastomosis between the ascending aorta *(arrow)* and the pulmonary artery *(arrowhead)*.

vere cases, both the atrial and ventricular portions of the septum around the valve origins are absent, a condition referred to as *complete atrioventricular canal.* This creates a common atrioventricular valve orifice with continuous, common atrioventricular valve leaflets. The deficient ostium primum atrial septum, inlet ventricular septum, and absent cardiac crux have been well demonstrated in several series (37,38).

VENTRICULOARTERIAL CONNECTIONS

In the primitive heart tube, blood flowing out passes through the primitive conus, which develops into the muscular outflow of the RV and into a single great artery, the truncus arteriosus. During development, the truncus arte-

riosus normally spirals and divides to form a separate pulmonary artery and aorta. Abnormal development of these structures can cause one or both of the great arteries to originate from the incorrect ventricle (discordant atrioventricular connection), stenosis or atresia of the origins of the great arteries, or persistence of a common arterial trunk. MRI is well suited for evaluating abnormalities of the ventriculoarterial connections. A great vessel is considered to be arising from a particular ventricle if more than 50% of the great vessel orifice is above that ventricle, a relationship displayed on axial MRI.

Ventriculoarterial connections can be concordant or discordant. Concordant connections are RV to pulmonary artery and LV to aorta. Discordant connections occur in a diverse group of anomalies in which either the great arteries

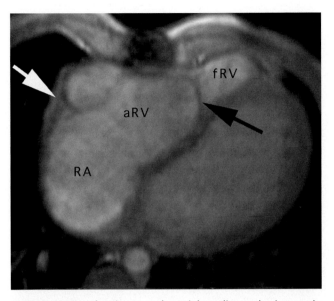

FIGURE 20.15. Ebstein anomaly. Axial gradient-echo images in a 16-year-old boy. The tricuspid valve leaflets *(black arrow)* have been displaced apically away from the atrioventricular groove *(white arrow)*, so that the right ventricle is divided into a functional right ventricle *(fRV)*, which still serves to pump blood to the pulmonary artery, and an atrialized right ventricle *(aRV)*, which has become thin-walled and is no longer functional. *RA*, right atrium.

are inverted (transposition), both great arteries arise predominantly from one of the ventricles (double-outlet ventricle), or a single large artery arises from the ventricle (truncus arteriosus). The ventriculoarterial connections and the arterial relationships are depicted on coronal and transverse MR images.

Complete Transposition of the Great Arteries/Atrioventricular Concordance and Ventriculoarterial Discordance

In this anomaly, the pulmonary artery arises from the LV and the aorta arises from the RV. The ventricles are in their usual location (Fig. 20.17). Therefore, the pulmonary and systemic circulations are in separate loops. A shunt lesion, usually a VSD, must be present for oxygenated blood to reach the systemic circulation (39).

This condition is sometimes called *complete transposition* to distinguish it from corrected transposition, or *D-transposition,* because the aorta is usually anterior to and to the right of the pulmonary artery. However, as discussed previously, the relationship of the great arteries does not always indicate the ventricular morphology, and the spatial orientation of the great vessels should be described separately from their ventriculoarterial connections (39).

Today, the preferred surgery for this anomaly is the Jatene (arterial switch) procedure. In this operation, the roots of the great arteries are transected and reattached to the opposite ventricle, so that the blood will flow from each ventricle into the appropriate artery. The size and thickness of the LV may be important for the success of this operation in older children.

Tetralogy of Fallot

In the original description, tetralogy of Fallot consisted of pulmonary stenosis, an overriding aorta, a perimembranous VSD, and resultant RV hypertrophy. The key feature of

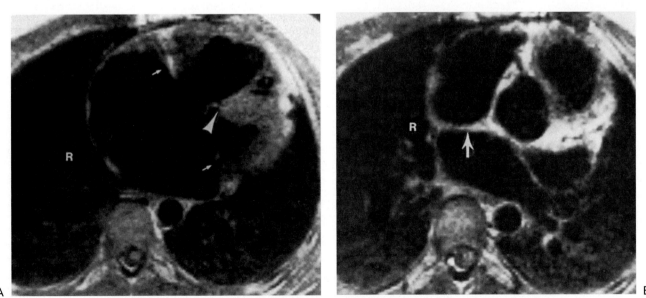

A   B

FIGURE 20.16. Atrioventricular septal defect. **A, B:** Axial T1-weighted spin-echo images show a shortened ventricular septum *(arrowhead)*. The components of a common atrioventricular valve *(small arrows)* are equidistant from the apex. A large primum atrial septal defect is present. The secundum portion of the atrial septum *(arrow in B)* is intact. *R*, right side of the body. (From Higgins CB. Congenital heart disease. In: Higgins CB, Hricak H, Helms CA, eds. *Magnetic resonance imaging of the body*, 3rd ed. Philadelphia: Lippincott–Raven Publishers, 1997:486, with permission.)

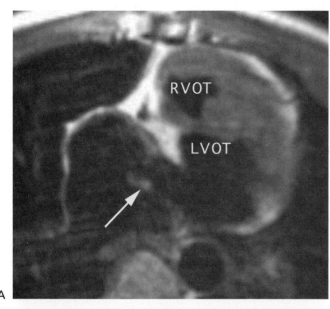

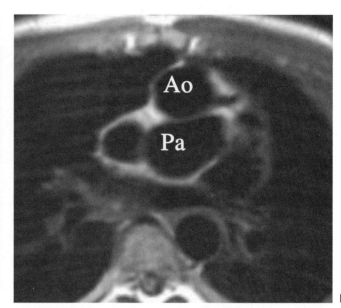

FIGURE 20.17. Complete transposition. **A:** Axial T1-weighted spin-echo images in a 13-year-old boy show the morphologic right ventricle defined by its muscular right ventricular outflow tract *(RVOT),* appropriately on the right side of the heart. The left ventricular outflow tract *(LVOT)* is on the left side. A surgical conduit has been placed *(arrow)* that diverts blood from the right atrium to the left side of the heart. **B:** A more superior image shows that the RVOT gives rise to the aorta *(Ao).* Note the left main coronary artery. The pulmonary artery *(PA)* is posterior to the aorta. **C:** A slightly more superior image shows that the aorta is anterior to and slightly to the right of the pulmonary artery. This spatial orientation, called *D-transposition,* is usually, although not invariably, present in complete transposition (ventriculoarterial discordance).

tetralogy is malalignment of the infundibular septum (40). The anteriorly displaced infundibular septum encroaches on the RV outflow, causing the RV outflow to be small and the aorta to override the VSD. These features are readily identified on MRI (Fig. 20.18). Sagittal and coronal MR images display the size and overriding position of the aorta and the narrowing of the RV outflow tract. Transverse images demonstrate the VSD and the locations of the pulmonary outflow and arterial stenoses.

Tetralogy of Fallot is usually repaired by relieving the pulmonic stenosis and closing the VSD. Stenosis of the main or branch arteries, the size of the RV outflow tract, and the size of the RV are important to assess in preoperative planning and are well delineated by MRI (41,42). Coronary anomalies may occur in patients with tetralogy of Fallot.

The most significant to the surgeon is an origin of the left anterior descending coronary artery from the right coronary artery. In this situation, the left anterior descending artery passes anterior to the RV outflow tract in the site of potential surgical repair (40).

Central pulmonary artery stenosis occurs commonly in tetralogy of Fallot. MRI is the modality of choice to depict pulmonary stenoses. Thin (3-mm) oblique tomograms parallel to the long axis of the right or left pulmonary artery are optimal to identify such stenoses. The oblique images can also be used to evaluate the stenoses after balloon angioplasty. Adequate sizes of the central pulmonary arteries and the presence of a central confluence may signify that the patient is a candidate for a Rastelli procedure connecting the RV to the pulmonary artery.

Pulmonary Atresia

Pulmonary atresia with VSD is an extreme form of tetralogy of Fallot in which a direct connection from the RV to the pulmonary arteries is lacking. On axial MRI, a solid layer of muscle in the region of the RV outflow tract indicates an infundibulum with a blind end. No connection between the RV and the pulmonary artery confluence (if present) can be followed on sequential images (Fig. 20.19A). The atresia can be focal, limited to the valve level, or more extensive. The length of the atresia can be determined by inspecting sequential axial tomograms. Focal membranous pulmonary atresia may be indistinguishable from severe stenosis on ax-

ial MR images because of partial volume averaging. The use of 3-mm-thick spin-echo images reduces partial volume effects, and cine MRI in the axial or sagittal planes can establish the presence or absence of flow across the valve. A markedly enlarged aorta is seen overriding a perimembranous VSD (Fig. 19B). Blood is usually delivered to the lungs via systemic-to-pulmonary collateral channels, which can be seen as abnormal vessels originating from the descending aorta and traveling toward the lungs or connecting with the pulmonary arteries (Fig. 19C).

The surgical correction of pulmonary atresia with VSD usually consists of placing a conduit from the RV to the central pulmonary arteries (if present) or to a surgically created

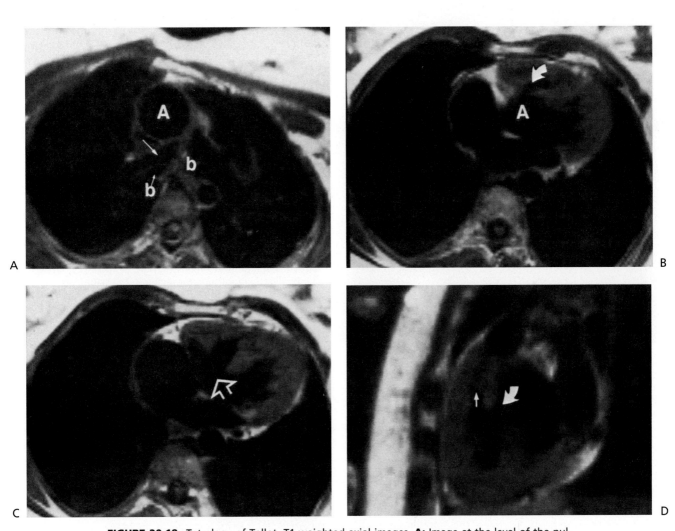

FIGURE 20.18. Tetralogy of Tallot. T1-weighted axial images. **A:** Image at the level of the pulmonary bifurcation shows a small right pulmonary artery *(small arrow)*. **B:** A more inferior image shows severe narrowing of the right ventricular outflow tract *(curved arrow)* caused by anterior displacement of the ventricular septum at this level. Note that the pulmonary outflow is smaller than and encroached upon by the aorta *(A)* at this level. **C:** Directly inferior to the aorta is a membranous ventricular septal defect *(open arrow)*. On these adjacent images, it can be seen that the aorta overrides the ventricular septal defect. **D:** Sagittal image shows infundibular stenosis of the right ventricular outflow tract *(small arrow)* and a ventricular septal defect *(curved arrow)*. A, aorta; b, bronchi. (From Higgins CB. Congenital heart disease. In: Higgins CB, Hricak H, Helms CA, eds. *Magnetic resonance imaging of the body*, 3rd ed. Philadelphia: Lippincott–Raven Publishers, 1997:477, with permission.)

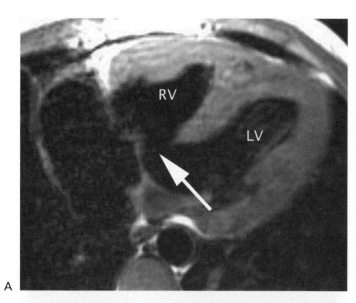

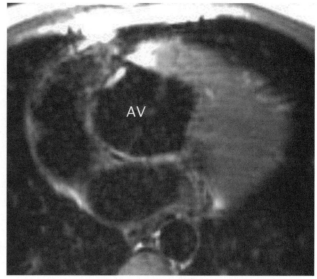

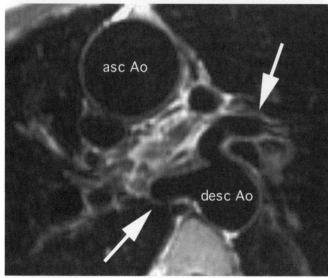

FIGURE 20.19. Pulmonary atresia with ventricular septal defect. **A:** T1-weighted axial spin-echo images show a large ventricular septal defect *(arrow)*. *RV,* right ventricle; *LV,* left ventricle. **B:** Slightly more superior image in the same patient shows that the aortic valve *(AV)* overrides the ventricular septal defect. Note that no pulmonary artery is seen. **C:** More superior image shows prominent bronchial collaterals *(arrows)* originating from the descending thoracic aorta *(desc Ao)*. *asc Ao,* ascending thoracic aorta.

confluence of pulmonary arteries and larger systemic-to-pulmonary collateral vessels (unifocalization procedure). Therefore, it is important for the surgeon to know whether a native confluence of the pulmonary arteries is present, its size, and the number and size of collateral vessels. Axial spin-echo MRI is excellent for defining the main pulmonary arteries (43–45). The collateral channels are especially well seen on contrast-enhanced MRA (Fig. 20.20).

It is important to assess the sizes of the central pulmonary arteries in patients who have tetralogy of Fallot with severe stenosis or pulmonary atresia. Thin (3-mm) axial MR images can readily depict the sizes of the main, right, and left pulmonary arteries. The right pulmonary artery is observed on the image that contains the right main bronchus, coursing in front of the right bronchus, and the left pulmonary artery passes over the left main bronchus and is seen on the image containing the left bronchus or on the one just above.

The identification of central pulmonary arteries and of a central confluence of the right and left pulmonary arteries is a unique capability of MRI, and opacification of the vessels with contrast medium is not required. The pulmonary arteries are frequently hypoplastic, or the central or peripheral arteries may contain one or more stenoses.

Cine MRI can be used to identify the blood supply to the lungs. Pulmonary and bronchial arteries have bright signal on cine MRI. On axial images at the level of the carina, pulmonary arteries can be differentiated from bronchial arteries. Bronchial arteries arise from the aorta or its branches and are usually located dorsal to the bronchi, whereas pulmonary arteries are ventral to the bronchi. On occasion, a bronchial artery originating from a subclavian artery can be seen ventral to the bronchi.

A VSD is not identified in the form of pulmonary atresia with intact ventricular septum. In this variety of pulmonary

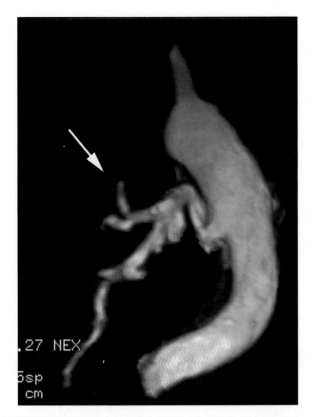

FIGURE 20.20. Systemic–pulmonary collaterals. Posterior view of a volume-rendered reconstruction of gadolinium MRA shows a large collateral vessel *(arrow)* arising from the left side of the descending thoracic aorta.

atresia, MRI is effective for demonstrating the size of the RV, which varies from markedly hypoplastic to dilated. The pulmonary arteries are usually normal or nearly normal in size and do not contain stenoses.

Double-Outlet Right Ventricle

The definition of double-outlet RV has been debated. Some authors include any situation in which more than 50% of the orifice of both great vessels is over the RV. Others further stipulate that the aortic valve and mitral valve must lack their normal fibrous continuity (46) (Fig. 20.21).

A VSD is always present in double-outlet RV (46). The location of the VSD, especially its relationship to the great arteries, is important in determining the type of surgical repair to be performed (47). On axial MRI, the location can be determined by identifying the great vessels on images and then inspecting the images immediately inferior to determine which arterial outflow tract is confluent with the VSD. Usually, the infundibular portion of the septum separates one of the valves from the VSD (48). In the most common form of double-outlet RV, the VSD is related to the aorta (subaortic), and in these cases, the surgical repair usually involves the creation of an intraventricular tunnel from the VSD to the aorta. If the VSD is on the pulmonic side of the

infundibular septum (subpulmonic), the surgical options are more variable (47). Double-outlet RV with a subpulmonic defect is often referred to as the *Taussig-Bing heart* (47). If the VSD is immediately inferior to both great vessels, it is said to be *doubly committed,* and if distant from both, it is said to be *noncommitted.* Both of these are less common.

Axial MRI can depict the relationship of the great arteries at the level of the ventriculoarterial valves. In double-outlet RV, the great arteries usually have a side-by-side relationship at the base of the heart, but in some cases, the aorta is anterior to the pulmonary artery and slightly to the left or right of the pulmonary artery. MR images can show the origins of the great vessels from the RV outflow tract. The location of the VSD can also be seen on axial MR images. MRI shows that neither ventriculoarterial valve is in direct fibrous continuity with the mitral valve. A complete ring of myocardium is present between the two ventriculoarterial valves and the two atrioventricular valves.

Other important aspects of double-outlet RV are valvular and subvalvular obstructions. A wide variety of associated anomalies have been reported. Of note, coarctation of the aorta is frequently found in patients with subpulmonic VSDs.

Truncus Arteriosus

If the primitive truncus arteriosus does not divide, the aorta and pulmonary artery do not develop normally, and a single arterial trunk forms over both ventricles. A VSD is always present.

Truncus arteriosus was initially classified by Collet and Edwards (49) based on the origin of the pulmonary artery from the common arterial trunk. In type I, a septum divides the origin of the aorta and pulmonary trunk. In type II, the right and left pulmonary arteries are close to each other but arise separately from the pulmonary trunk. In type III, right and left pulmonary arteries arise further laterally. In type IV, no pulmonary vessels arise from the aorta, but branches from the descending thoracic aorta supply the pulmonary vasculature. However, this classification has been criticized, primarily because the lesion labeled type IV truncus is in fact pulmonary atresia with VSD rather than truncus arteriosus.

Axial, sagittal, and coronal MR images at the base of the heart can show the truncus arteriosus aligned over the VSD. The origins of the main pulmonary artery from the truncus in type I can be delineated with MRI. Axial images can show the relative sizes of the ventricles. Because it can demonstrate a small infundibular chamber in pulmonary atresia, MRI can be used to distinguish truncus arteriosus from pulmonary atresia.

The relative sizes and confluence of the pulmonary arteries are useful information to the surgeon because surgical treatment involves excision of the pulmonary arteries from the common trunk and the creation of a conduit from the

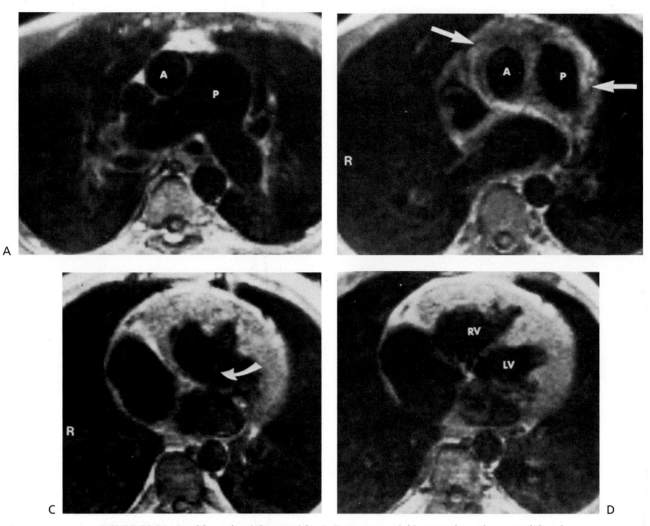

FIGURE 20.21. Double-outlet right ventricle. **A:** Transverse axial images show the aorta *(A)* and pulmonary artery *(P)*. **B:** A more inferior image shows that both have complete muscular rings *(arrows)*. Therefore, muscle is interposed between the aortic and mitral valves, and this case meets the strictest criteria for double-outlet right ventricle. **C,D:** More inferiorly located is a ventricular septal defect *(curved arrow)* that the aorta slightly overrides and that connects the right ventricle *(RV)* and left ventricle *(LV)*. R, right side of the body. (From Higgins CB. Congenital heart disease. In: Higgins CB, Hricak H, Helms CA, eds. *Magnetic resonance imaging of the body,* 3rd ed. Philadelphia: Lippincott–Raven Publishers, 1997:473, with permission.)

RV to the pulmonary arteries. Also important for surgical planning is the proximity of the pulmonary artery origins to the coronary arteries, the presence of aortic arch abnormalities, and the presence of truncal valve regurgitation. All these features can be demonstrated with MRI (11,27) (Fig. 20.22).

INTRACARDIAC SHUNTS

Ventricular Septal Defect

Perimembranous Ventricular Septal Defect

VSDs are classified according to the affected part of the ventricular septum. The ventricular septum is a complex, three-dimensional structure. Inferiorly, the ventricular septum runs parallel to the plane between the cardiac apex and base. Superiorly, the ventricular septum curves around the RV outflow tract.

The membranous part of the ventricular septum is a small area just inferior to the root of the aorta, nestled between the right coronary cusp and the noncoronary cusp (5) (Fig. 20.23). Most VSDs in this region extend beyond the anatomic membranous ventricular septum and so are often called *perimembranous*. The embryologic development of the membranous ventricular septum is complex, with contributions from several primitive structures, and it is one of the last parts of the interventricular septum to form (15). For this reason, it is the most frequent location for a VSD.

Supracristal Ventricular Septal Defect

The crista supraventricularis is a muscular ridge that defines the outlet part of the RV. The crista supraventricularis can be difficult to see on axial images because it runs parallel to the scan plane (Fig. 20.24A). However, the supracristal part of the ventricular septum can be defined as the part of the ventricular septum that is inferior to the right and left coronary cusps (50) (Fig. 24B). Note that this is the infundibular part of the ventricular septum and is anterior and superior to the membranous septum. A supracristal VSD is located just below the pulmonary valve and the aortic valve and so sometimes is called *subaortic* (Fig. 20.25). One of the complications of a supracristal VSD is prolapse of the right coronary cusp into the septal defect, which results in aortic insufficiency (51).

Muscular Ventricular Septal Defect

The muscular septum is the largest part of the septum; it is more apical in location than the membranous part (Fig. 20.26). VSDs here can be multiple. Because of the trabeculation on the right side of the heart, they are often difficult to visualize at surgery and must be clearly delineated by imaging.

Atrial Septal Defect

Ostium Primum Atrial Septal Defect

The atrial septum is derived from several structures that together divide the primitive atria into two chambers. During this process, several septa and ostia form and involute in the development of the final interatrial septum. ASDs are usu-

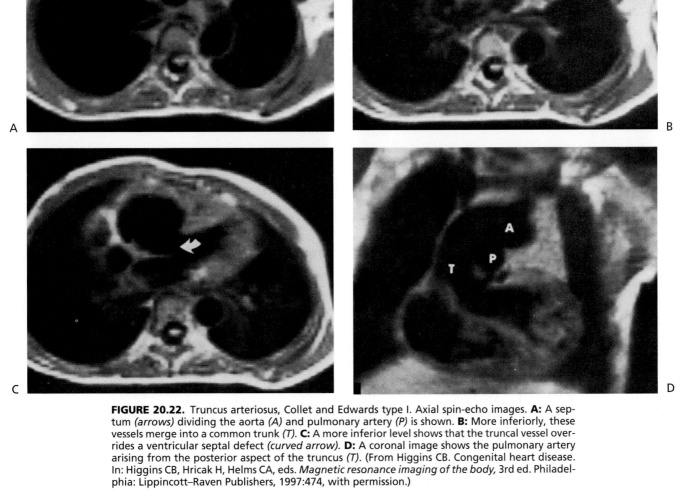

FIGURE 20.22. Truncus arteriosus, Collet and Edwards type I. Axial spin-echo images. **A:** A septum *(arrows)* dividing the aorta *(A)* and pulmonary artery *(P)* is shown. **B:** More inferiorly, these vessels merge into a common trunk *(T)*. **C:** A more inferior level shows that the truncal vessel overrides a ventricular septal defect *(curved arrow)*. **D:** A coronal image shows the pulmonary artery arising from the posterior aspect of the truncus *(T)*. (From Higgins CB. Congenital heart disease. In: Higgins CB, Hricak H, Helms CA, eds. *Magnetic resonance imaging of the body*, 3rd ed. Philadelphia: Lippincott–Raven Publishers, 1997:474, with permission.)

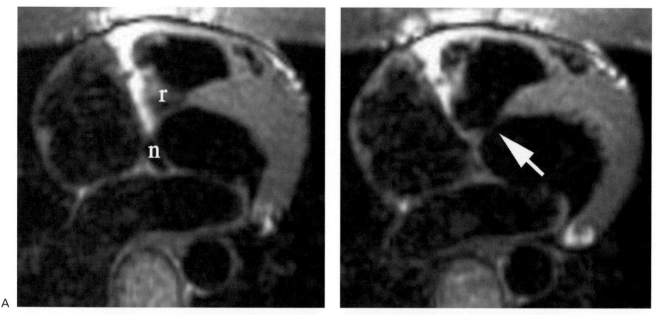

FIGURE 20.23. Membranous ventricular septum. **A:** Thin-section (3 mm with 0.5-mm skip) T1-weighted axial spin-echo images. The inferior aspect of the right sinus of Valsalva *(r)* and noncoronary sinus of Valsalva *(n)* are seen. The left sinus of Valsalva superior to the plane of the image is not included. **B:** A slightly more inferior level shows the membranous portion of the ventricular septum *(arrow)*, which is situated between and inferior to the right and noncoronary sinuses of Valsalva.

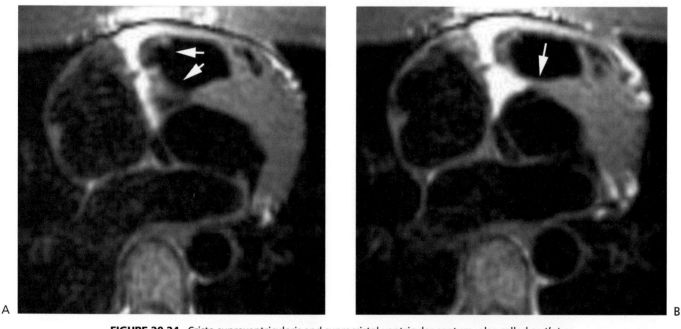

FIGURE 20.24. Crista supraventricularis and supracristal ventricular septum, also called *outlet* or *infundibular septum.* Axial T1-weighted spin-echo images. **A:** The crista supraventricularis is a muscular ridge that runs parallel to the axial plane *(arrows)*. It separates the body of the right ventricle from the right ventricular outflow. **B:** A slightly more superior image in the same patient shows the supracristal part of the interventricular septum *(arrow)*. This is between the right and left coronary sinuses. Defects in this area angle slightly inferiorly so that they enter the left ventricle just below the aortic valve.

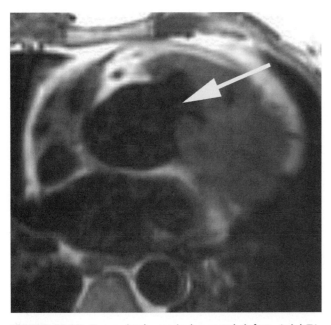

FIGURE 20.25. Supracristal ventricular septal defect. Axial T1-weighted spin-echo image shows a ventricular septal defect *(arrow)* in the right ventricular outflow tract, between the right and left sinuses of Valsalva.

ally named according to the embryologic septal communications that fail to close normally. The first such ostium to form is called the *ostium primum,* which is defined by the first interatrial septum, called the *septum primum.* Persistence of the ostium primum causes a defect in the interatrial septum at the junction of the atrial and ventricular septa, which is appropriately called an *ostium primum septal defect.* This defect is part of the spectrum of atrioventricular septal defects described above (52) (Fig. 20.16).

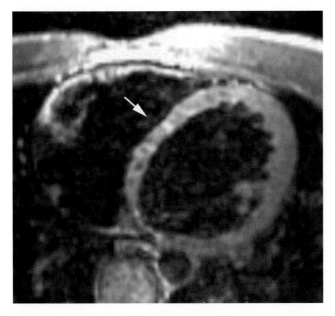

FIGURE 20.26. Muscular ventricular septum. Axial spin-echo image shows the muscular ventricular septum *(arrow).*

Ostium Secundum Atrial Septal Defect

After the septum primum forms, a second primitive septum develops, the septum secundum, which eventually forms the posterior and inferior part of the interatrial septum, including the foramen ovale. Deficiencies of this part of the septum are the most common type of ASD (Fig. 20.27). A patent foramen ovale is at the same site (52).

Sinus Venosus Atrial Septal Defect

The sinus venosus is formed from the confluence of systemic veins with the RA and constitutes the smooth, posterior wall of the RA. Deficient incorporation of the sinus venosus creates an ASD near the junction of the RA with the superior vena cava (Fig. 20.28). This portion of the interatrial septum also normally creates part of the separation of the superior right pulmonary vein from the LA, so that when a sinus venosus ASD is present, the right superior pulmonary vein inserts into the RA (52).

THORACIC AORTIC ANOMALIES

MRI has been shown to be effective for the assessment of thoracic aortic anomalies, and it is the procedure of choice to evaluate such anomalies. In most aortic abnormalities, MRI yields complete diagnostic information that can be substituted for angiography.

Coarctation of the Aorta

Coarctation of the aorta is a congenital narrowing of the aorta. The stenosis can be long or short and involve any part of the aorta, but most commonly, it is a focal narrowing just inferior to the origin of the left subclavian artery. When discovered in infants, the coarctation is usually severe, the blood flow to the lower extremities depends on the patent ductus arteriosus, and cardiac anomalies are usually associated. Patients who present later in life, typically in childhood and young adulthood, tend to have a less severe, more focal narrowing and usually present with signs and symptoms of hypertension in the head and upper extremities.

MRI has been shown to be effective for the preoperative assessment of coarctation and for postoperative monitoring. To evaluate coarctation, spin-echo sequences are obtained in the axial, sagittal, and oblique sagittal planes. The diameter of the narrowing is accurately measured with MRI, especially with the use of thin (3-mm) sections through the lesion. Thin oblique sagittal images through the plane of the aorta (a plane comparable with a left anterior oblique projection of conventional angiography) show the diameter of the stenosis and yield an accurate measurement of its length (Fig. 20.29). Thin axial images can also display the coarctation, but measurement of the stenosis may be inaccurate because

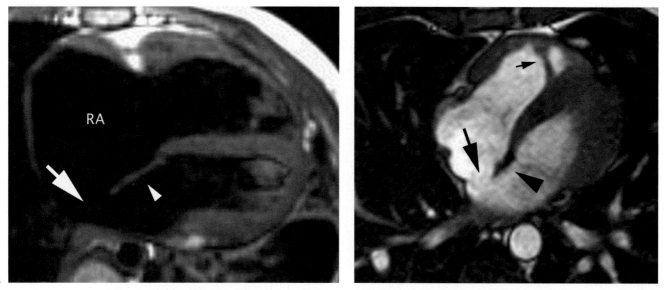

FIGURE 20.27. Secundum atrial septal defect. **A:** Axial T1-weighted spin-echo image shows a defect in the posterior, inferior atrial septum *(arrow)*, which is the secundum portion of the atrial septum. The residual septum primum is well seen *(arrowhead)*. Note the dilation of the right atrium *(RA)* from the left-to-right shunt. **B:** Axial gradient-echo cine image from a different patient shows the atrial septal defect in a similar location *(large arrow)*. Again note the residual septum primum *(arrowhead)*. The moderator band *(small arrow)*, a feature of the normal morphologic right ventricle, is well seen.

of the effects of partial volume averaging. It is important to measure the diameter of the distal arch because it can influence the type of surgery. MRI can be used to display the entire thoracic aorta on a single image with the use of maximum intensity projection or volume-rendering reconstruction techniques (Fig. 20.30). Gadolinium-enhanced MRA is also effective for demonstrating collateral vessels (Fig. 20.30). Because it precisely depicts the diameter of a stenosis and is non-invasive, MRI has long been considered the gold standard for evaluating coarctation of the aorta (53–55).

More recently, MRI techniques have been developed for directly determining the functional significance of a stenosis in aortic coarctation. In patients with aortic coarctation, a collateral supply to the descending thoracic aorta develops from the internal mammary artery and other branches of the subclavian arteries and intercostal arteries. The development

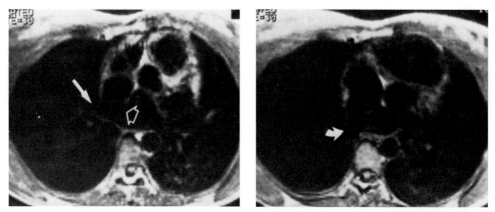

FIGURE 20.28. Sinus venosus atrial septal defect. **A:** Axial T1-weighted spin-echo image shows a defect *(open arrow)* in the superior aspect of the atrial septum, near the insertion of the superior vena cava. Note that the defect is at the site of insertion of the right superior pulmonary vein *(closed arrow)*, so that it causes this vein to insert into the right atrium. **B:** A more inferior image again shows the insertion of the pulmonary vein into the right atrium *(curved arrow)*. Note the intact secundum portion of the atrial septum. (From Higgins CB. Congenital heart disease. In: Higgins CB, Hricak H, Helms CA, eds. *Magnetic resonance imaging of the body,* 3rd ed. Philadelphia: Lippincott–Raven Publishers, 1997:497, with permission.)

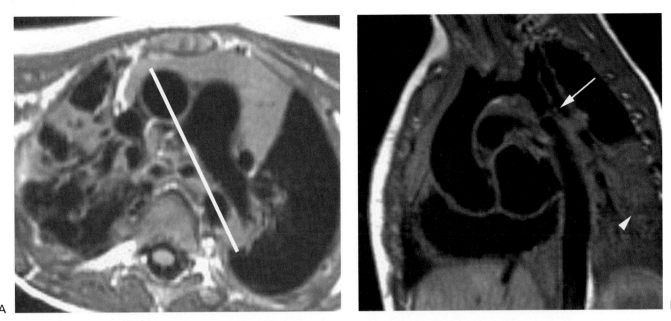

FIGURE 20.29. Coarctation of the aorta in an infant. **A:** Axial spin-echo image. A plane through the ascending and descending aorta is selected *(line)*. **B:** The resultant plane displays the aorta in a single image. Note the discrete narrowing of the aorta *(arrow)* distal to origin of the left sub-clavian artery. Atelectasis in the bases *(arrowhead)* is frequently seen in small children, who undergo the MRI examination with anesthesia.

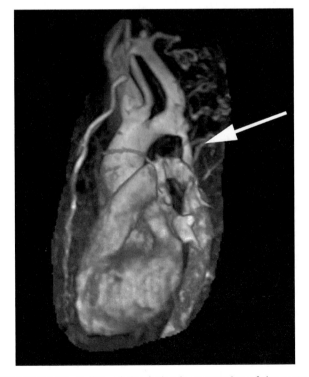

FIGURE 20.30. Collateral circulation in coarctation of the aorta. Volume-rendered image from gadolinium MRA shows a long segment of narrowing in the descending thoracic aorta *(arrow)* and numerous collateral vessels connecting branches of the subclavian arteries to the descending thoracic aorta.

of these collateral vessels is a marker for the hemodynamic significance of the narrowing. The collaterals can often be visualized directly on gadolinium MRA (Fig. 20.30). With velocity-encoded cine techniques (described below), the volume of the collateral circulation can be quantified (27,56) (Fig. 20.31). The presence of collateral flow should be taken as an indicator of the hemodynamic significance of a stenosis, and the volume of collateral flow is significantly related to the severity of a stenosis.

MRI can be used to evaluate restenosis, aneurysm, or pseudoaneurysm after patch repair or balloon angioplasty.

Abnormal Branching of the Aorta/Vascular Rings

The aortic arch supplies the head and arms via four main arteries: the right and left common carotid arteries and the right and left subclavian arteries. In most persons, these vessels arise via three arch vessels: the brachiocephalic (innominate) artery, which divides into the right-sided arteries, and the left common carotid and left subclavian arteries, each of which arises directly from the aortic arch. However, many variations in the branching patterns are possible, some of which create vascular rings and cause symptoms of tracheal and esophageal compression. MRI can be used to identify arch anomalies, including right aortic arch with retroesophageal left subclavian artery and double aortic arch. Gadolinium-enhanced MRA also may be effective for evaluating arch anomalies (57,58).

true ring that causes tracheal and esophageal compression. The aberrant vessel can be readily identified and its diameter measured on axial MR images. Often, a focal dilation of the proximal portion of the retroesophageal left subclavian artery exacerbates the airway compression. The tracheal compression is generally best seen on sagittal images (Fig. 20.33). The aortic arch usually crosses to the left of midline in the upper thorax, but the location of the crossover is variable and can be identified with MRI.

Double Aortic Arch

In double aortic arch, the ascending aorta divides into two arches, each of which gives rise to a common carotid and subclavian artery. Axial and coronal MRI display the anomaly; the trachea and esophagus are surrounded on four sides, so that a complete ring is formed (Fig. 20.34). The right-sided arch is larger and higher in 80% of cases. Surgical ligation of the smaller arch is the treatment of choice. Axial and sagittal images can be used for preoperative measurement of the two arches.

FUNCTION

In addition to the depiction of morphology, technologic improvements have made possible the use of MRI for reliable, and in many cases unique, measurements of function. The two main techniques for functional evaluation are cine gradient-echo and phase-contrast velocity imaging.

Cine Gradient-Echo Imaging

Gradient-echo sequences can be referenced to the ECG to produce multiple acquisitions through a cardiac cycle. Retrospective gating of these acquisitions over several cycles creates a series of images corresponding to multiple phases of the cardiac cycle. These can be played in a cine loop to show

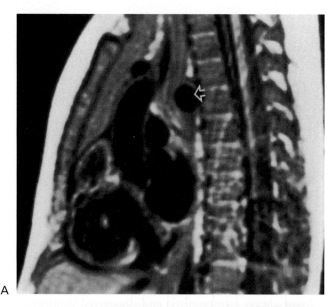

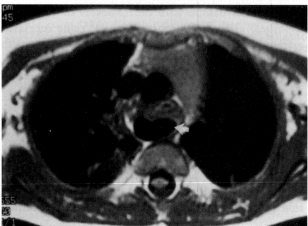

A

B

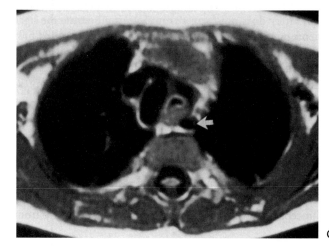

C

FIGURE 20.33. Right aortic arch with aberrant left subclavian artery. **A:** Sagittal spin-echo image shows compression of the trachea and esophagus by the posterior aberrant subclavian artery *(open arrow).* **B,C:** Axial spin-echo images show the aberrant left subclavian artery *(arrow)* originating from a focal dilation of the descending thoracic aorta. (From Higgins CB. Congenital heart disease. In: Higgins CB, Hricak H, Helms CA, eds. *Magnetic resonance imaging of the body,* 3rd ed. Philadelphia: Lippincott–Raven Publishers, 1997:503, with permission.)

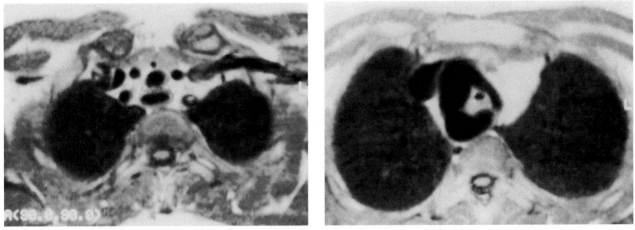

FIGURE 20.34. Double aortic arch. Axial spin-echo images at the level of the cervicothoracic junction **(A)** and aortic arch **(B)** show that the right arch is slightly superior to and larger than the left. Arch branches are arranged symmetrically on each side of the trachea and esophagus. Note the compression of the trachea at the site of the double arch. (From Higgins CB. Congenital heart disease. In: Higgins CB, Hricak H, Helms CA, eds. *Magnetic resonance imaging of the body*, 3rd ed. Philadelphia: Lippincott–Raven Publishers, 1997:502, with permission.)

cardiac motion, so that wall motion, contractility, and wall thickening can be evaluated qualitatively and quantitatively. Volumes and mass can be measured precisely without assumptions about geometry. Such measurements are especially helpful in cases with functionally univentricular hearts, in which the ventricles may have unusual geometry and in which both the performance of the larger, more functional ventricle and that of the smaller, rudimentary ventricle are important in determining prognosis and planning surgery (59).

Ventricular Volumes/Ejection Fraction

Cine images in the short-axis plane (Fig. 20.35) are used to quantify ventricular volumes, ejection fraction, and ventricular mass. For each short-axis image, an end-diastolic image is selected, and a region-of-interest (ROI) is created by tracing the inner (endocardial) border of the myocardium. The area of the ROI is multiplied by the slice thickness. Repeating this process for all the end-diastolic images and summing them yields the end-diastolic volume. The same process is performed for all the end-systolic images to calculate end-systolic volume (Fig. 20.36). The ejection fraction can then be calculated without any assumptions about ventricular geometry for either the LV or RV.

Ventricular Mass

To measure the ventricular mass, an ROI is traced around the outer (epicardial) border of the myocardium to define an area that includes the myocardium and ventricular cavity. A second ROI is drawn along the endocardial border of the myocardium. Subtraction of the latter area from the former

yields the area of the myocardium on each image. The area of myocardium on each slice is multiplied by the slice thickness, and the areas obtained from all slices encompassing the heart are summed to obtain the myocardial volume. This volume is multiplied by the density of myocardium, 1.05 g/mL (27), to calculate the myocardial mass.

Phase-Contrast Velocity/Flow Measurements

In phase-contrast imaging, the signal intensity signifies the velocity of blood at each pixel. ECG-gated phase-contrast images can be produced in which each image shows the velocity at a different time in the cardiac cycle. Because these are cine images, they are referred to as velocity-encoded cine (VEC) MR images. An ROI drawn around a blood vessel will give the mean velocity within the vessel at that point in the cardiac cycle. The cross-sectional area of the vessel can be multiplied by the spatial mean velocity to obtain the flow in the blood vessel (27).

Assessment of Functional Severity of Coarctation of the Aorta and Measurement of Collateral Flow

The functional severity of a coarctation can be estimated with VEC MRI (60,61) (Fig. 4.2). VEC MRI sequences are ideally prescribed from an oblique sagittal image in the plane of the aortic arch. The VEC MRI acquisition should be performed in a plane orthogonal to the direction of blood flow. To quantify the collateral circulation, blood flow is estimated at two different locations, one at the proximal aorta just distal to the coarctation site and the other in the de-

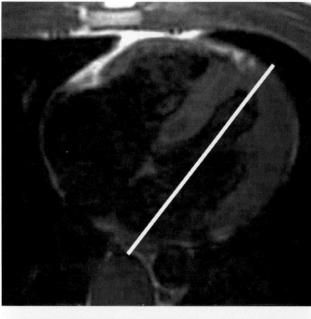

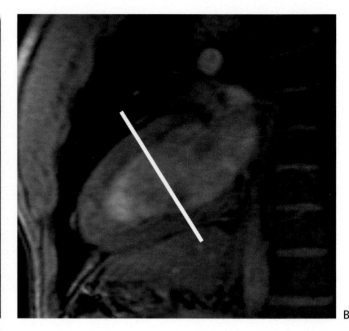

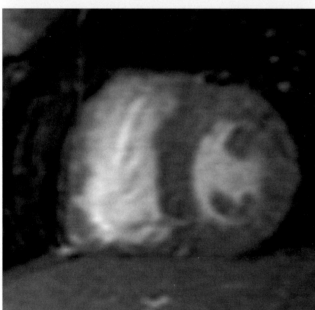

FIGURE 20.35. Short-axis MR images. **A:** From the axial images, a plane is selected that connects the left ventricular apex to the middle of the mitral valve *(line)*. This produces an image in the cardiac long axis **(B)**. From the long-axis image, a plane is selected perpendicular to the lumen of the left ventricle *(line)*. This in turn produces the short-axis plane **(C)**.

scending aorta at the level of the diaphragm (61). Flow is greater in the proximal descending aorta than in the distal aorta in normal persons. However, in coarctation, blood flow may be greater distally, indicating retrograde collateral flow into the aorta through the intercostal arteries and other branches of the thoracic aorta. To calculate the collateral blood flow, the aortic flow distal to the coarctation site is subtracted from the flow at level of the diaphragm. The degree of collateral flow may be an important factor in operative planning. The pressure gradient across the coarctation is another important parameter in surgical planning. The peak flow velocity can be estimated by performing VEC MRI through the narrowest segment of the aorta (60), and

the pressure gradient can be calculated with the modified Bernoulli equation: $\Delta P = 4v^2$, where ΔP is the pressure gradient in millimeters of mercury and v is the peak flow velocity in meters per second.

Quantification of Shunts

Studies have established the usefulness of VEC MRI for quantifying the pulmonary-to-systemic flow ratio (Q_p/Q_s), and the correlation with oximetry at cardiac catheterization is good (62,63). VEC MRI is also useful for monitoring changes in the volume of the shunt over time (63).

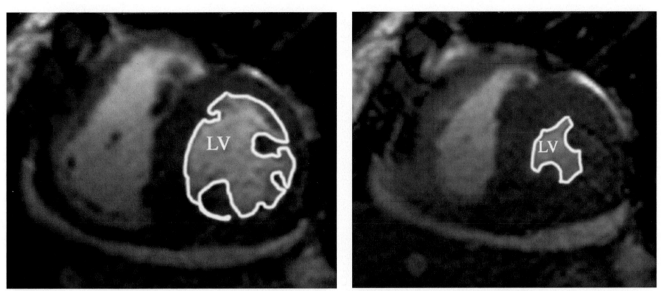

FIGURE 20.36. Ejection fraction. A region-of-interest is traced along the endocardial surface in **(A)** end-diastole and **(B)** end-systole. For each image, the end-diastolic area is multiplied by the slice thickness, and the resultant volumes are summed to give the end-diastolic volume of the heart. The same process is repeated for the end-systolic images to give the end-systolic volume. From these volumes, the ejection fraction (end-systolic volume divided by end-diastolic volume) is calculated. *LV,* left ventricle.

Two primary methods are used to quantify shunts with cine MRI. Both of these approaches rely on a comparison of the RV and LV stroke volumes. Because the presence of aortic or pulmonic valvular regurgitation leads to an inaccurate determination of the stroke volume, coexisting valvular insufficiency can result in a miscalculation of shunt volume unless the estimated stroke volume is reduced by the volume of regurgitation.

In the first technique for shunt quantification, cine MRI is used to measure the ventricular volumes and calculate the total stroke volumes for the RV and LV according to the method described in the previous section (64). In a normal subject, the stroke volumes in the two ventricles are equal. In the presence of a left-to-right shunt at the atrial level (ASD or partial anomalous pulmonary venous connection), the RV stroke volume is greater than the LV stroke volume by a quantity equal to the volume of the shunt (65). For a left-to-right shunt through a patent ductus arteriosus, the shunt volume can be calculated by subtracting the RV stroke volume from the LV stroke volume. This method of estimating shunt size is not applicable in persons with a VSD. For right-to-left shunts, similar calculations can be made by substituting RV stroke volume for LV stroke volume, and vice versa.

In the second method of shunt quantification, VEC MRI is used to ascertain the effective stroke volume (Fig. 4.3). VEC MRI flow measurements are obtained in both the ascending aorta and main pulmonary artery (63). In a normal subject, blood flow is equal in these two vessels. If a patient has a left-to-right shunt with an ASD, VSD, or partial anomalous pulmonary venous connection, flow in the pulmonary artery will be greater than aortic flow by the quantity of the shunt. On the other hand, with a patent ductus arteriosus, aortic flow is greater than pulmonary blood flow, and shunt volume is calculated by subtracting pulmonary flow from aortic flow. The opposite relationships are true in patients with a right-to-left shunt.

Measurement of Pulmonary Flow

VEC MRI has the unique capability to measure differential flow in the right and left pulmonary arteries (65). VEC MRI can therefore provide important information about patients with a disparity of blood flow between the right and left pulmonary arteries. Such disparity of flow can occur in patients with tetralogy of Fallot, pulmonary atresia with VSD, pulmonary artery hypoplasia, or pulmonary sling; it can also occur after surgery—for example, after a Jatene (arterial switch) repair of transposition of the great arteries.

Pulmonary Regurgitation

Pulmonary regurgitation frequently occurs in patients who have undergone a right ventriculoplasty or Rastelli procedure to repair tetralogy of Fallot. VEC MRI can be used to measure the volume of pulmonic regurgitation in these cases (66) (Figs. 4.5 and 20.37). It has been shown that the volume of pulmonary regurgitation measured at VEC MRI closely correlates with the difference in stroke volume indices of the ventricles and with the RV end-diastolic volume (66) (Fig. 20.37).

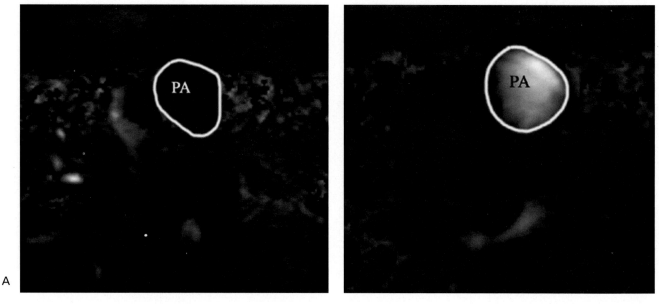

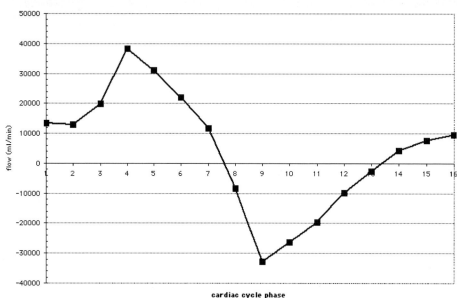

FIGURE 20.37. Regurgitant fraction. **A:** Cine phase-contrast image through the plane of the main pulmonary artery. A region-of-interest has been drawn around the main pulmonary artery *(PA)*. In this image, black pixels indicate forward flow in the pulmonary artery. **B:** A second image later in the cardiac cycle shows white pixels in the main pulmonary artery, which indicate that the flow, previously encoded by black pixels, has reversed. **C:** Graph of flow in the pulmonary artery shows reversal of flow. Multiplying the area by the mean velocity for each phase of the cardiac cycle gives the area under the curve. The total forward flow and regurgitant flow can be measured and the regurgitant fraction calculated.

SUMMARY

MRI is useful for demonstrating the anatomy in a wide variety of congenital cardiac lesions. The large field of view and flexible imaging planes allow the depiction of complex lesions, such as abnormalities of situs or complicated three-dimensional relations of cardiac chambers. MRI also can be used to obtain quantitative functional information, such as ventricular volumes, ejection fractions, and flow measurements.

REFERENCES

1. Freedom RM. The "anthropology" of the segmental approach to the diagnosis of complex congenital heart disease. *Cardiovasc Intervent Radiol* 1984;7:121–123.
2. Van Praagh R. Diagnosis of complex congenital heart disease: morphologic-anatomic method and terminology. *Cardiovasc Intervent Radiol* 1984;7:115–120.
3. Freedom RMM, Yoo SJ, Benson LN. The segmental and sequential approach to congenital heart disease. In: Freedom RMM, Yoo SJ, Benson LN, eds.*Congenital heart disease: a text-*

book of angiocardiography, vol 1. Armonk, NY: Futura Publishing, 1997:95–120.

4. Kersting-Sommerhoff BA, Diethelm L, Teitel DF, et al. Magnetic resonance imaging of congenital heart disease: sensitivity and specificity using receiver operating characteristic curve analysis. *Am Heart J* 1989;118:155–161.

5. Williams PLW, Dyson M, Bannister LH. The heart. In: Williams PLW, Dyson M, Bannister LH, eds. *Gray's anatomy.* New York: Churchill Livingstone, 1989:696–726.

6. Mazzucco A, Bortolotti U, Stellin G, et al. Anomalies of the systemic venous return: a review. *J Card Surg* 1990;5:122–133.

7. Applegate KE, Goske MJ, Pierce G, et al. Situs revisited: imaging of the heterotaxy syndrome. *Radiographics* 1999;19:837–852; discussion 853–854.

8. Peoples WM, Moller JH, Edwards JE. Polysplenia: a review of 146 cases. *Pediatr Cardiol* 1983;4:129–137.

9. Julsrud PRF. Anomalous pulmonary venous connection. In: Baum S, ed. *Abrams' angiography,* vol 1. Boston: Little, Brown and Company, 1997:868–890.

10. Masui T, Seelos KC, Kersting-Sommerhoff BA, et al. Abnormalities of the pulmonary veins: evaluation with MR imaging and angiography and echocardiography. *Radiology* 1991;181: 645–649.

11. Donnelly LF, Higgins CB. MR imaging of conotruncal abnormalities. *AJR Am J Roentgenol* 1996;166:925–928.

12. Ferrari VA, Scott CH, Holland GA, et al. Ultrafast three-dimensional contrast-enhanced magnetic resonance angiography and imaging in the diagnosis of partial anomalous pulmonary venous drainage. *J Am Coll Cardiol* 2001;37:1120–1128.

13. Van Praagh R. Terminology of congenital heart disease. Glossary and commentary [Editorial]. *Circulation* 1977;56:139–143.

14. Angelini P. Embryology and congenital heart disease. *Tex Heart Inst J* 1995;22:1–12.

15. Netter FH. Embryology. In: Netter FH, ed. *The Ciba collection of medical illustrations: a compilation of pathological and anatomical paintings,* vol 5. Summit, NJ: Ciba Pharmaceutical Products, 1981:112–130.

16. Amplatz KM. Congenitally corrected transposition of the great vessels: L-transposition of the great vessels. In: Amplatz KM, ed. *Radiology of congenital heart disease.* St. Louis: Mosby–Year Book, 1993:709–726.

17. Freedom RMM, Yoo SJ, Benson LN. Corrected transposition of the great arteries (atrioventricular and ventriculoarterial discordance). In: Freedom RMM, Yoo SJ, Benson LN, eds. *Congenital heart disease: a textbook of angiocardiography,* vol 2. Armonk, NY: Futura Publishing, 1997:1071–1117.

18. Kersting-Sommerhoff BA, Diethelm L, Stanger P, et al. Evaluation of complex congenital ventricular anomalies with magnetic resonance imaging. *Am Heart J* 1990;120:133–142.

19. Graham TP Jr, Bernard YD, Mellen BG, et al. Long-term outcome in congenitally corrected transposition of the great arteries: a multi-institutional study. *J Am Coll Cardiol* 2000;36:255–261.

20. Anderson RH, Ho SY. What is a ventricle? *Ann Thorac Surg* 1998;66:616–620.

21. Anderson RH, Ho SY. Which hearts are unsuitable for biventricular correction? *Ann Thorac Surg* 1998;66:621–626.

22. Fletcher BD, Jacobstein MD, Abramowsky CR, et al. Right atrioventricular valve atresia: anatomic evaluation with MR imaging. *AJR Am J Roentgenol* 1987;148:671–674.

23. Orie JD, Anderson C, Ettedgui JA, et al. Echocardiographic-morphologic correlations in tricuspid atresia. *J Am Coll Cardiol* 1995;26:750–758.

24. Amplatz KM. Tricuspid atresia with normally related great vessels. In: Amplatz KM, ed. *Radiology of congenital heart disease.* St. Louis: Mosby–Year Book, 1993:607–623.

25. Pearl JMP, Laks H. Tricuspid atresia. In: Baue AEG, Hammond GL, Laks H, et al., eds. *Glenn's thoracic and cardiovascular surgery,* vol 2. Stamford, CT: Appleton & Lange, 1996:1431–1449.

26. Kurosawa H. Current strategies of the Fontan operation. *Ann Thorac Cardiovasc Surg* 1998;4:171–177.

27. Reddy GP, Higgins CB. Congenital heart disease: measuring physiology with MRI. *Semin Roentgenol* 1998;33:228–238.

28. Fellows KE, Fogel MA. MR imaging and heart function in patients pre- and post-Fontan surgery. *Acta Paediatr Suppl* 1995; 410:57–59.

29. Bharati S, Lev M. The surgical anatomy of the heart in tubular hypoplasia of the transverse aorta (preductal coarctation). *J Thorac Cardiovasc Surg* 1986;91:79–85.

30. Freedom RMM, Yoo SJ, Benson LN. Aortic atresia and variants. In: Freedom RMM, Yoo SJ, Benson LN, eds. *Congenital heart disease: a textbook of angiocardiography,* vol 2. Armonk, NY: Futura Publishing, 1997:731–765.

31. Fogel MA, Hubbard AM, Fellows KE, et al. MRI for physiology and function in congenital heart disease: functional assessment of the heart preoperatively and postoperatively. *Semin Roentgenol* 1998;33:239–251.

32. Kondo C, Hardy C, Higgins SS, et al. Nuclear magnetic resonance imaging of the palliative operation for hypoplastic left heart syndrome. *J Am Coll Cardiol* 1991;18:817–823.

33. Anderson KR, Zuberbuhler JR, Anderson RH, et al. Morphologic spectrum of Ebstein's anomaly of the heart: a review. *Mayo Clin Proc* 1979;54:174–180.

34. Freedom RMM, Yoo SJ, Benson LN. Ebstein's malformation. In: Freedom RMM, Yoo SJ, Benson LN, eds. *Congenital heart disease: a textbook of angiocardiography,* vol 1. Armonk, NY: Futura Publishing, 1997:349–366.

35. Eustace S, Kruskal JB, Hartnell GG. Ebstein's anomaly presenting in adulthood: the role of cine magnetic resonance imaging in diagnosis. *Clin Radiol* 1994;49:690–692.

36. Freedom RMM, Yoo SJ, Benson LN. Atrioventricular septal defect. In: Freedom RMM, Yoo SJ, Benson LN, eds. *Congenital heart disease: a textbook of angiocardiography,* vol 1. Armonk, NY: Futura Publishing, 1997:133–188.

37. Parsons JM, Baker EJ, Anderson RH, et al. Morphological evaluation of atrioventricular septal defects by magnetic resonance imaging. *Br Heart J* 1990;64:138–145.

38. Jacobstein MD, Fletcher BD, Goldstein S, et al. Evaluation of atrioventricular septal defect by magnetic resonance imaging. *Am J Cardiol* 1985;55:1158–1161.

39. Amplatz KM. Complete transposition of the great vessels. In: Amplatz KM, ed. *Radiology of congenital heart disease.* St. Louis: Mosby–Year Book, 1993:675–708.

40. Freedom RMM, Yoo SJ, Benson LN. Tetralogy of Fallot and pulmonary atresia and ventricular septal defect. In: Freedom RMM, Yoo SJ, Benson LN, eds. *Congenital heart disease: a textbook of angiocardiography,* vol 1. Armonk, NY: Futura Publishing, 1997: 493–533.

41. Beekman RP, Beek FJ, Meijboom EJ. Usefulness of MRI for the pre-operative evaluation of the pulmonary arteries in tetralogy of Fallot. *Magn Reson Imaging* 1997;15:1005–1015.

42. Holmqvist C, Hochbergs P, Bjorkhem G, et al. Pre-operative evaluation with MR in tetralogy of Fallot and pulmonary atresia with ventricular septal defect. *Acta Radiol* 2001;42:63–69.

43. Gomes AS, Lois JF, Williams RG. Pulmonary arteries: MR imaging in patients with congenital obstruction of the right ventricular outflow tract. *Radiology* 1990;174:51–57.

44. Kersting-Sommerhoff BA, Sechtem UP, Higgins CB. Evaluation of pulmonary blood supply by nuclear magnetic resonance imaging in patients with pulmonary atresia. *J Am Coll Cardiol* 1988; 11:166–171.

45. Powell AJ, Chung T, Landzberg MJ, et al. Accuracy of MRI

evaluation of pulmonary blood supply in patients with complex pulmonary stenosis or atresia. *Int J Card Imaging* 2000;16: 169–174.

46. Freedom RMM, Yoo SJ, Benson LN. Double-outlet right ventricle. In: Freedom RMM, Yoo SJ, Benson LN, eds. *Congenital heart disease: a textbook of angiocardiography,* vol 2. Armonk, NY: Futura Publishing, 1997:1119–1169.

47. Starnes VAPTW. Double-outlet right ventricle and double-outlet left ventricle. In: Baue AEG, Hammond GL, Laks H, et al., eds. *Glenn's thoracic and cardiovascular surgery,* vol 2. Stamford, CT: Appleton & Lange, 1996:1417–1429.

48. Yoo SJ, Lim TH, Park IS, et al. MR anatomy of ventricular septal defect in double-outlet right ventricle with situs solitus and atrioventricular concordance. *Radiology* 1991;181:501–505.

49. Collett RW, Edwards JE. Persistent truncus arteriosus: a classification according to anatomic types. *Surg Clin North Am* 1949; 1949:1245.

50. Bremerich J, Reddy GP, Higgins CB. MRI of supracristal ventricular septal defects. *J Comput Assist Tomogr* 1999;23:13–15.

51. Amplatz KM. Ventricular septal defect with aortic insufficiency or aortic stenosis. In: Amplatz KM, ed. *Radiology of congenital heart disease.* St. Louis: Mosby–Year Book, 1993:273–277.

52. Freedom RMM, Yoo SJ, Benson LN. Atrial septal defect. In: Freedom RMM, Yoo SJ, Benson LN, eds. *Congenital heart disease: a textbook of angiocardiography,* vol 1. Armonk, NY: Futura Publishing, 1997:125–132.

53. Baker EJ, Ayton V, Smith MA, et al. Magnetic resonance imaging of coarctation of the aorta in infants: use of a high field strength. *Br Heart J* 1989;62:97–101.

54. Rees S, Somerville J, Ward C, et al. Coarctation of the aorta: MR imaging in late postoperative assessment. *Radiology* 1989;173: 499–502.

55. Boxer RA, LaCorte MA, Singh S, et al. Nuclear magnetic resonance imaging in evaluation and follow-up of children treated for coarctation of the aorta. *J Am Coll Cardiol* 1986;7: 1095–1098.

56. Steffens JC, Bourne MW, Sakuma H, et al. Quantification of collateral blood flow in coarctation of the aorta by velocity-encoded cine magnetic resonance imaging. *Circulation* 1994;90:937–943.

57. Bisset GS III, Strife JL, Kirks DR, et al. Vascular rings: MR imaging. *AJR Am J Roentgenol* 1987:149:251–256.

58. Kersting-Sommerhoff BA, Sechtem UP, Fisher MR, et al. MR imaging of congenital anomalies of the aortic arch. *AJR Am J Roentgenol* 1987:149:9–13.

59. Fogel MA, Hubbard AM, Fellows KE, et al. MRI for physiology and function in congenital heart disease: functional assessment of the heart preoperatively and postoperatively. *Semin Roentgenol* 1998;23:239–251.

60. Mohiaddin RH, Kilner PT, Rees S, et al. Magnetic resonance volume flow and jet velocity mapping in aortic coarctation. *J Am Coll Cardiol* 1993;22:1515–1521.

61. Steffens JC, Bourne MW, Sakuma H, et al. Quantitation of collateral blood flow in coarctation of the aorta by velocity-encoded cine magnetic resonance imaging. *Circulation* 1994;90:937–943.

62. Brenner LD, Caputo GR, Mostbeck G, et al. Quantification of left-to-right atrial shunts with velocity-encoded cine nuclear magnetic resonance imaging. *J Am Coll Cardiol* 1992;20: 1246–1250.

63. Edelman RR, Mattle HP, Kjeefield J, et al. Quantification of blood flow with dynamic MR imaging and presaturation bolus tracking. *Radiology* 1989;171:551–556.

64. Sechtem U, Pflugfelder P, Cassidy MC, et al. Ventricular septal defect: visualization of shunt flow and determination of shunt size by cine magnetic resonance imaging. *AJR Am J Roentgenol* 1987; 149:689–691.

65. Higgins CB. Congenital heart disease. In: Higgins CB, Hricak H, Helms CA, eds. *Magnetic resonance imaging of the body,* 3rd ed. Philadelphia: Lippincott–Raven Publishers, 1997:461–518.

66. Rebergen SA, Chin JGJ, Ottenkamp J, et al. Pulmonary regurgitation in the late postoperative follow-up of tetralogy of Fallot: volumetric quantification by MR velocity mapping. *Circulation* 1993;88:2257–2266.

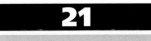

21

POSTOPERATIVE FUNCTIONAL EVALUATION OF CONGENITAL HEART DISEASE

ARNO A. W. ROEST
WILLEM A. HELBING
ERNST E. VAN DER WALL
ALBERT DE ROOS

The population of patients with adult congenital heart disease (CHD) is growing at a rapid pace of 5% per year. The number of patients in the United States alone is now approximately 1 million (1). Improved survival after surgery has largely contributed to the growth rate of the population with corrected adult CHD. Traditionally, these patients have been monitored over time by clinical assessment, electrocardiography, echocardiography, and catheter-based x-ray angiography. The trend in the last 10 years is the increasing acceptance of MRI as an important imaging tool for assessing postoperative cardiovascular anatomy and function in adult patients with corrected or palliated CHD.

Several categories of patients with corrected congenital defects are now referred for MRI to assess morphology, ventricular function, and flow. The most common referrals for MRI are discussed in Chapter 22. Many clinical issues in these patients center around the assessment of right ventricular (RV) function and pulmonary flow. A particular strength of MRI is that the modality has exquisite capabilities to measure RV function and pulmonary flow with a high rate of technical success in comparison with echocardiography (2). The focus of this chapter is the potential role of MRI in assessing heart function in postoperative CHD.

The MRI techniques that are available are constantly improving. Recently, significant advances have been made in black blood imaging for assessing morphology and in gradient-echo sequences for functional evaluation. True fast imaging with steady-state free precession (FISP) or balanced fast-field echo (FFE) sequences in combination with the new sensitivity-encoded (SENSE) technology are now in wide use because of their capability to provide remarkable improvements in image quality, which are of particular advantage in imaging the RV.

First, the technical options that are available with MRI for studying the heart are reviewed. Then, the use of these tools for the functional evaluation of patients after repair of tetralogy of Fallot, transposition of the great arteries, and patients with a Fontan circulation is discussed in some detail.

TECHNICAL OPTIONS

Black Blood Imaging

Traditionally, spin-echo MR sequences have been used to study the morphology of the heart. These sequences provide a high level of contrast between the heart wall and the blood pool. The blood pool appears black because of the flow of blood during acquisition of the images. This feature provides detailed anatomic images, although flow artifacts sometimes degrade their diagnostic quality. The spin-echo sequence is triggered by the electrocardiogram and acquires data over multiple heart beats, so that motion artifacts may be caused by residual cardiac motion and respiration.

Recently, improved black blood imaging was introduced. This technique uses a double-inversion pulse to suppress further the signal from the blood pool and can be performed during breath-holding to minimize motion artifacts.

A. A. W. Roest and W. A. Helbing: Department of Pediatric Cardiology, Leiden University Medical Center, Leiden, The Netherlands.

E. E. van der Wall: Department of Cardiology, Leiden University Medical Center, Leiden, The Netherlands.

A. de Roos: Department of Radiology, Leiden University Medical Center, Leiden, The Netherlands.

Anatomic imaging is performed in multiple directions, and images may be acquired along intrinsic axes of the aorta or pulmonary vessels for optimal depiction of the morphology. Thin-slice (3- to 5-mm) imaging is preferred to avoid partial volume effects. The assessment of focal stenosis (e.g., in coarctation or pulmonary artery stenosis) is best accomplished with a 3-mm slice thickness in oblique planes along the course of the vessel of interest. In addition, three-dimensional (3D) MRA has advantages in demonstrating focal stenosis because it provides a 3D display of the vasculature.

Balanced Gradient-Echo Imaging and Sensitivity-Encoded Technology

Another recent technical advance has been the introduction of true FISP or balanced FFE sequences for evaluating cardiac function. Balanced FFE is a fast gradient-echo pulse sequence that generates a steady-state free-precession signal. The resulting tissue contrast characteristics are quite different from those of the existing T1 or T2 contrast-producing methods. The method has been known for several years in the literature but has only recently become operational owing to the advent of strong gradients that allow short repetition times (TRs), in the order of 4 milliseconds or less. The pulse sequence is characterized by the balanced time integrated area over one TR between any two radiofrequency excitation pulses of each gradient waveform. *Balanced* means zero net result of the time integrated area. This is accomplished for all functional gradient directions, including slice selection, frequency readout, and phase encoding. Together with the alternating phase of the excitation pulse, this implementation ensures that both signals (free induction decay and echo) are measured. The resulting images reveal very high signal for tissues with a high T2-to-T1 ratio independently of the absolute values of T1 and T2 and independently of the TR. For a T2-to-T1 ratio of 1, which is the highest possible ratio, the magnitude of the signal approaches one-half of what could be observed in a nonenhanced gradient-echo experiment at infinitely long TRs. This magnitude is much greater than what is possible with T1- or T2-enhanced fast-field echo schemes at practical TRs.

A major advantage of balanced FFE is its low sensitivity to flow disturbances owing to the zero integrated area condition, which means that the large steady-state signal of fluids with a high T2-to-T1 ratio is hardly diminished by slow flow. These advantages are very useful to optimize functional cine imaging of the heart. The blood pool produces a very bright and homogeneous signal that is independent of flow and motion, and an excellent contrast with the myocardium is achieved. The myocardium appears with relatively very low signal intensity in comparison with the high-signal blood pool. A high degree of spatial resolution in combination with a short scan time is usually achieved by using a reduced scan percentage, whereas the resolution in the readout direction remains 100% but is reduced in the phase-encoding direction to save scan time. For the application of this sequence, it is important to keep the TR as short as possible and to use automatic volume shim to achieve absolute homogeneity.

True FISP of heart function allows better automated contour detection for functional analysis than does the conventional gradient-echo pulse sequence (3). In the implementation of true FISP imaging, the steady state builds up in both the longitudinal and transverse directions, and with balancing of the gradients in all three directions, a maximum recovery of the transverse magnetization is ensured. Newer generations of this pulse sequence are under development and will probably further improve image quality, so that more and more operator-independent analysis of the functional data will be possible.

Another major recent advance has been the introduction of parallel signal acquisition with multiple coil elements to enhance the speed of imaging (4). This so-called SENSE technology allows a considerable reduction of scan time in most MRI techniques, including black blood and balanced FFE imaging. Simultaneously operated coils are utilized for improving the signal-to-noise ratio, and also for spatial signal encoding complementary to common gradient switching. Theoretically, SENSE reconstruction may achieve reduction factors up to the number of coils used (e.g., a six-element cardiac array), although in practice the geometry of the used coil arrangement is a limiting factor.

Measurements of Blood Flow

MR velocity mapping is an indispensable tool to assess flow velocity and volume in both large and small vascular structures (5). MR velocity mapping as an addition to MRI is comparable to Doppler techniques as an addition to echocardiography, although the applications of MR velocity mapping are more versatile than those of Doppler flow imaging. MR velocity mapping is based on the phase-shift method, in which a phase change is proportional to velocity. Phase is a component of the MR signal of flowing protons, and the phase angle will change in proportion to their velocity if an MR gradient is applied in the direction of flow. The technical background of MR velocity mapping is described in greater detail in Chapter 10.

In the evaluation of CHD, velocity mapping has proved valuable for assessing vascular and valvular flow, especially in territories that are difficult to measure by ultrasonography, such as the pulmonary artery. In patients who have undergone surgery, transthoracic echocardiography may be limited by the complexity of the anatomy and postsurgical distortions. MRI and transthoracic echocardiography have been shown to provide complementary information in this group of patients (6). Transthoracic echocardiography has advantages for evaluating intracardiac structures, whereas the strength of MRI is in the evaluation of morphology and flow in extracardiac vascular structures and conduits. Overall, the advantages of MR velocity mapping include the following: accurate flow measurements per pixel when the vessel of interest is interrogated in a plane perpendicular to the vector of flow (peak and mean velocities); free choice of the imaging plane, either perpendicular to or along the vessel of interest; unrestricted windows of access, even for deep-lying vascular structures that are beyond the reach of the ultrasound beam; and highly accurate measurements of volume flow made possible by the simultaneous acquisition of mean velocity and the cross-sectional area of the vessel.

Contrast-Enhanced MRA

Three-dimensional gadolinium-enhanced MRA is a valuable adjunct to gradient-echo and black blood techniques for assessing the morphology of the aorta and pulmonary vasculature (Fig. 21.1). Gadolinium-enhanced MRA, performed during a single breath-hold at peak enhancement, provides a high-resolution 3D data set that can be used for projection angiography and multiplanar re-formation (7). Timing of the data acquisition is aimed at collecting the central section of k-space during peak arterial enhancement to optimize the effect of the contrast medium (Fig. 21.1). This angiographic technique allows a more complete assessment of complex 3D anatomy.

MRI Stress Testing

Stress testing, either pharmacologic or physical, may reveal abnormalities of ventricular function that are not evident under resting conditions. Pharmacologic stress testing in

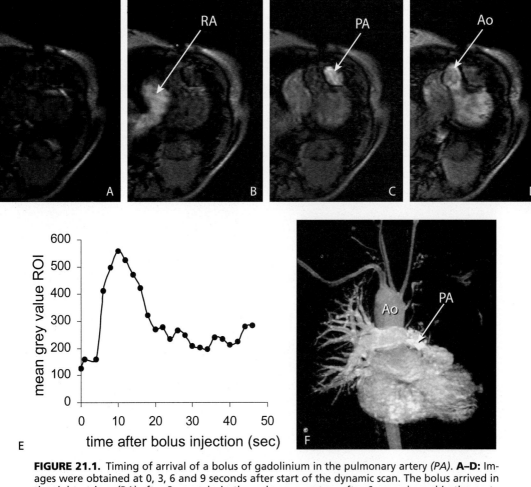

FIGURE 21.1. Timing of arrival of a bolus of gadolinium in the pulmonary artery *(PA)*. **A–D:** Images were obtained at 0, 3, 6 and 9 seconds after start of the dynamic scan. The bolus arrived in the right atrium *(RA)* after 3 seconds, in the pulmonary artery after 6 seconds, and in the aorta *(Ao)* after 9 seconds. A region of interest can be placed in the pulmonary artery, and **(E)** the graph represents the increase in signal within the region of interest at the arrival of the bolus. **F:** A three-dimensional gadolinium-enhanced MR angiogram of tetralogy of Fallot in a patient after palliative shunt placement (between left subclavian artery and left pulmonary artery) and subsequent total repair is shown. Fifteen years after total repair of tetralogy of Fallot, the left pulmonary artery is obstructed, and a hypoperfusion of the left lung is observed.

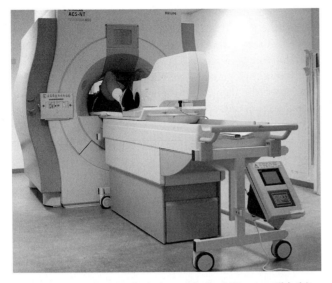

FIGURE 21.2. MRI exercise setup with the MR-compatible bicycle ergometer (Lode BV, Groningen, The Netherlands) fitted to the table top and positioned in the scanner (Philips Gyroscan ACS/NT, 1.5-tesla MR scanner, Philips Medical Systems, Best, The Netherlands.)

combination with MRI is now successfully applied in the evaluation of ischemic heart disease (8). In patients with CHD, pharmacological stress testing is mainly performed in combination with nuclear imaging techniques (9,10).

Physical stress testing in the MRI machine poses special practical problems, especially space limitations in the scanner and the induction of motion-related artifacts when bicycle exercise is performed; the latter may degrade image quality. The use of an MR-compatible bicycle ergometer (11) (Fig. 21.2) and a dedicated exercise protocol makes it possible to measure large-vessel flow in response to exercise (12). Recently, the feasibility of using MRI to measure the biventricular response to bicycle exercise was demonstrated in healthy young adults (13). Ultrafast MRI was applied to study possible changes in ventricular volumes at rest and at individualized workloads corresponding to 60% of the maximal oxygen uptake. A complete volumetric evaluation of both ventricles was performed during exercise breaks and short breath-holding. In all subjects, images of good quality could be obtained with accurate volume determination (Fig. 21.3). The responses of both the left ventricle (LV) and RV

Rest

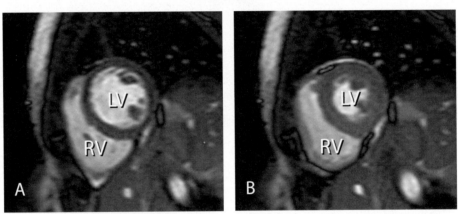

Exercise

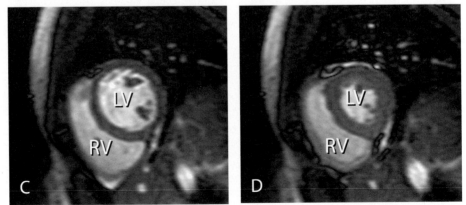

FIGURE 21.3. Short-axis images of the left ventricle *(LV)* and right ventricle *(RV)* at rest and with exercise at end-diastole **(A,C)** and end-systole **(B,D)** in a healthy subject obtained with a balanced FFE (fast-field echo) MR sequence and SENSE (sensitivity encoding).

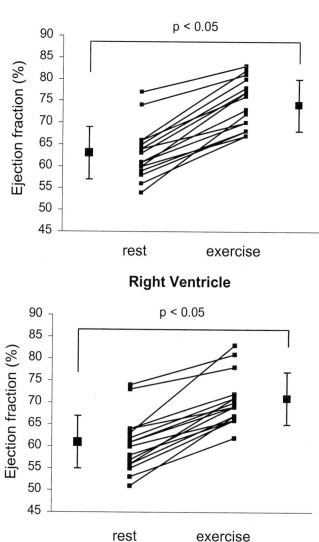

FIGURE 21.4. Change in ejection fraction from rest to stress of the left ventricle *(upper chart)* and right ventricle *(lower chart).* A significant increase from rest to stress was found for both the left and right ventricles. (From Roest AA, Kunz P, Lamb HJ, et al. Biventricular response to supine physical exercise in young adults assessed with ultrafast magnetic resonance imaging. *Am J Cardiol* 2001;87:601–605, with permission.)

were evaluated, and physiologic information on changes in ventricular volume during stress was obtained (Fig. 21.4). In these young healthy adults, the LV stroke volume increased because of a decrease in end-systolic volume, whereas the end-diastolic volume remained unchanged. The response of the LV appears to be an age-dependent phenomenon because in older patients, the physiologic response seemed to be caused by an increase in end-diastolic volume. In a similar fashion, the physiologic response of the RV was observed during bicycle stress MRI (13). Again, observed increases in RV stroke volume and ejection fraction were the consequence of a decrease in end-systolic ventricular volumes, not of a change in end-diastolic volumes.

Another application of exercise MRI is in the evaluation of cardiac recovery after physical exercise (14). With multiple turbo-field echo-planar MR flow velocity measurements of the ascending aorta, it is possible to cover changes in the function of the systemic ventricle in response to exercise and during the recovery period. In healthy subjects, recovery of the heart rate is characterized by an exponential decrease to 10% above the resting level for up to 8 minutes after exercise (15,16). The recovery of LV stroke volume in healthy subjects is characterized by an increase during the first minute after exercise and a subsequent decrease toward resting levels (15,17).

HEART FUNCTION IN SPECIFIC ENTITIES

Tetralogy of Fallot

Tetralogy of Fallot is one of the most common types of cyanotic CHD, accounting for approximately 5.5% of all patients with CHD (18). Anterior displacement of the outflow septum is the primary defect; this in turn results in a ventricular septal defect (VSD), overriding of the aorta, obstruction of the RV outflow tract, and RV hypertrophy (19). In 1955, Lillehei et al. (20) introduced intracardiac repair of tetralogy of Fallot, which aims at closure of the VSD and relief of the obstruction of the RV outflow tract by resection or patch placement. This surgical approach has been refined and is now performed in many centers early in childhood, preferably between 3 to 11 month after birth, without prior placement of palliative shunts (21). Long-term survival is excellent (22). However, despite improved surgical management and good survival rates, complications, residua, and sequelae after tetralogy of Fallot repair are common. Pulmonary valve insufficiency is a common finding after intracardiac repair and influences the clinical outcome of patients with corrected tetralogy of Fallot (23). Long-standing volume overload of the RV is associated with biventricular dysfunction (24–26), ventricular arrhythmias (27), and impaired exercise capacity (28–31). Additionally, a recurrent or residual VSD and central or peripheral pulmonary stenosis can be observed after correction of tetralogy of Fallot.

The timely detection and monitoring of these morphologic and functional abnormalities require accurate and preferably noninvasive imaging methods.

Intracardiac and extracardiac large-vessel anatomy can be well displayed by spin-echo MRI (32). In these patients, RV hypertrophy, RV outflow obstruction, and pulmonary vessel size are depicted in great detail, especially with the recently introduced black blood imaging techniques (Fig. 21.5).

The ability of conventional imaging techniques, such as echocardiography and nuclear imaging, to quantify the volume of pulmonary regurgitation is limited, so that comparisons of clinical studies of the effects of pulmonary regurgitation have been hampered. Pulmonary regurgitation can be quantified by MRI in two different approaches. First, pul-

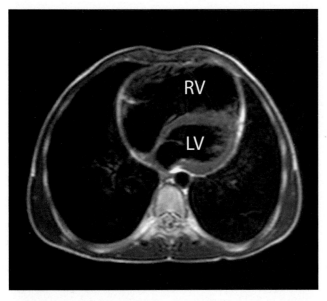

FIGURE 21.5. Transverse MR image of a patient with corrected tetralogy of Fallot obtained with improved black blood imaging and a double-inversion pulse for further suppression of the signal from the blood pool. Note the marked right ventricular *(RV)* dilation caused by regurgitant diastolic flow through an insufficient pulmonary valve. *LV,* left ventricle.

monary regurgitation can be assessed by determining the difference between LV and RV stroke volumes with short-axis gradient-echo MRI. Net output values for the LV and RV should be equal, so the regurgitant volume through the pulmonary valve can be calculated by subtracting LV stroke volume from RV stroke volume (33). The advantage of using this approach is that additional information is obtained about biventricular function. A disadvantage, however, is that in the presence of additional atrioventricular or aortic valve regurgitation, it is not reliable. A direct measurement of pulmonary regurgitation is possible with phase-contrast MRI in the pulmonary artery, which is an accurate technique for quantifying pulmonary regurgitation in patients with surgically repaired tetralogy of Fallot (33) (Fig. 21.6).

To evaluate biventricular function after correction of tetralogy of Fallot, gradient-echo MRI of the RV and LV can be performed. Because of the chronic volume overload, end-systolic and end-diastolic RV volumes are significantly increased, and ejection fraction is decreased (33) (Fig. 21.7). Additionally, LV end-systolic volume, stroke volume, and ejection fraction were impaired in a study of 19 children with moderate to severe pulmonary regurgitation after correction of tetralogy of Fallot (26). The increased RV myocardial mass observed in this study indicates that RV hypertrophy may persist despite successful repair.

The diastolic filling of a ventricle is a complicated process that depends on atrial pressure, ventricular pressure, myocardial compliance, myocardial relaxation, and other factors, and abnormalities of diastolic filling may precede systolic dysfunction (34). In patients with tetralogy of Fallot,

the importance of RV diastolic function has been well established (35), and diastolic function can be assessed by analyzing the flow characteristics of the atrioventricular valves with Doppler echocardiography (36) or phase-contrast MRI (37). However, in the presence of pulmonary regurgitation, diastolic filling of the RV cannot be assessed adequately by examination of the tricuspid valve flow alone. Phase-contrast MRI of both the tricuspid valve and pulmonary valve provides information on the diastolic filling pattern of the RV in the presence of pulmonary regurgitation and allows the construction of an RV time–volume curve (38). The RV time–volume curve of patients with corrected tetralogy of Fallot and pulmonary regurgitation has been used to demonstrate impaired relaxation and restriction to filling as markers of abnormal RV diastolic function (38). In children, these abnormalities have been related to a diminished exercise capacity (38,39).

An indication for closure of a recurrent or residual VSD is a shunt ratio of flow through the pulmonary circulation (Q_p) to flow through the systemic circulation (Q_s) of more than 1.5:1, clinical symptoms, or an increased risk for endocarditis. Particularly in older patients, detection of a recurrent or residual VSD by transthoracic echocardiography may be difficult, and quantification of the left-to-right shunt may be not reliable. Gradient-echo MRI identifies a recurrent or residual VSD by displaying a signal void at the site of turbulent flow through the VSD. Turbulent flow causes dephasing of the protons within the jet, which results in a local loss of signal intensity observed as a signal void on gradient-echo MR images (Fig. 21.8 A,B).

In addition to its use in localizing a residual VSD, measurement of the ratio of Q_p to Q_s is important for other reasons, and the ratio can be assessed with both phase-contrast and gradient-echo MRI. The shunt volume can be derived by comparing either flow volumes through the ascending aorta and pulmonary artery (40,41) (Fig. 21.8C) or RV and LV stroke volumes (42). The accuracy of measuring left-to-right shunt volume by flow velocity MRI was recently confirmed in 50 pediatric patients with a mean age of 6.2 years (range, 1.1 to 17.7 years) (43).

Gadolinium-enhanced MRI is becoming an attractive technique to visualize the pulmonary vessels in an angiographic format (Fig. 21.1) and is currently performed with sedation in patients under 6 years old and with breath-holding in older patients (44). In a subset of patients before and after correction or palliation of a congenital heart defect, including tetralogy of Fallot, the diameter of the pulmonary artery was evaluated, and excellent correlation between gadolinium-enhanced MRA and conventional angiography was observed (44). Furthermore, the sensitivity (93%), specificity (96%), and overall accuracy (95%) of MRA in detecting pulmonary branch stenoses were excellent (44) (Fig. 21.9).

One of the major issues in the clinical management of pulmonary regurgitation and concomitant RV dysfunction

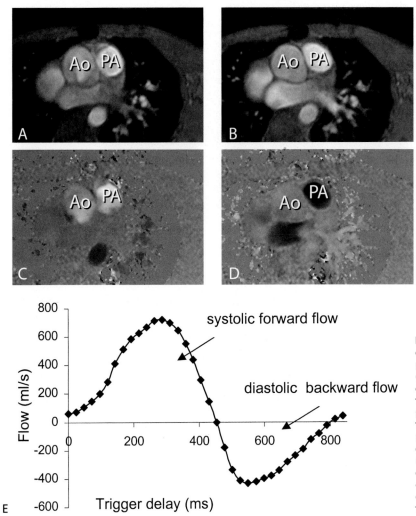

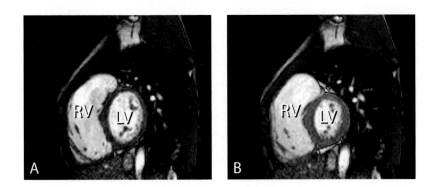

FIGURE 21.6. Gradient-echo **(A,B)** and phase-contrast **(C,D)** MR images perpendicular to the pulmonary artery *(PA)* obtained during systole (A,C) and diastole (B,D) from a patient with an incompetent pulmonary valve after correction of tetralogy of Fallot. The bright white signal in the pulmonary artery during systole represents systolic forward flow, whereas the black signal in the pulmonary artery during diastole is caused by regurgitant flow through the incompetent pulmonary valve. **E:** Graphic reproduction of one cardiac cycle of flow in the pulmonary artery obtained with phase-contrast MRI. The area under the curve provides quantification of regurgitant flow. *Ao,* ascending aorta.

after correction of tetralogy of Fallot is whether or not to replace the pulmonary valve and the timing of replacement (45). Several studies indicate improved cardiac function and exercise capacity after pulmonary valve replacement (46–48). In one study, MRI measurements of pulmonary regurgitation and biventricular function were performed before and 1 year after pulmonary valve replacement for pulmonary valve regurgitation after tetralogy of Fallot repair (47). Decreases in RV end-diastolic and end-systolic vol-

umes were observed after pulmonary valve replacement (47). Therrien et al. (45), however, observed no improvement in RV function after pulmonary valve replacement in patients with corrected tetralogy of Fallot, and the authors state that pulmonary valve implantation should be considered before RV function deteriorates.

The evaluation of pulmonary regurgitation and biventricular function in patients with corrected tetralogy of Fallot during exercise may reveal cardiac dysfunction that is not

FIGURE 21.7. Short-axis images at end-diastole **(A)** and end-systole **(B)** obtained with a balanced FFE (fast-field echo) MR sequence in a patient after correction of tetralogy of Fallot. Note the marked right ventricular *(RV)* dilation. *LV,* left ventricle.

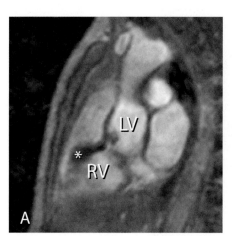
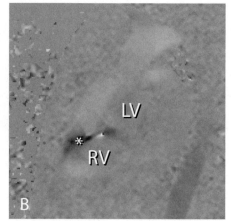

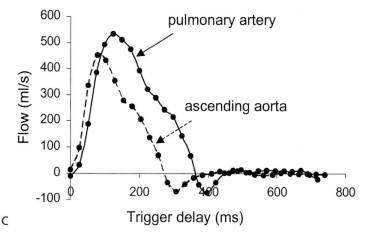

C

FIGURE 21.8. Gradient-echo **(A)** and phase-contrast **(B)** MR images of a ventricular septal defect. The black void *(*)* on the gradient-echo MR image (A) is caused by the dephasing of spins in the turbulent left-to-right shunt. The bright white pixels within the black shunt flow (B) indicate high velocities (>250 cm/s) through a restrictive ventricular septal defect. Flow volume measurements of the pulmonary artery and ascending aorta, obtained by phase-contrast MRI, can accurately quantify the amount of left-to-right shunt by subtraction of both volumes **(C)**. *LV,* left ventricle; *RV,* right ventricle. (From Roest AA, Helbing WA, van der Wall EE, de Roos A. Postoperative evaluation of congenital heart disease by magnetic resonance imaging. *J Magn Reson Imaging* 1999;10: 656–666, with permission.)

apparent at rest (49). However, the quantitative assessment of pulmonary regurgitation during exercise has not been possible so far. Furthermore, the noninvasive assessment of biventricular function at rest or during exercise is limited when radionuclide angiography (50) or echocardiography (2) is used.

The recent introduction of exercise MRI to evaluate the biventricular response to exercise (13) has made it possible to evaluate changes in pulmonary regurgitation and biven-

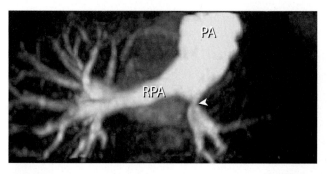

FIGURE 21.9. Three-dimensional gadolinium-enhanced MR angiogram from a patient with tetralogy of Fallot and a proximal stenosis of the left pulmonary artery *(arrowhead)*. *PA,* pulmonary artery; *RPA,* right pulmonary artery.

tricular volumes and function (51). In that study, the RV ejection fraction at rest was normal in 80% of the patients, who had undergone surgical repair at a mean age of 2.1 years. Exercise MRI, however, revealed an abnormal RV response to exercise in most of the patients with corrected tetralogy of Fallot. Furthermore, the RV end-diastolic volume increased with exercise, whereas the RV end-systolic volume did not change. This abnormal ventricular response to supine exercise is normally seen in older healthy subjects (52) and patients with ischemic heart disease (53).

These abnormalities are most likely related to long-standing volume overload and underline the importance of preventing pulmonary regurgitation at corrective surgery or implementing strategies to restore pulmonary valve competence early. Furthermore, exercise MRI may prove to be an important imaging tool in the timing of reintervention after correction of tetralogy of Fallot by detecting early RV dysfunction in these patients when they have normal resting RV function.

Transposition of the Great Arteries

Transposition of the great arteries, defined as a normal atrial situs, a normal (concordant) relation between atria and ven-

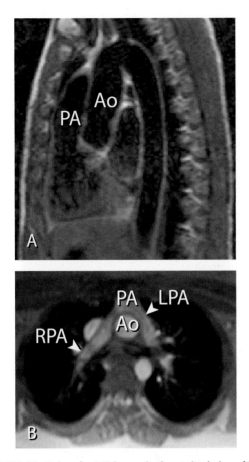

FIGURE 21.10. Spin-echo MR image in the sagittal plane **(A)** visualizes the typical anteroposterior position of the pulmonary artery *(PA)* relative to the ascending aorta *(Ao)*. Gradient-echo MR image in the transverse plane **(B)** shows the typical morphology of transposition of the great arteries after the arterial switch operation. *RPA*, right pulmonary artery; *LPA*, left pulmonary artery. (From Roest AA, Helbing WA, van der Wall EE, de Roos A. Postoperative evaluation of congenital heart disease by magnetic resonance imaging. *J Magn Reson Imaging* 1999;10:656–666, with permission.)

dure is the operation of choice in the large majority of centers because normal anatomic relations are restored (Fig. 21.10) and good intermediate (54) and long-term (55) results have been reported. The sequelae most frequently reported after the arterial switch operation are dilation of the aortic root (56), RV outflow tract obstruction, and central or peripheral stenosis of the pulmonary arteries (55). In a study of the Congenital Heart Surgeons Society, 2 years after the arterial switch operation, right-sided obstruction (both central and peripheral) occurred at a rate of 1% per year, and a risk-adjusted base incidence of 0.5% per year after reintervention for right-sided obstruction was observed (57).

Several reports have addressed the noninvasive assessment of pulmonary arterial stenosis after the arterial switch operation (58–60). MRI proved to be better than transthoracic echocardiography in detecting stenoses in the great vessels, especially in the branch pulmonary arteries (58–60). Information on specific hemodynamic changes in the great vessels after the arterial switch procedure can be obtained with cine MRI (61). With this technique, transient stenoses were observed, especially in the right pulmonary artery, that were caused by expansion of the ascending aorta during systole (61). Furthermore, the hemodynamic significance of pulmonary artery stenoses can be evaluated with MR velocity mapping. In patients who had undergone the arterial switch operation for transposition of the great arteries, good correlations were found between pressure gradients in the pulmonary arteries estimated with MRI and those obtained with Doppler echocardiography and cardiac catheterization (61). Gadolinium-enhanced MRI is also useful to evaluate the pulmonary arteries after surgical correction of transposition of the great arteries (44) and can detect pulmonary branch artery stenoses with excellent sensitivity and specificity (see preceding section on tetralogy of Fallot).

Before the arterial switch operation was introduced in 1975 (62), transposition of the great arteries was corrected at the atrial level; systemic venous blood was redirected from the superior and inferior venae cavae to the LV and pulmonary venous blood to the RV (Fig. 21.11) with the use of either artificial or pericardial tissue (Mustard technique) or atrial tissue (Senning technique). Although a

tricles, and an abnormal (discordant) ventriculoarterial junction, accounts for 4.5% of all congenital cardiac malformations (18). Because the pulmonary circulation is isolated from the systemic circulation, transposition of the great arteries is a life-threatening CHD requiring correction early in life. Currently, the Jatene or arterial switch proce-

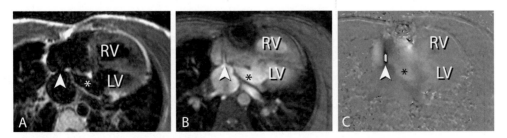

FIGURE 21.11. Spin-echo **(A)**, gradient-echo **(B)**, and phase-contrast **(C)** MR images in the transverse plane from a patient with a Mustard repair for transposition of the great arteries. A stenosis in the pulmonary venous conduit was observed *(arrowheads in A and B)* causing high-flow velocities during systole *(arrowhead in C)*. *LV*, left ventricle; *RV*, right ventricle; *, systemic venous conduit.

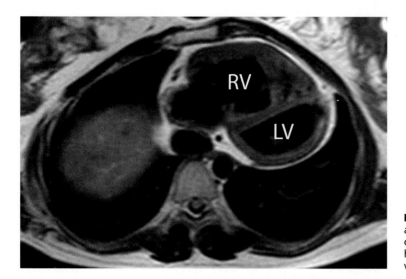

FIGURE 21.12. Transverse MR image of a patient after atrial correction of transposition of the great arteries obtained with black blood imaging. Note the marked hypertrophy of the systemic right ventricle *(RV)*. *LV,* left ventricle.

"physiologic" correct circulation is created, the normal anatomic relations are not restored, and the RV remains subject to systemic loading conditions, so that RV failure occurs in up to 10% of patients with an atrial redirection operation (63).

The systolic RV function of patients with an atrial redirection can be evaluated with gradient-echo MRI. Several studies observed an enlarged RV and depressed ejection fraction in these patients in comparisons with controls (37,64). In atrially corrected patients with arrhythmias, an observed significant increase in the ratio of right to left end-diastolic diameter, assessed with MRI, suggested RV enlargement (65). Furthermore, an observed correlation between RV end-diastolic dimension and maximum QRS duration on the electrocardiogram may have reflected a mechano-electric relation after atrial correction of transposition of the great arteries (65).

Gradient-echo MRI can also be used to measure ventricular wall mass. After atrial correction of transposition of the great arteries, a significantly increased RV wall mass and a decreased LV wall mass were observed in comparisons with normal subjects (64) (Fig. 21.12).

Diastolic dysfunction may precede systolic dysfunction of the RV (34), and therefore flow characteristics of the tricuspid valve, obtained by phase-contrast MRI, may reveal abnormal filling of the RV in patients after atrial redirection. In children 11 years after atrial repair, abnormal peak filling rates and a decreased atrial contribution to RV filling were observed, possibly related to reduced myocardial compliance of the hypertrophied RV (37).

Exercise MRI is another approach to detecting ventricular dysfunction, which may not be apparent at rest. Flow velocity MRI was used to evaluate the response of the stroke volume of the systemic ventricle to supine bicycle exercise and changes in stroke volume during recovery after exercise in patients who had undergone atrial correction of transposition of the great arteries (14). In that study, the increase in RV stroke volume in response to bicycle exercise was significantly smaller than that in controls (Fig. 21.13). Furthermore, the recovery of stroke volume was significantly pro-

Stroke volume recovery

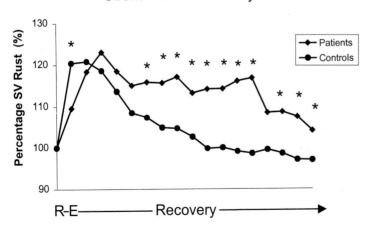

FIGURE 21.13. Stroke volume at rest, with exercise, and during recovery from exercise in patients with atrially corrected transposition of the great arteries and healthy subjects. The stroke volume of the patients shows a significantly smaller increase in response to exercise but remains significantly elevated for up to 8 minutes after exercise, whereas the stroke volume of the controls returns to resting level 4.5 minutes after exercise (*p* <.05). (From Roest AA, Kunz P, Helbing WA, et al. Prolonged cardiac recovery from exercise in asymptomatic adults late after atrial correction of transposition of the great arteries: evaluation with magnetic resonance flow mapping. *Am J Cardiol* 2001;88(9): 1011–1017, with permission.)

longed after exercise (Fig. 21.13) and returned to resting levels 8 minutes after exercise, whereas in the controls, the stroke volume returned to resting levels 4.5 minutes after exercise (14).

Besides RV failure, other postoperative complications can occur that are related to the pulmonary venous pathway, systemic venous pathway, and constructed baffle. Venous pathway obstruction and baffle leakage are frequently reported (63,66), and therefore noninvasive follow-up of these aspects is just as essential as the follow-up of ventricular function. MRI has proved to be a successful tool for this purpose (67–69). Turbulent flow patterns within the atria or ventricles, caused by stenosis of the venous pathways, leakage of the baffle, or incompetence of the atrioventricular valves, result in a signal void on gradient-echo MR images. The differentiation between stenosis, leakage, and valve incompetence on gradient-echo MRI images is based on the location of the signal void within the atria or ventricles (68) (Fig. 21.11).

Fontan Circulation

In 1971, Fontan and Baudet (70) introduced a surgical correction of tricuspid atresia. This type of operation has become the treatment of choice for a heterogeneous group of congenital cardiac malformations characterized by the presence of a single (functional) ventricle. The procedure is intended to establish a circulation in which the systemic venous return directly enters the pulmonary arteries. Different types of connections can be used, including total cavopulmonary connection, atriopulmonary connection, and atrioventricular pulmonary connection.

In patients who have undergone construction of a Fontan circulation, the dimensions of the right and left pulmonary arteries are expressed as a McGoon ratio, which is one of the most powerful risk factors for death or takedown of the Fontan operation (71). Therefore, in patients who are being considered for a Fontan circulation, visualization of the pulmonary arteries and pulmonic and systemic veins is of particular importance. Spin-echo MRI and gadolinium-enhanced MRA can visualize these structures with great accuracy; in the past, they could be assessed only by angiography (44,72,73).

The postsurgical management of patients with a Fontan circulation is concerned with evaluation of the Fontan circulation itself and the function of the single ventricle (74,75).

Because of their retrosternal location, the various connections used in the Fontan circulation are difficult to assess with transthoracic echocardiography and angiography. MRI makes it possible to visualize conduits and other selected structures in ways that are limited with the other imaging modalities (76). Spin-echo MRI has proved successful in detecting conduit obstruction later confirmed by angiography

and operation. In adult patients, a conduit diameter of less than 15 mm on spin-echo MRI suggests that a significant pressure gradient can be expected within the conduit, whereas a diameter of more then 20 mm is regarded as optimal (77).

Phase-contrast MRI can be used to provide information on flow patterns within the different types of Fontan connections (37,78,79). In patients with an atriopulmonary connection, a biphasic forward flow was observed in the pulmonary arteries, reflecting the expected venous flow pattern. In 50% of the patients with an atrioventricular connection, a systolic arterial flow pattern was found in the pulmonary arteries, which indicated that the RV was significantly sustaining pulmonary blood flow. In the other half of these patients, the contribution of the RV contraction seemed to be of minor importance because a venous biphasic flow pattern was observed (37). In patients with a total cavopulmonary connection, phase-contrast MRI indicated that shear stress in the pulmonary arteries was greater than in patients with an atriopulmonary connection and in healthy controls (79). However, when multidimensional phase-velocity MRI was used, Be'eri et al. (78) observed a more organized and uniform blood flow pattern in patients with a total cavopulmonary connection than in patients with an atriopulmonary pathway, and the authors speculated that a total cavopulmonary connection may result in a more hemodynamically efficient circulation than an atriopulmonary connection because of differences in pathway dimension and uniformity. Another method to evaluate flow in a Fontan circulation and the ascending aorta is MR blood tagging (80,81), which provides detailed information on flow pattern and velocity. Using a novel MRI sequence, including the application a presaturation pulse, Fogel et al. (82) observed that in Fontan patients with a total cavopulmonary connection, blood in the superior caval vein is directed toward the right pulmonary artery, and blood in the inferior caval vein is directed toward the left pulmonary artery.

The state of a functional single ventricle is important in presurgical planning because ventricular hypertrophy and abnormal wall motion negatively influence surgical outcome (83). Furthermore, ventricular function may deteriorate postoperatively with time and should therefore be carefully followed (84,85). Gradient-echo MRI is ideally suited to assess the complex morphology of a single (functional) ventricle and the ventricular function before and after construction of a Fontan circulation (86,87). Fogel et al. (85) successfully used gradient-echo MRI to assess ventricular dimensions, mass, and wall motion in 35 patients with a functional single ventricle both before and after complete Fontan surgery. Between 1 and 2 years after the Fontan operation, important changes in ventricular volume and wall motion were observed, and the ejection fraction was reduced in comparison with the preoperative data (85).

FUTURE APPLICATIONS

Future applications of MRI in the setting of CHD include new sequences, integration in algorithms for clinical decision making in corrected or palliated patients with CHD, and the emerging field of interventional MRI.

The new MRI techniques may provide more detailed information on cardiac function and increase our understanding of cardiac dysfunction in patients with CHD (88). Furthermore, ultrafast or real-time MRI makes it possible to assess dynamic processes, such as the cardiac response to exercise (89) and changes in cardiac function during recovery from exercise (14). The new MRI techniques may also help in the early detection of cardiac dysfunction, which is important in the management of patients with CHD.

Besides detecting abnormalities in individual patients with excellent sensitivity and specificity, MRI may play a role in clinical decision making in various groups of patients with CHD. For example, the timing of pulmonary valve replacement after total correction of tetralogy of Fallot is an important and still unresolved question (45,47). MRI performed during rest and exercise may play a key role in solving this complicated problem.

Interventional MRI is an exciting field, and the unique advantages of MR-guided therapy may be widely applicable in such forms of CHD as (re)coarctation of the aorta and pulmonary artery stenosis (90).

REFERENCES

1. Brickner ME, Hillis LD, Lange RA. Congenital heart disease in adults. First of two parts. *N Engl J Med* 2000;342:256–263.
2. Helbing WA, Bosch HG, Maliepaard C, et al. Comparison of echocardiographic methods with magnetic resonance imaging for assessment of right ventricular function in children. *Am J Cardiol* 1995;76:589–594.
3. Barkhausen J, Ruehm SG, Goyen M, et al. MR evaluation of ventricular function: true fast imaging with steady-state precession versus fast low-angle shot cine MR imaging: feasibility study. *Radiology* 2001;219:264–269.
4. Weiger M, Pruessmann KP, Leussler C, et al. Specific coil design for SENSE: a six-element cardiac array. *Magn Reson Med* 2001; 45:495–504.
5. Mohiaddin RH, Pennell DJ. MR blood flow measurement. Clinical application in the heart and circulation. *Cardiol Clin* 1998; 16:161–187.
6. Hirsch R, Kilner PJ, Connelly MS, et al. Diagnosis in adolescents and adults with congenital heart disease. Prospective assessment of individual and combined roles of magnetic resonance imaging and transesophageal echocardiography. *Circulation* 1994;90: 2937–2951.
7. Ho VB, Prince MR. Thoracic MR aortography: imaging techniques and strategies. *Radiographics* 1998;18:287–309.
8. de Roos A, Niezen RA, Lamb HJ, et al. MR of the heart under pharmacologic stress. *Cardiol Clin* 1998;16:247–265.
9. Lubiszewska B, Gosiewska E, Hoffman P, et al. Myocardial perfusion and function of the systemic right ventricle in patients after atrial switch procedure for complete transposition: long-term follow-up. *J Am Coll Cardiol* 2000;36:1365–1370.
10. Millane T, Bernard EJ, Jaeggi E, et al. Role of ischemia and infarction in late right ventricular dysfunction after atrial repair of transposition of the great arteries. *J Am Coll Cardiol* 2000;35: 1661–1668.
11. Niezen RA, Doornbos J, van der Wall EE, et al. Measurement of aortic and pulmonary flow with MRI at rest and during physical exercise. *J Comput Assist Tomogr* 1998;22:194–201.
12. Pedersen EM, Kozerke S, Ringgaard S, et al. Quantitative abdominal aortic flow measurements at controlled levels of ergometer exercise. *Magn Reson Imaging* 1999;17:489–494.
13. Roest AA, Kunz P, Lamb HJ, et al. Biventricular response to supine physical exercise in young adults assessed with ultrafast magnetic resonance imaging. *Am J Cardiol* 2001;87:601–605.
14. Roest AA, Kunz P, Helbing WA, et al. Prolonged cardiac recovery from exercise in asymptomatic adults late after atrial correction of transposition of the great arteries: evaluation with magnetic resonance flow mapping. *Am J Cardiol* 2001;88(9):1011–1017.
15. Goldberg DI, Shephard RJ. Stroke volume during recovery from upright bicycle exercise. *J Appl Physiol* 1980;48:833–837.
16. Imai K, Sato H, Hori M, et al. Vagally mediated heart rate recovery after exercise is accelerated in athletes but blunted in patients with chronic heart failure. *J Am Coll Cardiol* 1994;24: 1529–1535.
17. Kano H, Koike A, Yajima T, et al. Mechanism of overshoot in cardiac function during recovery from submaximal exercise in man. *Chest* 1999;116:868–873.
18. Hoffman JI. Incidence of congenital heart disease: I. Postnatal incidence. *Pediatr Cardiol* 1995;16:103–113.
19. Anderson RH, Tynan M. Tetralogy of Fallot—a centennial review. *Int J Cardiol* 1988;21:219–232.
20. Lillehei CW, Cohen M, Warden HE, et al. Direct vision intracardiac surgical correction of the tetralogy of Fallot, pentalogy of Fallot and pulmonary atresia defects: report of the first ten cases. *Ann Surg* 1955;142:418–445.
21. Van Arsdell GS, Maharaj GS, Tom J, et al. What is the optimal age for repair of tetralogy of Fallot? *Circulation* 2000;102: III123–III129.
22. Murphy JG, Gersh BJ, Mair DD, et al. Long-term outcome in patients undergoing surgical repair of tetralogy of Fallot [see Comments]. *N Engl J Med* 1993;329:593–599.
23. Gatzoulis MA, Balaji S, Webber SA, et al. Risk factors for arrhythmia and sudden cardiac death late after repair of tetralogy of Fallot: a multicentre study. *Lancet* 2000;356:975–981.
24. Bove EL, Byrum CJ, Thomas FD, et al. The influence of pulmonary insufficiency on ventricular function following repair of tetralogy of Fallot. Evaluation using radionuclide ventriculography. *J Thorac Cardiovasc Surg* 1983;85:691–696.
25. Waien SA, Liu PP, Ross BL, et al. Serial follow-up of adults with repaired tetralogy of Fallot. *J Am Coll Cardiol* 1992;20:295–300.
26. Niezen RA, Helbing WA, van der Wall EE, et al. Biventricular systolic function and mass studied with MR imaging in children with pulmonary regurgitation after repair for tetralogy of Fallot. *Radiology* 1996;201:135–140.
27. Gatzoulis MA, Till JA, Somerville J, et al. Mechanoelectrical interaction in tetralogy of Fallot. QRS prolongation relates to right ventricular size and predicts malignant ventricular arrhythmias and sudden death [see Comments]. *Circulation* 1995;92:231–237.
28. Rowe SA, Zahka KG, Manolio TA, et al. Lung function and pulmonary regurgitation limit exercise capacity in postoperative tetralogy of Fallot. *J Am Coll Cardiol* 1991;17:461–466.
29. Carvalho JS, Shinebourne EA, Busst C, et al. Exercise capacity after complete repair of tetralogy of Fallot: deleterious effects of residual pulmonary regurgitation. *Br Heart J* 1992;67:470–473.
30. Norgard G, Bjorkhaug A, Vik-Mo H. Effects of impaired lung

function and pulmonary regurgitation on maximal exercise capacity in patients with repaired tetralogy of Fallot. *Eur Heart J* 1992;13:1380–1386.

31. Kondo C, Nakazawa M, Kusakabe K, et al. Left ventricular dysfunction on exercise long-term after total repair of tetralogy of Fallot. *Circulation* 1995;92:II250–II255.

32. Duerinckx AJ, Wexler L, Banerjee A, et al. Postoperative evaluation of pulmonary arteries in congenital heart surgery by magnetic resonance imaging: comparison with echocardiography. *Am Heart J* 1994;128:1139–1146.

33. Rebergen SA, Chin JG, Ottenkamp J, et al. Pulmonary regurgitation in the late postoperative follow-up of tetralogy of Fallot. Volumetric quantitation by nuclear magnetic resonance velocity mapping. *Circulation* 1993;88:2257–2266.

34. Nishimura RA, Housmans PR, Hatle LK, et al. Assessment of diastolic function of the heart: background and current applications of Doppler echocardiography. Part I. Physiologic and pathophysiologic features. *Mayo Clin Proc* 1989;64:71–81.

35. Gatzoulis MA, Clark AL, Cullen S, et al. Right ventricular diastolic function 15 to 35 years after repair of tetralogy of Fallot. Restrictive physiology predicts superior exercise performance. *Circulation* 1995;91:1775–1781.

36. Nishimura RA, Abel MD, Hatle LK, et al. Assessment of diastolic function of the heart: background and current applications of Doppler echocardiography. Part II. Clinical studies. *Mayo Clin Proc* 1989;64:181–204.

37. Rebergen SA, Helbing WA, van der Wall EE, et al. MR velocity mapping of tricuspid flow in healthy children and in patients who have undergone Mustard or Senning repair. *Radiology* 1995;194:505–512.

38. Helbing WA, Niezen RA, Le Cessie S, et al. Right ventricular diastolic function in children with pulmonary regurgitation after repair of tetralogy of Fallot: volumetric evaluation by magnetic resonance velocity mapping. *J Am Coll Cardiol* 1996;28:1827–1835.

39. Singh GK, Greenberg SB, Yap YS, et al. Right ventricular function and exercise performance late after primary repair of tetralogy of Fallot with the transannular patch in infancy. *Am J Cardiol* 1998;81:1378–1382.

40. Brenner LD, Caputo GR, Mostbeck G, et al. Quantification of left to right atrial shunts with velocity-encoded cine nuclear magnetic resonance imaging. *J Am Coll Cardiol* 1992;20:1246–1250.

41. Rebergen SA, van der Wall EE, Helbing WA, et al. Quantification of pulmonary and systemic blood flow by magnetic resonance velocity mapping in the assessment of atrial-level shunts [see Comments]. *Int J Card Imaging* 1996;12:143–152.

42. Mohiaddin RH, Underwood R, Romeira L, et al. Comparison between cine magnetic resonance velocity mapping and first-pass radionuclide angiocardiography for quantitating intracardiac shunts. *Am J Cardiol* 1995;75:529–532.

43. Beerbaum P, Korperich H, Barth P, et al. Noninvasive quantification of left-to-right shunt in pediatric patients: phase-contrast cine magnetic resonance imaging compared with invasive oximetry. *Circulation* 2001;103:2476–2482.

44. Kondo C, Takada K, Yokoyama U, et al. Comparison of three-dimensional contrast-enhanced magnetic resonance angiography and axial radiographic angiography for diagnosing congenital stenoses in small pulmonary arteries. *Am J Cardiol* 2001;87:420–424.

45. Therrien J, Siu SC, McLaughlin PR, et al. Pulmonary valve replacement in adults late after repair of tetralogy of Fallot: are we operating too late? *J Am Coll Cardiol* 2000;36:1670–1675.

46. Bove EL, Kavey RE, Byrum CJ, et al. Improved right ventricular function following late pulmonary valve replacement for residual pulmonary insufficiency or stenosis. *J Thorac Cardiovasc Surg* 1985;90:50–55.

47. Hazekamp MG, Kurvers MM, Schoof PH, et al. Pulmonary valve insertion late after repair of Fallot's tetralogy. *Eur J Cardiothorac Surg* 2001;19:667–670.

48. Warner KG, Anderson JE, Fulton DR, et al. Restoration of the pulmonary valve reduces right ventricular volume overload after previous repair of tetralogy of Fallot. *Circulation* 1993;88:II189–II197.

49. Gibbons RJ, Lee KL, Cobb FR, et al. Ejection fraction response to exercise in patients with chest pain, coronary artery disease and normal resting ventricular function. *Circulation* 1982;66:643–648.

50. Beier J, Wellnhofer E, Oswald H, et al. Accuracy and precision of angiographic volumetry methods for left and right ventricle. *Int J Cardiol* 1996;53:179–188.

51. Roest AA, Helbing WA, Kunz P, et al. Exercise MR imaging in the assessment of pulmonary regurgitation and biventricular function in patients after tetralogy of Fallot repair. *Radiology* 2002;223(1):204–211.

52. Stratton JR, Levy WC, Cerqueira MD, et al. Cardiovascular responses to exercise. Effects of aging and exercise training in healthy men. *Circulation* 1994;89:1648–1655.

53. Newman GE, Rerych SK, Upton MT, et al. Comparison of electrocardiographic and left ventricular functional changes during exercise. *Circulation* 1980;62:1204–1211.

54. Kirklin JW, Blackstone EH, Tchervenkov CI, et al. Clinical outcomes after the arterial switch operation for transposition. Patient, support, procedural, and institutional risk factors. Congenital Heart Surgeons Society [see Comments]. *Circulation* 1992; 86:1501–1515.

55. Haas F, Wottke M, Poppert H, et al. Long-term survival and functional follow-up in patients after the arterial switch operation. *Ann Thorac Surg* 1999;68:1692–1697.

56. Hourihan M, Colan SD, Wernovsky G, et al. Growth of the aortic anastomosis, annulus, and root after the arterial switch procedure performed in infancy. *Circulation* 1993;88:615–620.

57. Williams WG, Quaegebeur JM, Kirklin JW, et al. Outflow obstruction after the arterial switch operation: a multiinstitutional study. Congenital Heart Surgeons Society. *J Thorac Cardiovasc Surg* 1997;114:975–987.

58. Beek FJ, Beekman RP, Dillon EH, et al. MRI of the pulmonary artery after arterial switch operation for transposition of the great arteries. *Pediatr Radiol* 1993;23:335–340.

59. Blakenberg F, Rhee J, Hardy C, et al. MRI vs. echocardiography in the evaluation of the Jatene procedure. *J Comput Assist Tomogr* 1994;18:749–754.

60. Hardy CE, Helton GJ, Kondo C, et al. Usefulness of magnetic resonance imaging for evaluating great-vessel anatomy after arterial switch operation for D-transposition of the great arteries. *Am Heart J* 1994;128:326–332.

61. Gutberlet M, Boeckel T, Hosten N, et al. Arterial switch procedure for D-transposition of the great arteries: quantitative midterm evaluation of hemodynamic changes with cine MR imaging and phase-shift velocity mapping—initial experience. *Radiology* 2000;214:467–475.

62. Jatene AD, Fontes VF, Paulista PP, et al. Anatomic correction of transposition of the great vessels. *J Thorac Cardiovasc Surg* 1975;72:364–370.

63. Williams WG, Trusler GA, Kirklin JW, et al. Early and late results of a protocol for simple transposition leading to an atrial switch (Mustard) repair. *J Thorac Cardiovasc Surg* 1988;95:717–726.

64. Lorenz CH, Walker ES, Graham TP Jr, et al. Right ventricular performance and mass by use of cine MRI late after atrial repair of transposition of the great arteries. *Circulation* 1995;92:233–239.

65. Gatzoulis MA, Walters J, McLaughlin PR, et al. Late arrhythmia

in adults with the Mustard procedure for transposition of great arteries: a surrogate marker for right ventricular dysfunction? *Heart* 2000;84:409–415.

66. Park SC, Neches WH, Mathews RA, et al. Hemodynamic function after the Mustard operation for transposition of the great arteries. *Am J Cardiol* 1983;51:1514–1519.

67. Rees S, Somerville J, Warnes C, et al. Comparison of magnetic resonance imaging with echocardiography and radionuclide angiography in assessing cardiac function and anatomy following Mustard's operation for transposition of the great arteries. *Am J Cardiol* 1988;61:1316–1322.

68. Sampson C, Kilner PJ, Hirsch R, et al. Venoatrial pathways after the Mustard operation for transposition of the great arteries: anatomic and functional MR imaging. *Radiology* 1994;193:211–217.

69. Theissen P, Kaemmerer H, Sechtem U, et al. Magnetic resonance imaging of cardiac function and morphology in patients with transposition of the great arteries following Mustard procedure. *Thorac Cardiovasc Surg* 1991;39(Suppl 3):221–224.

70. Fontan F, Baudet E. Surgical repair of tricuspid atresia. *Thorax* 1971;26:240–248.

71. Fontan F, Fernandez G, Costa F, et al. The size of the pulmonary arteries and the results of the Fontan operation. *J Thorac Cardiovasc Surg* 1989;98:711–719.

72. Fogel MA, Donofrio MT, Ramaciotti C, et al. Magnetic resonance and echocardiographic imaging of pulmonary artery size throughout stages of Fontan reconstruction. *Circulation* 1994;90:2927–2936.

73. Julsrud PR, Ehman RL, Hagler DJ, et al. Extracardiac vasculature in candidates for Fontan surgery: MR imaging. *Radiology* 1989;173:503–506.

74. DeLeon SY, Ilbawi MN, Idriss FS, et al. Fontan type operation for complex lesions. Surgical considerations to improve survival. *J Thorac Cardiovasc Surg* 1986;92:1029–1037.

75. Driscoll DJ, Offord KP, Feldt RH, et al. Five- to fifteen-year follow-up after Fontan operation. *Circulation* 1992;85:469–496.

76. Bornemeier RA, Weinberg PM, Fogel MA. Angiographic, echocardiographic, and three-dimensional magnetic resonance imaging of extracardiac conduits in congenital heart disease. *Am J Cardiol* 1996;78:713–717.

77. Sampson C, Martinez J, Rees S, et al. Evaluation of Fontan's operation by magnetic resonance imaging. *Am J Cardiol* 1990;65:819–821.

78. Be'eri E, Maier SE, Landzberg MJ, et al. *In vivo* evaluation of Fontan pathway flow dynamics by multidimensional phase-ve-

locity magnetic resonance imaging. *Circulation* 1998;98:2873–2882.

79. Morgan VL, Graham TP Jr, Roselli RJ, et al. Alterations in pulmonary artery flow patterns and shear stress determined with three-dimensional phase-contrast magnetic resonance imaging in Fontan patients. *J Thorac Cardiovasc Surg* 1998;116:294–304.

80. Fogel MA, Weinberg PM, Hoydu A, et al. The nature of flow in the systemic venous pathway measured by magnetic resonance blood tagging in patients having the Fontan operation. *J Thorac Cardiovasc Surg* 1997;114:1032–1041.

81. Fogel MA, Weinberg PM, Hoydu AK, et al. Effect of surgical reconstruction on flow profiles in the aorta using magnetic resonance blood tagging. *Ann Thorac Surg* 1997;63:1691–1700.

82. Fogel MA, Weinberg PM, Rychik J, et al. Caval contribution to flow in the branch pulmonary arteries of Fontan patients with a novel application of magnetic resonance presaturation pulse. *Circulation* 1999;99:1215–1221.

83. Akagi T, Benson LN, Green M, et al. Ventricular performance before and after Fontan repair for univentricular atrioventricular connection: angiographic and radionuclide assessment. *J Am Coll Cardiol* 1992;20:920–926.

84. Chin AJ, Franklin WH, Andrews BA, et al. Changes in ventricular geometry early after Fontan operation. *Ann Thorac Surg* 1993;56:1359–1365.

85. Fogel MA, Weinberg PM, Chin AJ, et al. Late ventricular geometry and performance changes of functional single ventricle throughout staged Fontan reconstruction assessed by magnetic resonance imaging. *J Am Coll Cardiol* 1996;28:212–221.

86. Fogel MA, Weinberg PM, Fellows KE, et al. Magnetic resonance imaging of constant total heart volume and center of mass in patients with functional single ventricle before and after staged Fontan procedure. *Am J Cardiol* 1993;72:1435–1443.

87. Altmann K, Shen Z, Boxt LM, et al. Comparison of three-dimensional echocardiographic assessment of volume, mass, and function in children with functionally single left ventricles with two-dimensional echocardiography and magnetic resonance imaging. *Am J Cardiol* 1997;80:1060–1065.

88. Fogel MA, Weinberg PM, Hubbard A, et al. Diastolic biomechanics in normal infants utilizing MRI tissue tagging. *Circulation* 2000;102:218–224.

89. Weiger M, Pruessmann KP, Boesiger P. Cardiac real-time imaging using SENSE. SENSitivity Encoding scheme. *Magn Reson Med* 2000;43:177–184.

90. Lardo AC. Real-time magnetic resonance imaging: diagnostic and interventional applications. *Pediatr Cardiol* 2000;21:80–98.

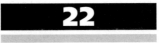

ADULT CONGENITAL HEART DISEASE

PHILIP J. KILNER

This chapter considers the uses of MRI and MRA in the assessment of adolescents and adults with congenital heart disease (CHD), an important group of patients whose numbers are increasing year by year, largely because of the success of surgical and catheter interventions. The effects of congenital disease, surgery, and acquired disease may combine to create varied and challenging pathology (1–5). Residual structural and functional abnormalities generally must be followed on a lifelong basis, preferably at a specialist referral center. Appropriate imaging facilities represent a key aspect of such a center. Cardiovascular MR can make outstanding contributions to the assessment of CHD in adults, in whom body size and the results of surgery tend limit echocardiographic access. The costs of imaging should be weighed against the potential costs of inappropriate management, which can entail complicated repeated surgery and extended hospitalization.

Imaging specialists need not be deterred by the anatomic variability found in these patients. Discussion with the CHD specialist can clarify questions to be answered, and the comprehensive anatomic coverage offered by MRI almost always provides useful diagnostic information. Variations of anatomy and function do, however, mean that decisions on cine imaging planes and sequences generally must be made during acquisition. It is not only anatomic structures that vary; surgical techniques have also evolved and changed. Operations for conditions such as transposition of the great arteries and "single"-ventricle heart have changed radically during the last few decades, and those investigating older patients need to be aware of both previous and current surgical practices. Certain people—technicians, radiologists, and cardiologists—should therefore take an interest and gain experience in the rewarding field of cardiovascular imaging. A number of reviews have been published (6–9), and information on the investigation and management of malformations has been put together by the Canadian Consensus Conference on Adult Congenital Heart Disease (10), conveniently accessible through the Web site of the Canadian Adult Congenital Heart Network.*

The diagnostic contributions of MRI, such as the evaluation of extracardiac vessels, tend to complement those of transesophageal echocardiography (11), which can be more effective than MRI for imaging thin, mobile intracardiac structures such as the atrial septum, components of valves, and the vegetations of endocarditis. Diagnostic catheterization is rarely needed, and interventional catheterization is expedited after MRI and transesophageal echocardiography, but adequate assessments of coronary artery stenoses or pulmonary vascular resistance still rely on invasive investigations.

Because many adults with CHD have a complex clinical history with multiple complementary investigations, collaborative presentation and discussion can be important, allowing a comprehensive picture to be built up that can clarify questions of clinical management and further the process of learning. At such meetings, MR images should be shown interactively by a computer linked to a projector, with programs for the display and interrogation of multislice, cine, velocity, and three-dimensional (3D) MRA acquisitions, although such programs may prove surprisingly difficult to implement. We use a program called *CMRTools* (Royal Brompton Hospital and Imperial College, London, United Kingdom) that is Digital Imaging and Communications in Medicine (DICOM)-compatible and runs on personal computers. The computer may also be used to display digitally stored catheter and echocardiographic studies, in addition to any prepared text on patient history.

P. J. Kilner: Royal Brompton and Harefield National Health Service Trust, London, United Kingdom.

*www.cachnet.org is a web link to the Canadian Adult Congenital Heart Network, with information on managing congenital heart defects.

Cardiovascular MR can provide functional as well as anatomic information, including the location and severity of stenoses (e.g., aortic coarctation or pulmonary artery stenosis), severity of regurgitation (e.g., pulmonary regurgitation), size and function of the heart chambers (the right as well as the left ventricle), and measurements of shunt flow. In adults with CHD, the underlying cardiac anatomy is likely to have been assessed previously. Although it is important to understand the descriptions, they should not necessarily be assumed to be correct and should be reviewed in the light of new information. The terminology used for malformed cardiovascular anatomy is described in Chapter 20, and further examples are shown in Figures 22.1 and 22.2.

TECHNIQUES

Multislice Imaging

Spin-echo imaging [echo time (TE) = 20 to 40 milliseconds] has been widely used for multislice acquisition. Struc-

tures of the chest are imaged in multiple parallel slices, and loss of the signal from flowing blood provides distinct contrast between blood and tissue (Fig. 22.1, *images left and center*). Contemporary cardiac-dedicated MRI systems allow alternative, faster approaches to multislice imaging. For example, in half-Fourier acquisition single-shot turbo spin-echo (HASTE) sequences, dark blood contrasts with tissue signal, as in conventional spin-echo imaging. True fast imaging with steady-state free precession (FISP), on the other hand, is a variant of gradient-echo imaging in which protons are repeatedly energized to achieve a steady state of magnetization. The technique depends on the rapid switching of magnetic gradients and the homogeneity of a well-shimmed magnetic field. Its advantages are speed of acquisition and contrast between bright blood and gray tissue that is relatively independent of blood flow velocity. Blood and other aqueous fluids, whether static or flowing, appear brighter than surrounding tissues (Fig. 22.2). The speed of acquisition allows clinically useful 2D images to be acquired at a speed of about 200 milliseconds per image following a

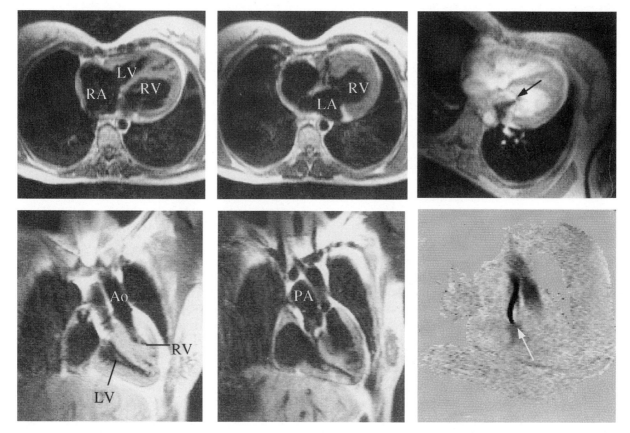

FIGURE 22.1. Unoperated congenitally corrected transposition of the great arteries with subpulmonary stenosis in an adult. Atrioventricular discordance can be identified in the transaxial spin-echo and cine images *(above).* Ventriculoarterial discordance is seen in the coronal images *(below).* The left-sided right ventricle has thick apical trabeculations. Gradient-echo cine imaging (echo time = 14 milliseconds) *(above right),* shows signal void from a jet of tricuspid regurgitation. Phase velocity mapping, vertically encoded *(below right),* shows the jet past the subpulmonary stenosis directed from the right-sided left ventricle to the pulmonary artery (peak velocity = 4.5 m/s). These are all non–breath-hold, cardiac-gated acquisitions obtained at 0.5 T. *LA,* left atrium; *RA,* right atrium; *LV,* left ventricle; *RV,* right ventricle; *PA,* pulmonary artery; *Ao,* aorta.

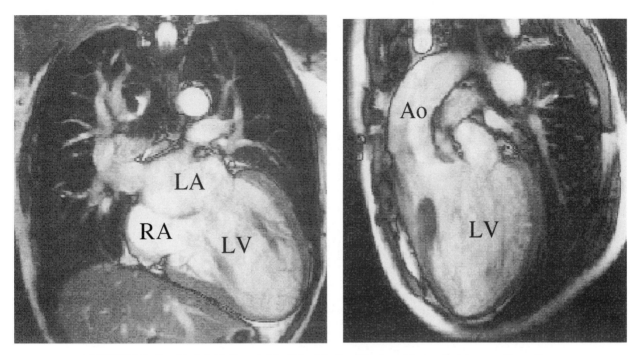

FIGURE 22.2. Double-inlet left ventricle *(LV)* with discordant ventriculoarterial connections, the aorta *(Ao)* arising anteriorly above a rudimentary right ventricular outlet chamber (unoperated), by cine true fast imaging with steady-state precession (FISP) acquired during 10-second breath-holds in a 1.5-T magnet. *LA,* left atrium; *RA,* right atrium.

preparatory excitation of about 200 milliseconds to achieve the steady state of magnetization. This means that adjacent slices can be acquired in consecutive heart beats, so that 20 or more slices can be acquired in a single breath-hold. Each image in a stack then represents the same cardiac phase, it is free from the blurring caused by respiratory motion, and the location of its structures can be used for accurate subsequent alignment of breath-hold cine acquisitions, provided that the chest and diaphragm are maintained in similar positions.

Cine Imaging

Gradient-echo sequences and their variants, which include fast low-angle shot (FLASH), FISP, and echo-planar imaging (EPI), allow short echo times and rapid repetition for cine imaging. Contemporary cardiac-dedicated systems allow high-quality cine images with 20 or more frames per cardiac cycle to be acquired in about 10 heart beats, or in real time on some systems. True FISP cine imaging provides good blood–tissue contrast and is well suited for imaging and measuring ventricular function and mass and for visualizing valve leaflets. However, sequences of this type with a short echo time (TE = 1.6 milliseconds) show less signal loss from turbulent jets than do gradient-echo acquisitions with longer TEs (Fig. 21.3). However, true FISP cine imaging can outline a coherent jet core, if present, because of the localized loss of signal from shear layers, and rapid acquisition makes it possible to interrogate a jet area precisely and

repeatedly. The approach of "cross-cutting"—locating an orthogonal slice though a partially visualized feature such as a valve orifice or jet—is an effective way of "homing in" on a jet with MRI (Fig. 22.4). Flow appearances depend on several aspects of sequence design and also on fluid dynamic factors. Turbulent flow results in a marked loss of signal in gradient-echo images with relatively long echo times (e.g., TE = 14 milliseconds), which can be useful for locating turbulent jet lesions.

Phase Velocity Mapping

Phase-shift velocity mapping, if correctly implemented, is an accurate and versatile means of visualizing and measuring flow (12–14). Its capacity for measuring flow at any location and in any direction through the heart and great vessels is unrivaled, and it can make valuable contributions to the assessment of adults with CHD. The recovery of signal from flowing blood is a prerequisite of velocity mapping, so that gradient-echo sequences, with the refinement of even-echo rephasing, are used with shorter TEs for higher-velocity flows. Phase-shift velocity mapping is based on the frequency changes experienced by nuclei moving relative to applied magnetic gradients (12). The direction, steepness, and timing of the applied gradients can be chosen, so that flows with a range of velocities, from low-velocity venous to high-velocity post-stenotic flows, can be measured accurately. Clinical uses include measurements of cardiac output (15), shunt flow (16), collateral flow (17), regurgitant flow (18),

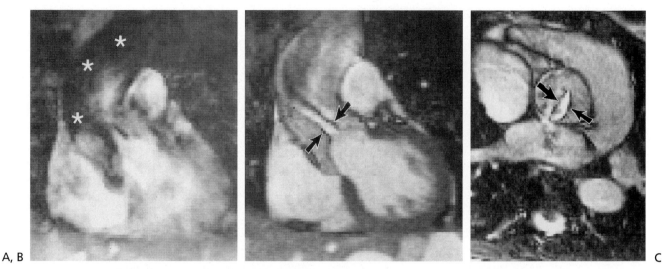

FIGURE 22.3. Systolic jet of moderate aortic stenosis shown by gradient-echo imaging (echo time = 14 milliseconds) **(A)** and true fast imaging with steady-state precession (FISP) (echo time = 1.6 milliseconds) **(B,C)** in the same coronal plane **(A,B)** and transecting the jet and aortic root **(C)**. *Asterisks* mark signal loss from turbulent flow. The *arrows* point to lines of signal loss caused by shear, outlining the jet core in the true FISP images.

and jet velocities through stenoses (14). However, for successful clinical application, the operator should have an understanding not only of the anatomy and pathophysiology of operated CHD, but also of the available technical choices for velocity mapping. It is necessary to select a plane, TE, velocity-encoding direction, and sensitivity appropriate for a particular investigation.

Velocity can be encoded in directions that lie either in or through an image plane. The mapping of velocities through a plane transecting a vessel (velocity encoded in the direction of the slice-selection gradient) allows the measurement of flow volume. The cross-sectional area of the lumen and the mean axially directed velocity within that area are measured for each phase through the heart cy-

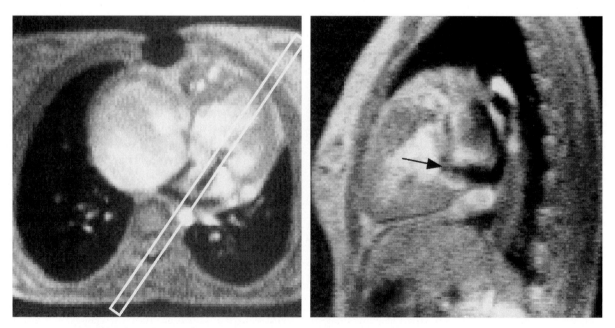

FIGURE 22.4. The jet of mitral regurgitation *(dark)* in a patient after Fontan operation for tricuspid atresia by gradient-echo imaging at 0.5 T (echo time = 14 milliseconds). The white grid *(left)* shows the location of an orthogonal cut providing an oblique sagittal image aligned with the regurgitant jet *(arrow, right)*.

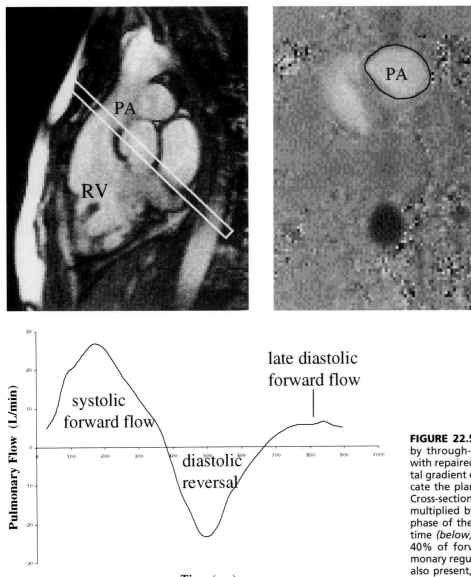

FIGURE 22.5. Pulmonary regurgitation measured by through-plane velocity mapping in a patient with repaired tetralogy of Fallot. The oblique sagittal gradient echo image *(above left)* was used to locate the plane for velocity mapping *(above right)*. Cross-sectional area of the pulmonary artery *(PA)* multiplied by mean velocity in that area for each phase of the cycle gives the curve of flow against time *(below)*; in this case, diastolic reverse flow is 40% of forward flow, which indicates free pulmonary regurgitation. Late-diastolic forward flow is also present, driven by rising pressure in the right side of the heart in this phase.

cle. From these data, a flow curve is plotted, and systolic forward flow and any diastolic reversed flow are computed by integration (Fig. 22.5). Such flow measurements are accurate only if phase shifts are caused by velocities and not by other factors, such as eddy currents in receiver coils, motion artifacts, and background noise. Appropriate sequences must be used and, if necessary, postprocessing to minimize artifacts.

To calculate shunt flow, both aortic and pulmonary artery flows are measured. Two separate acquisitions are generally needed, except in cases of transposition of the great arteries, in which the aorta and pulmonary trunk usually run almost parallel to each other. For aortic flow measurement, a suitable plane transects the aortic root at the level of the sinotubular junction, and for pulmonary flow measurement, a suitable plane transects the pulmonary trunk proximal to its bifurcation. Pulmonary regurgitation is common

after repair of tetralogy of Fallot, and in such cases, the repaired outflow tract and pulmonary trunk are tethered by scarring. However, if the mobility of the aortic and pulmonary valves is normal, especially in cases in which the root is dilated, the diastolic regurgitant flow can be significantly underestimated because of compliance and movement of the arterial root relative to the imaging plane. A potential solution to this problem is movement of the acquisition plane to follow valve movement through the heart cycle, "motion tracking."

Through-plane velocity mapping can be used to delineate an atrial septal defect (19) and measure the velocities and cross-sectional areas of jets through stenotic orifices (20). It can be helpful to map velocities in a plane aligned with the direction of flow, with velocity encoded in the read gradient direction, which must also be aligned with the direction of jet flow (21,14). This allows depiction of the jet

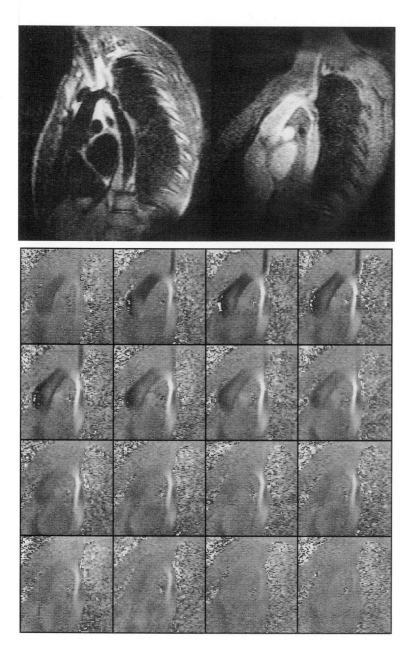

FIGURE 22.6. Aortic re-coarctation imaged by spin-echo *(above left)*, gradient-echo *(above right)*, and phase velocity mapping *(16 frames below)* (echo time = 3.6 milliseconds). The velocity maps show a narrow jet with prolongation of forward flow into diastole and a peak velocity of 3.5 m/s, indicative of significant re-coarctation.

in relation to upstream and downstream regions (Fig. 22.6). It is necessary, however, to locate the image plane correctly by cross-cutting (Fig. 22.4).

Jet velocity mapping can be particularly valuable for assessing stenoses in which ultrasonic access is limited, such as in aortic coarctation (native or repaired) (22), ventriculopulmonary conduits (23), pulmonary artery branch stenoses, and obstructions at the atrial or atriopulmonary level following a Mustard, Senning, or Fontan operation. When a jet is flat in cross section, either because its orifice is slitlike or it is attached to a surface, clearer images of the jet can be obtained with voxels parallel to the larger rather than the smaller diameter of the jet—that is, with the slice at a right angle to the plane of the flattened jet. In this orientation, the jet appears narrower and is more clearly delineated

than when the image plane coincides with the plane of the jet.

Three-Dimensional Angiography

Although 3D MRA by time-of-flight or phase-contrast techniques does not require the injection of a contrast agent, gadolinium-enhanced angiography combines fast acquisition with good resolution and allows one or more 3D angiographic data sets to be acquired in a single breath-hold. MRA is useful for depicting branches of the pulmonary artery and aorta and for assessing aortic coarctation or re-coarctation when a tortuous narrow segment or collateral vessels must be visualized. The presence of metallic stents, sternal wires, or arterial clips can cause a localized loss of signal in an angiogram and lead to a false impression of stenosis.

Measurement of Right Ventricular Function and Mass

Ventricular measurements have been described in greater detail elsewhere. In CHD, measurements of the right ventricle (RV) are at least as important as those of the left ventricle (LV), but they pose particular challenges (24,25). The RV cavity is crossed by coarse trabeculations, particularly near the apex. These become thickened and significant in summed volume when the RV is hypertrophied. But even if clearly visualized, trabeculations are difficult to outline individually because of their complex structure. Furthermore, the base of the RV tends to be more difficult to delineate that that of the LV. After repair of tetralogy of Fallot, the RV outflow tract can be dilated and dyskinetic and may have no effective pulmonary valve. All these factors can make it difficult to decide on the limits of the RV. In our unit, we count a dilated or aneurysmal outflow tract as part of the RV, so that the measurement of the ejection fraction is lower than measurements that exclude the noncontracting region. A particular unit or research protocol must establish reproducible methods for the measurement of RV function, which, despite difficulties, are likely to prove more reliable than those obtained by any other imaging modality.

Measurement of the RV mass is equally challenging. We adopt the approach of measuring the mass of the free wall of the RV only, attempting to include trabecular mass if the RV is hypertrophied but counting the septum as part of the mass of the LV (24 25).

APPLICATIONS OF MRI/MRA IN SPECIFIC DISEASES

Aortic Coarctation, Recoarctation, and Aneurysm

Aortic coarctation consists of narrowing or occlusion of the proximal descending thoracic aorta, in most cases just distal to the left subclavian artery branch, but occasionally proximal to it. The geometry of the aorta is highly variable in adults with aortic coarctation, especially after different types of repair. The risks associated with repaired aortic coarctation are related to systemic hypertension in the upper body, which may be exacerbated by any residual coarctation; rupture of an aneurysm or false aneurysm is also a risk. In this setting, a resting peak velocity of 3 m/s is significant, particularly if associated with a diastolic prolongation of forward flow (diastolic "tail"), which is a useful indicator of the obstructive significance of coarctation (Fig. 22.6).

When aortic coarctation is investigated in an adult (unoperated, balloon-dilated, or operated), a number of questions must be considered:

- Is blood pressure high in one or both arms?
- To what extent is it caused by obstruction resulting from coarctation?
- If operated, what type of surgery?
- Is diastolic prolongation of forward flow present?
- Do blood pressure and "gradient" rise markedly with exercise?
- Is associated aortic valve disease present?
- Is the LV hypertrophied?
- How extensive is the collateral flow?
- What is the location and severity of the coarctation?
- Of what type is it (e.g., membrane or narrow segment)?
- What is the geometry of the aorta and its branches in the vicinity of the coarctation?
- Is dissection, aneurysm, or false aneurysm present?

No single modality answers all questions, but MRI with cine imaging and velocity mapping can generally determine the nature and severity of coarctation (26–28) and identify any dissecting or false aneurysms (29). Gadolinium-enhanced MRA can provide additional information if a narrow, tortuous segment or collateral vessels must be visualized, but it may not reliably assess severity if the obstruction is caused by a relatively thin membrane; appropriately located cine imaging and velocity mapping are better for this purpose.

Post-stenotic dilation is common. It appears as fusiform dilation beyond a stenosed or previously stenosed region and is usually distinguishable by its location and smooth contours from more sinister aneurysmal dilation, which may require reoperation or protection with a lined stent. True or false aneurysms may complicate repairs, particularly those incorporating patches of noncompliant fabric, such as Dacron (Fig. 22.7). We recommend that patients with such patches be followed regularly with MRI examinations. Leakage of blood through a false aneurysm can lead to hemoptysis. In such cases, paraaortic hematoma is generally well visualized by MRI (30), appearing bright, usually with diffuse edges, on spin-echo images (Fig. 22.7). Postoperative hematoma is common, however, and sometimes leaves a region of signal adjacent to the aorta, which may be distinguished from a developing false aneurysm only if a comparison of images over time is possible. For this reason, it is worth acquiring baseline postoperative images in adults who have undergone repeated surgery for coarctation. Dissecting aneurysm can result from attempted balloon dilation (31,32). Repeated surgery for coarctation can be made difficult and complicated by the presence of adhesions and weakness of the aortic wall in the previously repaired region. It carries a considerably higher risk than the initial operation, so that the relative risks of operative or interventional approaches must be weighed against the expected risk of leaving an aneurysm or residual stenosis.

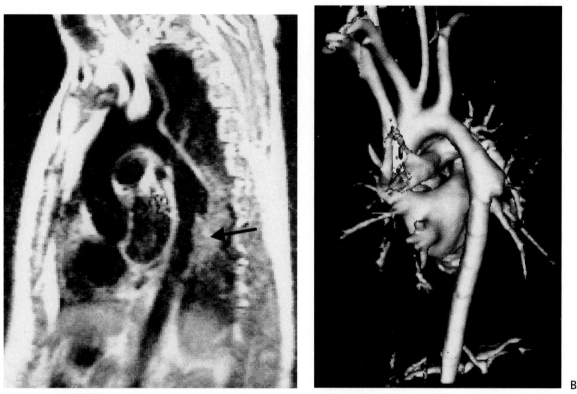

FIGURE 22.7. Aneurysm formation after Dacron patch repair of aortic coarctation. **A:** On the spin-echo image, signal from the hematoma of a leak or false aneurysm is indicated by an *arrow*. **B:** Surface rendering of a gadolinium-enhanced MR angiogram shows the location and shape of the true aneurysm.

Patent Ductus Arteriosus

Patent ductus arteriosus is identifiable by MRI if sought. Flow through a patent ductus arteriosus, usually directed anteriorly in the top of the left pulmonary artery close to the pulmonary artery bifurcation, is detectable on cine images, especially if a relatively long TE of 14 milliseconds is used to provide sensitivity to turbulence. Shunting can be assessed by measuring flow in the pulmonary trunk and aorta. Ascending aortic flow will be greater than pulmonary artery flow if duct flow is from the aorta to the pulmonary artery bifurcation. If true FISP imaging is used for multislice assessment of the anatomy, pericardial fluid in interstices above the pulmonary artery bifurcation can cause a spot of bright signal that can be mistaken for a patent ductus arteriosus unless cine imaging is also used.

Atrial and Ventricular Septal Defects

Although atrial septal defects (ASDs) and ventricular septal defects (VSDs) can often be assessed satisfactorily by echocardiography, MRI offers unrestricted access and makes it possible to determine shunt flow from the difference between measurements of flow in the pulmonary artery and aorta (33).

Right Ventricular Outflow Tract and Conduit Obstruction

The RV outflow tract and conduits from the RV to the pulmonary artery are rarely visualized adequately by ultrasonography, so MRI can make important contributions in this region (23). For cine imaging and in-plane velocity mapping, an oblique sagittal slice located with respect to transaxial scouts is usually suitable. In some cases, it is also helpful to orient the plane with respect to coronal scouts. It is important to identify the level of stenosis. The level of the pulmonary valve can usually be identified on cine imaging by visualizing the valve cusps as they close at the onset of diastole—for example, by the location of a regurgitant jet at the moment of valve closure. Obstruction may be subvalvar or supravalvar—for example, at the distal suture line of a homograft conduit. An important variant is double-chambered RV (34), in which the RV obstruction is subinfundibular, resulting from hypertrophied muscular ridges or bands beneath an infundibulum that is not hypertrophied and a pulmonary valve that is not stenosed (Fig. 22.8). This can be corrected by surgical resection without the need for incision or replacement of the pulmonary valve.

Repaired Tetralogy of Fallot

After repair of tetralogy of Fallot, particularly with a transannular patch, pulmonary regurgitation is common (35) (Fig. 22.5). It is generally well tolerated but can eventually lead to RV dilation and life-threatening arrhythmias. Stenosis of the right or left pulmonary artery may occur, particularly where a previous surgical shunt may have been closed, and pulmonary artery branch stenosis exacerbates the regurgitation. Interestingly, free pulmonary regurgitation is only about 40% (diastolic reversed flow as a percentage of forward flow) but may be made worse by the presence of branch stenoses (36). The long-term follow-up of patients with a repaired tetralogy of Fallot should include measurement of the pulmonary regurgitant fraction by through-plane velocity mapping, measurement of the RV volume and ejection fraction, visualization of the pulmonary arteries, and measurement of any aortic dilation.

Ebstein Anomaly

Ebstein anomaly is a malformation of the tricuspid valve, with displacement of the septal and posterolateral leaflets toward the apex from their usual position at the atrioventricular junction (37). This is associated with "atrialization" of part of the RV and varying degrees of tricuspid regurgitation. Depending on the severity of the malformation, the right atrium (RA) may become grossly enlarged. An ASD, VSD, tricuspid stenosis, or pulmonary stenosis may be present. In adults, MRI can be useful to assess the degree of RA dilation, the size and function of the RV, and the severity of tricuspid regurgitation. It can also demonstrate how partial compression by the distended right side of the heart may compromise LV filling in diastole. A four-chamber view should be acquired, aligned with the long axis of the LV and tilted down anteriorly to pass through the abnormal tricuspid orifice (Fig. 22.9). Cine imaging in additional planes through the tricuspid valve and RV outflow tract may be helpful when it must be decided whether the tricuspid valve can be repaired surgically. Although echocardiography may better define the valve leaflets, MRI has the advantage of providing wide fields of view across the enlarged volume of the heart.

Transposition of the Great Arteries

In complete transposition of the great arteries, the usual relations between the atria and ventricles are preserved, but the aorta and pulmonary artery are transposed with respect to the ventricles (Fig. 22.10). About two-thirds of such patients have no major additional malformations ("simple" transposition); the other third have associated abnormalities, such as a VSD and pulmonary or subpulmonary stenosis. Because unoperated simple transposition is not compatible with long-term survival, patients seen as adults are likely to have undergone surgery. The current surgical approach to simple transposition is usually to switch the great arteries with respect to the ventricles in the first years of life (Fig.

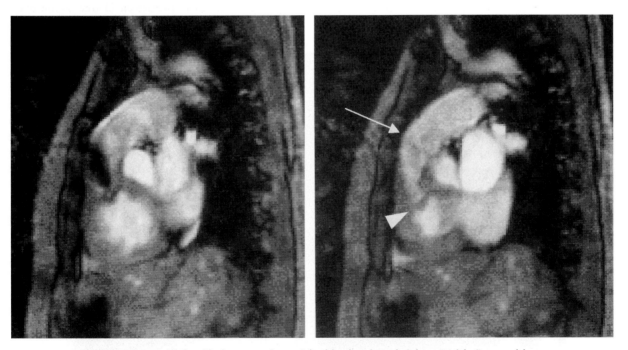

FIGURE 22.8. Subinfundibular stenosis, or "double-chambered right ventricle," caused by a subinfundibular muscle band *(arrowhead)*. The pulmonary valve is not stenosed *(white arrow)*. Systolic image *(left)* and diastolic image *(right)* by gradient-echo cine imaging (echo time = 14 milliseconds).

crease as its capabilities in the assessment of ischemic heart disease are developed and validated. As a result, systems very well suited to assessing adults with CHD will become more widely available. Advances that will increase the usefulness of cardiovascular MRI include greater speed and automation in the measurement of ventricular function and in the analysis and acquisition of data. Such measurements will be incorporated into databases on which decisions regarding reoperations or interventions can be based in a range of conditions.

Free-breathing acquisition has been replaced by more rapid breath-hold acquisition in recent years. However, we may see a trend back to free breathing for the acquisition of comprehensive data sets, with the integration of registration and adjustment for respiratory chest deformation into highly sophisticated sequences of acquisition/reconstruction.

Measurements of flow may become more inclusive, so that "comprehensive" flow data acquired within minutes will represent flow in any direction through the volume of the heart and great vessels. The term *comprehensive flow data* indicates the measurement of all three directional components of velocity for all voxels distributed throughout a 3D volume (47), with sufficient temporal resolution to repre-

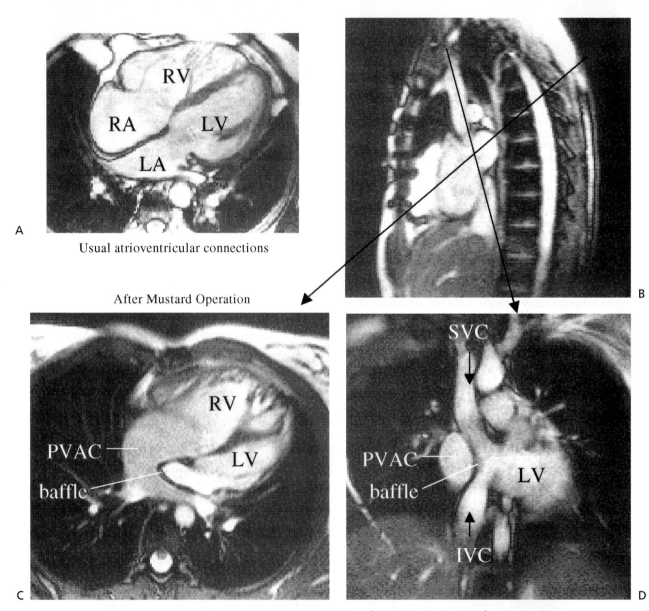

FIGURE 22.12. Surgically reconstructed atrial anatomy after Mustard operation for transposition of the great arteries **(B–D)** compared with the usual anatomy **(A)**. Lines across the sagittal image (B) show the location of the oblique transaxial (C) and oblique coronal (D) planes used to visualize reconstructed atrial pathways in this patient, who had a good result after the Mustard operation. Outflow tracts are as shown in the left panel of Figure 22.9. *PVAC*, pulmonary venous atrial compartment. *LV*, left ventricle; *RV*, right ventricle; *RA*, right atrium; *LA*, left atrium; *IVC*, inferior vena cava; *SVC*, superior vena cava.

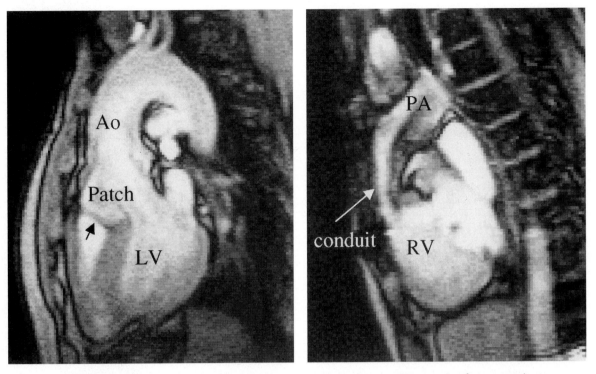

FIGURE 22.13. Reconstructed ventriculoarterial anatomy after Rastelli operation for transposition of the great arteries with ventricular septal defect and pulmonary stenosis. The patch *(black arrow)* is positioned to direct flow from the left ventricle to the aorta via the ventricular septal defect. The right ventricle-to-pulmonary artery conduit *(white arrow)* is located retrosternally. In this case, it is mildly narrowed, with a peak velocity of 2.8 m/s. The native pulmonary valve was closed at surgery. *Ao,* aorta, *LV,* left ventricle; *RV,* right ventricle; *PA,* pulmonary artery.

sent 20 or more phases through the cardiac cycle. Once this technology has been achieved, postprocessing for the visualization and analysis of flow will be a formidable challenge that is nonetheless well worth surmounting. Blood is virtually incompressible, so that once velocity acquisition becomes comprehensive, the laws of conservation of volume can be applied between adjacent voxels in a flow field and localized artifacts recognized and corrected. As a result, measurements of flow through parts of the flow field (e.g., veins, heart valves, arteries) should become more robust than when obtained by current methods that map only one component of velocity through a 2D plane. Furthermore, all major valves and vessels will be covered in a single acquisition. A large part of the challenge will lie in the identification, segmentation, and measurement of parts of the flow field during postprocessing. It is possible that postprocessing will eventually be automated, with valves or vessels recognized by their positions in respect to overall patterns of converging, swirling, and branching flows.

It is likely that effective 3D angiography within the chest will become possible without the need for contrast injection with the use of sequences that provide a high degree of spatial resolution and contrast between blood and tissue. Stress MRI and functional measurement may come into regular clinical use (48), as may assessments of perfusion of the

lungs and RV and LV myocardium. Furthermore, the MRI guidance of catheter-mounted interventional devices may become a clinical reality in adult CHD sooner than in pediatric or ischemic heart disease because the relevant structural lesions are relatively large.

SUMMARY

Cardiovascular MRI and MRA offer unrestricted access to structures throughout the chest, including the RV and great arteries. They therefore have very important contributions to make in the diagnosis and follow-up of adults with CHD. Examples of the principal applications have been provided. However, investigations can be costly and time-consuming in regard to both acquisition and analysis. These costs should be weighed against the potential expense of incomplete assessment and inappropriate management. Variations of underlying anatomy and surgical procedures between patients mean that planes and sequences must be selected during acquisition. It is therefore important for imaging specialists to gain experience in the growing subspeciality of adult CHD, and in this field, collaboration between specialists is essential. Acquisition and analysis are likely to become more rapid, automated, and comprehensive in the coming years.

REFERENCES

1. Somerville J. Congenital heart disease in adults and adolescents. *Br Heart J* 1986;56:395–397.
2. Somerville J. The physician's responsibilities: residua and sequelae. *J Am Coll Cardiol* 1991;18:325–327.
3. Perloff JK. Congenital heart disease in adults: a new cardiovascular subspeciality. *Circulation* 1991;84:1881–1890.
4. Warnes C. Establishing an adult congenital heart disease clinic. *Am J Card Imaging* 1995;9:11–14.
5. Moodie DS. Adult congenital heart disease. *Curr Opin Cardiol* 1995;10:92–98.
6. de Roos A, Rebergen SA, van der Wall EE. Congenital heart disease assessed with magnetic resonance techniques. In: Skorton DJ, Schelbert HR, Wolf GL, et al., eds. *Marcus' cardiac imaging: a companion to Braunwald's heart disease.* Philadelphia:W.B. Saunders, 1996:671–691.
7. Kilner PJ. Imaging of adults with congenital heart disease. In: Lima JAC, ed. *Diagnostic imaging in clinical cardiology.* London: Martin Dunitz, 1998.
8. Nienaber CA, Rehders TC, Fratz S. Detection and assessment of congenital heart disease by magnetic resonance techniques. *J Cardiovasc Magn Reson* 1999;1:169–184.
9. de Roos A, Roest AA. Evaluation of congenital heart disease by magnetic resonance imaging. *Eur Radiol* 2000;10:2–6.
10. Therrien J, Warnes C, Daliento L, et al. Canadian Cardiovascular Society Consensus Conference 2001 update: recommendations for the management of adults with congenital heart disease part III. *Can J Cardiol* 2001;17(11):1135–1158.
11. Hirsch R, Kilner PJ, Connelly MS, et al. Diagnosis in adolescents and adults with congenital heart disease. Prospective assessment of individual and combined roles of magnetic resonance imaging and transesophageal echocardiography. *Circulation* 1994;90: 2937–2951.
12. Firmin DN, Nayler GL, Kilner PJ, et al. The application of phase shifts in NMR for flow measurement. *Magn Reson Med* 1990; 14:230–241.
13. Mohiaddin RH, Longmore DB. Functional aspects of cardiovascular nuclear magnetic resonance imaging. Techniques and application. *Circulation* 1993;88:264–281.
14. Kilner PJ, Manzara CC, Mohiaddin RH, et al. Magnetic resonance jet velocity mapping in mitral and aortic valve stenosis. *Circulation* 1993;87:1239–1248.
15. Hundley WG, Li HF, Hillis LD, et al. Quantitation of cardiac output with velocity-encoded, phase-difference magnetic resonance imaging. *Am J Cardiol* 1995;75:1250–1255.
16. Hundley WG, Li HF, Lange RA, et al. Assessment of left-to-right intracardiac shunting by velocity-encoded, phase-difference magnetic resonance imaging: a comparison with oximetric and indicator dilution techniques. *Circulation* 1995;91:2955–2960.
17. Steffens JC, Bourne MW, Sakuma H, et al. Quantification of collateral blood flow in coarctation of the aorta by velocity encoded cine magnetic resonance imaging. *Circulation* 1994;90: 937–943.
18. Rebergen SA, Chin JGJ, Ottenkamp J, et al. Pulmonary regurgitation in the late postoperative follow-up of tetralogy of Fallot—volumetric quantitation by nuclear magnetic resonance velocity mapping. *Circulation* 1993;88:2257–2266.
19. Holmvang G, Palacios IF, Vlahakes GJ, et al. Imaging and sizing of atrial septal defects by magnetic resonance. *Circulation* 1995; 92:3473–3480.
20. Sondergard L, Stahlberg F, Thomsen C, et al. Accuracy and precision of MR velocity mapping in measurement of stenotic cross sectional area, flow rate and pressure gradient. *J Magn Reson Imaging* 1993;3:433–437.
21. Kilner PJ, Firmin DN, Rees RS, et al. Valve and great vessel stenosis: assessment with MR jet velocity mapping. *Radiology* 1991;178:229–235.
22. Kilner PJ, Shinohara T, Sampson C, et al. Repaired aortic coarctation in adults—MRI with velocity mapping shows distortions of anatomy and flow. *Cardiol Young* 1996;6:20–27.
23. Martinez JE, Mohiaddin RH, Kilner PJ, et al. Obstruction in extracardiac ventriculopulmonary conduits: value of nuclear magnetic resonance imaging with velocity mapping and Doppler echocardiography. *J Am Coll Cardiol* 1992;20:338–344.
24. Lorenz CH, Walker ES, Morgan VL, et al. Normal human right and left ventricular mass, systolic function, and gender differences by cine magnetic resonance imaging. *J Cardiovasc Magn Reson* 1999;1:7–21.
25. Lorenz CH, Walker ES, Graham TP Jr, et al. Right ventricular performance and mass by use of cine MRI late after atrial repair of transposition of the great arteries. *Circulation* 1995;92:233–239.
26. Kilner PJ, Shinohara T, Samson C, et al. Repaired aortic coarctation in adults—magnetic resonance imaging with velocity mapping shows distortions of anatomy and flow. *Cardiol Young* 1996;6:20–27.
27. Greenberg SB, Marks LA, Eshaghpour EE. Evaluation of magnetic resonance imaging in coarctation of the aorta: the importance of multiple imaging planes. *Pediatr Cardiol* 1997;18:345–349.
28. Riquelme C, Laissy JP, Menegazzo D, et al. MR imaging of coarctation of the aorta and its postoperative complications in adults: assessment with spin-echo and cine-MR imaging. *Magn Reson Imaging* 1999;17:37–46.
29. Therrien J, Thorne S, Wright A, et al. Repaired coarctation: a "cost effective" approach to identify complications in adults. *J Am Coll Cardiol* 2000;35:997–1002.
30. Lo SSS, Kilner PJ, Somerville J. Leaking aortic aneurysm after repair of aortic coarctation—the significance of MRI. *Cardiol Young* 1997;7:340–343.
31. Fawzy ME, von Sinner W, Rifai A, et al. Magnetic resonance imaging compared with angiography in the evaluation of intermediate-term result of coarctation balloon angioplasty. *Am Heart J* 1993;126:1380–1384.
32. Hamaoka K, Satou H, Sakata K, et al. Three-dimensional imaging of aortic aneurysm after balloon angioplasty for coarctation of the aorta. *Circulation* 1999;100:1673–1674.
33. Rebergen SA, van der Wall EE, Helbing WA, et al. Quantification of pulmonary and systemic blood flow by magnetic resonance velocity mapping in the assessment of atrial-level shunts [see Comments]. *Int J Card Imaging* 1996;12:143–152.
34. McElhinney DB, Chatterjee KM, Reddy VM. Double-chambered right ventricle presenting in adulthood. *Ann Thorac Surg* 2000;70:124–127.
35. Niezen RA, Helbing WA, van der Wall EE, et al. Biventricular systolic function and mass studied with MR imaging in children with pulmonary regurgitation after repair for tetralogy of Fallot. *Radiology* 1996;201:135–140.
36. Chaturvedi RR, Kilner PJ, White PA, et al. Increased airway pressure and simulated branch pulmonary artery stenosis increase pulmonary regurgitation after repair of tetralogy of Fallot: real-time analysis using a conductance catheter technique. *Circulation* 1997;3:643–649.
37. Giuliani ER, Fuster V, Brandenburg RO, et al. Ebstein's anomaly: the clinical features and natural history of Ebstein's anomaly of the tricuspid valve. *Mayo Clin Proc* 1979;54:163–173.
38. Beek FJ, Beekman RP, Dillon EH, et al. MRI of the pulmonary artery after arterial switch operation for transposition of the great arteries. *Pediatr Radiol* 1993;23:335–340.

39. Hardy CE, Helton GJ, Kondo C, et al. Usefulness of magnetic resonance imaging for evaluating great-vessel anatomy after arterial switch operation for D-transposition of the great arteries. *Am Heart J* 1994;128:326–332.
40. Gutberlet M, Boeckel T, Hosten N, et al. Arterial switch procedure for D-transposition of the great arteries: quantitative midterm evaluation of hemodynamic changes with cine MR imaging and phase-shift velocity mapping—initial experience. *Radiology* 2000;214:467–475.
41. Myridakis DJ, Ehlers KH, Engle MA. Late follow-up after venous switch operation (Mustard procedure) for simple and complex transposition of the great arteries. *Am J Cardiol* 1994;74:1030–1036.
42. Vouhe PR, Tamisier D, Leca F, et al. Transposition of the great arteries, ventricular septal defect and right ventricular outflow tract obstruction: Rastelli or Lecompte procedure? *J Thorac Cardiovasc Surg* 1992;103:4.
43. Girod DA, Fontan F, Deville C, et al. Long-term results after the Fontan operation for tricuspid atresia. *Circulation* 1987;75:605–610.
44. Rebergen SA, Ottenkamp J, Doornbos J, et al. Postoperative pulmonary flow dynamics after Fontan surgery: assessment with nuclear magnetic resonance velocity mapping. *J Am Coll Cardiol* 1993;21:123–131.
45. Fogel MA, Weinberg PM, Hoydu AK, et al. Effect of surgical reconstruction on flow profiles in the aorta using magnetic resonance blood tagging. *Ann Thorac Surg* 1997;63:1691–1700.
46. de Leval M, Kilner PJ, Gewillig M, et al. Total cavo-pulmonary connection: a logical alternative to atrio-pulmonary connection for complex Fontan patients. *J Thorac Cardiovasc Surg* 1988;96:682–695.
47. Firmin DN, Gatehouse PD, Konrad JP, et al. Rapid 7-dimensional imaging of pulsatile flow. *Comput Cardiol* 1993:353–356.
48. Pedersen EM, Kozerke S, Ringgaard S, et al. Quantitative abdominal aortic flow measurements at controlled levels of ergometer exercise. *Magn Reson Imaging* 1999;17:489–494.

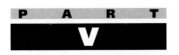

P A R T
V

VASCULAR DISEASES

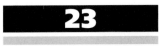

23

MRI AND MRA OF THORACIC AORTA

ROSSELLA FATTORI

In the past few years, considerable interest in aortic diseases has been shown in the medical literature. The prevalence of aortic disease appears to be increasing in the Western population, likely corresponding to aging of the population in addition to heightened clinical awareness. The continuous advances in our understanding of aortic pathology have been based on molecular and cellular studies elucidating the mechanisms of many pathologic conditions of the aorta and the complex interaction of this vessel with the cardiovascular system. However, increased clinical observations of aortic disease, demonstrated in epidemiologic studies, and a more appropriate definition of its pathologic substrate, reported in recent literature, may also reflect concurrent outstanding progress in imaging techniques. Among the imaging modalities, MRI offers the greatest versatility. With its ability to delineate the intrinsic contrast between blood flow and vessel walls and acquire images in multiple planes with a wide field of view, MRI provides a high degree of reliability in the diagnosis of aortic diseases, both acute and chronic. MRI is totally noninvasive and can be repeated, so that the progression of disease over time can be evaluated. Functional information can be obtained by gradient-echo sequences and phase mapping, which quantify blood flow volume and velocity, so that our knowledge of aortic function can be expanded. The new MRA techniques have enhanced the noninvasive evaluation of vascular pathology, providing a high degree of spatial and contrast resolution and in many instances making invasive x-ray angiography an obsolete procedure for the detection of aortic diseases. In addition, the ability to differentiate tissue structures at a power of resolution in the order of micrometers provides incomparable accuracy in the analysis of atherosclerotic plaque. At present, MRI microscopy, intravascular MRI,

and spectroscopy are emerging techniques that will be used to understand atherosclerotic disease and its contributing pathogenic mechanisms more clearly.

MRI TECHNIQUES

Spin-Echo MRI

Conventional spin-echo T1-weighted imaging provides the best anatomic detail of the tissue of the aortic wall and is still the basis of any aortic study (1,2). With the spin-echo technique, a presaturation pulse is used to null the signal of the blood pool. The "signal void" produced by flowing blood throughout most of the cardiac cycle provides a natural contrast between the lumen and the layers of the vessel wall. Electrocardiographic (ECG) triggering is essential to minimize motion and pulsatility artifacts. An echo time (TE) of 20 to 30 milliseconds is standard, and the repetition time (TR) is determined from the R-R' interval of the ECG. Slices thickness of 3 to 8 mm and high-resolution parameters (matrix size and signal average) ensure a detailed definition of the morphology of the aorta and surrounding structures. T1-weighted ECG-gated spin-echo images reveal the anatomic details of the aortic wall and pathologic conditions, such as atheromatous plaque, intimal flaps, and intramural hemorrhage (Fig. 23.1). In spin-echo imaging, each section corresponds to a different cardiac phase. Diastolic slow flow and entry or exit slice phenomena may produce high signal intensity in the aortic lumen that can mask underlying luminal pathology or erroneously simulate mural plaque or thrombosis. A shorter acquisition time can be achieved with fast spin-echo pulse sequences. In a fast spin-echo sequence, a long train of echoes is acquired by using a series of 180-degree radiofrequency (RF) pulses; as a result, washout effects are even more substantial than those obtained with conventional spin-echo techniques. A superior black blood effect is achieved by using preparatory pulses

R. Fattori: Cardiovascular Unit, Department of Radiology, S. Orsola University Hospital, Bologna, Italy.

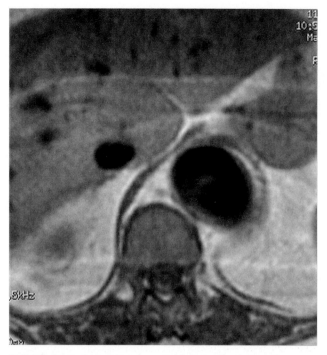

FIGURE 23.1. Fast spin-echo axial image of a large atheromatous plaque protruding into the lumen of the descending aorta.

(3). Preparatory pulses such as presaturation, dephasing gradients, and preinversion pulses involve the application of one or more additional RF pulses outside the plane to suppress the signal intensity of in-flowing blood and nullify the blood signal. The replacement of conventional spin-echo sequences with fast spin-echo sequences has resulted in substantial savings of time and improvements in image quality. Conventional T2-weighted spin-echo sequences are of little utility in the study of the thoracic aorta. Because of the low signal-to-noise ratio and long acquisition time, image quality is affected, mainly by motion artifacts. On the contrary, with fast spin-echo techniques, it is possible to obtain high-resolution T2-weighted images that provide a further option for evaluating the aortic wall. With a short acquisition time, respiratory motion can be suppressed by means of a breath-hold technique.

Usually, a conventional study of the thoracic aorta is first acquired in the axial plane (Table 23.1) for a display of the orientation of the great arteries and the optimal visualization of mural lesions perpendicular to their long axes. Images in additional planes, depending on the anatomy and diagnostic problems, are then acquired; for example, the oblique sagittal view shows the entire extent of the thoracic aorta and the supraaortic vessels in a single image. Fast spin-echo sequences allow the acquisition of high-quality T2 images, useful in tissue characterization of the aortic wall and blood components.

TABLE 23.1. GENERAL STRATEGY OF MR STUDY OF THE THORACIC AORTA

Congenital anomalies (coarctation, aortic arch anomalies)		
Spin-echo MRI		*axial* (slice thickness 5–7mm)
		sagittal (coarctation)
		coronal (aortic arch anomalies)
GRE/flow mapping (coarctation)		
MRA		
Marfan syndrome		
Spin-echo MRI		*axial* (slice thickness 5–7 mm)
		sagittal (slice thickness 3–5 mm)
GRE/flow mapping		*axial, ascending aorta* (aortic distensibility)
Chronic aortic disease (aneurysm, postoperative)		
Spin-echo MRI		*sagittal* thoracic; slice thickness 3–7 mm)
		axial (region-of-interest; slice thickness 5–7 mm, black blood, high-resolution parameters)
MRA		(thoracic and abdominal)
Acute aortic disease		
Trauma	Spin-echo MRI	*sagittal* (slice thickness 3–5 mm)
	MRA	(thoracic)
Dissection	Spin-echo MRI	*axial* (slice thickness 7–10 mm)
		sagittal (slice thickness 3–5 mm)
	GRE/flow mapping	*coronal* (aortic valve, entry site)
	MRA	(thoracic and abdominal)

GRE, gradient-echo MRI.

Gradient-Echo MRI

Gradient-echo techniques provide dynamic and functional information, although with fewer details of the vessel wall. In gradient-echo imaging, data are acquired with monitoring of the ECG such that multiple images at the same slice are reconstructed to represent multiple phases of the cardiac cycle. The bright signal of the blood pool on gradient-echo images results from flow-related enhancement obtained by applying RF pulses to saturate a volume of tissue. With a short TR (20 to 40 milliseconds) and a low flip angle (30 to 40 degrees), maximal signal is emitted by blood flowing in the voxel. An ECG signal is acquired with the imaging data so that the images are reconstructed in the different phases of the cardiac cycle. Gradient-echo images are acquired with a high degree of temporal resolution throughout the cardiac cycle (8 to 16 frames per second) and can be displayed in cine format. Flow-related enhancement is produced by the inflow of unsaturated blood exposed to only one RF pulse. As result, the laminar moving blood displays bright signal in contrast to stationary tissues. Signal can be reduced if the rate of flow is low, as in aortic aneurysms. Mural thrombi can be identified by persistently low signal intensity in different phases of the cardiac cycle. Turbulent flow produces rapid spin dephasing and results in a signal void. This phenomenon makes it possible to detect anomalous turbulence, such as aortic or mitral insufficiency or jetlike communication between the true lumen and false lumen in aortic dissection. Despite the use of flow compensation, turbulent flow can also be observed in the normal aorta, especially on the inner wall of the aortic arch. Recently, high-performance gradient systems with even faster acquisition (TE, 2 to 3 milliseconds; TR, 4 to 8 milliseconds; flip angle, 20 degrees), have provided high-quality images of the entire aorta at 15 to 25 different levels in less than 10 minutes. Gradient-echo images can provide additional information in many pathologic conditions, such as coarctation, aortic valve insufficiency, and aortic aneurysm and dissection (4). Particularly in aortic dissection, the detection of entry and reentry sites is a special capability of functional MRI that can be helpful in planning both surgical and endovascular therapy.

Flow Mapping

Gradient-echo imaging permits the semiquantitative measurement of flow turbulence by sizing the signal void in the heart chambers and great vessels. However, various imaging parameters can influence this measurement and produce erroneous results. Accurate quantitative information on blood flow is obtained from modified gradient-echo sequences with parameter reconstruction from the phase rather than the amplitude of the MR signal, known as *flow mapping* or *velocity-encoded cine MRI* (5–7). Most of the MR methods of measuring flow velocity are based on the flow dependence of the MR signal. In each pixel of velocity images, the phase of the signal is related to the velocity component in the direction of a bipolar velocity phase-encoding gradient. In the phase image, the velocity of blood flow can be determined for any site of the vascular system. Flow velocity is calculated with a formula in which velocity is proportional to the change in phase angle of the protons in motion. MR maps of flow velocity are obtained two-dimensionally, which is particularly important in profiles of nonuniform flow, such as that in the great vessels. On phase images, the gray value of a pixel depends on velocity and direction with respect to the imaging plane. Signals below a defined range are considered noise and are eliminated by a subtraction process. Quantitative data on flow velocity and flow volume are obtained from the velocity maps through a region of interest. The mean blood flow is estimated by multiplying the spatial mean velocity and the cross-sectional area of the vessel.

MR velocity mapping has been validated both *in vivo* and *in vitro* as an accurate technique for detecting flow patterns. The accurate analysis of aortic elastic properties provides specific information on alterations in aortic wall structure. Vector mapping has been used to describe flow patterns in various physiologic conditions (e.g., patterns in the normal aorta as a function of age) and aortic diseases (e.g., Marfan syndrome, coarctation, hypertension, aneurysm, dissection) (8–10).

MRA

The "gold standard" for studying many manifestations of vascular disease, especially arterial occlusive disease, has long been catheter angiography, which is an invasive, costly, and potentially hazardous procedure. MRA may represent an alternative, noninvasive approach. A variety of MRA techniques, including various pulse sequences, methods of data acquisition, and postprocessing, have been developed (11).

Bright blood techniques, which constitute the basis of MRA, can be subcategorized as time-of-flight (TOF) and phase-contrast techniques. All bright blood MRA techniques rely on the visualization of flowing blood for luminal imaging of the vessel. The essence of MRA is the ability to portray blood vessels in a projective format, similar to that of conventional angiography, with the use of postprocessing methods such as the maximum intensity projection (MIP) algorithm. In an MIP algorithm, the brightest pixels along a user-defined direction are extracted to create a projection image. In the TOF method, flow signal is enhanced by inflow effects, whereas the background (stationary tissue) is saturated by the rapidly repeated application of RF pulses. To provide a flow signal before phase dispersion, the TE is kept very short (<10 milliseconds) and the 180-degree refocusing pulse is eliminated. Fresh blood flowing into the plane of imaging produces a bright signal on a dark background. Venous signal, which can confuse the arterial image, can be eliminated with presaturation pulses. The use of a segmented gradient-echo sequence with cardiac triggering is helpful to eliminate arterial pulsation artifacts. TOF images can be acquired in two-dimensional (2D) or three-dimensional (3D) fashion. Two-dimensional TOF imaging is very fast but its resolution is low, whereas high-resolution 3D images require 10 to 20 minutes of acquisition time. The advantages of both the 2D and 3D techniques are gained with a series of thin-slab 3D acquisitions. The sequential 3D [multiple overlapping thin-slab acquisition (MOTSA)] technique provides better flow enhancement than single-slab 3D techniques and causes less dephasing than 2D techniques. However, with sequential 2D or 3D acquisitions, even slight movements by the patient can generate discontinuities in the vessel contour.

The basis for phase-contrast MRA is that the flow of blood along a magnetic field gradient causes a shift in the phase of the MR signal. In this technique, information about flow direction and velocity is encoded in the image data set. With phase contrast, pairs of images are acquired that have different sensitivities to flow. These are then subtracted to cancel background signal, so that only signal from flowing blood is left. Phase-contrast MRA requires a determination of the range of velocities in the vessel of interest, and this information strongly affects image quality. In patients with aneurysm or dissection with nonlaminar, turbulent flow, this technique is often not effective.

The recent implementation of faster gradient systems has made possible the development of 3D contrast-enhanced MRA (12–18), in which bright blood images are not strictly dependent on blood flow. Gadolinium diethylenetriamine pentaacetic acid (Gd-DTPA) is infused during data acquisition. The technique relies on the T1-shortening effects of the contrast medium, and saturation problems with slow flow or turbulence-induced signal voids are avoided. During the short intravascular phase, the paramagnetic contrast agent provides signal in the arterial or venous system, enhancing the vessel-to-background contrast-to-noise ratio irrespective of flow patterns and velocity. Flow-induced artifacts are mostly eliminated. Pulsatility artifacts are minimized, even in the ascending aorta, and ECG gating is not required. Contrast-enhanced MR aortography is performed following the acquisition of axial localizer images to determine the maximum anterior and posterior extension of the thoracic and abdominal aorta and the left and right borders. If the main area of interest is limited to the thoracic aorta, a sagittal acquisition is advisable. The paramagnetic contrast agent (0.2 mmol/kg of body weight) is generally administered via an intravenous catheter placed in the antecubital vein. It is necessary to time the gadolinium bolus so that peak enhancement occurs during the middle of the MR acquisition. The flow rate should be adjusted to ensure that the contrast volume is injected in a period not exceeding the acquisition time. Imperfectly timed acquisitions can result in variable degrees of venous enhancement in the MR aortogram. Improved gradient systems allow a considerable reduction of the minimum TRs and TEs and the acquisition of complex 3D data

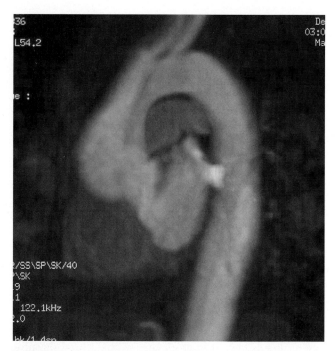

FIGURE 23.2. Gadolinium-enhanced MRA in a patient with type A dissection (maximum intensity projection algorithm). The intimal flap is visible in the ascending aorta.

sets within a breath-hold interval under 30 seconds. With the support of MIP images and 3D multiplanar re-formation, this technique delineates all the morphologic details of the aorta and its side branches in any plane in a 3D format (Figs. 23.2 and 23.3). Ultrafast 3D acquisition in conjunction with fast table feeds also makes it possible to chase the contrast bo-

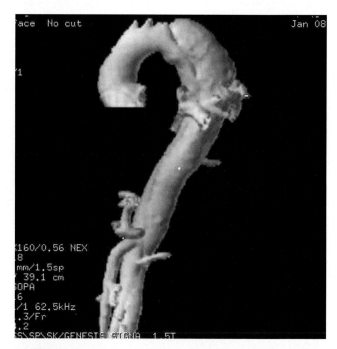

FIGURE 23.3. Gadolinium-enhanced MRA in a patient with type B dissection (surface-shaded display algorithm). The intimal flap is visible in the thoracic and abdominal aorta.

lus through several vascular districts. Because aortic aneurysm and dissection are mainly related to atherosclerotic vascular disease, a noninvasive concomitant assessment of the entire vascular system is advisable before surgical planning.

ACQUIRED DISEASES OF THE THORACIC AORTA

Aortic Dissection

Aortic dissection is characterized by a laceration of the aortic intima and inner layer of the aortic media that allows blood to course through a false lumen in the outer third of the media. Dissection can occur throughout the length of the aorta, and the two most common classifications are based on the anatomic location and extension of the intimal flap. According to the DeBakey classification, in type I dissection, the intimal tear originates in the ascending aorta and the intimal flap extends below the origin of the left subclavian artery; type II dissection is confined to the ascending aorta, and in type III dissection, the entry tear develops after the origin of the subclavian artery and extends distally. The Stanford classification simply classifies an aortic dissection, irrespective of the site of the entry tear, as type A if the ascending aorta is involved and as type B if the ascending aorta is spared. The Stanford classification is fundamentally based on prognostic factors; type A dissection requires urgent surgical repair, whereas most type B dissections can be successfully managed with medical therapy.

Acute aortic dissection is a life-threatening condition requiring prompt diagnosis and treatment (19). The 14-day period after onset has been designated as an acute phase because the rates of morbidity and mortality are highest during this period. The estimated mortality rate of untreated aortic dissection is 1% to 2% per hour in the first 24 hours after onset and 80% within 2 weeks. Early and accurate detection of the dissection and a delineation of its anatomic details are critical for successful management. However, because physical findings may be absent or misleading and symptoms may mimic those of other disorders, such as myocardial ischemia and stroke, the diagnosis of aortic dissection is often missed at the initial evaluation (20,21). The anatomic characteristics of the dissection indicate the type of surgical technique and affect both the surgical success rate and long-term results. Thus, in dissection, the diagnostic goal, regardless of the imaging modality used, is a clear delineation not only of the intimal flap and its extension but also of the entry and reentry sites, presence and degree of aortic insufficiency, and flow in the aortic branches (22). Transcatheter endovascular reconstruction of type B aortic dissection is a new option for the treatment of both acute and chronic dissection (23,24). In endovascular techniques, the success of the procedure is strictly related to a detailed anatomic definition of the features of the dissected aorta. The identification of the entry and reentry sites, the relationship between the true and false lumina and the visceral vessels, and any involvement of the iliac arteries is crucial in patient selection and design of the stent graft (Fig. 23.4).

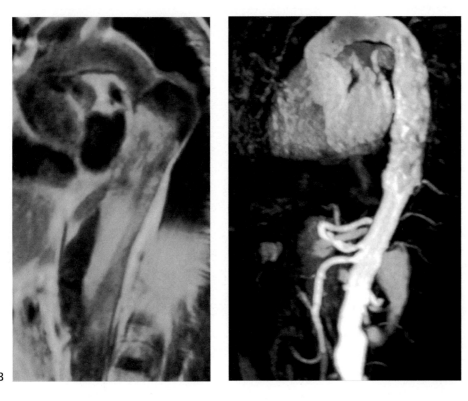

FIGURE 23.4. A: Spin-echo sagittal image of type B dissection; the double aortic lumen is 4 cm below the left subclavian artery. The false lumen (high signal intensity) is severely dilated. **B:** MRA of the same patient after placement of a stent graft reveals aortic remodeling with complete thrombosis of the false lumen. The metallic structure of the stent graft produces minimal artifacts in the upper portion of the descending aorta.

A,B

TABLE 23.2. MR STUDY MODALITY IN ACUTE AORTIC SYNDROMES

Sequence/Plane	Diagnostic Findings	Anatomic Details
Aortic dissection		
Spin-echo axial/sagittal	Intimal flap/true-false lumen	Periaortic hematoma Pericardial effusion
Gradient-echo axial/sagittal	Intimal flap/true-false lumen Aortic insufficiency	Thrombosis false lumen/entry and reentry sites
MRA	Intimal flap/true-false lumen	Origin/perfusion of supraaortic, coronary, abdominal vessels
Intramural hematoma		
Spin-echo axial/sagittal T1-weighted	Abnormal wall thickness, crescentic shape, high signal intensity (T1)	Periaortic hematoma Pericardial effusion
Spin-echo axial T2-weighted	High signal intensity (recent) Low signal intensity (old)	Pericardial, pleural, mediastinal effusion: increased signal intensity
MRA	No utility	
Penetrating aortic ulcer		
Spin-echo axial/sagittal	Crater-like outpouching/circumscribed dissection/intramural hemorrhage	Periaortic hematoma/pleural effusion Diffuse aortic wall atherosclerosis
Gradient-echo sagittal	No utility	
MRA	Crater-like outpouching/saccular pseudoaneurysm	Relationship with aortic arch or abdominal vessels

Standard MRI Technique

In a suspected case of aortic dissection, the standard examination should begin with spin-echo sequences acquired with high-resolution parameters and preparatory pulses to nullify the blood signal and obtain a better definition of the aortic wall structures (Table 23.2). In the axial plane, the intimal flap is detected as a straight linear image inside the aortic lumen. The true lumen can be differentiated from the false lumen by the anatomic features and flow pattern. The true lumen shows a signal void, whereas the false lumen has a higher signal intensity. In addition, the visualization of remnants of the dissected media as cobwebs adjacent to the outer wall of the lumen may help to identify the false lumen. The leakage of blood from the descending aorta into the periaortic space, which can appear with high signal intensity and result in a left-sided pleural effusion, is usually better visualized on axial images. A high signal intensity of a pericardial effusion indicates a bloody component and is considered a sign of impending rupture of the ascending aorta into the pericardial space. A detailed anatomic map must indicate the type and extension of the dissection and also distinguish the origin and perfusion of branch vessels (arch branches; celiac, superior mesenteric, and renal arteries; possibly coronary arteries) from the true and false channels. Therefore, a further spin-echo sequence in the sagittal plane should be performed to define the extension of the dissection in the thoracic and abdominal aorta and in the aortic arch branches (Fig. 23.5).

Adjunctive gradient-echo sequences or phase-contrast images can be instrumental in identifying aortic insufficiency and entry or reentry sites (Fig. 23.6) and in differentiating slow flow from thrombus in the false lumen (25,26). However, because the diagnosis of aortic dissection does not depend on functional gradient-echo images, these sequences should be reserved for clinically stable patients.

The third step in the diagnosis of an aortic dissection and the definition of its anatomic detail relies on the use of gadolinium-enhanced 3D MRA. Because 3D MRA is rapidly acquired without any need for ECG triggering, this technique may be used even in severely ill patients. Because it is not nephrotoxic and causes no other adverse effects, gadolinium can be used in patients with renal failure or low

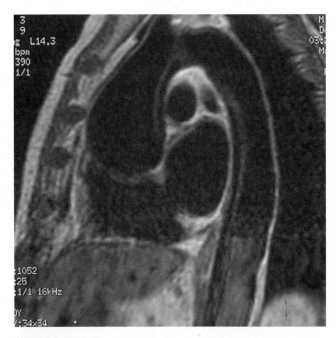

FIGURE 23.5. Spin-echo sagittal image of type A dissection. The intimal flap is visible as a subtle linear image in the ascending and descending aorta.

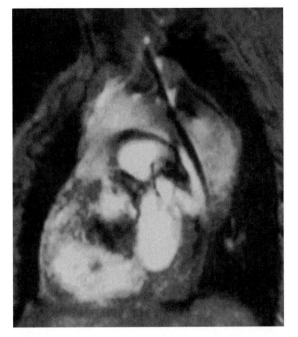

FIGURE 23.6. Gradient-echo sagittal image of type B dissection. Flow turbulence (signal void) in the descending aorta indicates the entry site.

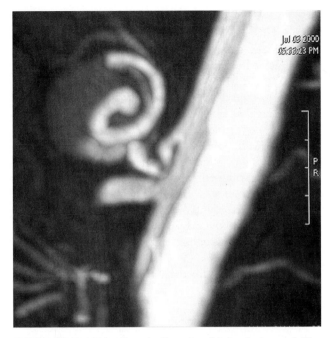

FIGURE 23.7. MRA of aortic dissection (abdominal aorta). The celiac and mesenteric arteries originate from the anterior true lumen.

cardiac output. With spin-echo sequences, artifacts caused by imperfect ECG gating, respiratory motion, or a slow blood pool can result in intraluminal signal simulating or obscuring an intimal flap. In gadolinium-enhanced 3D MRA, the intimal flap is easily detected and the relationship with aortic vessels clearly depicted (Fig. 23.7). Entry and reentry sites appear as a segmental interruption of the linear intimal flap on axial or sagittal images (Fig. 23.8). The analysis of MRA images should not be limited to viewing MIP images or surface-shaded displays; it should also include a complete evaluation of reformatted images in all three planes to confirm or improve spin-echo information and exclude artifacts. In MRA postprocessing displays, the appearance of the dissected aorta is similar to that on conventional catheter angiograms, but diagnostic information, such as the intimal flap, can be masked. Combining the spin-echo with the MRA images completes the diagnosis and anatomic definition (27). Two cases of intramural hematoma missed by MRA (18) should raise concern about using MRA as the sole modality for evaluating suspected aortic dissection.

Comparison with Other Imaging Modalities

At present, MRI is the most accurate tool for detecting aortic dissection. A high degree of spatial resolution and contrast and the capability for multiplanar acquisition provide excellent sensitivity and specificity, which approach 100% in published series (27–30). With modern scanners, a comprehensive study of the entire aorta can be completed in less than 10 minutes, and the patient's ECG, blood pressure,

and oxygen saturation can be monitored even during assisted ventilation. The implementation of open systems may soon allow a wider use of MRI, even in acute pathology.

Aortography has long been considered the method of choice in suspected aortic dissection, despite the risks associated with catheter manipulation and the injection of flow contrast in a dissected aorta. With the advent of noninvasive

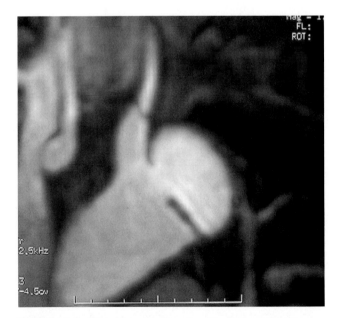

FIGURE 23.8. MRA of aortic dissection (thoracic aorta). The entry site is visible as a segmental interruption of the linear intimal flap.

imaging modalities, its low rate of accuracy has been demonstrated; the reported sensitivity is 77% to 90%, and the specificity is 90% to 100%. The superiority of transesophageal echocardiography (TEE), computed tomography (CT), and MRI in comparison with angiography has been widely reported in the literature (20–22,28).

In general, TEE is a reliable method that has excellent sensitivity, and a great advantage is that it can be performed at the bedside in patients too unstable to be moved. However, artifacts and "blind areas," such as the distal portion of the ascending aorta, can influence the specificity in an operator-dependent manner. Because the information provided by TEE is limited to the thoracic aorta, sometimes with an additional suboptimal display of the aortic arch, a second imaging modality encompassing the entire aorta is advisable in stable patients.

The role of CT in the diagnostic workup for aortic dissection is both difficult and crucial. According to the results of the International Registry of Acute Aortic Dissection (31), CT is the initial modality to confirm a clinically suspected aortic dissection in most cases because of its widespread availability. The accuracy of standard CT is moderate, particularly in the ascending aorta, because of respiratory and pulsation artifacts. Streak artifacts from the vena cava or pulsatility may also affect spiral CT and produce false-positive results. Furthermore, CT cannot provide information on aortic insufficiency and the location of entry sites, which is essential in planning the surgical strategy. The recent advent of multislice, ECG-gated, spiral CT represents a further important advance of CT technology in the study of cardiac and aortic disease, with potentially optimal characteristics in the evaluation of aortic dissection.

Intramural Hematoma

Intramural hematoma was first described in 1920 as "dissection without intimal tear" (32), but it was rarely recognized in the clinical setting before the advent of high-resolution imaging modalities. Spontaneous rupture of the vasa vasorum of the aortic media is considered the initiating process, which is confined to the aortic wall without intimal tear. This results in a circumferentially oriented blood-containing space seen on tomographic imaging studies. Intramural hematoma may occur spontaneously or as the consequence of a penetrating aortic ulcer in an intrinsically diseased media; it has also been described following blunt chest trauma (33). As in aortic dissection, arterial hypertension is the most frequent predisposing factor. The clinical signs and symptoms and the prognosis do not differ from those of classic aortic dissection, and intramural hematoma should be regarded as a variant of dissection with similar or more serious prognostic and therapeutic implications (34). Typical complications of dissection, such as fluid extravasation with pericardial, pleural, and periaortic hematoma, may also occur in intramural hematoma. In a retrospective

analysis of the Yale experience of 214 patients with acute aortic syndromes, Coady et al. (35) found a 47.1% rate of aortic rupture for intramural hematoma, higher than that for classic type A (7.5%) or type B (4.1%) dissection. However, after the acute phase, the evolution of intramural hematoma may also be favorable; in the series described by Yamada et al. (35A), 9 of 10 survivors of the initial presentation showed complete resolution of the aortic hematoma within 1 year.

Imaging Findings

The diagnosis of intramural hematoma relies on the visualization of intramural blood that is manifested as a locally thickened aortic wall. The abnormal wall thickness, symmetric or asymmetric, can vary from 3 mm to more than 1 cm. The mural involvement can encompass the entire aortic circumference. However, with all the imaging modalities, intramural hematoma can be confused with clot or plaque, especially if localized in the descending aorta. In particular with TEE, the differentiation of an intramural hematoma from an aortic atherosclerotic plaque may be difficult, and false-positive and false-negative results have been reported (36,37). The displacement of intimal calcification represents a useful marker for distinguishing intramural hematoma from mural thrombus or plaque on both TEE and CT. Intramural hematoma is best depicted on precontrast CT images as subtle areas that can be masked following contrast administration. A concentric area of high density around the aortic lumen with calcium dislodgment is the most characteristic feature on precontrast CT images.

In a comparison of the various imaging modalities, MRI demonstrated the best sensitivity for the detection of intramural hematoma (37). T1-weighted images reveal a crescent-shaped area of abnormal signal intensity within the aortic wall (Fig. 23.9). Moreover, MRI is the only imaging method that allows an assessment of the age of a hematoma on the basis of the different degradation products of hemoglobin. In the acute phase (0 to 7 days after the onset of symptoms) on T1-weighted spin-echo images, oxyhemoglobin shows intermediate signal intensity, whereas in the subacute phase (>8 days), methemoglobin shows high signal intensity. However, when the signal intensity is medium to low, it can be difficult to distinguish intramural hematoma from mural thrombus. T2-weighted spin-echo sequences may help in differentiating the two entities; signal intensity is high in recent hemorrhage but low in chronic thrombosis. In a retrospective study of 22 cases, Murray et al. (38) described three cases with recurrent symptoms and unfavorable evolution in which the MR signal intensity changed consistently with recurrent bleeding. The progression of intramural hematoma to overt dissection and rupture has been reported in 32% of cases, in particular cases with involvement of the ascending aorta (Fig. 23.10). Instability of the hematoma and recurrent bleeding, which can be

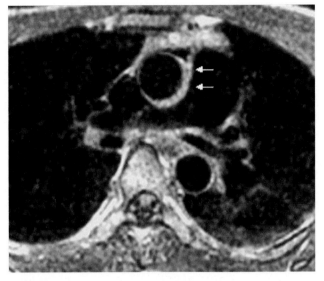

FIGURE 23.9. Spin-echo axial image of intramural hematoma of the ascending aorta. The abnormal wall thickening *(arrows)* exhibits high signal intensity (recent hematoma).

detected by MRI, are important parameters in assessing the need for surgical repair.

Aortic Ulcers

In 1934, Shennan (38A) was the first to describe penetrating atheromatous ulcers of the thoracic aorta. In elderly, hypertensive patients with severe atherosclerotic involvement of the aortic wall, usually in the descending aorta, a plaque may ulcerate into the media. Aortic ulcer is characterized by rupture of the atheromatous plaque and disruption of the internal elastic lamina. Extension of the ulcerated atheroma into the media may result in an intramural hematoma or lo-

calized intramedial dissection, or the plaque may break through to the adventitia and form a saccular pseudoaneurysm. The adventitia may also rupture, in which case only the surrounding mediastinal tissues contain the hematoma. Aortic ulcers occur almost exclusively in the descending aorta, but locations in the aortic arch and ascending aorta have occasionally been reported. The clinical features of penetrating atherosclerotic ulcers may be similar to those of aortic dissection, but the ulcers should be considered a distinct entity with a different management and prognosis. Hypertension, advanced age, and systemic atherosclerosis are common predisposing factors. Persistent pain, hemodynamic instability, and signs of expansion should trigger surgical treatment, whereas asymptomatic patients can be managed medically and monitored with imaging follow-up. Movsowitz et al. (39) analyzed 45 cases of aortic ulcers reported in the medical literature and found an incidence of transmural rupture of 8%. Different prognostic profiles were reported by Coady et al. (35); among 19 patients with a diagnosis of penetrating ulcer, the ulcers of 8 (42%) ruptured before surgical treatment. Because penetrating ulcer is much less common than classic dissection and imaging findings may be subtle, careful awareness of its insidious behavior is particularly important for successful management.

The MRI diagnosis of aortic ulcer is based on the visualization of a crater-like ulcer in the aortic wall (Fig. 23.11). Mural thickening with high or intermediate signal intensity on spin-echo sequences may indicate extension of the ulcer into the media and the formation of an intramural hematoma. MRA is particularly suitable for depicting aortic ulcers (Fig. 23.12), along with the irregular aortic wall profile seen in diffuse atherosclerotic involvement (40). The aortic ulcer is easily recognized as a contrast-filled outpouching of variable extent with jagged edges, which may

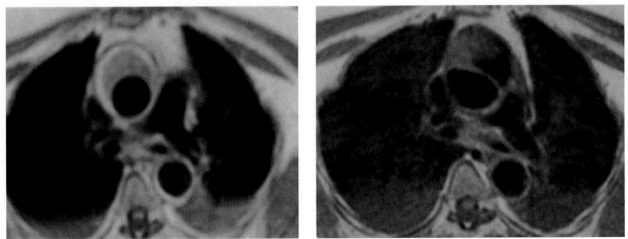

A   B

FIGURE 23.10. Spin-echo axial images of intramural hematoma evolving in classic dissection in the acute (A) and chronic (B) phases. **A:** The high signal intensity of hematoma is visible in the ascending and descending aorta. **B:** Three months later, the hematoma exhibits low signal intensity and a partial area of reabsorption; an intimal flap is visible.

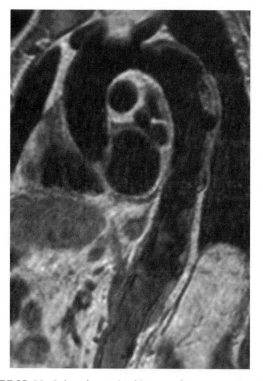

FIGURE 23.11. Spin-echo sagittal image of severe aortic atheromatous plaques and multiple penetrating ulcers of the descending aorta.

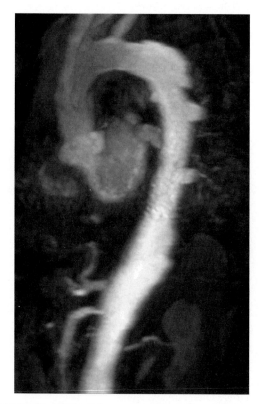

FIGURE 23.12. MRA of the same patient. The ulcers appear as contrast-filled outpouchings protruding from the vessel profile.

even form a large pseudoaneurysm (41). The disadvantage of MRI with respect to CT is its failure to visualize dislodgment of the intimal calcifications that are very frequently observed in aortic ulcers.

Postoperative Evaluation of Aortic Dissection

The objective of surgical treatment in aortic dissection is to prevent aortic rupture in the proximal portion of the ascending aorta. Early and accurate detection by new imaging modalities and an aggressive surgical approach have contributed to a decrease in operative mortality, from 40% to 50% in the 1970s to 5% to 7% in recent series (42,43). Nevertheless, survivors after initial repair remain at considerable risk for future complications. A persistent distal false lumen has been reported in 75% to 100% of cases. Second entry tears in the descending aorta or aortic arch, which are common, are responsible for patency of the distal dissection, which is associated with an unfavorable prognosis. It is recognized that dilation with subsequent rupture of the distal aorta is the most common cause of death in patients after surgery for aortic dissection. Prosthetic graft degeneration or infection (Fig. 23.13) and malfunction of the prosthetic aortic valves are additional causes of postoperative complications. Therefore, every patient who undergoes repair of an aortic dissection must be carefully monitored with imaging according to a strict schedule, and the timing is crucial. Heinemann et al. (44) suggest a first imaging session at discharge so that a relatively normal baseline postoperative image of the new anatomic situation is available. Afterward,

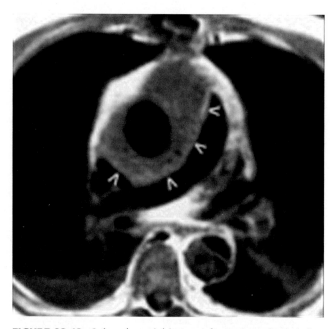

FIGURE 23.13. Spin-echo axial image of a periprosthetic infective collection *(arrows)* in a patient who underwent surgery for aortic dissection.

the subsequent examinations are scheduled on the basis of the absolute diameter (<5 cm, once per year; >5 cm, every 6 months) and expansion rate on two subsequent follow-up imaging sessions. Rupture is often preceded by a period of rapid aneurysm expansion, and detection of this phenomenon can identify patients at high risk for rupture, thereby decreasing the risk-to-benefit ratio of prophylactic surgical repair. The reported expansion rate for dissected segments ranges from 1.2 to 4.3 mm per year. However, a yearly expansion rate of 5.6 mm has been reported by Bonser et al. (45) in aneurysms with a diameter of more than 60 mm. The presence of partial thrombosis in the false lumen seems to protect against dilation; an aortic growth rate of 3.4 mm/y has been observed in dissection with partial thrombosis of the false lumen, versus an increase of 5.6 mm/y in dissection with no thrombosis of the false lumen (46). Therefore, in patients who have undergone surgery for aortic dissection, an appropriate imaging follow-up should take into account an accurate measurement of the residual aorta to identify high-risk patients early.

MRI is recognized as the imaging modality of choice in postoperative evaluation (47–50). MRI measurements of parameters are highly reproducible, and reproducibility is an essential component of serial examinations, in which minimal changes in dimension may represent a prognostic finding or indicate a need for preventive surgical strategies. Residual dissection is easily detected on spin-echo images, and gradient-echo sequences or phase-display images can be used to distinguish thrombosis of the false lumen from slow flow.

Slight thickening around the graft is a common finding that is caused by perigraft fibrosis (50,51). However, large or asymmetric thickening around the tube graft may represent a localized hematoma caused by an anastomotic leakage. Suture detachment with leakage has been reported in particular after composite graft replacement of the ascending aorta. Reoperation for bleeding at the site of repair has been reported after composite graft operation in 8% of patients after 30 days and 4% of patients after 1 year. A higher incidence of bleeding has been reported at the site of reimplanted coronary arteries. Gadolinium-enhanced MRI with standard spin-echo sequences can provide detailed information on suture detachment (52); the site of bleeding appears as high signal intensity within the hematoma. Moreover, gadolinium-enhanced MRA is particularly effective in depicting the complex postoperative anatomy and elucidating the prosthetic tube, distal and proximal anastomoses, and residual distal dissection and eventually dilated segments (Fig. 23.14). Reimplanted coronary arteries or reimplanted supraaortic vessels can also be visualized by MRA, and particular attention should be paid to evaluating these sites for possible postoperative weakness. Aneurysm of a reimplanted coronary ostium has been reported after composite graft replacement of the ascending aorta with the Bentall technique. In the Cabrol technique, intraoperative thrombosis or dis-

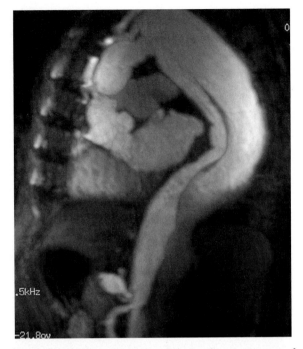

FIGURE 23.14. MRA of a patient who underwent surgery for type A dissection. The prosthetic tube is visible in the ascending aorta and aortic arch. Residual dissection is seen in the descending aorta with dilation of the false lumen.

tortion of the prosthetic limb connecting the right coronary artery to the main prosthetic tube may cause myocardial infarction. Contrast-enhanced MRA can visualize the proximal segment of a reimplanted coronary artery and detect and monitor proximal coronary aneurysms (Fig. 23.15).

Aortic Aneurysms

An aortic aneurysm is a localized or diffuse dilation involving all layers of the aortic wall and exceeding the expected aortic diameter by a factor of 1.5 or more. Aortic aneurysms are the 13th most common cause of death in United States. Because of the increasing age of the population and environmental factors, it is expected that aortic aneurysms will occur more frequently in the near future.

Thoracic Aneurysm

Between 1951 and 1980, the incidence of thoracic aortic aneurysm was estimated to be 3.5 cases per 100,000 person-years. Recently, a population-based study of thoracic and thoracoabdominal aortic aneurysm reported an incidence of 10.9 cases per 100,000 person-years, revealing an increased rate of occurrence of the disorder (53). This phenomenon is not completely explained; the complex multifactorial mechanism, which leads to an alteration of the media and the formation of an aneurysm, is still under investigation. Most aneurysms are atherosclerotic in nature, usually fusiform and long. Saccular false aneurysms may also develop in pa-

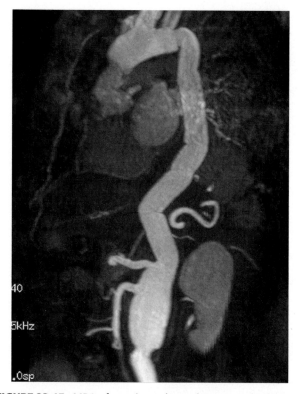

FIGURE 23.15. MRA of a patient who underwent multiple operations for type A dissection. In the ascending aorta, the origins of the reimplanted coronary arteries are well depicted. The right coronary artery is visible up to its distal portion.

tients with atherosclerosis who have penetrating ulcers. The natural history is quite diverse, reflecting a broad spectrum of underlying causes. Although many studies have identified risk factors related to the formation and progression of aortic aneurysms, none has fully explained the etiology of the disorder. Atherosclerosis is less commonly found in aneurysms of the ascending aorta than in those of the descending aorta. However, atherosclerosis should be considered a concomitant process and not a direct cause of aneurysm formation and growth. Aortic medial degeneration has been demonstrated in most aneurysms, regardless of their cause and location. The structural integrity of the adventitia is also lost as an aneurysm forms and expands. In the ascending aorta, gradual degenerative changes of the media can be related to congenital disorders of the extracellular matrix associated with an alteration of the elastic fibers, such as Marfan syndrome (Fig. 23.16). Moreover, families with a genetic predisposition to the development of thoracic and abdominal aneurysms, without evidence of collagen-vascular disease, have been documented.

The overall survival of patients with thoracic aortic aneurysms has improved significantly in the past few years. The estimated 5-year risk for rupture of a thoracic aneurysm with a diameter between 4 and 5.9 cm is 16%, but it rises to 31% for aneurysms with a diameter of 6 cm or more. Because the only well-documented risk factor for aortic rup-

ture is increasing size of an aneurysm, the major goal in the imaging evaluation of an aortic aneurysm is accurate measurement of its size (45).

MRI Findings

MRI is effective in identifying and characterizing thoracic and abdominal aortic aneurysms. Standard spin-echo sequences are helpful in evaluating alterations of the aortic wall and periaortic space. Periaortic hematoma and areas of high signal intensity within the thrombus may indicate instability of the aneurysm and are well depicted on spin-echo images. Atherosclerotic lesions are visualized as areas of increased thickness with high signal intensity and irregular profiles. Use of the sagittal plane allows assessment of the location and extent of an aneurysm and avoids partial volume effects. With fat suppression techniques, the outer wall of the aneurysm can be easily distinguished on MR images by the periadventitial fat tissue, so that the aneurysmal diameter can be accurately measured. The high level of reproducibility of MRI measurements ensures optimal reliability in monitoring the expansion rate (49). Gadolinium-enhanced T1-weighted MRI and MRA may play an important role in the preoperative evaluation. Contrast-enhanced 3D angiography can provide precise topographic information about the extent of an aneurysm and its relationship to the aortic branches (11,14,16,18). The homogeneous enhancement of flowing blood within the lumen facilitates the delineation of thrombus. Stenosis of the aortic branch arteries can be detected with a high rate of sensitivity, and x-ray angiography is not needed (54,55).

Postoperative neurologic deficit secondary to spinal cord ischemia is a serious and unpredictable complication of

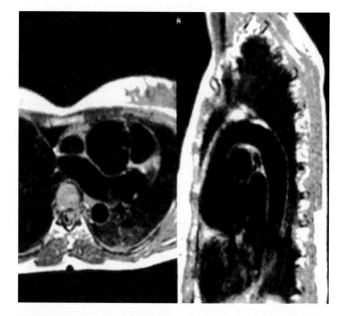

FIGURE 23.16. Spin-echo axial and sagittal images of the thoracic aorta of a patient with Marfan syndrome. The Valsalva sinuses are severely dilated.

surgery performed on the descending aorta. Because selective angiography of the spinal arteries is time-consuming, difficult, and potentially hazardous, preoperative evaluation of the artery of Adamkiewicz has been uncommon. The capability of contrast MRA to visualize the artery of Adamkiewicz reported in the literature represents an important advance in planning the surgical repair of a thoracic aneurysm (56).

Abdominal Aneurysm

The incidence of abdominal aneurysm is 3% in persons ages 50 years or more. As in thoracic aneurysm, atherosclerosis is considered the most common cause. A familial predisposition to the development of atherosclerotic aneurysms is under investigation. The causes are thought to be multifactorial, including genetic, environmental, and physiologic influences. The effects of normal aging, such as fragmentation of elastic fibers, decreases in the number of smooth-muscle cells, and alterations in collagen, are accelerated by hypertension and smoking. Since the initial studies in the 1960s, several trials have investigated the natural history of abdominal aortic aneurysms, and the results have been controversial. Large size is recognized as the major risk factor for aortic rupture and is the finding most relevant to the decision to intervene on a nonemergent basis. In a study of 300 patients by Guirguis and Barber (57), the 6-year cumulative incidence of rupture was 1% among patients with aneurysms smaller than 4.0 cm and 2% in patients with aneurysms 4.0 to 5.0 cm in size. For patients with aneurysms larger than 5.0 cm, the incidence of rupture was considerably higher, approaching 20%.

Abdominal aneurysms are usually monitored by ultrasonography or CT, both of which are accurate in depicting the dimensions of an aneurysm and its relationship to the renal or iliac arteries. However, the standard for preoperative evaluation has long been considered catheter angiography; it provides detailed information about the vessels of the abdomen and lower extremities, which are not always well defined even by spiral CT. The use of endovascular procedures to treat abdominal aneurysms has further increased the need for precise definition of these anatomic details, which is strictly related to procedural success (58). The distance of the aneurysm from the renal arteries, involvement of the iliac arteries, and angle of the aneurysm neck or iliac-femoral axis are crucial in planning an endovascular stent graft.

MRI Findings

MRI was ineffectively used in the evaluation of abdominal aneurysms before the recent advent of technical improvements. The implementation of inversion recovery fast spin-echo sequences has made possible T1-weighted breath-hold imaging with adequate suppression of the blood pool. Acquisition with this technique is rapid, so that ECG gating is unnecessary. The aortic wall, mural thrombus, and atheromatous plaques are well depicted in the axial plane, whereas the coronal plane allows definition of the diameter and longitudinal extent of an aneurysm. T1-weighted and T2-weighted spin-echo sequences are also effective in detecting inflammatory changes in the mural and periaortic space. Inflammatory abdominal aortic aneurysms are a variant of abdominal aneurysms characterized by a thickened aortic wall, periaortic fibrosis, and adhesion to local structures. This form is known to be associated with a higher rate operative mortality, and a specific operative technique is required. On spin-echo images, the periaortic cuff of an inflammatory aneurysm has intermediate signal intensity. After the intravenous administration of gadolinium, the periaortic cuff enhances significantly, so that intraluminal thrombus and the aortic wall are clearly defined, along with adjacent involved structures embedded in the inflammatory cuff. Gadolinium-enhanced MRA will eventually replace catheter angiography in the preoperative assessment of abdominal aortic aneurysms (59). The extent and morphology of the abdominal aorta are clearly depicted by 3D MRA. Postprocessing by surface rendering provides a 3D impression that can be helpful in planning surgical or endovascular therapy. Targeted coronal MIP images display the arterial anatomy and pathology of an aortic aneurysm and the abdominal vessels, so that vascular stenosis can be identified. Because the contrast agent is not nephrotoxic, contrast-enhanced MRA is the method of choice for detecting and monitoring abdominal aortic aneurysms.

Aortic Trauma

A traumatic aortic rupture is a lesion caused by trauma that extends from the intima to the adventitia. Trauma is the third leading cause of death in the United States and the leading cause of death in persons under the age of 40. Among lethal traumatic lesions, aortic rupture is secondary only to head trauma; one-fourth of the deaths resulting from motor vehicle accidents are associated with aortic rupture, which occurs in 8,000 victims per year in the United States. Air bags and seat belts do not protect against this type of injury, which can be expected to increase in the statistics on road traffic injuries; the frequency of lethal injuries in head-on collisions has been lowered by the mandatory use of restraints, which protect the victim from thoracic and head lesions but not from the mechanism producing aortic rupture. The aortic segment subjected to the greatest strain by rapid deceleration forces is just beyond the isthmus, where the relatively mobile thoracic aorta is joined by the ligamentum arteriosum. Aortic rupture occurs at this site 90% of the time in clinical series. In the ascending aorta, the segment close to the innominate artery or the proximal segment immediately superior to the aortic valve may be involved. Other less common locations of trauma are the distal segments of the descending aorta and the abdominal infrarenal segment. The lesion is transverse and involves all or part of the aortic circumference, penetrating the aortic layers to various degrees. Intimal hemorrhage without any laceration has been described in pathologic series but was not recognized in the clinical setting before the advent of high-resolution tomographic imaging modalities. When a laceration is present, it may extend through the media into the adventitia, with formation of a false aneurysm. Periaortic hemorrhage occurs irrespective of the type of lesion. Complete rupture causes immediate death in 85% of cases. If the aorta is not completely ruptured at the time of trauma, the continuity of the aortic wall is stabilized by the formation of a hematoma in the adventitia and surrounding structures. In such cases, effective intravenous therapy with vasodilators and beta blockers reduces aortic wall stress and the risk for rupture in the acute phase. Delayed surgery can be planned after other associated lesions have been treated (60). This type of management, reported in recent surgical series, has lowered the operative mortality to 0 to 10%, in comparison with the 20% to 50% mortality previously reported with emergency surgery.

Imaging Findings

Although the new surgical strategies are associated with low rates of spontaneous mortality in patients with traumatic aortic lesions observed in the clinical setting, traumatic aortic rupture must be considered a potentially evolving lesion. For this reason, a prompt and accurate diagnosis is necessary to initiate pharmacologic control of the arterial blood pressure and stratify the risk of delayed or emergency surgical repair. Chest x-ray is routinely performed in all victims of blunt thoracic trauma and plays an essential role in determining whether a traumatic aortic lesion should be suspected. On the basis of positive chest x-ray findings, several imaging modalities are currently available to confirm or exclude the presence of a lesion (61). Particularly in a patient with multiple trauma, aortography should be considered obsolete because its sensitivity is low, the information it provides is limited, and the approach is potentially dangerous. The choice of imaging strategy must take account of the patient's clinical condition. In cases of severe hemodynamic instability, TEE has the advantage that it can be performed at the bedside without interruption of resuscitative and therapeutic measures. In more stable patients, the ideal modalities are those that provide high-definition images of the aortic wall and information on the other organs and structures affected by the traumatic impact. With conventional CT, the detection of subtle aortic injuries is still a problem because a small intimal tear extending in the axial plane may be obscured by volume averaging with the normal aortic lumen. Spiral CT, with multiplanar reconstruction and better contrast enhancement, overcomes these limitations. Because it provides high-quality images with a drastic reduction of acquisition time and motion artifacts, spiral CT is a diagnostic method of great value. It is potentially the method

of first choice in the acute phase in the evaluation of patients with blunt chest trauma and suspected aortic injury, particularly patients with multiple lesions.

MRI Findings

A long examination time and difficult access to the patient have been considered the main limitations of MRI in acute aortic pathology. The development of fast MRI techniques have shortened the examination time to a few minutes, so that MRI can be used even in critically ill patients. The value of MRI in detecting traumatic aortic rupture in comparison with angiography and CT was reported in a series of 24 consecutive patients (62). The diagnostic accuracy of MRI was 100%, that of angiography was 84% (two false-negatives in two cases of limited partial lesion), and that of CT was 69% (two false-negatives and three false-positives). The potential of MRI to detect the hemorrhagic component of a lesion by its high signal intensity is beneficial in traumatized patients. On spin-echo images in the sagittal plane (Fig. 23.17), longitudinal visualization of the thoracic aorta makes it possible to distinguish a partial lesion (a tear limited to the anterior or posterior wall) from a lesion encompassing the entire aortic circumference. This discrimination is of prognostic significance because a circumferential lesion may be more likely to rupture (63). The presence of periadventitial hematoma and of pleural and mediastinal hemorrhagic effusion may also be considered a sign of instability (Fig. 23.18). In the same sequence

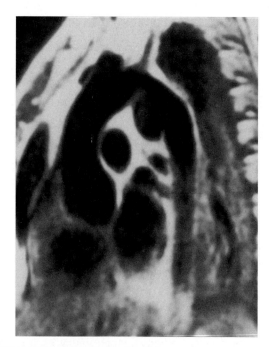

FIGURE 23.17. Spin-echo sagittal image of an acute traumatic aortic lesion. Partial laceration of the aortic wall results in a diverticular aneurysm.

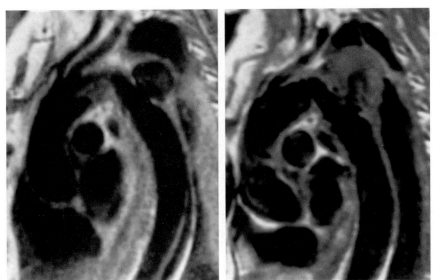

FIGURE 23.18. Spin-echo sagittal images of an unstable traumatic aortic lesion. **A:** Circumferential laceration with diverticular aneurysm and large periaortic hematoma. **B:** One week later, the diverticular aneurysm has enlarged.

used to evaluate the aortic lesion, without the need for any additional time, the wide field of view of MRI provides a comprehensive evaluation of chest trauma, such as lung contusion and edema, pleural effusion, and rib fractures. Furthermore, if delayed surgery is being considered, MRI can be used to monitor thoracic and aortic lesions because it is noninvasive and repeatable.

MRA provides an excellent display of the aortic lesion and its relationship with supraaortic vessels (Fig. 23.19). However, it does not add any diagnostic value to spin-echo

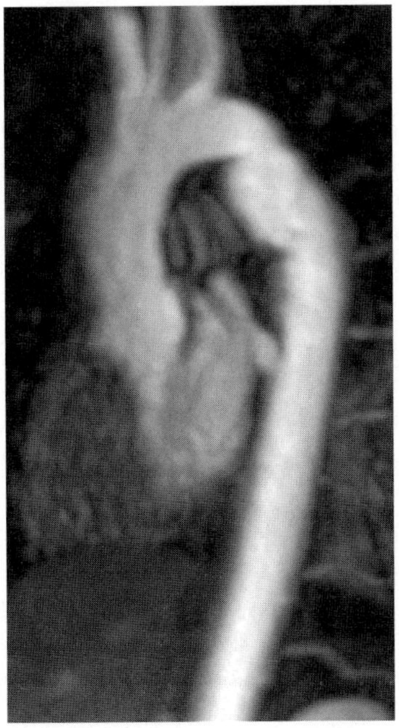

FIGURE 23.19. MRA of a traumatic aortic lesion. The relationship with arch vessels is well depicted.

MRI, and it cannot supply information on parietal lesions and hemorrhagic fluids outside the aortic vessel.

Aortitis

Inflammatory diseases of the aorta can be classified in two major subgroups: aortitis of nonspecific or unknown etiology (Takayasu aortitis, Behçet disease, giant cell aortitis, Kawasaki disease, ankylosing spondylitis), and specific aortitis, in which the aortitis is the consequence of an inflammatory disease of known origin (e.g., syphilitic aortitis). Strong ethnic differences have been observed in the epidemiologic distribution of nonspecific aortitis. It is common in Asian countries and rare in Caucasian populations, so that the hypothesis of a genetic transmission is supported. Histologically, marked irregular thickening of the aortic wall and a fibrous lesion are the result of an inflammatory process in the media. These alterations can lead to stenotic lesions (Takayasu disease), aneurysms of the aorta and its major branches, or aortic insufficiency as a consequence of dilation of the aortic root.

Imaging Findings

The diagnosis of aortitis is often difficult because nonspecific systemic symptoms are present in the early phase, when medical treatment may be more effective. Conventional angiography provides information mainly on late manifestations of the disease, such as vascular stenosis or localized aneurysms. Subtle changes of the aortic wall during the early phase of aortitis can be detected on spiral CT with contrast enhancement of the inflamed segments. However, the high density of contrast medium inside the vessel lumen may cause artifacts in the adjacent aortic wall, so that these images may be unsuitable for detecting early mural changes.

MRI Findings

Spin-echo images can detect mural thickening of the aorta. High signal intensity of the aortic wall has been observed in giant cell aortitis, whereas media with fibrotic replacement generally has lower signal intensity. Contrast-enhanced T1- and T2-weighted spin-echo MRI has been shown to be highly effective in the evaluation of Takayasu arteritis (64), even in the early phases, providing important information on the activity of the disease. Active inflammatory disease appears as variable thickening of the aortic wall that enhances after gadolinium administration. Choe et al. (64) reported 88% concordance between contrast-enhanced MRI and clinical and laboratory findings in 26 patients with active Takayasu arteritis; the chronic, quiescent stage is characterized by extensive perivascular fibrosis without contrast enhancement. MRA can replace invasive angiography in the study of aortic and branch vessel stenosis, allowing diagnostic assessment and follow-up (65). Avoidance of angiography is highly desirable in patients affected with aortitis because it carries a risk for pseudoaneurysm formation at the site of arterial puncture. Moreover, MRI can be useful in evaluating the response to medical treatment by depicting decreases in wall thickness of the involved arteries. In patients who undergo surgery for aortitis, recurrence of the inflammatory process is frequently reported that causes dehiscence of the sutures. Strict, life-long follow-up is therefore mandatory in patients with aortitis, both before and after surgery.

CONGENITAL AORTIC DISEASES

Aortic Arch Anomalies

During fetal life, six pairs of aortic arches form to join the two dorsal aortae with the aortic sac that will become the ascending aorta. At the end of development, some of the arches disappear, and the third, fourth, and sixth aortic arches give rise to the adult vascular structures. Aortic arch anomalies result either from abnormal regression of an embryonic arch that normally remains patent or from persistent patency of a structure that normally regresses (66) (Table 23.3).

Aberrant right subclavian artery, the most common type of vascular anomaly, affects 0.5% of the population. The reported prevalence ranges from 0.4% to 2%, with the condition occurring in approximately 1 in 200 births. The right subclavian artery arises from the left embryonic aortic arch. At the end of development, an aberrant right subclavian artery originates in the proximal portion of the descending aorta and passes posterior to the esophagus to form an incomplete vascular ring. The right subclavian artery may arise from an outpouching known as the *diverticulum of Kommerell,* which represents persistence of the most dis-

TABLE 23.3. ANOMALIES OF THE AORTIC ARCH COMPLEX

Anomalies of the course or composition of the aorta
  Double aortic arch
  Aberrant right subclavian artery
  Aberrant innominate or left common carotid arteries with or without trachea compression
  Subclavian steal
  Ductus arteriosum sling
  Circumflex retroesophageal aortic arch
  Right aortic arch with or without retroesophageal component

Anomalies of the length, size, or continuity of the aorta
  Cervical aorta
  Pseudocoarctation of the aorta
  Hypoplasia of the aorta
  Complete interruption of the aortic arch

tal portion of the embryonic right arch. Usually, an aberrant right subclavian artery does not cause any symptoms and is an incidental finding on MRI or CT of the chest. Sometimes, with aging, the right subclavian artery becomes tortuous and ectatic and may cause an esophageal indentation or obstruction (67).

A *right aortic arch* passes to the right of the trachea and may descend either to the right or to the left of the thoracic spine. It occurs in approximately 0.1% of adults. Two types of right aortic arch are described—right aortic arch with mirror image brachiocephalic branching and right aortic arch with *aberrant left subclavian artery.* The origin of the aberrant left subclavian artery may have a focal enlargement. Both types are frequently associated with other congenital cardiac anomalies. Usually, a right aortic arch with a left subclavian artery does not in itself cause any symptoms. However, if the ligamentum arteriosum is on the left side, a vascular ring is formed by the right aortic arch, anterior left common carotid artery, ligamentum arteriosum, and retroesophageal left subclavian artery.

Double aortic arch is characterized by the presence of both a left and a right aortic arch; these arise from a branching of the ascending aorta, pass on both sides of the trachea and esophagus, and join posteriorly to form the descending aorta, which may lie to the right or left of the vertebral column. The luminal size of the two arches in relation to each other varies considerably, and one of them, usually the left, may be partially or completely atretic. The double aortic arch is a vascular ring that can produce severe symptoms if it compresses the trachea and esophagus.

Cervical arch is a rare anomaly in which the aortic arch extends into the soft tissues of the neck before turning down on itself to form the descending aorta. The anomalous high position of the aortic arch may sometimes cause symptoms related to tracheal compression, such as stridor or dyspnea. The presence of a pulsatile neck mass is the most characteristic finding.

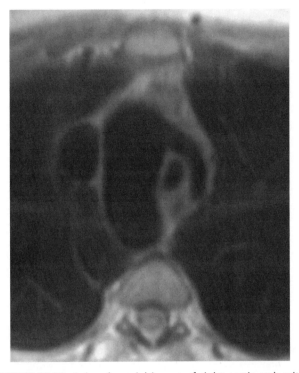

FIGURE 23.20. Spin-echo axial image of right aortic arch with aberrant left subclavian artery joining the trachea and esophagus.

MRI Findings

MRI is particularly valuable in detecting aortic arch anomalies because of its ability to image multiple projections with a large field of view. When an aortic arch anomaly is suspected, a systematic approach should be used to examine the anatomic structures in each subsequent slice. Spin-echo images in the axial plane can detect the abnormal vessel and its relationship with the esophagus and trachea (Fig. 23.20). Additional information can be derived by using the coronal and sagittal planes and thin slices to demonstrate the origin of the aberrant vessels. Kersting-Somerhoff et al. (67A) demonstrated the ability of spin-echo MRI to detect aortic arch anomalies in 16 patients. At present, contrast-enhanced MRA is the method of choice to assess aortic arch anomalies because it can provide an accurate overview of the aortic arch and associated vascular malformation noninvasively in a 3D format (68,69) (Fig. 23.21). Postprocessing with MIP and surface rendering provides a 3D impression that can be useful in understanding the abnormal mediastinal anatomy, which is particularly helpful in planning an optimal surgical approach. The combination of MRA and spin-echo MRI is more effective than catheter angiography in preoperative evaluations because MRI can display the abnormal aortic arch and arch vessels along with any compression of mediastinal structures.

Aortic Coarctation

Coarctation is a common congenital anomaly in which an abnormal plication of the tunica media of the posterior aortic wall proximal to the ligametum arteriosum causes a fibrous ridge to form that protrudes into the aorta and causes an obstructive lesion. The stenotic segment can be focal (aortic coarctation), diffuse (hypoplastic aortic isthmus), or complete (aortic arch interruption).

MRI Findings

Spin-echo sagittal images show the morphologic features of the coarctation. Obtaining a display of the extent and severity of the stenotic segment is the first important step in the diagnosis and quantification of the disease. Aortic coarctation is easier to identify in the sagittal plane; on axial images, partial volume effects may lead to an underestimation of the severity of coarctation. The aortic arch and arch vessels are also well depicted in the sagittal plane. By measuring the aortic diameter at the isthmus and above the diaphragm, morphologic indexes of coarctation can be determined. The severity of the stenosis is expressed as the ratio of the diameter or cross-sectional area at the isthmus to the same parameter measured in the abdominal aorta. However, although the detection of anatomic narrowing of the aorta establishes the diagnosis of coarctation, an assessment of its clinical significance depends on determining the hemodynamic effects. Cine MRI has been applied to evaluate flow turbulence across the coarctation; the severity of coarctation is quantified on the basis of the length of flow void. Further functional information can be provided by MR flow map-

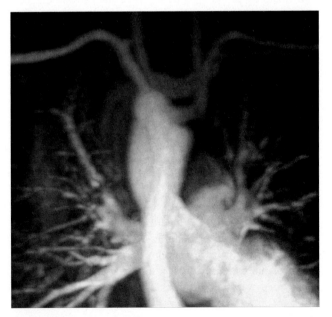

FIGURE 23.21. MRA of right aortic arch. The aberrant left subclavian artery arises from the right arch.

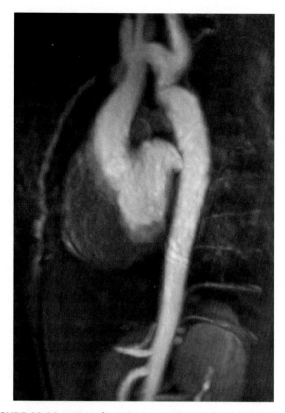

FIGURE 23.22. MRA of aortic coarctation. A focal stenotic segment is seen at the zone of the isthmus zone below a large left subclavian artery.

ping, which can define the severity of the stenosis by measuring velocity jets at the level of the coarctation. Moreover, flow mapping is able to quantify the flow pattern and volume of collateral flow in the descending aorta (70). The volume of collateral flow is another important parameter of the severity of coarctation, and this information may be crucial in the choice of surgical strategy. Three-dimensional MRA can display the extent and severity of the coarctation without partial volume errors and spin-dephasing artifacts (Fig. 23.22). Collateral vessels, which indicate the severity of the hemodynamic effects of the anatomic coarctation, are also displayed, and this information is also important in planning surgical repair.

Postoperative Findings

Several therapeutic strategies are available for the treatment of aortic coarctation, depending on the morphology of the aortic arch and coarctation and on the age and clinical condition of the patient. Surgery for aortic coarctation is recommended at an early age because long-term results appear to be better. Recently, interventional procedures and balloon angioplasty have come into wide use and provide good results, especially in mild or moderate cases. An accurate selection of favorable anatomy by high-resolution imaging

modalities is particularly important in interventional procedures to ensure a low rate of complications and restenosis (71).

Residual coarctation and aortic arch hypoplasia may be responsible for postoperative hypertension; these are more frequently associated with surgical techniques such as coarctation resection with end-to-end anastomosis. An increased risk for aneurysm formation at the site of repair has been reported after both synthetic patch aortoplasty and subclavian flap arterioplasty. Moreover, restenosis, aortic dissection, and pseudoaneurysm have been reported after balloon angioplasty. Therefore, careful follow-up is recommended for patients who have undergone repair of an aortic coarctation, regardless of the surgical technique used and the timing of the repair (72). Echocardiography is widely applied in the postoperative evaluation of aortic coarctation repair. With color Doppler, it can provide useful data on the gradient across the coarctation, which identifies restenosis. However, evaluation of the aortic arch anatomy can often be made difficult by limited acoustic windows, especially in adults. MRI has long been used in the follow-up of repaired aortic coarctation; it provides an optimal depiction of the thoracic aorta with multiplanar standard spin-echo sequences. Additional diagnostic information can be obtained with contrast-enhanced MRA. MRA better visualizes the aortic arch and proximal portion of the descending aorta, which may have a tortuous or kinked course. Postoperative complications, such as recoarctation, Dacron patch aneurysm (Figs. 23.23 and

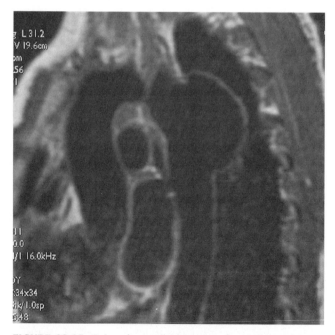

FIGURE 23.23. Spin-echo sagittal image of a patient who underwent surgery for aortic coarctation shows a large Dacron patch aneurysm.

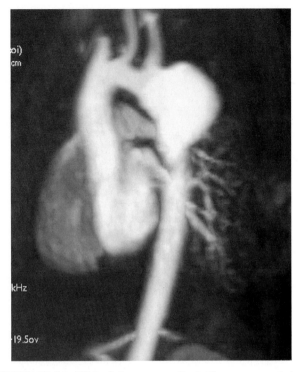

FIGURE 23.24. MRA of the same patient. The aneurysm is just below the left subclavian artery.

23.24), and anastomotic pseudoaneurysm, are well displayed by postprocessing methods (73). Because postoperative complications may not produce any symptoms, MRA of aortic coarctation after surgical repair should be recommended routinely.

Aortic Pseudo-coarctation

Pseudo-coarctation is a rare anomaly of the thoracic aorta that occurs when the third to seventh embryonic dorsal segments fail to fuse properly to form the aortic arch. It results in elongation of the aortic arch and first portion of the descending aorta, fixed by the ligamentum arteriosum, so that an abnormal kinking develops. Despite the abnormal tortuosity and morphologic aspects, similar to those of aortic coarctation, no significant gradient develops through the kinking. It is usually asymptomatic, but hypertension may be occasionally present. With aging, turbulent flow can cause progressive dilation of the pseudo-coarctation, and aortic dissection is frequently reported.

MRI is able to identify pseudo-coarctation and is particularly useful in differentiating it from true coarctation. On spin-echo images, the abnormal kinking may be visualized in the axial and sagittal planes. The morphology of the aortic tortuosity is similar to that of coarctation, but no fibrous ridge is present. The elongated and high position of the aortic arch and the absence of collateral vessels on MRA, and the absence of significant stenosis on reformatted images in

the axial and sagittal planes, are characteristic features diagnostic of pseudo-coarctation.

Aneurysms of the Sinuses of Valsalva

Aneurysm of a sinus of Valsalva is a rare congenital anomaly of the structural layers of the aortic wall characterized by the absence of the medial layer. This abnormality is usually limited to one of the Valsalva sinuses, most frequently the right coronary Valsalva sinus. Because of the absence of the elastic components of the medial layer, the Valsalva sinus is asymmetrically dilated, even in neonates. Aneurysm of a Valsalva sinus does not produce any symptoms, and a high incidence of aortic rupture has been reported in young patients in whom the disease was not suspected. In a neonate with severely dilated Valsalva sinuses, the differential diagnosis should include the neonatal variant of Marfan syndrome. The aortic abnormality is visible on spin-echo MR images and MR angiograms (74). The abnormal dilation of the aortic sinuses is typically asymmetric, whereas in Marfan syndrome, the dilation involves the aortic root uniformly. Rupture of a sinus aneurysm is usually into the right atrium; it creates a left-to-right shunt that can be visualized by gradient-echo sequences. Criteria for the timing of surgery to treat unruptured aneurysms have not been developed. Regardless the absolute size of an aneurysm, progressive enlargement on serial studies may be an indication for surgical repair.

MRI OF HUMAN ATHEROSCLEROTIC PLAQUE

Autopsy studies have shown that the amount of atherosclerotic plaque in the thoracic aorta is directly correlated with the degree of atherosclerotic disease in the coronary arteries. Thoracic aortic atherosclerosis is a stronger predictor of coronary artery disease than are conventional risk factors, and it is also a marker of an increased risk for mortality, stroke, and visceral thromboembolic events. Examination of the descending thoracic aorta by TEE and fast CT is used to predict cardiovascular risk. MRI is a noninvasive imaging modality that can visualize and characterize the composition of atherosclerotic plaque and differentiate tissue structure on the basis of proton magnetic properties (75–77). High-resolution MRI has been increasingly used to assessing the vascular wall and characterize atherosclerotic lesions. Continuous improvements in MR technology and software allow MR systems to achieve spatial resolutions in the order of micrometers and enable *in vivo* MR microscopy. The capability of MRI to distinguish tissue components with excellent soft-tissue contrast is unique for plaque characterization. The differences in composition of stable and unstable lesions can be detected by measuring T1, T2, and proton density changes (76). Lipid components present as hyperintense regions within the plaque on both T1- and proton density-weighted images and show hypointense signal on T2-weighted images. Fibrocellular components are defined as hyperintense regions of plaque on T1-, proton density-, and T2-weighted images. Calcium deposits can be appreciated as hypointense regions within the plaque on T1-, proton density-, and T2-weighted images. The fibrous cap and lipid core, organized thrombus and fresh thrombosis, and areas of calcification and necrosis have been imaged in studies performed both *in vitro* and *in vivo,* and atherosclerotic lesions have been assessed in the carotid arteries, coronary arteries, and thoracic aorta. MR methods for the direct noninvasive assessment of aortic atherosclerotic plaque thickness, extent, and composition allow serial evaluations of the progression and therapy-induced regression of atherosclerotic plaques.

Furthermore, MR spectroscopy with carbon 13 can provide information on the chemical constituents of the lipid pool as markers of the progression of atherosclerotic plaque (78). The advent of MR intravascular imaging devices further enhance the spatial resolution and homogeneity by providing close proximity between the imaging coil and vessel wall (79). The combination of tissue characterization and spectroscopy may have extraordinary potential in assessing the characteristics of plaque, so that new insight into plaque formation and evolution will be acquired.

REFERENCES

1. Urban BA, Bluemke DA, Johnson KM, et al. Imaging of thoracic aortic disease. *Cardiol Clin* 1999;17:659–682.
2. Reddy GP, Higgins CB. MR imaging of the thoracic aorta. *Magn Reson Imaging Clin N Am* 2000;8:1–15.
3. Stemerman DH, Krinsky GA, Lee VS, et al. Thoracic aorta: rapid black-blood MR imaging with half-Fourier rapid acquisition with relaxation enhancement with or without electrocardiographic triggering. *Radiology* 1999;213:185–191.
4. Sakuma H, Bourne MW, O'Sullivan M. et al. Evaluation of thoracic aortic dissection using breath-holding cine MRI. *J Comput Assist Tomogr* 1996;20:45–50.
5. Niezen RA, Doornbos J, van der Wall EE, et al. Measurement of aortic and pulmonary flow with MRI at rest and during physical exercise. *J Comput Assist Tomogr* 1998;22:194–201.
6. Powell AJ, Maier SE, Chung T, et al. Phase-velocity cine magnetic resonance imaging measurement of pulsatile blood flow in children and young adults: *in vitro* and *in vivo* validation. *Pediatr Cardiol* 2000;21:104–110.
7. Bogren HG, Buonocore MH. 4D magnetic resonance velocity mapping of blood flow patterns in the aorta in young vs. elderly normal subjects. *J Magn Reson Imaging* 1999;10:861–869.
8. Hopkins KD, Leheman ED, Gosling RG. Aortic compliance measurements: a noninvasive indicator of atherosclerosis. *Lancet* 1994;334:1447.
9. Groenink M, de Roos A, Mulder BJM, et al. Changes in aortic distensibility and pulse wave velocity assessed with magnetic resonance imaging following beta-blocker therapy in the Marfan syndrome. *Am J Cardiol* 1998;82:203–208.
10. Fattori R, Bacchi Reggiani L, et al. MRI evaluation of aortic elastic properties as early expression of Marfan syndrome. *J Cardiovasc Magn Reson* 2000;4:43–48.
11. Debatin JF, Hany TF. MR-based assessment of vascular morphology and function. *Eur Radiol* 1998;8:528–539.
12. Sodickson DK, McKenzie CA, Li W, et al. Contrast-enhanced 3D MR angiography with simultaneous acquisition of spatial harmonics: a pilot study. *Radiology* 2000;217:284–289.
13. Lee VS, Martin D J, Krinsky GA, et al. Gadolinium-enhanced MR angiography: artifacts and pitfalls. *AJR Am J Roentgenol* 2000;175:197–205.
14. Neimatallah MA, Ho VB, Dong Q, et al. Gadolinium-enhanced 3D magnetic resonance angiography of the thoracic vessels. *J Magn Reson Imaging* 1999;10:758–770.
15. Goyen M, Ruehm SG, Debatin JF. MR-angiography: the role of contrast agents. *Eur J Radiol* 2000;34:247–256.
16. Prince MR, Narasimham DL, Jacoby WT, et al. Three dimensional gadolinium-enhanced MR angiography of the thoracic aorta. *AJR Am J Roentgenol* 1996;166:1387–1397.
17. Krinsky G, Rofsky N, Flyer M, et al. Gadolinium-enhanced three dimensional MR angiography of acquired arch vessels disease. *AJR Am J Roentgenol* 1996;167:981–987.
18. Krinsky G, Rofsky N, De Corato DR, et al. Thoracic aorta: comparison of gadolinium-enhanced three dimensional MR angiography with conventional MR imaging. *Radiology* 1997;202:183–193.
19. Coady MA, Rizzo JA, Goldstein LJ, et al. Natural history, pathogenesis and etiology of thoracic aneurysms and dissection. *Cardiol Clin* 1999;17:615–633.
20. Bansal RC, Krishnaswamy C, Ayala K, et al. Frequency and explanation of false negative diagnosis of aortic dissection by aortography and transesophageal echocardiography. *J Am Coll Cardiol* 1995;25:1393–1401.
21. Spittel PC, Spittel JA, Joyce W, et al. Clinical features and differential diagnosis of aortic dissection: experience with 236 cases (1980 through 1990). *Mayo Clin Proc* 1993;68:642–651.
22. Cigarroa JE, Isselbacher EM, De Sanctis RW, et al. Diagnostic imaging in the evaluation of suspected aortic dissection. Old standard and new direction. *N Engl J Med* 1993;328:35–43.
23. Nienaber CA, Fattori R, Lund G, et al. Nonsurgical reconstruction of thoracic aortic dissection by stent-graft placement. *N Engl J Med* 1999;140:1338–1345.
24. Dake MD, Kato N, Mitchell RS, et al. Endovascular stent-graft placement for the treatment of acute aortic dissection. *N Engl J Med* 1999;140:1546–1552.
25. Nitatori T, Yokoyama K, Hachiya J, et al. Fast dynamic MRI of aortic dissection: flow assessment by subsecondal imaging. *Radiat Med* 1999;17:9–14.
26. Chang JM, Friese K, Caputo GR, et al. MR measurement of blood flow in the true and false channel in chronic aortic dissection. *J Comput Assist Tomogr* 1991;15:418–423.
27. Bogaert J, Meyns B, Rademakers FE, et al. Follow-up of aortic dissection: contribution of MR angiography for evaluation of the abdominal aorta and its branches. *Eur Radiol* 1997;7:695–702.
28. Nienaber CA, von Kodolitsch Y, Nikolas V, et al. The diagnosis of thoracic aortic dissection by noninvasive imaging procedures. *N Engl J Med* 1993;328:1–9.
29. Sommer T, Fehske W, Holzknecht, et al. Aortic dissection: a comparative study of diagnosis with spiral CT, multiplanar transesophageal echocardiography and MR imaging. *Radiology* 1996;199:347–352.
30. Fisher U, Vossherich R, Kopka L, et al. Dissection of the thoracic aorta: pre- and postoperative findings of turbo-FLASH MR images in the plane of the aortic arch. *AJR Am J Roentgenol* 1994;163:1069–1072.

31. Hagan PG, Nienaber CA, Isselbacher EM, et al. The International Registry of Acute Aortic Dissection (IRAD): new insight into an old disease. *JAMA* 2000;283:897–903.

32. Krukemberg E. Beiträge zur Frage des Aneurysma dissecans. *Beitr Pathol Anat Allg Pathol* 1920;67:329–351.

33. Fattori R, Bertaccini P, Celletti F, et al. Intramural posttraumatic hematoma of the ascending aorta in a patient with a double aortic arch. *Eur Radiol* 1997;7:51–53.

34. Nienaber CA, von Kodolitsch Y, Petersen B, at al. Intramural hemorrhage of the thoracic aorta. Diagnostic and therapeutic implications. *Circulation* 1995;92:1465–1472.

35. Coady MA, Rizzo JA, Elefteriades JA. Pathological variants of thoracic aortic dissection. Penetrating aortic ulcers and intramural hematomas. *Cardiol Clin* 1999;17:637–657.

35A. Yamada T, Takamiya M, Naito H, et al. Diagnosis of aortic dissection without intimal rupture by x-ray computed tomography. *Nippon Acta Radiol* 1985;45:699–710.

36. Keren A, Kim CB, Hu BS, et al. Accuracy of multiplane transesophageal echocardiography in diagnosis of typical acute aortic dissection and intramural hematoma. *J Am Coll Cardiol* 1996;28:627–636.

37. Moore A, Oh J, Bruckman D, et al. Transesophageal echocardiography in the diagnosis and management of aortic dissection. An analysis of data from the International Registry of Aortic Dissection (IRAD). *J Am Coll Cardiol* 1999;33-2(A):470A.

38. Murray JG, Manisali M, Flamm SD, et al. Intramural hematoma of the thoracic aorta: MR imaging findings and their prognostic implications. *Radiology* 1997;204:349–355.

38A. Shennan T. Dissecting aneurisms. *Medical Research Council Special Report* Series no. 193:1934.

39. Movsowitz HD, Lampert C, Jacobs LE, et al. Penetrating atherosclerotic aortic ulcers. *Am Heart J* 1994;128:1210–1217.

40. Hayashi H, Matsuoka Y, Sakamoto I, et al. Penetrating atherosclerotic ulcer of the aorta: imaging features and disease concept. *Radiographics* 2000;20:995–1005.

41. Yucel EK, Steinberg FL, Egglin TK, et al. Penetrating atherosclerotic ulcers: diagnosis with MR imaging. *Radiology* 1990;177:779–781.

42. Fann JI, Smith JA, Miller CD, et al. Surgical management of aortic dissection during a 30 years period. *Circulation* 1995;92 (Suppl II):110–121.

43. Svensson LG, Crawford SE. Statistical analyses of operative results. In: *Cardiovascular and vascular disease of the aorta.* Philadelphia: WB Saunders, 1997:432–455.

44. Heinemann M, Laas J, Karck M, et al. Thoracic aortic aneurysms after acute type A aortic dissection: necessity for follow-up. *Ann Thorac Surg* 1990;49:580–584.

45. Bonser RS, Pagano D, Lewis ME, et al. Clinical and pathoanatomical factors affecting expansion of thoracic aortic aneurysms. *Heart* 2000;84:277–283.

46. Fattori R, Bacchi Reggiani ML, Bertaccini P, et al. Evolution of aortic dissection after surgical repair. *Am J Cardiol* 2000;86:868–872.

47. Moore NR, Parry AJ, Trottman-Dickenson B, et al. Fate of the native aorta after repair of acute type A dissection: a magnetic resonance imaging study. *Heart* 1996;75:62–66.

48. Mesana TG, Caus T, Gaubert J, et al. Late complications after prosthetic replacement of the ascending aorta: what did we learn from routine magnetic resonance imaging follow-up? *Eur J Cardiothorac Surg* 2000;18:313–320.

49. Kawamoto S, Bluemke DA, Traill TA, et al. Thoracoabdominal aorta in Marfan syndrome: MR imaging findings of progression of vasculopathy after surgical repair. *Radiology* 1997;203:727–732 .

50. Gaubert J, Moulin G, Mesana T, et al. Type A dissection of the thoracic aorta. Use of MR imaging for long-term follow-up. *Radiology* 1995;196:363–369.

51. Loubeyre P, Delignente A, Boneloy L, et al. MRI evaluation of the ascending aorta after graft-inclusion surgery: comparison between an ultra-fast contrast-enhanced MR sequence and conventional cine-MRI. *J Magn Reson Imaging* 1996;6:478–483.

52. Fattori R, Descovich B, Bertaccini P, et al. Composite graft replacement of the ascending aorta: leakage detection with gadolinium-enhanced MR imaging. *Radiology* 1999;212:573–577.

53. Clouse WD, Hallett JW, Shaff HV, et al. Improved prognosis of thoracic aortic aneurysm: a population based study. *JAMA* 1998;280:1926–1929.

54. Weishaupt D, Ruhm SG, Binkert CA, et al. Equilibrium-phase MR angiography of the aortoiliac and renal arteries using a blood pool contrast agent. *AJR Am J Roentgenol* 2000;175:189–195.

55. Holland AE, Barentsz JO, Skotnicki S, et al. Preoperative MRA assessment of the coronary arteries in an ascending aortic aneurysm. *J Magn Reson Imaging* 2000;11:324–326.

56. Yamada N, Okita Y, Minatoya K, et al. Preoperative demonstration of the Adamkiewicz artery by magnetic resonance angiography in patients with descending or thoracoabdominal aortic aneurysms. *Eur J Cardiothorac Surg* 2000;18:104–111.

57. Guirguis EM, Barber GG. The natural history of abdominal aortic aneurysm. *Am J Surg* 1991;162:481–483.

58. Hilfiker PR, Quick HH, Pfammatter T, et al. Three-dimensional MR angiography of a nitinol-based abdominal aortic stent graft: assessment of heating and imaging characteristics. *Eur Radiol* 1999;9:1775–1780.

59. Grist TM. MRA of the abdominal aorta and lower extremities. *J Magn Reson Imaging* 2000;11:32–43.

60. Pate JW, Fabian TC, Walker W. Traumatic rupture of the aortic isthmus: an emergency? *World J Surg* 1995;19:119–126.

61. Mirvis SE, Shanmuganathan K. MR imaging of thoracic trauma. *Magn Reson Imaging Clin N Am* 2000;8:91–104.

62. Fattori R, Celletti F, Bertaccini P, et al. Delayed surgery of traumatic aortic rupture: role of magnetic resonance imaging. *Circulation* 1996;94:2865–2870.

63. Fattori R, Celletti F, Descovich B, et al. Evolution of post traumatic aneurysm in the subacute phase: magnetic resonance imaging follow-up as a support of the surgical timing. *Eur J Cardiothorac Surg* 1998;13:582–587.

64. Choe YH, Kim DK, Koh EM, et al. Takayasu arteritis: diagnosis with MR imaging and MR angiography in acute and chronic active stages. *J Magn Reson Imaging* 1999;10:751–757.

65. Berkmen T. MR angiography of aneurysms in Behçet disease: a report of four cases. *J Comput Assist Tomogr* 1998;22:202–206.

66. Thiene G, Frescura C. Etiology and pathology of aortic arch malformations. In: Nienaber CA, Fattori R, eds. *Diagnosis and treatment of aortic diseases.* New York: Kluwer Academic Publisher, 1999:225–269.

67. Bakker DA, Berger RM, Witsenburg M, et al. Vascular rings: a rare cause of common respiratory symptoms. *Acta Paediatr* 1999;88:947–952.

67A. Kersting-Somerhoff BA, Sechtem V, Fisher MR, Higgins CB. MR Imaging of congenital anomalies of the aortic arch. *AJR AM J Roentgenol* 1987;149:9.

68. Delabrousse E, Kastler B, Bernard Y, et al. MR diagnosis of a congenital abnormality of the thoracic aorta with an aneurysm of the right subclavian artery presenting as a Horner's syndrome in an adult. *Eur Radiol* 2000;10:650–652.

69. Carpenter JP, Holland GA, Golden MA, et al. Magnetic resonance angiography of the aortic arch. *J Vasc Surg* 1997;25:145–151.

70. Julsrud PR, Breen JF, Felmlee JP, et al. Coarctation of the aorta: collateral flow assessment with phase-contrast MR angiography. *AJR Am J Roentgenol* 1997;169:1735–1742.

71. Paddon AJ, Nicholson AA, Ettles DF, et al. Long-term follow-up of percutaneous balloon angioplasty in adult aortic coarctation. *Cardiovasc Intervent Radiol* 2000;23:364–367.

72. Therrien J, Thorne SA, Wright A, et al. Repaired coarctation: a "cost-effective" approach to identify complications in adults. *J Am Coll Cardiol* 2000;35:997–1002.

73. Bogaert J, Kuzo R, Dymor Kovski S, et al. Follow-up of patients with previous treatment for coarctation of the thoracic aorta: comparison between contrast-enhanced MR angiography and fast spin-echo MR imaging. *Eur Radiol* 2000;10:1047–1054.

74. Baur LH, Vliegen HW, van der Wall EE, et al. Imaging of an aneurysm of the sinus of Valsalva with transesophageal echocardiography, contrast angiography and MRI. *Int J Card Imaging* 2000;16:35–41.

75. Fayad ZA, Fallon JT, Shinnar M, et al. Noninvasive *in vivo* high-resolution magnetic resonance imaging of atherosclerotic plaque in genetically engineered mice. *Circulation* 1998;98:1541–1547.

76. Fayad ZA, Nahar T, Fallon JT, at al. *In vivo* magnetic resonance evaluation of atherosclerotic plaques in the human thoracic aorta: a comparison with transesophageal echocardiography. *Circulation* 2000;101:2503–2509.

77. Worthley SG, Helft G, Fuster V, et al. Serial *in vivo* MRI documents arterial remodeling in experimental atherosclerosis. *Circulation* 2000;101:586–589.

78. Toussaint J, Southern JF, Fuster V, et al. ^{13}C-NMR spectroscopy of human atherosclerotic lesions. Relation between fatty acid saturation, cholesteryl ester content and luminal obstruction. *Circulation* 1994;14:1951–1957.

79. Zimmermann-Paul GG, Quick HH, Vogt P, et al. High-resolution intravascular magnetic resonance imaging. Monitoring of plaque formation in heritable hyperlipidemic rabbits. *Circulation* 1999;99:1054–1061.

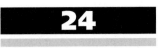

MRA OF ABDOMINAL AORTA AND
RENAL AND MESENTERIC ARTERIES

QIAN DONG
SHALINI G. CHABRA
MARTIN R. PRINCE

One of the earliest and simplest cardiovascular applications of MRI was imaging the abdominal aorta. Because of its large size and relative absence of cardiac motion, the abdominal aorta is one of the easiest arteries in the body to image. Coronal and axial spin-echo (black blood) images can reveal the size and extent of an abdominal aortic aneurysm, the most common pathology. Slow flow in the abdominal aorta often results in an incomplete flow void in older patients or patients with aortic pathology. However, a superior black blood effect can be achieved with longer echo times (i.e., 20 to 30 milliseconds) or the use of preparatory pulses to null the blood signal (1), although the relatively low level of resolution and low signal-to-noise ratio (SNR) of black blood MRI make it poorly suited for evaluating luminal detail or aortic branch vessels.

To obtain a higher SNR and superior resolution, a number of bright blood techniques can be utilized. The most basic bright blood technique, two-dimensional time-of-flight (2D TOF), can image the abdominal aorta in either the axial or coronal plane. Sagittal 2D TOF does not work well because of in-plane saturation. In patients with normal fast flow, a 3D TOF or 3D phase-contrast (PC) technique can evaluate the aortic branch vessels. For patients with slow flow, including older patients and those with aneurysmal disease, congestive heart failure, or atherosclerosis, gadolinium-enhanced MRA is the bright blood technique of choice

for comprehensively evaluating the abdominal aorta and branch vessels.

ABDOMINAL AORTIC ANEURYSM

Patients with aneurysmal disease fall into two categories: those in whom an aneurysm is being followed to measure its growth, and those in whom an aneurysm has reached a point at which intervention is required and detailed mapping of the luminal anatomy is necessary in preparation for surgical repair or stent grafting (2–16). For measuring the aortic diameter, coronal and axial black blood MRI, such as T1-weighted spin-echo MRI, is sufficient. However, for preoperative planning, coronal 3D MRA followed by axial 2D TOF after the administration of gadolinium at contiguous 3-mm intervals (or 4-mm intervals with 1-mm overlap) is necessary to obtain measurements for stent graft sizing and positioning. Axial 2D TOF after gadolinium is optimized by the use of respiratory-ordered phase encoding (ROPE) to eliminate respiratory motion artifacts. It may also be useful to perform 3D PC MRA of the celiac, superior mesenteric, and renal arteries to obtain a more comprehensive assessment, particularly if these arteries are not optimally seen on 3D gadolinium-enhanced MRA.

The images must then be analyzed to determine the aortic diameter at the level of the celiac and renal arteries, just above the aneurysm, and at the level of the maximal dilation; the diameters of the common iliac and common femoral arteries must also be determined. Additional measurements required include the distance from each renal artery to the beginning of the aneurysm, the length of the

Q. Dong: Department of Radiology, University of Michigan, Ann Arbor, Michigan.
S. G. Chabra and M. R. Prince: Department of Radiology, Weill Medical College of Cornell University, New York, New York.

aneurysm, and the exact location of the end of the aneurysm in the aorta or iliac arteries.

After placement of a stent graft, MRA can be used to detect changes in aneurysmal diameter and leaks in stents made of nitinol or other nonferromagnetic alloys. Ideally, the diameter of the aneurysm should decrease following stent placement, or at least should not increase further. In addition, no evidence of gadolinium enhancement within the aneurysmal sac outside the stent should be seen on delayed images after gadolinium. To maximize the detection of subtle leaks, precontrast images can be subtracted from postcontrast images to eliminate background signal.

RENAL ARTERY MRA

With MRA, it is now possible to perform an accurate evaluation of patients in whom renal artery stenosis is suspected without nephrotoxic contrast agents, ionizing radiation, or arterial catheterization and their associated risks. In addition to screening for renal artery stenosis, MRA can map the vascular anatomy when renal revascularization is being planned, assess renal bypass grafts, image renal transplant anastomoses, and evaluate vascular involvement by renal tumors. The renal arteries can also be evaluated after stent placement if the stent is made of platinum, nitinol, or another nonferromagnetic alloy. A variety of techniques provide complementary information about kidney morphology, arterial anatomy and blood flow, and renal function/excretion. This chapter reviews the techniques more commonly used. The emphasis is on combining 3D gadolinium-enhanced MRA with several other sequences to obtain a comprehensive renal MRA examination.

Early in the clinical course of renal artery stenosis, when the narrowing is focal and less than 50%, the hemodynamic effects are of little consequence, and opening the renal artery provides no benefit to the patient. When the stenosis exceeds 70% of the luminal diameter, reduced flow to the kidney results in renal ischemia and then to an elevation of blood pressure, mediated by the renin–angiotensin system. With time, progression of the stenosis leads to occlusion. Furthermore, controlling the blood pressure in the presence of significant renal artery stenosis reduces renal perfusion and function and accelerates the loss of nephrons. If the hypertension is poorly controlled, the ischemic kidney suffers less damage, but hypertensive nephropathy may develop in the contralateral normal kidney, and other tissues throughout the body are also damaged by the hypertension. Early revascularization can result in a nearly full recovery of renal function. If a chronic occlusion is allowed to develop, the kidney atrophies and nephrons are destroyed until little function is left to restore. For these reasons, an early diagnosis of renal artery stenosis is necessary to prevent permanent renal damage.

The importance of hypertension as a public health concern (17) and the devastating consequences of renal failure have motivated a search for a safe, noninvasive, and relatively inexpensive method to diagnose renal artery stenosis. In a recent metaanalysis in which conventional angiography was used as the "gold standard" reference (18), gadolinium-enhanced MRA was more accurate than ultrasonography and captopril renography and just as accurate as computed tomographic (CT) angiography in evaluating the main renal arteries. For a diagnosis of main renal artery stenosis by MRA, the area under the receiver operator curve was 0.99, indicating a very high rate of accuracy. Thus, MRA is a safe and accurate method to diagnose renal artery stenosis.

In the past, because of the risks associated with iodinated contrast material and arterial catheterization, the definitive diagnosis of renal artery stenosis by conventional renal arteriography was limited to patients in whom the clinical index of suspicion was high. Indications for the procedure were hypertension in children and young adults, poorly controlled hypertension, new-onset or newly worsening hypertension, renal failure induced by angiotensin-converting enzyme inhibitors, and peripheral vascular disease. With the availability of simpler, safer, less expensive, but still accurate MR contrast arteriography (18–22), screening for renal artery stenosis can be expanded to a broader spectrum of patients.

Recent studies of renal MRA with high-dose gadolinium have reported sensitivities and specificities of more than 90% for the detection of renal artery stenosis when conventional x-ray angiography was used as the reference standard. However, these studies were based on a highly simplified scheme in which renal artery stenosis was usually graded as 0, 50% or less, more than 50%, or more than 75%. Even with state-of-the-art MRI systems, the maximum spatial resolution is about 1 mm^3. On the other hand, the spatial resolution of x-ray angiography is still much higher. For this reason, an overestimation of the morphologic degree of stenosis on 3D gadolinium-enhanced MRA, particularly in higher-grade stenoses, is common.

Because of the limited spatial resolution of MRA, the hemodynamic and functional significance of a stenosis should be assessed in addition to its morphologic degree (23–27). Clinicians must know if a renal artery stenosis is hemodynamically significant so that they can decide whether a patient is likely to benefit from renal revascularization. The functional information available from several different MR sequences can help make this determination by identifying hemodynamically significant stenoses. A hemodynamically significant stenosis tends to exhibit spin dephasing on 3D PC images, and flow velocity curves show diminished and delayed systolic peak by cine PC. Additional functional consequences include asymmetry of kidney size, enhancement, and excretion and a loss of corticomedullar differentiation. A variety of MR pulse sequences provide functional data that can be integrated into the workup of a patient with renal artery stenosis to determine its significance, but a technically and clinically feasible comprehensive MR examination must be performed and analyzed in a standardized, reproducible fashion. The standardization must be applied to the acquisition, reconstruction, analysis, and interpretation of image data (27). In this process, numerous projections can be reconstructed from a single 3D volume of data collected after a single contrast injection to obtain perpendicular and optimized views of each renal artery (28–33). This capability is an inherent advantage of MRA over conventional digital subtraction angiography.

Suggested MRA Techniques

Several flow-based MRA techniques, including TOF and PC, have been used to image the renal arteries and veins directly (34–49) (Table 24.1). However, these techniques have limitations, including the following: turbulence-induced signal loss at stenoses (30,50,51); in-plane saturation (51); nonvisualization of small-caliber vessels, including distal renal arteries and accessory renal arteries; and poor-quality images as a result of slow flow in patients who have cardiac disease or aortic aneurysm or are older. Accordingly, contrast-enhanced MR arteriography with a high-dose gadolinium contrast agent and a high-resolution 3D spoiled gradient-echo pulse sequence is preferred (50–58). Gadolinium can be used safely, even at high doses, in patients with

renal failure (59). Three-dimensional gadolinium-enhanced MRA depicts the renal arteries along with the entire abdominal aorta, iliac arteries, and mesenteric arteries in a 15- to 30-second acquisition that can be performed during breath-holding. The renal vein and inferior vena cava (IVC) can be evaluated by repeating the examination during the venous and equilibrium phases. A delayed image can assess the symmetry of gadolinium excretion.

It must be pointed out that a morphologic assessment of the arterial lumen by 3D gadolinium-enhanced MRA is not sufficient for a complete evaluation of a suspected case of renal artery stenosis. Evaluating the hemodynamic significance of any stenosis identified is necessary to determine whether the patient will benefit from a renal revascularization procedure. Various MR techniques that have been proposed for evaluating the hemodynamic significance of renal artery stenoses include the following: (a) measurement of renal blood flow with 2D cine PC imaging (24); (b) identification of turbulence-induced dephasing at hemodynamically significant stenoses on 3D PC imaging (25,60); (c) evaluation of asymmetry of the temporal pattern of renal enhancement (61); (d) evaluation of the differential excretion of gadolinium (22); (e) determination of the effect of angiotensin-converting enzyme inhibition on MR measurements of renal artery flow (62) or gadolinium clearance rates (63). Many of these approaches are difficult to implement because reliable electrocardiographic (ECG) gating and challenging postprocessing are required. However, 3D PC

TABLE 24.1. ACCURACY OF RENAL MRA WITH TIME-OF-FLIGHT AND PHASE-CONTRAST TECHNIQUE

Investigator	Year	No. Patients	Technique	Sensitivity (%)	Specificity (%)
Kim et al. (34)	1990	25	2D TOF	100	90
Kent et al. (36)	1991	23	2D TOF	100	94
Debatin et al. (35)[a]	1991	33	2D PC	80	91
			2D TOF	53	97
Gedroyc et al. (37)	1992	50	3D PC	83	95
Grist (38)	1993	35	3D PC+2D TOF	89	95
Yucel et al. (39)	1993	16	2D+3D TOF	100	93
Servois et al. (42)	1994	21	2D TOF	70	78
Hertz et al. (40)	1994	16	2D TOF	91	94
Loubeyre et al. (41)	1994	53	3D TOF	100	76
De Cobelli et al. (82)	2000	50	3D PC	94	94
Silverman et al. (47)	1996	37	Cine PC	100	93
De Haan et al. (45)	1996	38	3D PC	93	95
Loubeyre et al. (46)	1996	46	3D TOF+3D PC	100	90
Schoenberg et al. (24)	1997	23	2D PC flow	100	93
Duda et al. (48)	1997	22	2D TOF	73	47
			3D PC	78	76
Hahn et al. (83)	1999	32	3D PC	93	81
Westenberg et al. (84)	1999	17	3D PC-PSL	Corr. coefficient = .90	
Nelson et al. (85)	1999	5	3D TOF	71	95
Lee et al. (62)[a]	2000	35	Cine PC	50	78
			+ ACE	67	84

[a]Two different MRA techniques were compared in the same patient.
TOF, time-of-flight; PC, phase-contrast; 2D, two-dimensional; 3D, three-dimensional; PSL, post-stenotic signal loss; ACE, angiotensin-converting enzyme.

pulse sequences are widely available, easy to perform, and do not require ECG gating; furthermore, postprocessing is not difficult. In addition, 3D PC MRA image quality is substantially improved following the administration of high-dose gadolinium, so that it is an excellent complementary sequence after 3D gadolinium-enhanced MRA.

A comprehensive imaging approach should be designed to obtain a contrast arteriogram and a hemodynamic characterization of renal artery stenosis in a single MR examination (Table 24.2). Generally, a 1.5-tesla (T) imaging system with high-performance gradients and some mechanism for timing the gadolinium bolus is required. Although the data can be acquired by the technologist without monitoring, the radiologist should perform the postprocessing to ensure accurate interpretation, especially if any of the imaging is of poor quality.

Preparing the Patient

The administration of oxygen helps patients who are short of breath to suspend their breathing during the entire 3D gadolinium MRA acquisition (64). Torso or body phased-array coils obtain a higher SNR in thinner patients, although the bright, near-field artifact from tissue close to the coil can be a problem. Placing 1 to 2 cm of foam between the patient and the coil can reduce the near-field artifact. The body coil is preferred in obese patients and has the advantage of a large field of view (FOV) with homogeneous signal. A landmark is placed on the lower margin of the rib cage along the axillary line to center imaging on the kidneys.

Localizer

A black blood sequence, such as a T1-weighted spin-echo or HASTE (half-Fourier acquisition single-shot turbo spin-echo) technique, gives a black blood effect useful for locat-ing arteries and organs simultaneously (Fig. 24.1A). Single-shot fast spin-echo (SSFSE) can be used even without breath-holding, although breath-holding is preferred (Fig. 24.1B). We prefer the sagittal plane for the black blood localizer. Alternatively, a fast 2D TOF bright blood locator can be obtained in the axial plane.

Axial T2-Weighted Images

Axial fast spin-echo T2-weighted images with fat saturation are useful to characterize any masses that are present. Simple renal cysts can be distinguished on T2-weighted images from more complex lesions that are suspected of being malignant. The entire length of the kidneys is covered in this sequence. Using sufficient averages and repetition time (TR) to make this sequence at least 4 to 5 minutes long allows enough time to set up the more complex 3D gadolinium MRA sequence, which is performed next.

Three-Dimensional Gadolinium MRA

Use a 3D spoiled gradient-echo volume including the entire abdominal aorta, renal arteries, and iliac arteries in the coronal plane. In selecting the specific parameters, it is important to realize that faster is better for 3D gadolinium MRA acquisition. Faster scans allow the same dose of gadolinium to be injected over a shorter scan time. The faster injection rate produces a higher arterial concentration of gadolinium, which in turn produces arteriograms with a high SNR. Fast scans also are subject to less motion artifact and make it easier for patients to suspend their breathing. To make the scan fast, use the shortest possible TR, a short echo time (TE), and the fewest number of slices that are sufficient to cover the arterial anatomy with adequate resolution. However, avoid using too wide a bandwidth. Widening the bandwidth makes the scan faster but reduces the SNR. Also, take

TABLE 24.2. RENAL MRA IMAGING PARAMETERS

	Spin Echo Location	SSFSE Locator	Axial T2	3D Gd MRA	3D PC	3D Gd Delay*
Plane	Sagittal	Sagittal	Axial	Coronal	Axial	Coronal
TE	Minimum full	180	102	Minimum	5–10	Minimum
TR	275	∝	2,920	5	18	5
Flip angle	—	—	—	45	35	45
Bandwidth	15.6	31.25	16	62	16	62
Frequency	256	256	256	512	256	512
Phase	192	256	256	192 (128–256)	192	192
Averages	2	1	3	1 (0.5–1)	1	1
FOV	40 (32–48)	40 (32–48)	32 (26–44)	34 (30–44)	28 (26–40)	32 (32–36)
Slice thickness	10	9	8 (8–12)	2.6 (2–4)	2.5 (2–3)	3 (2.6–3)
Spacing	Interleaved	0	2 (2–3)	—	0	0
No. slices	20	24	18	30 (28–44)	28 (28–60)	32 (30–36)
Scan time (min:s)	3:59	0:56	4:46	0:30	7:23	35

*Delay 10 minutes after Gd injection, if no excretion of Gd observed. Give 10–20 mg lasix and repeat.
SSFSE, single-shot fast spin-echo; 3D, three-dimensional; PC, phase-contrast; Gd, gadolinium; TE, echo time; TR, repetition time; FOV, field of view.

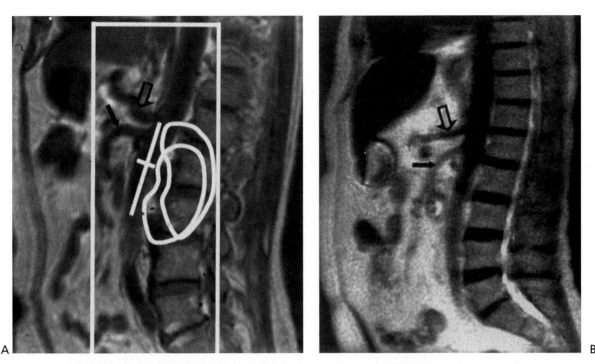

FIGURE 24.1. Abdominal aorta and origins of the celiac artery *(open arrows)* and superior mesenteric artery *(arrows)* are revealed on **(A)** a sagittal T1-weighted spin-echo image or **(B)** a single-shot fast spin-echo image for localizer purposes. The position of the 3D volume for gadolinium MRA is the black rectangular box (A), which includes the abdominal aorta and most of kidneys *(curved white outlines)*. The tracker for automatic triggering is placed on the aorta at the level of the superior mesenteric artery. (From Dong Q, Schoenberg SO, Carlos RC, et al. Diagnosis of renal vascular disease with MR angiography. *Radiographics* 1999;19:1540, with permission.)

into consideration that bolus timing is difficult with scans that are 30 seconds or shorter but relatively easy with scans that are 40 seconds and longer.

It is important to make the TE less than 3 milliseconds to avoid excessive spin dephasing, especially from the swirling jet flow distal to a stenosis. Selecting a TE in which fat and water are out of phase (~2.5 milliseconds at 1.5 T) helps to suppress fat but may create artifacts at boundaries between fat and organs. This is important because fat is the brightest background tissue. Obtaining a 3D data set before gadolinium administration to use for digital subtraction can also reduce the background tissue signal.

In theory, the flip angle should be tuned for optimal T1 contrast based on the TR and expected blood concentration of gadolinium. However, we have found in practice that the technique is not particularly dependent on the flip angle, and an angle of 30 to 45 degrees works well in nearly all cases. The flip angle can be larger for higher doses of gadolinium and a longer TR or smaller for lower doses and a shorter TR.

When prescribing the 3D spoiled gradient-echo image volume, first estimate how long the patient can suspend breathing. Then, adjust the coverage, slice thickness, and number of phase-encoding steps so that the data acquisition covers the aorta and renal arteries and can still be completed within the patient's breath-hold capacity. Cor-

rectly estimating the breath-hold capacity of the patient is essential (65). Usually, older patients, smokers, and patients with cardiopulmonary disease can suspend breathing for 20 to 25 seconds at most. Younger patients, nonsmokers, and those without cardiopulmonary disease can easily hold their breath for 30 to 40 seconds or longer. Adjust the slice thickness, number of slices, and number of phase-encoding steps to ensure that the acquisition time is short enough for the patient to suspend breathing for the entire scan. However, if the patient is very short of breath and unable to suspend breathing at all, it is better to make the scan duration 1 minute long and have the patient breathe freely.

Prescribe the image volume from anterior to the abdominal aorta to posterior to the middle of the kidney with a slice thickness of 2 to 3 mm (Fig. 24.1A). Zero padding or zero filling by a factor of 2 in the slice direction is useful because it doubles the number of slices without increasing scanner time. Set the top of the imaging volume 2 to 3 cm above the celiac axis. Use an FOV that is about as large as the patient is wide to avoid wrap-around artifact. Typically, 30 to 36 cm is sufficient and will ensure that the iliac arteries are included inferiorly. It is also helpful to elevate the patient's arms with cushions, exclude them within Faraday cages, or elevate them over the chest or head to prevent wrap-around of the arms into the imaging volume.

Timing the gadolinium bolus is critical. The moment of peak renal artery enhancement must be synchronized with the acquisition of central k-space data. This can be accomplished by using a gadolinium-detection pulse sequence, such as SmartPrep (GE Medical Systems, Milwaukee, WI) or CARE bolus (Siemens, Erlangen, Germany), or a test bolus (66–68). It can also be done empirically based on the patient's age and cardiovascular status. Typically, a delay of 10 seconds between the start of the injection and the start of scanning works for the majority of patients when sequential phase encoding and a 40- to 50-second scan are used. Shorter scans are more difficult to time consistently without a test bolus or gadolinium-detection pulse sequence.

The gadolinium dose is one of the most important determinants of image quality. In general, the higher the dose, the better the image quality. At our institution, a dose of 30 to 40 mL is given to most patients to simplify a standard pattern of hand injection with an injection rate of 2 mL/s. It is necessary to flush the gadolinium through the intravenous tubing and veins with at least 20 mL of normal saline solution to ensure delivery of the entire gadolinium dose and rapid venous return. It is helpful to use a standardized intravenous tubing set with an automatic mechanism for switching between contrast infusion and flush without delay, such as SmartSet (TopSpins, Ann Arbor, Michigan).

For the further characterization of renal function, the rate of contrast medium transit in the kidney should be assessed. This can be accomplished by obtaining repeated data sets during the arterial, venous, and equilibrium phases with three separate breath-holds. Alternatively, several 3D data sets can be acquired in a single breath-hold with ultrafast multiphase 3D gadolinium MRA (57). For this, the scan time for each 3D data set must be reduced to 5 to 10 seconds to allow the depiction of minor changes in the temporal evolution of the renal enhancement (Fig. 24.2).

Three-Dimensional Phase Contrast

For the further characterization of the renal arteries and any stenoses, an axial 3D PC image can be acquired immediately after the dynamic gadolinium-enhanced acquisition. This is useful in the evaluation of the functional significance of a renal artery stenosis and improves the evaluation of the distal renal artery. The velocity encoding should be set at 50 cm/s for patients with normal renal blood flow. It can be reduced to 30 cm/s in patients with heart failure, renal failure (creatinine >2.0 mg/dL), or aortic aneurysm and in patients 70 years old or more. Young (<30 years of age) or athletic patients may require velocity encoding of 60 cm/s. The renal blood flow can be quantified precisely with ECG-gated 2D cine PC measurements. In this technique, multiple 2D images are obtained at a single location perpendicular to the long axis of the renal artery; these show the cross-sectional renal blood flow with a high level of temporal resolution over the cardiac cycle (Fig. 24.3).

Delayed Excretory-Phase Imaging

After 10 minutes have elapsed, a repeated coronal 3D spoiled gradient-echo pulse sequence with a relatively large

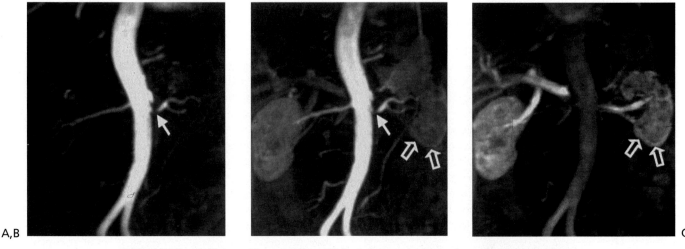

A,B   C

FIGURE 24.2. Multiphase 3D gadolinium MRA of the renal arteries (repetition time = 3.2 ms, echo time = 1.1, field of view = 27 × 36 cm, slab thickness = 8 cm, number of reconstructed slices = 44, acquisition time per phase = 6.3 seconds. **A:** In the early arterial phase, the renal arteries are completely enhanced, showing a proximal high-grade stenosis *(arrows)* on the left and a normal right renal artery. No parenchymal enhancement is seen. **B:** In the late arterial phase, delayed enhancement of the shrunken left kidney is seen *(open arrows)*. **C:** The early venous phase demonstrates equal bilateral enhancement. (From Schoenberg SO, Knopp MV, Bock M, et al. MRI of the kidneys: new diagnostic strategies. *Der Radiologe* 1999;39:373–385, with permission.)

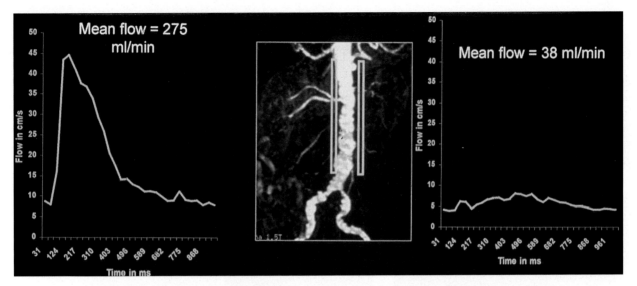

FIGURE 24.3. Diagram of renal blood flow measurements obtained with 2D cine phase-contrast flow technique performed bilaterally perpendicular to each renal artery. The right renal artery has a normal flow profile with an early systolic peak. Mean flow is 275 mL/min. The left renal artery has a flattened flow profile with loss of the systolic velocity components. Mean flow is only 38 mL/min. A hemodynamically and functionally significant stenosis of the left renal artery was diagnosed.

flip angle of at least 45 degrees can show the excreted gadolinium in the collecting system ureters and bladder. Asymmetry in excretion can reflect functional asymmetry. Make sure the TE is as short as possible. It may be necessary to use the widest bandwidth available to obtain a TE short enough to avoid dephasing from highly concentrated gadolinium in the collecting system. To make the ureters and collecting system fill out more completely, it may be useful to inject 10 mg of furosemide.

IMAGE ANALYSIS

Measurement of Renal Size and Cortical Thickness

The kidney length, corticomedullary differentiation, and parenchymal thickness can be determined on sagittal T1-weighted images (Fig. 24.4A). Alternatively, equilibrium phase 3D gadolinium MRA images can be used, especially if the renal axis is unusual (Fig. 24.4 B,C). The kidney length

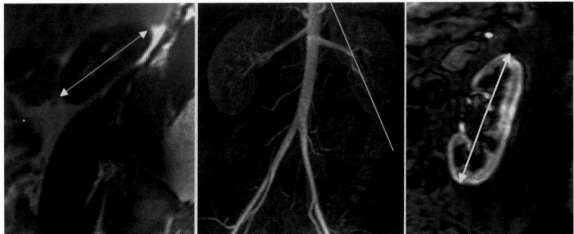

A,B　　　　　　　　　　　　　　　　　　　　　　　　C

FIGURE 24.4. A: Sagittal T1-weighted spin-echo image shows the right kidney with normal size and parenchymal thickness. **B,C:** Kidney length can also be measured on oblique re-formation of the 3D gadolinium MRA arterial phase, which is the long axis of the kidney.

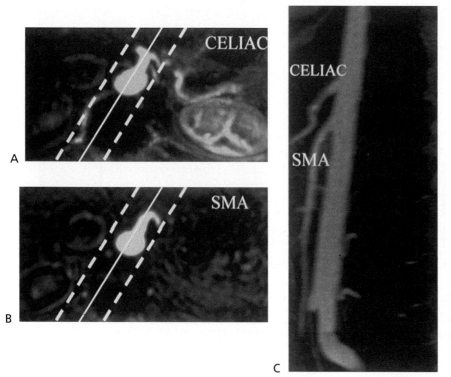

FIGURE 24.5. Use of axial re-formations of the celiac artery **(A)** and superior mesenteric artery **(B)** origins to guide the reconstruction of a sagittal subvolume maximum intensity projection **(C)**. This 3D gadolinium MR angiogram shows normal celiac, superior mesenteric, and inferior mesenteric arteries.

and parenchymal thickness are reduced in patients with long-standing renal artery stenosis.

Characterization of Renal Masses

The axial T2-weighted images help identify and characterize any renal masses or other abdominal pathologies. Any suspect lesion can also be evaluated by examining the 3D gadolinium MRA source images, which are analogous to contrast-enhanced CT. Do not analyze masses on maximum intensity projections (MIPs) because important details and sometimes the entire mass may be obscured.

Reconstructing and Reformatting

After the 3D MRA data have been acquired, postprocessing requires an additional 10 to 20 minutes on a computer workstation. MIPs and re-formations should be obtained to optimize visualization of the abdominal aorta, each renal artery, the celiac axis, the superior mesenteric artery (Fig. 24.5), and the common iliac arteries. Renal artery subvolume MIPs are performed encompassing each renal artery in the coronal oblique and axial oblique planes so that each renal artery origin is evaluated with perpendicular views (Fig. 24.6). Volume rendering may also be useful.

Assessing the Severity of Renal Artery Stenosis

A renal artery stenosis can be graded based on its appearance on 3D gadolinium MRA and the presence of dephasing on 3D PC MRA (Fig. 24.7 and Table 24.3). The consideration of additional factors can further refine the determination of the hemodynamic significance. The hemodynamic significance can be assessed semiquantitatively by looking at the change of the cine PC flow profile, particularly any delay or loss of the early systolic peak. In addition, functional changes in the renal parenchyma can be identified by a loss of corticomedullary differentiation, delayed renal enhancement, and an asymmetric concentration of gadolinium in the collecting systems, and reduced kidney length and parenchymal thickness. Post-stenotic dilation is also associated with hemodynamically significant stenosis.

SPECTRUM OF RENAL MRA FINDINGS
Normal Findings, Pitfalls, and Anatomic Variations

The typical normal kidney ranges in length from 11 to 13 cm. The right kidney is typically a little shorter (about 1 cm) than the left. One renal MRA study showed the renal parenchyma thickness to be 1.7 ± 0.3 cm for kidneys supplied by widely patent renal arteries (25). A reduction in parenchymal thickness can be determined by a comparison with a contralateral normal kidney. Patients with normal renal function have bright cortical enhancement with corticomedullary differentiation and bright arterial signal on 3D PC MRA. With the combination of 3D PC MRA and 3D gadolinium MRA, the entire renal artery up to the first level of branching in the renal hilum can usually be evaluated (Fig. 24.7A). Given the prevalence of artifacts, when either

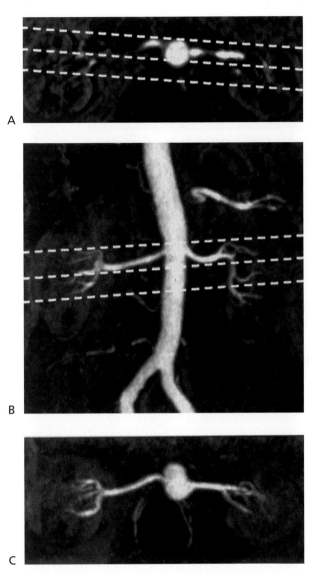

FIGURE 24.6. Use of an axial re-formation **(A)** to guide subvolume for coronal oblique subvolume maximum intensity projection **(B)** of each renal artery. A second maximum intensity projection in an axial oblique orientation **(C)** may be reconstructed by using (B). This provides two perpendicular images of the renal artery to help identify eccentric atherosclerotic plaque. (From Dong Q, Schoenberg SO, Carlos RC, et al. Diagnosis of renal vascular disease with MR angiography. *Radiographics* 1999;19:1545, with permission.)

the 3D PC or 3D gadolinium angiogram shows a normal renal artery, the artery is considered to be normal.

The most common pitfalls are related to poor image quality resulting from failure to suspend breathing, poor timing of the bolus, or administration of an inadequate dose of gadolinium. In these instances, the 3D PC sequence may be the best one for evaluating the renal arteries. However, 3D PC imaging is limited in patients with slow flow or renal failure, and when the velocity encoding is not closely matched to the renal flow velocity. Also, 3D PC images commonly exhibit artifactual dephasing at the renal artery origins. Three-dimensional PC MRA is particularly severely affected by surgical clip and stent artifacts. These may be identified on source images as an area of signal dropout adjacent to an extremely bright spot related to mismapping of signal.

Many pitfalls are also associated with image reconstruction. Eccentric disease may be identified on only one view, so that it is important to look at the renal arteries on multiple views. When the renal artery overlaps enhancing cortex or a renal vein on an MIP, an artifactual appearance of stenosis may result if the MIP is too thick. If the MIP is too thin, artifactual stenosis or occlusion may result if the artery is not entirely within the MIP volume. One last pitfall to be aware of is ringing artifact from errors of bolus timing, which can mimic dissection (65). Ringing artifact occurs when the injection rate is variable or the duration of the injection is too short or poorly timed so that the concentration of gadolinium changes during the acquisition of central k-space data.

It is important to be aware of the possibility of accessory or aberrant renal arteries, which occur in an estimated 30% of patients (69). Most accessory renal arteries originate from the abdominal aorta (Fig. 24.8). However, rarely, an accessory renal artery may arise from a common iliac artery. Accessory renal arteries are found especially frequently in cases of horseshoe kidney (Fig. 24.9). The left renal vein usually passes anterior to the aorta just behind the superior mesenteric artery. It may course behind the aorta, in which case it is called a *retroaortic renal vein* (Fig. 24.10). The presence of both a preaortic vein and a retroaortic vein is referred to as

TABLE 24.3. GRADING OF RENAL ARTERY STENOSIS BASED ON THREE-DIMENSIONAL GADOLINIUM MRA AND THREE-DIMENSIONAL PHASE-CONTRAST MRA

Grade	3D Gd MRA	3D PC
Normal (0–24%)	Normal	Normal
Mild (25–49%)	Mild stenosis	Normal
Moderate (50–75%)	Stenotic	Stenosis ± dephasing
Severe (75–99%)	Stenosis >75%	Severe dephasing
Occlusion	Image quality excellent but cannot find renal artery	Image quality excellent but cannot find renal artery

3D, three-dimensional; Gd, gadolinium; PC, phase-contrast.

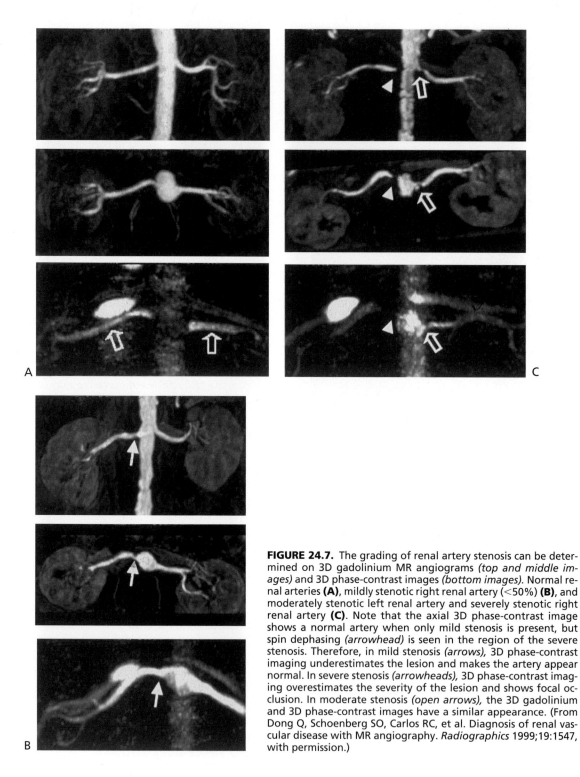

FIGURE 24.7. The grading of renal artery stenosis can be determined on 3D gadolinium MR angiograms *(top and middle images)* and 3D phase-contrast images *(bottom images)*. Normal renal arteries **(A)**, mildly stenotic right renal artery (<50%) **(B)**, and moderately stenotic left renal artery and severely stenotic right renal artery **(C)**. Note that the axial 3D phase-contrast image shows a normal artery when only mild stenosis is present, but spin dephasing *(arrowhead)* is seen in the region of the severe stenosis. Therefore, in mild stenosis *(arrows)*, 3D phase-contrast imaging underestimates the lesion and makes the artery appear normal. In severe stenosis *(arrowheads)*, 3D phase-contrast imaging overestimates the severity of the lesion and shows focal occlusion. In moderate stenosis *(open arrows)*, the 3D gadolinium and 3D phase-contrast images have a similar appearance. (From Dong Q, Schoenberg SO, Carlos RC, et al. Diagnosis of renal vascular disease with MR angiography. *Radiographics* 1999;19:1547, with permission.)

circumaortic renal vein. Duplication of the right renal vein is also common.

Renal Artery Stenosis

Atherosclerotic stenosis is the most common form of renal arterial pathology (Fig. 24.11). Usually, atherosclerotic renal artery stenosis is a manifestation of generalized atherosclerosis that also involves the coronary, cerebral, and peripheral vessels, although in 15% to 20% of all cases, it is not associated with disease elsewhere. In patients with renovascular hypertension, atherosclerosis is usually present in the aorta and typically compromises the ostium or proximal 1 to 2 cm of one or both renal arteries. In rare cases,

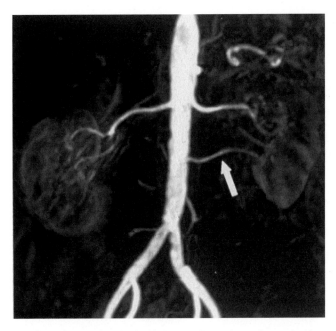

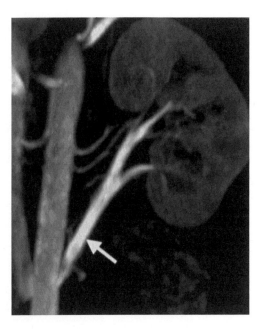

FIGURE 24.8. Coronal subvolume maximum intensity projection of 3D gadolinium MRA shows normal renal arteries bilaterally, with an accessory left renal artery *(arrow)* arising from the aorta. (From Dong Q, Schoenberg SO, Carlos RC, et al. Diagnosis of renal vascular disease with MR angiography. *Radiographics* 1999;19: 1548, with permission.)

FIGURE 24.10. Coronal subvolume maximum intensity projection of 3D gadolinium MRA during equilibrium phase shows a retroaortic left renal vein *(arrow)* with its characteristic inferior insertion on the inferior vena cava. (From Dong Q, Schoenberg SO, Carlos RC, et al. Diagnosis of renal vascular disease with MR angiography. *Radiographics* 1999;19:1548, with permission.)

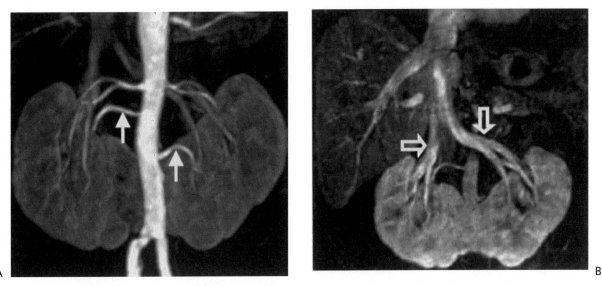

FIGURE 24.9. A: Coronal subvolume maximum intensity projection of 3D gadolinium MRA shows main left and right renal arteries in the expected location in addition to bilateral accessory renal arteries *(arrows)* during the arterial phase. **B:** Both renal veins *(open arrows)* are demonstrated, and fusion of the lower poles (horseshoe kidneys) is confirmed during the venous phase. (From Dong Q, Schoenberg SO, Carlos RC, et al. Diagnosis of renal vascular disease with MR angiography. *Radiographics* 1999;19:1548, with permission.)

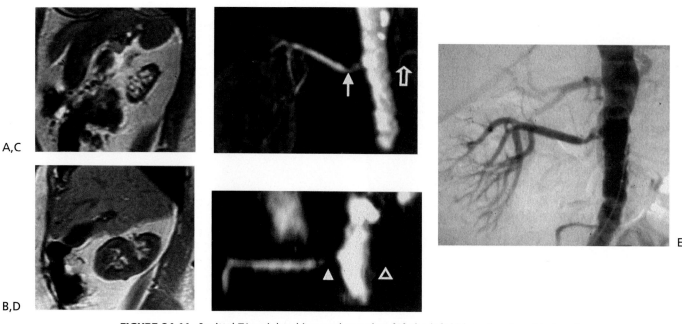

A,C

B,D

E

FIGURE 24.11. Sagittal T1-weighted image shows that **(A)** the left kidney is reduced in length with parenchymal thinning and **(B)** the right kidney is normal in size. **C:** Coronal subvolume maximum intensity projection of 3D gadolinium MRA shows atherosclerotic changes of the abdominal aorta, stenosis of the right renal artery *(arrow),* and occlusion *(open arrow)* of the left renal artery. **D:** Axial maximum intensity projection of 3D phase-contrast image shows dephasing *(arrowhead)* in the region of stenosis. No signal corresponds to the occluded left renal artery *(open arrowhead).* **E:** Conventional arteriogram confirms MRA findings and demonstrates a pressure gradient of 60 mm Hg across the right renal artery stenosis. (From Dong Q, Schoenberg SO, Carlos RC, et al. Diagnosis of renal vascular disease with MR angiography. *Radiographics* 1999;19:1549, with permission.)

atherosclerosis may be isolated to the distal renal artery or renal artery branches. When left untreated, it progresses to renal artery occlusion and permanent loss of renal parenchyma (Fig. 24.11A).

For this reason, in patients with renovascular hypertension or renal insufficiency, it is important to detect and treat renal artery stenosis early. The sensitivity and specificity data in Table 24.4 show the accuracy of 3D gadolinium MRA in detecting renal artery stenosis. Several studies have reported on functional changes indicative of the severity of stenosis, including the following: significant differences in parenchymal enhancement and cortical thickness (25), signal dropout at the region of stenosis on 3D PC MRA (25,26), and reduction of mean flow and the early systolic peak on MR cine PC flow measurements (24). MR determination of the gadolinium extraction fraction and glomerular filtration rate (63) and the feasibility of captopril-sensitized dynamic MRI in patients with renovascular hypertension (70) have also been reported.

Fibromuscular dysplasia is a distant second-most-common cause of renal artery stenosis. This is a nonatheromatous vascular lesion that occurs in medium-sized and small arteries (71). Fibromuscular dysplasia may involve the distal renal, internal carotid, and intracerebral arteries. It has been reported in other arterial beds, including the subclavian, axillary, mesenteric, hepatic, splenic, and iliac arteries, but involvement of these sites is rare. The majority of patients are female, and fibromuscular dysplasia almost always presents at a young age (<40 years of age). The histologic classification is based on the angiographic appearance and the layer of arterial wall that is primarily affected. In this way, lesions can be categorized as intimal fibroplasia, medial fibromuscular dysplasia, and perimedial (adventitial) fibroplasia. Medial fibromuscular dysplasia is the most common type and is further subdivided into medial fibroplasia (common), medial hyperplasia, and perimedial dysplasia (both rare). The angiographic findings of the most common type, medial fibroplasia, are a characteristic of "string-of-beads" appearance in which areas of weblike stenoses alternate with small fusiform or saccular aneurysms. Usually, fibromuscular dysplasia spares the proximal renal artery and involves only the distal two-thirds of the main renal artery. Sometimes, it extends into segmental vessels. When the proximal renal artery is involved, the form is more likely to be intimal fibroplasia. Bilateral involvement is common. MRA may not always detect the subtle irregularities of the distal main renal arteries associated with fibromuscular dysplasia if the spatial resolution is inadequate (Fig. 24.12).

TABLE 24.4. ACCURACY OF RENAL MRA WITH THREE-DIMENSIONAL GADOLINIUM MRA TECHNIQUE

Investigator	Year	No. Patients	Technique	Sensitivity (%)	Specificity (%)
Prince et al. (12)	1995	19	3D Gd	100	93
Grist[a]	1996	35	3D Gd	89	95
Snidow et al. (52)	1996	47	3D Gd	100	89
Holland (19)	1996	63	3D Gd	100	100
Steffens et al. (56)	1997	50	3D Gd	96	95
Rieumont et al. (31)	1997	30	3D Gd	100	71
De Cobelli et al. (21)	1997	55	3D Gd	100	97
Bakker et al. (22)	1998	50	3D Gd	97	92
Hany et al. (32)	1998	103	3D Gd	93	90
Thornton et al. (86)	1999	62	3D Gd	88	98
Schoenberg et al. (87)	1999	26	3D Gd	94–100	96–100
Thornton et al. (88)	1999	42	3D Gd	100	98
Cambria et al. (89)	1999	25	3D Gd + PC	97	100
Ghantous et al. (90)	1999	12	3D Gd	NA	100
Marchand et al. (91)	2000	NA	3D Gd	88–100	71–100
Shetty et al. (92)	2000	51	3D Gd	96	92
Winterer et al. (93)	2000	23	3D Gd	100	98
Weishaupt et al. (94)	2000	20	Blood pool 3D	82	98
Bongers et al. (95)[b]	2000	43	3D Gd	100	94
			Captopril renogram	85	71
Volk et al. (96)	2000	40	Time-resolved 3D Gd	93	83
Oberholzer et al. (97)	2000	23	3D Gd at 1 T	96	97
Korst et al. (98)	2000	38	3D Gd	100	85
De Cobelli et al. (99)[b]	2000	45	3D Gd	94	93
			Doppler US	71	93
Qanadli et al. (109)	2001	41	3D Gd	95	82
			Doppler with captopril	79	80
			Captopril scintigraphy	47	88
Voiculescu et al. (110)	2001	36	3D Gd	96	86
Mittal et al. (111)	2001	26	3D Gd	96	93
		TOTAL = 1,005	WEIGHTED MEAN = 95%		92%
			MIN–MAX	(82–100)	(64–100)

[a]Preliminary data presented on Proceedings of the Twelfth Annual Meeting of the Society of Magnetic Resonance in Medicine. New York, 1996.
[b]Three-dimensional gadolinium MRA compared with another technique.
3D, three-dimensional; Gd, gadolinium; PC, phase-contrast; T, tesla; US, ultrasonography.

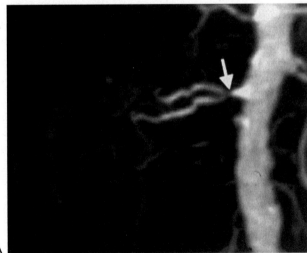
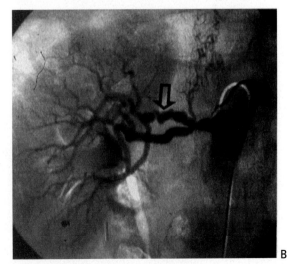

A   B

FIGURE 24.12. A: Coronal subvolume maximum intensity projection of 3D gadolinium MRA optimized for the right renal artery shows severe stenosis *(arrow)*. This stenosis was thought to be atherosclerotic on the basis of MRA. **B:** However, at conventional digital subtraction angiography, it was found to be fibromuscular dysplasia with much more extensive involvement of the artery *(open arrow)*. Note that the accuracy of MRA in diagnosing of fibromuscular dysplasia is not established. (From Dong Q, Schoenberg SO, Carlos RC, et al. Diagnosis of renal vascular disease with MR angiography. *Radiographics* 1999;19:1550, with permission.)

Dissection

Aortic dissection occurs when blood dissects into the media of the aortic wall through an intimal tear. It is related to degeneration of an aging aorta and may be accelerated in patients with hypertension or underlying mural defects, including those associated with Marfan syndrome, Ehlers-Danlos syndrome, relapsing polychondritis, coarctation, Turner syndrome, and aortic valve replacement. Renal artery flow can be compromised in patients with an aortic dissection that extends into the abdominal aorta (Fig. 24.13). The dissection may extend into a renal artery. The intimal dissection flap may move between systole and diastole and intermittently cover the origin of the renal artery. Reduced perfusion pressure and collapse of the true lumen may also reduce renal blood flow despite patency of the renal artery (72).

Renal Artery Aneurysm

Aneurysms associated with atherosclerosis usually occur in the infrarenal aorta and common iliac arteries. However,

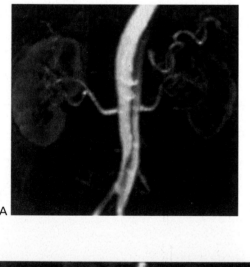

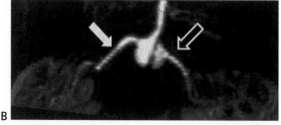

FIGURE 24.13. Coronal subvolume maximum intensity projection **(A)** and axial subvolume maximum intensity projection **(B)** of 3D gadolinium MRA images show that aortic dissection extends distally to the level of the aortic bifurcation. The superior mesenteric artery axis and right renal artery arise from the true lumen *(arrow)*, and the left renal artery arises from the false lumen *(open arrow)*. (From Dong Q, Schoenberg SO, Carlos RC, et al. Diagnosis of renal vascular disease with MR angiography. *Radiographics* 1999;19:1550, with permission.)

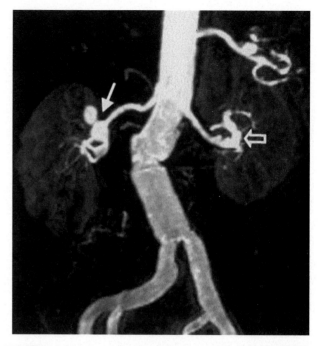

FIGURE 24.14. Coronal subvolume maximum intensity projection of 3D gadolinium MR angiogram shows a right renal artery saccular aneurysm *(arrow)* and a left renal artery fusiform aneurysm *(open arrow)*. (From Dong Q, Schoenberg SO, Carlos RC, et al. Diagnosis of renal vascular disease with MR angiography. *Radiographics* 1999;19:1551, with permission.)

they also occur in the renal arteries (Fig. 24.14). Most aneurysms of the renal artery have been found in persons between 50 and 70 years of age (73). Renal artery aneurysms are subject to the same complications as aneurysms elsewhere, including rupture, thrombosis, embolization, and dissection. Because of its 3D nature, MRA is helpful in evaluating the anatomic characteristics of an aneurysm, its relationship to other vascular structures, diameter in all orientations, and type, such as saccular or fusiform.

Transplanted Renal Arteries

Whenever the serum creatinine level rises in a patient with a renal transplant, the possibility of a stenosis in the transplanted renal artery should be considered. Typically, stenoses occur at the surgical anastomosis connecting the transplanted artery to the iliac artery. This may be an end-to-end anastomosis to the internal iliac artery or an end-to-side anastomosis to the external iliac artery. Atherosclerotic narrowing of the iliac artery proximal to the transplanted arterial anastomosis may also develop (Fig. 24.15). Sometimes, this occurs at the site where a surgical clamp was placed on the iliac artery at the time of transplantation. If the transplanted renal artery is widely patent, renal enhancement is minimal, and no gadolinium is excreted, then the kidney has probably been rejected. The sensitivity and specificity data in Table 24.5 show the accuracy of 2D and

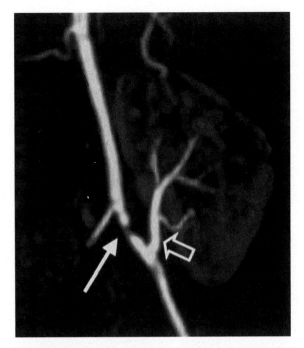

FIGURE 24.15. Coronal subvolume maximum intensity projection of 3D gadolinium MR angiogram shows a stenosis of the left external iliac artery *(arrow)* and a normal transplanted renal artery *(open arrow)*. This external iliac stenosis compromised flow to the transplanted kidney and caused hypertension and elevated serum creatinine, which improved after balloon angioplasty. (From Dong Q, Schoenberg SO, Carlos RC, et al. Diagnosis of renal vascular disease with MR angiography. *Radiographics* 1999;19:1551, with permission.)

3D MRA with or without gadolinium in detecting stenosis in a transplanted renal artery.

Renal Vein and Caval Invasion by Renal Cell Carcinoma

Renal cell carcinoma tends to involve the renal vein and grow upward along the IVC. The extent of tumor invasion of the IVC may be difficult to assess on ultrasonography and even on contrast-enhanced CT (74), and MR evaluation has been shown to have 100% sensitivity for the detection of tumor

thrombus beyond the distal renal vein. T1- and T2-weighted spin-echo sequences, in combination with axial TOF images, provide a comprehensive assessment of patients presenting with solid renal masses. Tumor enhancement and the renal vein extension can be demonstrated during the arterial and equilibrium phases of 3D gadolinium MRA (Fig. 24.16).

MESENTERIC ARTERY MRA

MRA has the potential to become a definitive noninvasive test for the diagnosis of chronic mesenteric ischemia. It can provide information about patency and stenosis in mesenteric vessels (Fig. 24.17) and is becoming a modality of choice in the selection of patients suspected of having mesenteric ischemia who may benefit from surgery (Fig. 24.18). MRI can also provide functional information, including blood flow and venous oxygen saturation.

Chronic mesenteric ischemia is characterized by symptoms of postprandial abdominal pain, weight loss, and food aversion. A demonstration of stenosis or occlusion in at least two of the three major mesenteric vessels is used to confirm the diagnosis of chronic mesenteric ischemia (Figs. 24.19 and 24.20). However, this diagnostic criterion is imperfect because even chronic stenosis and occlusion of all three mesenteric arteries may not cause any abdominal symptoms. Thus, the clinical diagnosis of chronic mesenteric ischemia is difficult to make.

Functional Measurements

Mesenteric blood flow can be measured accurately and noninvasively with a cine PC technique. Flow in the superior mesenteric vein and superior mesenteric artery normally increases postprandially, but this increase is diminished in patients with mesenteric ischemia (75–80).

In Vivo MR Oximetry

The estimation with MRI of the percentage of oxygenated hemoglobin in the superior mesenteric vein (SMV% HbO$_2$)

TABLE 24.5. TRANSPLANT RENAL MRA: SINGLE TECHNIQUE

Investigator	Year	No. Patients	Technique	Sensitivity (%)	Specificity (%)
Gedroyc et al. (101)	1992	50		83	97
Smith et al. (102)	1993	34	3D TOF	100	95
Johnson et al. (103)	1997	11	Gd MRA	67	88
			3D PC	60.3	76
			2D TOF	47	81
			Gd/PC	100	100
Ferreiros et al. (104)	1999	24	Gd 3D	100	98
Luk et al. (105)	1999	9	3D Gd	NA	100
Chan et al. (100)	2001	17	3D Gd	100	75

TOF, time-of-flight; Gd, gadolinium; 3D, three-dimensional; 2D, two-dimensional; PC, phase-contrast.

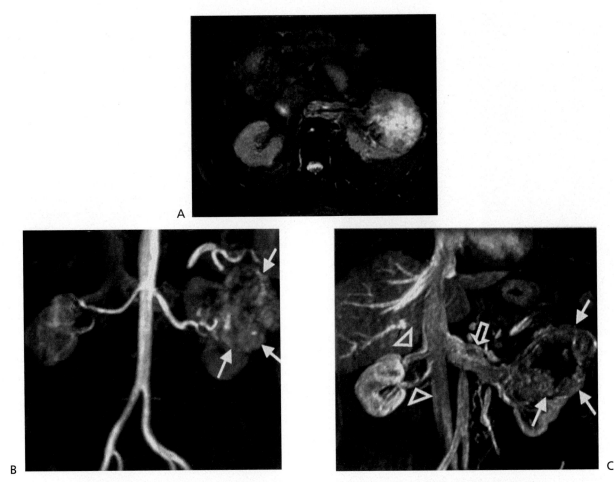

FIGURE 24.16. Axial T2-weighted **(A)** subvolume maximum intensity projection image during the arterial phase **(B)** and reformatted image from 3D gadolinium MRA during the venous phase **(C)** in a patient with a large renal cell carcinoma show a heterogeneously enhancing mass within the left kidney *(solid arrows)* with tumor extension into the left renal vein *(open arrows)*. Two right renal veins are also demonstrated *(arrowheads)*. (From Dong Q, Schoenberg SO, Carlos RC, et al. Diagnosis of renal vascular disease with MR angiography. *Radiographics* 1999;19:1552, with permission.)

is useful in studying the mesenteric circulation. The SMV% HbO_2 can be determined *in vivo* with flow-independent T2-weighted measurements of the venous blood. Measurements of the mesenteric arteriovenous difference in oxygen saturation can be an even more accurate method of diagnosing mesenteric ischemia than measurements of blood flow. Fasting and postprandial blood changes are used to predict mesenteric ischemia. Normally, oxygen saturation in the superior mesenteric vein increases postprandially. A decrease in SMV% HbO_2 after a standard meal is an indicator of chronic mesenteric ischemia (81).

Contrast-Enhanced Three-Dimensional MRA

Gadolinium-enhanced ultrafast 3D spoiled gradient-echo MRI (Table 24.6) has been used instead of or in addition to

conventional contrast-enhanced angiography in patients with symptoms of mesenteric ischemia, especially those who are at risk for reactions related to the administration iodinated contrast media.

With fast gradient systems, abdominal sections can be obtained during breath-holding to eliminate respiratory motion. The 3D volume obtained from a single acquisition can be reformatted at the workstation, so that the vascular anatomy can be viewed in any projection. MRA is also useful to evaluate aberrant arteries, vessel thrombosis, and dissection, and to evaluate the portal venous system.

SUMMARY

MRA is useful for evaluating a wide spectrum of abdominal aortic, renal, and mesenteric vascular pathology. The

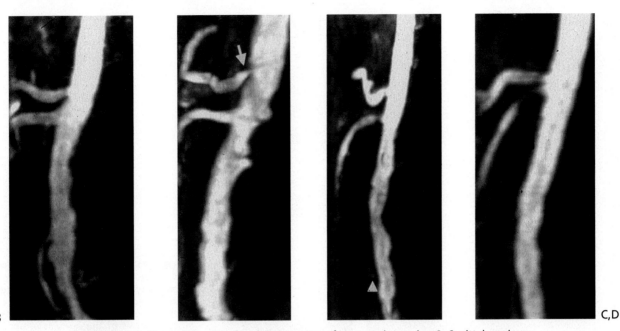

FIGURE 24.17. Three-dimensional gadolinium MRA of mesenteric arteries. **A:** Sagittal maximum intensity projection reconstruction shows widely patent celiac, superior mesenteric, and inferior mesenteric arteries. **B:** The celiac artery *(arrow)* is severely stenotic at origin. **C:** Mild superior mesenteric artery stenosis *(black arrow)* with severe inferior mesenteric artery stenosis *(white arrowhead)*. **D:** Moderate superior mesenteric artery stenosis *(up arrow)* with moderate to severe inferior mesenteric artery stenosis *(black arrowhead)*.

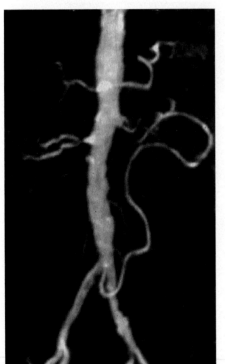

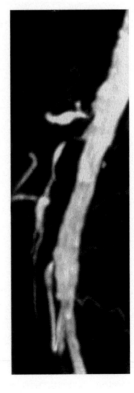

FIGURE 24.18. Coronal 3D gadolinium-enhanced MRA **(A)** and sagittal maximum intensity projection reconstruction **(B)** show widely patent splenorenal graft *(arrows)* with abdominal aortic aneurysm. The celiac and superior mesenteric arteries are widely patent.

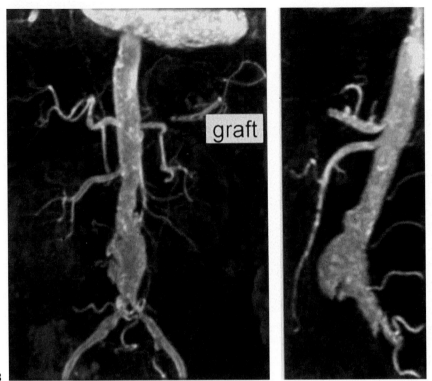

FIGURE 24.19. A,B: Mesenteric ischemia. MRA shows severe stenosis at origin of the celiac artery and moderate to severe stenosis of the superior mesenteric artery and origin of the inferior mesenteric artery. Severe atherosclerosis of the aorta is present. The coronal maximum intensity projection MR image (A) shows the prominent meandering marginal artery that is typical of this condition, which is associated with the development of extensive collaterals.

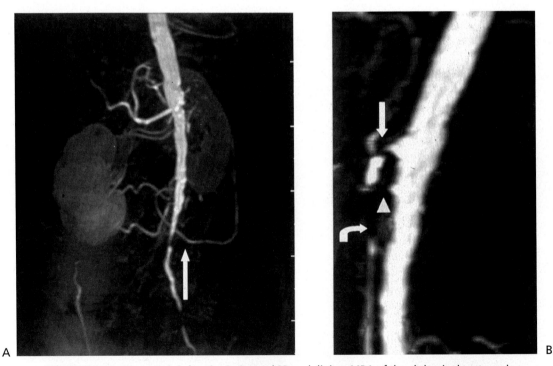

FIGURE 24.20. Mesenteric ischemia. **A:** Coronal 3D gadolinium MRA of the abdominal aorta and mesenteric arteries shows atherosclerotic abdominal aorta with prominent marginal artery *(up arrow)*. **B:** Sagittal maximum intensity projection reconstruction shows severe proximal stenosis of the celiac artery *(down arrow)*. The superior mesenteric artery *(triangular arrow)* is occluded at the origin and reconstitutes 2 cm beyond the origin. The inferior mesenteric artery *(curved arrow)* is occluded.

TABLE 24.6. ACCURACY OF MRA FOR MESENTERIC VESSELS

Investigator	Year	No. Patients	Technique	Sensitivity (%)	Specificity (%)
Carlos et al. (58)	2002	26	3D Gd	96	95
Meaney et al. (106)	1997	14	3D Gd	100	95
Miyazaki et al. (107)	1995	100	2D TOF	80	33
Prince et al. (12)	1995	43	3D Gd	94	98
Durham J et al. (108)	1993	28	2D TOF	60	96

Gd, gadolinium; TOF, time-of-flight; 3D, three-dimensional; 2D, two-dimensional.

comprehensive examination should include multiple sequences to assess the renal luminal morphology and the functional significance of any lesions identified, and to detect the presence of any renal or retroperitoneal masses.

REFERENCES

1. Edelman RR, Chien D, Kim D. Fast selective black blood MR imaging. *Radiology* 1991;187:655–660.
2. Arlart IP, Gerlach A, Kolb M, et al. MR angiography using Gd-DTPA in staging of abdominal aortic aneurysm: a correlation with DSA and CT [in German]. *Rofo Fortschr Geb Rontgenstr Neuen Bildgeb Verfahr* 1997;167:257–263.
3. Atkinson DJ, Vu B, Chen DY, et al. First pass MRA of the abdomen: ultrafast, non–breath-hold time-of-flight imaging using Gd-DTPA bolus. *J Magn Reson Imaging* 1997;7:1159–1162.
4. Gilfeather M, Holland GA, Siegelman ES, et al. Gadolinium-enhanced ultrafast three-dimensional spoiled gradient-echo MR imaging of the abdominal aorta and visceral and iliac vessels [published erratum appears in *Radiographics* 1997;17:804]. *Radiographics* 1997;17:423–432.
5. Hany TF, Pfammatter T, Schmidt M, et al. Ultrafast contrast-enhanced 3D MR angiography of the aorta and renal arteries in apnea [in German]. *Rofo Fortschr Geb Rontgenstr Neuen Bildgeb Verfahr* 1997;166:397–405.
6. Kaufman JA, Geller SC, Petersen MJ, et al. MR imaging (including MR angiography) of abdominal aortic aneurysms: comparison with conventional angiography. *AJR Am J Roentgenol* 1994;163:203–210.
7. Kelekis NL, Semelka RC, Molina PL, et al. Immediate postgadolinium spoiled gradient-echo MRI for evaluating the abdominal aorta in the setting of abdominal MR examination. *J Magn Reson Imaging* 1997;7:652–656
8. Laissy JP, Soyer P, Tebboune D, et al. Abdominal aortic aneurysms: assessment with gadolinium-enhanced time-of-flight coronal MR angiography (MRA). *Eur J Radiol* 1995;20:1–8.
9. Leung DA, Hany TF, Debatin JF. Three-dimensional contrast-enhanced MR angiography of the abdominal arterial system. *Cardiovasc Intervent Radiol* 1998;21:1–10.
10. Petersen MJ, Cambria RP, Kaufman JA, et al. Magnetic resonance angiography in the preoperative evaluation of abdominal aortic aneurysms. *J Vasc Surg* 1995;21:891–898; discussion 899.
11. Prince MR, Narasimham DL, Stanley JC, et al. Breath-hold gadolinium-enhanced MR angiography of the abdominal aorta and its major branches. *Radiology* 1995;197:785–792.
12. Prince MR, Narasimham DL, Stanley JC, et al. Gadolinium-enhanced magnetic resonance angiography of abdominal aortic aneurysms. *J Vasc Surg* 1995;21:656–669.
13. Shetty AN, Shirkhoda A, Bis KG, et al. Contrast-enhanced three dimensional MR angiography in a single breath-hold: a novel technique. *AJR Am J Roentgenol* 1995;165:1290–1292.
14. Sivananthan UM, Ridgway JP, Bann K, et al. Fast magnetic resonance angiography using turbo-FLASH sequences in advanced aortoiliac disease. *Br J Radiol* 1993;66:1103–1110.
15. Snidow JJ, Johnson MS, Harris VJ, et al. Three-dimensional gadolinium-enhanced MR angiography for aortoiliac inflow assessment plus renal artery screening in a single breath-hold. *Radiology* 1996;198:725–732.
16. Yucel EK. MR angiography for evaluation of abdominal aortic aneurysm: has the time come? *Radiology* 1994;192:321–323.
17. Lewin A, Blaufox MD, Castle H, et al. Apparent prevalence of curable hypertension in the Hypertension Detection and Follow-up Program. *Arch Intern Med* 1985;145:424–427.
18. Boudewijn G, Vasbinder C, Nelemans PJ, et al. Diagnostic tests for renal artery stenosis in patients suspected of having renovascular hypertension: a meta-analysis. *Ann Intern Med* 2001;135:401–411.
19. Holland BA, Dougherty L, Carpenter JP, et al. Breath-hold ultrafast three-dimensional gadolinium-enhanced MR angiography of the aorta and the renal and other visceral abdominal arteries. *AJR Am J Roentgenol* 1996;166:971–981.
20. Hany TF, Debatin JF, Leung DA, et al. Evaluation of the aortoiliac and renal arteries: comparison of breath-hold, contrast-enhanced, three-dimensional MR angiography with conventional catheter angiography. *Radiology* 1997;204:357–362.
21. De Cobelli F, Vanzulli A, Sironi S, et al. Renal artery stenosis: evaluation with breath-hold, three-dimensional, dynamic, gadolinium-enhanced versus three-dimensional, phase-contrast MR angiography. *Radiology* 1997;205:689–695.
22. Bakker J, Beek FJ, Beutler JJ, et al. Renal artery stenosis and accessory renal arteries: accuracy of detection and visualization with gadolinium-enhanced breath-hold MR angiography. *Radiology* 1998;207:497–504.
23. Walsh P, Rofsky NM, Krinsky GA, et al. Asymmetric signal intensity of the renal collecting systems as a sign of unilateral renal artery stenosis following administration of gadopentetate dimeglumine. *J Comput Assist Tomogr* 1996;20:812–814.
24. Schoenberg SO, Knopp MV, Bock M, et al. Renal artery stenosis: grading of hemodynamic changes with cine phase-contrast MR blood flow measurements. *Radiology* 1997;203:45–53.
25. Prince MR, Schoenberg SO, Ward JS, et al. Hemodynamically significant atherosclerotic renal artery stenosis: MR angiographic features. *Radiology* 1997;205:128–136.
26. Wasser MN, Westenberg J, van der Hulst VP, et al. Hemodynamic significance of renal artery stenosis: digital subtraction angiography versus systolically gated three-dimensional phase-contrast MR angiography. *Radiology* 1997;202:333–338.
27. Prince MR. Renal MR angiography: a comprehensive approach. *J Magn Reson Imaging* 1998;8:511–516.
28. Prince MR. Gadolinium-enhanced MR aortography. *Radiology* 1994;191:155–164.
29. Prince MR, Grist TM, Debatin JF. *Three-dimensional contrast MR angiography*, 2nd edition. Berlin:Springer-Verlag, 1998.

30. Leung DA, McKinnon GC, Davis CP, et al. Breath-hold, contrast-enhanced, three-dimensional MR angiography. *Radiology* 1996;200:569–571.

31. Rieumont MJ, Kaufman JA, Geller SC, et al. Evaluation of renal artery stenosis with dynamic gadolinium-enhanced MR angiography. *AJR Am J Roentgenol* 1997;169:39–44.

32. Hany TF, Leung DA, Pfammatter T, et al. Contrast-enhanced magnetic resonance angiography of the renal arteries. Original investigation. *Invest Radiol* 1998;33:653–665.

33. Gilfeather M, Yoon HC, Siegelman ES, et al. Renal artery stenosis: evaluation with conventional angiography versus gadolinium-enhanced MR angiography. *Radiology* 1999;210:367–372

34. Kim D, Edelman RR, Kent KC, et al. Abdominal aorta and renal artery stenosis: evaluation with MR angiography. *Radiology* 1990;174:727–731.

35. Debatin JF, Spritzer CE, Grist TM, et al. Imaging of the renal arteries: value of MR angiography. *AJR Am J Roentgenol* 1991; 157:981–990.

36. Kent KC, Edelman RR, Kim D, et al. Magnetic resonance imaging: a reliable test for the evaluation of proximal atherosclerotic renal arterial stenosis. *J Vasc Surg* 1991;13:311–318.

37. Gedroyc WM, Negus R, al-Kutoubi A, et al. Magnetic resonance angiography of renal transplants. *Lancet* 1992;339:789–791.

38. Grist TM. Magnetic resonance angiography of the aorta and renal arteries. *Magn Reson Imaging Clin N Am* 1993;1:253–269.

39. Yucel EK, Kaufman JA, Prince M, et al. Time of flight renal MR angiography: utility in patients with renal insufficiency. *Magn Reson Imaging* 1993;11:925–930.

40. Hertz SM, Holland GA, Baum RA, et al. Evaluation of renal artery stenosis by magnetic resonance angiography. *Am J Surg* 1994;168:140–143.

41. Loubeyre P, Revel D, Garcia P, et al. Screening patients for renal artery stenosis: value of three-dimensional time-of-flight MR angiography. *AJR Am J Roentgenol* 1994;162:847–852.

42. Servois V, Laissy JP, Feger C, et al. Two-dimensional time-of-flight magnetic resonance angiography of renal arteries without maximum intensity projection: a prospective comparison with angiography in 21 patients screened for renovascular hypertension. *Cardiovasc Intervent Radiol* 1994;17:138–142.

43. Fellner C, Strotzer M, Geissler A, et al. Renal arteries: evaluation with optimized 2D and 3D time-of-flight MR angiography. *Radiology* 1995;196:681–687.

44. Borrello JA, Li D, Vesely TM, et al. Renal arteries: clinical comparison of three-dimensional time-of-flight MR angiographic sequences and radiographic angiography. *Radiology* 1995;197: 793–799.

45. de Haan MW, Kouwenhoven M, Thelissen GR, et al. Renovascular disease in patients with hypertension: detection with systolic and diastolic gating in three-dimensional, phase-contrast MR angiography. *Radiology* 1996;198:449–456.

46. Loubeyre P, Trolliet P, Cahen R, et al. MR angiography of renal artery stenosis: value of the combination of three-dimensional time-of-flight and three-dimensional phase-contrast MR angiography sequences. *AJR Am J Roentgenol* 1996;167:489–494.

47. Silverman JM, Friedman ML, Van Allan RJ. Detection of main renal artery stenosis using phase-contrast cine MR angiography. *AJR Am J Roentgenol* 1996;166:1131–1137.

48. Duda SH, Schick F, Teufl F, et al. Phase-contrast MR angiography for detection of arteriosclerotic renal artery stenosis. *Acta Radiol* 1997;38:287–291.

49. Gedroyc WM, Neerhut P, Negus R, et al. Magnetic resonance angiography of renal artery stenosis. *Clin Radiol* 1995;50:436–439.

50. Prince MR. Body MR angiography with gadolinium contrast agents. *Magn Reson Imaging Clin N Am* 1996;4:11–24

51. Maki JH, Chenevert TL, Prince MR. Contrast-enhanced MR angiography. *Abdom Imaging* 1998;23:469–484.

52. Snidow JJ, Johnson MS, Harris VJ, et al. Three-dimensional gadolinium-enhanced MR angiography for aortoiliac inflow assessment plus renal artery screening in a single breath-hold. *Radiology* 1996;198:725–732.

53. Dong Q, Schoenberg SO, Carlos RC, et al. Diagnosis of renal vascular disease with MR angiography. *RadioGraphics* 1999;19:1535–1554.

54. Schoenberg SO, Knopp MV, Prince MR, et al. Arterial-phase three-dimensional gadolinium magnetic resonance angiography of the renal arteries. Strategies for timing and contrast media injection: original investigation. *Invest Radiol* 1998;33:506–514.

55. Schoenberg SO, Prince MR, Knopp MV, et al. Renal MR angiography. *Magn Reson Imaging Clin N Am* 1998;6:351–370.

56. Steffens JC, Link J, Grassner J, et al. Contrast-enhanced, k-space-centered, breath-hold MR angiography of the renal arteries and the abdominal aorta. *J Magn Reson Imaging* 1997;7:617–622.

57. Schoenberg SO, Bock M, Knopp MV, et al. Renal arteries: optimization of three-dimensional gadolinium-enhanced MR angiography with bolus-timing-independent fast multiphase acquisition in a single breath-hold. *Radiology* 1999;211:667–679.

58. Carlos RC, Stanley JC, Stafford-Johnson D, Prince MR. Interobserver variability in the evaluation of chronic mesenteric ischemia with gadolinium-enhanced MR angiography. *Acad Radiol* 2001;8:879–887.

59. Prince MR, Arnoldus C, Frisoli JF. Nephrotoxicity of high-dose gadolinium compared to iodinated contrast. *J Magn Reson Imaging* 1996;6:162–166.

60. Bass JC, Prince MR, Londy FJ, et al. Effect of gadolinium on phase-contrast MR angiography of the renal arteries. *AJR Am J Roentgenol* 1997;168:261–266.

61. Ros PR, Gauger J, Stoupis C, et al. Diagnosis of renal artery stenosis: feasibility of combining MR angiography, MR renography, and gadopentetate-based measurements of glomerular filtration rate. *AJR Am J Roentgenol* 1995;165:1447–1451.

62. Lee VS, Rofsky NM, Ton AT, et al. Angiotensin-converting enzyme inhibitor-enhanced phase-contrast MR imaging to measure renal artery velocity waveforms in patients with suspected renovascular hypertension. *AJR Am J Roentgenol* 2000;174:499–508.

63. Niendorf ER, Grist TM, Lee FT, et al. Rapid *in vivo* measurement of single-kidney extraction fraction and glomerular filtration rate with MR imaging. *Radiology* 1998;206:791–798.

64. Marks B, Mitchell DG, Simelaro JP. Breath-holding in healthy and pulmonary-compromised populations: effects of hyperventilation and oxygen inspiration. *J Magn Reson Imaging* 1997;7:595–597.

65. Maki JH, Chenevert TL, Prince MR. The effects of incomplete breath-holding on 3D MR imaging quality. *J Magn Reson Imaging* 1997;7:1132–1139.

66. Prince MR, Chenevert TL, Foo TK, et al. Contrast-enhanced abdominal MR angiography: optimization of imaging delay time by automating the detection of contrast material arrival in the aorta. *Radiology* 1997;203:109–114.

67. Wilman AH, Riederer SJ, King BF, et al. Fluoroscopically triggered contrast-enhanced three-dimensional MR angiography with elliptical centric view order: application to the renal arteries. *Radiology* 1997;205:137–146.

68. Rofsky NM, DeCorato DR, Krinsky GA, et al. Hepatic arterial-phase dynamic gadolinium-enhanced MR imaging: optimization with a test examination and a power injector. *Radiology* 1997;202:268–273.

69. Kadir S. *Atlas of normal and variant angiographic anatomy.* Philadelphia: WB Saunders, 1991:388.

70. Grenier N, Trillaud H, Combe C, et al. Diagnosis of renovascular hypertension: feasibility of captopril-sensitized dynamic MR imaging and comparison with captopril scintigraphy. *AJR Am J Roentgenol* 1996;166:835–843.

71. Lüscher TF, Lie JT, Stanson AW, et al. Arterial fibromuscular dysplasia. *Mayo Clin Proc* 1987;62:931–952.

72. Williams DM, Lee DY, Hamilton BH, et al. The dissected aorta. Part III. Anatomy and radiologic diagnosis of branch-vessel compromise. *Radiology* 1997;203:37–44.

73. Kincaid OW. *Renal angiography.* Chicago: Year Book, 1966:124–125.

74. Kallman DA, King BF, Hattery RR, et al. Renal vein and inferior vena cava tumor thrombus in renal cell carcinoma: CT, US, MRI, and venacavography. *J Comput Assist Tomogr* 1992;16:240–247.

75. Li KC, Whitney WS, McDonnell CH, et al. Chronic mesenteric ischemia: evaluation with phase-contrast cine MR imaging. *Radiology* 1994;190:175–179.

76. Li KC, Dalman RL, Ch'en IY, et al. Chronic mesenteric ischemia: use of *in vivo* MR imaging measurements of blood oxygen saturation in the superior mesenteric vein for diagnosis. *Radiology* 1997;204:71–77.

77. Li KC, Pelc LR, Dalman RL, et al. *In vivo* magnetic resonance evaluation of blood oxygen saturation in the superior mesenteric vein as a measure of the degree of acute flow reduction in the superior mesenteric artery: findings in a canine model. *Acad Radiol* 1997;4:21–25.

78. Dalman RL, Li KC, Moon WK, et al. Diminished postprandial hyperemia in patients with aortic and mesenteric arterial occlusive disease. Quantification by magnetic resonance flow imaging. *Circulation* 1996;94(9 Suppl):II206–II210.

79. Li KC, Hopkins KL, Dalman RL, et al. Simultaneous measurement of flow in the superior mesenteric vein and artery with cine phase-contrast MR imaging: value in diagnosis of chronic mesenteric ischemia. Work in progress. *Radiology* 1995;194:327–330.

80. Li KC, Whitney WS, McDonnell CH, et al. Chronic mesenteric ischemia: evaluation with phase-contrast cine MR imaging. *Radiology* 1994;190:175–179.

81. Li KC, Wright GA, Pelc LR, et al. Oxygen saturation of blood in the superior mesenteric vein: *in vivo* verification of MR imaging measurements in a canine model. Work in progress. *Radiology* 1995;194:321–325.

82. De Cobelli F, Venturini M, Vanzulli A, et al. Renal arterial stenosis: prospective comparison of color Doppler US and breath-hold, three-dimensional, dynamic, gadolinium-enhanced MR angiography. *Radiology* 2000;214:373–380.

83. Hahn U, Miller S, Nagele T, et al. Renal MR angiography at 1.0 tesla: three-dimensional (3D) phase contrast techniques versus gadolinium enhanced 3D fast low angle shot breath-hold imaging. *AJR Am Roentgenol* 1999:172:1501–1508.

84. Westenberg JJ, Van der Geest RJ, Wasser MN, et al. Stenosis quantification from post-stenotic signal loss in phase-contrast MRA data sets of flow phantoms and renal arteries. *Int J Card Imaging* 1999;15:483–493.

85. Nelson HA, Gilfeather M, Holman JM, et al. Gadolinium-enhanced breath-hold three-dimensional time-of-flight renal MR angiography in the evaluation of potential renal donors. *J Vasc Interv Radiol* 1999;10(2 Pt1):175–181.

86. Thornton MJ, Thornton F, O'Callaghan J, et al. Evaluation of dynamic gadolinium-enhanced breath-hold MR angiography in the diagnosis of renal artery stenosis. *AJR Am J Roentgenol* 1999;173:1279–1283.

87. Schoenberg SO, Essig M, Bock M, et al. Comprehensive MR evaluation of renovascular disease in five breath holds. *J Magn Reson Imaging* 1999;10:347–356.

88. Thornton J, O'Callaghan J, Walshe J, et al. Comparison of digital subtraction angiography with gadolinium-enhanced magnetic resonance angiography in the diagnosis of renal artery stenosis. *Eur Radiol* 1999;9:930–934.

89. Cambria RP, Kaufman JL, Brewster DC, et al. Surgical renal artery reconstruction without contrast arteriography: the role of clinical profiling and magnetic resonance angiography. *J Vasc Surg* 1999;29:1012–1021.

90. Ghantous VE, Eisen TD, Sherman Ah, et al. Evaluating patients with renal failure for renal artery stenosis with gadolinium-enhanced magnetic resonance angiography. *Am J Kidney Dis* 1999;33:36–42.

91. Marchand B, Hernandez-Hoyos M, Orkisz M, et al. Diagnosis of renal artery stenosis with magnetic resonance angiography and stenosis quantification [Review; 36 references; in French]. *J Mal Vasc* 2000;25:312–320.

92. Shetty AN, Bis KG, Kirsch M, et al. Contrast-enhanced breath-hold three-dimensional magnetic resonance angiography in the evaluation of renal arteries: optimization of technique and pitfalls. *J Magn Reson Imaging* 2000;12:912–923.

93. Winterer JT, Strey C, Wolffram C, et al. Preoperative examination of potential kidney transplantation donors: value of gadolinium-enhanced 3D MR angiography in comparison with DSA and urography [in German]. *Fortschritte auf dem Gebiete der Rontgenstrahlen und der Neuen Bildgebenden Verfahren* 2000;172:449–457.

94. Weishaupt D, Ruhm SG, Binkert CA, et al. Equilibrium-phase MR angiography of the aortoiliac and renal arteries using a blood pool contrast agent. *AJR Am J Roentgenol* 2000;175:189–195.

95. Bongers V, Bakker J, Beutler JJ, et al. Assessment of renal artery stenosis: comparison of captopril renography and gadolinium-enhanced breath-hold MR angiography. *Clin Radiol* 2000;55:346–353.

96. Volk M, Strotzer M, Lenhart M, et al. Time-resolved contrast-enhanced MR angiography of renal artery stenosis: diagnostic accuracy and interobserver variability. *AJR Am J Roentgenol* 2000;174:1583–1588.

97. Oberholzer K, Kreitner KF, Kalden P, et al. Contrast-enhanced MR angiography of abdominal vessels using a 1 tesla system [in German]. *Rofo Fortschr Geb Rontgenstr Neuen Bildgeb Verfahr* 2000;172:134–138.

98. Korst MB, Joosten FB, Postma CT, et al. Accuracy of normal-dose contrast-enhanced MR angiography in assessing renal artery stenosis and accessory renal arteries. *AJR Am J Roentgenol* 2000;174:629–634.

99. De Cobelli F, Venturini M, Vanzulli A, et al. Renal arterial stenosis: prospective comparison of color Doppler US and breath-hold, three-dimensional, dynamic, gadolinium-enhanced MR angiography. *Radiology* 2000;214:373–380.

100. Chan YL, Leung CB, Yu SC, et al. Comparison of non-breath-hold high-resolution gadolinium-enhanced MRA with digital subtraction angiography in the evaluation on allograft renal artery stenosis. *Clin Radiol* 2001;56:127–132.

101. Gedroyc WM, Negus R, al-Kutoubi A, et al. Magnetic resonance angiography of renal transplants. *Lancet* 1992;339:789–791.

102. Smith HJ, Bakke SJ. MR angiography of in situ and transplant renal arteries. Early experience using a three-dimensional time-of-flight technique. *Acta Radiol* 1993:34:150–155.

103. Johnson DB, Lerner CA, Prince MR, et al. Gadolinium-enhanced magnetic resonance angiography of renal transplants. *Magn Reson Imaging* 1997;15:13–20.

104. Ferreiros J, Mendea R, Jorquera M, et al. Using gadolinium-enhanced three-dimensional MR angiography to assess arterial in-

flow stenosis after kidney transplantation. *AJR Am J Roentgenol* 1999;172:751–757.

105. Luk SH, Chan JH, Kwan TH, et al. Breath-hold 3D gadolinium-enhanced subtraction MRA in the detection of transplant renal artery stenosis. *Clin Radiol* 1999; 54:651–654.

106. Meaney JF, Prince MR, Nostrant TT, et al. Gadolinium-enhanced MR angiography of visceral arteries in patients with suspected chronic mesenteric ischemia. *J Magn Reson Imaging* 1997;7:171–176.

107. Miyazaki T, Yamashita Y, Shinzato J, et al. Two-dimensional time-of-flight magnetic resonance angiography in the coronal plane for abdominal disease: its usefulness and comparison with conventional angiography. *Br J Radiol* 1995;68:351–357.

108. Durham JR, Hackworth CA, Tober JC, et al. Magnetic resonance angiography in the preoperative evaluation of abdominal aortic aneurysm. *Am J Surg* 1993;166:173–177.

109. Qanadli SD, Souliz G, Therasse E, et al. Detection of renal artery stenosis: prospective comparison of captopril enhanced Doppler sonography, captopril enhanced scintigraphy and MR angiography. *AJR Am J Roentgenol* 2001;177:1123–1129.

110. Voiculescu A, Hofer M, Hetzel GR, et al. Noninvasive investigation for renal artery stenosis: contrast-enhanced MRA and color Doppler sonography as compared to DSA. *Clin Exp Hypertens* 2001;23:521–531.

111. Mittal TK, Evans C, Perkins T, et al. Renal arteriography using gadolinium enhanced 3D MR angiography—clinical experience with the technique, its limitations and pitfalls. *Br J Radiol* 2001;74:495–502.

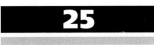

MRA OF PERIPHERAL ARTERIES

MARTIN N. WASSER

As the average age of the population in the industrialized world increases, atherosclerotic disease of the peripheral vessels is gaining importance. Although atherosclerotic lesions occur in all vascular territories, the lower limbs are affected in 90% of cases. Presently, atherosclerosis in the lower limbs accounts for 50,000 to 60,000 percutaneous angioplasties, the implantation of 110,000 vascular prostheses, and 100,000 amputations annually in the United States (1).

Before therapeutic actions can be planned, detailed information on the localization, extent, and severity of disease is essential. Conventional angiography has long served as the imaging modality of choice in this respect. However, x-ray angiography has definite risks and limitations, including the possibility of a severe reaction to the contrast medium, even when nonionic agents are used (2). Also, because approximately 70% of patients with severe occlusive peripheral disease have evidence of impaired renal function (3), contrast-induced renal insufficiency is a matter of concern. Therefore, noninvasive alternatives such as duplex ultrasonography and MRA are increasingly used in the diagnostic workup of patients with peripheral arterial disease.

Contrast-enhanced MRA has rapidly emerged as an attractive alternative to conventional angiography. The reason for this rapid acceptance in the "vascular community" is the close resemblance of images obtained with contrast-enhanced MRA to those obtained with conventional angiography. It has been shown that the contrast agent Gd-DTPA (gadolinium diethylenetriamine pentaacetic acid) in the doses used for MRA is not nephrotoxic (4). This means that patients with impaired renal function can also be examined with contrast-enhanced MRA.

Unlike phase-contrast (PC) MRA and time-of-flight (TOF) MRA, which are older MRA techniques, contrast-enhanced MRA does not suffer from artifacts caused by turbulence and in-plane saturation. For this reason, contrast-enhanced MR angiograms are easier to interpret than PC or TOF MR angiograms. Also, the lack of in-plane saturation makes it possible to image in the coronal plane, so that much larger anatomic regions can be covered. In general, the most important advantage of contrast-enhanced MRA in comparison with conventional MRA is the enormous reduction in examination time. An important reason for the long acquisition times in conventional MRA is the need to obtain images in the transverse plane to circumvent in-plane saturation. Because the flow pattern in the peripheral vessels is triphasic (diastolic flow reversal), cardiac triggering must be performed in conventional MRA to prevent erroneous signal loss (5). Such cardiac triggering further lengthens the study.

Two studies have directly compared the best conventional MRA technique, cardiac-triggered two-dimensional (2D) TOF MRA, with contrast-enhanced MRA (6,7). These two studies were included in a metaanalysis in which the results of 21 studies of peripheral MRA published from January 1991 through June 1999 were evaluated (8). In 11 of the other 19 studies, only 2D TOF MRA was applied, and in 8 of the 19, only 3D gadolinium-enhanced MRA was used.

The sensitivity for detecting hemodynamically significant stenosis (>50% luminal reduction) was between 64% and 100% for 2D TOF MRA and between 92% and 100% for 3D contrast-enhanced MRA. The specificity was between 68% and 96% for 2D TOF MRA and between 91% and 99% for 3D contrast-enhanced MRA. These figures indicate that 3D contrast-enhanced MRA is superior to 2D TOF MRA for the detection of peripheral arterial disease. Especially for imaging the proximal vessels in the legs, 2D TOF MRA appears to be less reliable (sensitivity, 83% to 100%; specificity, 23% to 98%). In tortuous, elongated iliac arteries, false-positive results of 2D TOF MRA may be caused by in-plane saturation or saturation of the arterial signal by the venous presaturation slab. Short segments of

M. N. Wasser: Department of Radiology, Leiden University Medical Center, Leiden, The Netherlands.

signal void may be caused by either a short occlusion or a severe stenosis. Also, retrograde flow may not be recognized because of the venous presaturation slab.

From the only two of the 10 studies included in the meta-analysis in which 3D contrast-enhanced MRA was evaluated, data were extracted describing the accuracy of contrast-enhanced MRA in detecting disease in the femoropopliteal and infrapopliteal regions. In these regions, contrast-enhanced MRA also appeared to perform better than 2D TOF MRA. The sensitivity was between 88% and 92% for 2D TOF MRA and between 94% and 100% for contrast-enhanced MRA in evaluation of the femoropopliteal region (specificity, 82% to 98% vs. 97% to 99%). For the infrapopliteal vessels, the sensitivity and specificity were 89% to 98% and 91% to 95%, respectively, for 2D TOF MRA, and they were 91% to 94% and 100%, respectively, for contrast-enhanced MRA. Contrast-enhanced MRA is therefore the best MRA technique for evaluating arterial disease in the lower limbs in terms of time savings and accuracy.

No data are available for the accuracy of MRA in evaluating arterial disease in the upper limbs. Although conventional MRA and contrast-enhanced MRA have not been compared, there is no reason to doubt that contrast-enhanced MRA is also the best technique for studying arteries in this territory. Like the arteries in the lower extremities, arteries in the arms show a triphasic, high-resistance flow pattern with identical artifacts on conventional MRA.

This chapter provides an overview of the techniques and indications for contrast-enhanced MRA of the peripheral arteries in both the legs and arms. Although atherosclerosis is the major cause of peripheral arterial disease, other abnormalities are also addressed.

TECHNIQUES FOR PERIPHERAL CONTRAST-ENHANCED MRA

Basics

The basic principle behind contrast-enhanced MRA is imaging the arterial first pass of paramagnetic contrast agent in the vessels after intravenous injection (9). The injected contrast agent causes a pronounced shortening of the T1 relaxation time of blood. This results in high signal intensity of the arteries on T1-weighted spoiled gradient-echo images. The delay between arterial and venous enhancement provides a time window for purely arterial imaging. This time window depends not only on the rate of injection of the contrast agent but also on the anatomic region being imaged. In the upper limbs, venous return is much faster than in the lower limbs, so that a much shorter measurement time is required. Because the technique depends on imaging of the first pass of contrast agent, correct timing of the start of image acquisition after the injection is essential. Various techniques have been developed to calculate this so-called scan delay, which are explained below.

The quality of MRA images with regard to selective arterial visualization, resolution, and volume-of-interest depends both on the sequence parameters used and on the geometry of the bolus of contrast medium. Arterial enhancement depends on individual physiologic parameters, such as cardiac output and blood volume, and also on parameters of contrast agent application, which can be manipulated (flow rate, dose, and volume of saline flush). The T1 shortening of blood depends on the intravascular concentration of the contrast agent, which in its turn depends on the rate of injection. In general, the faster the injection rate, the higher the concentration will be, although rates exceeding 5 mL/s do not result in further increases in signal intensity. In fact, the intravascular signal may become lower at rates faster than 6 mL/s (10). On the other hand, a faster infusion rate results in faster venous return and a shorter bolus length, so that a shorter measurement time is required. A compromise between imaging time, resolution, and the arterial–venous time window must always be sought. The scan duration for imaging of the relatively large subclavian and brachial arteries can be relatively short because the scan volume can be moderately small and spatial resolution does not have to be optimized. Therefore, in the upper limbs, a flow rate of 2 to 3 mL/s is recommended. The arterial–venous time window is much longer in the lower limbs than in the upper limbs, so that longer imaging times are possible. These longer scan times are required anyway because the level of spatial resolution must be high to depict the small infrapopliteal arteries. Therefore, in the lower extremities, injection rates of 0.5 to 1.5 mL/s are used.

A heavily T1-weighted spoiled gradient-echo sequence [short TR (repetition time)/TE (echo time), flip angle of 25 to 50 degrees] is used in which the achievable field of view, matrix size, scan volume, and number of partitions are determined by the arterial–venous time interval. Subtraction of precontrast and postcontrast images is performed to visualize only the arteries for greater ease of image interpretation and reduction of artifacts (6) (Fig. 25.1). The obtained volumetric data set containing the high-intensity voxels corresponding to arteries can be postprocessed with the maximum intensity projection (MIP) algorithm. For a superior diagnostic performance, review of the individual source images or reformatting of images in the transverse plane is required.

Timing of Image Acquisition

In contrast-enhanced MRA, adequate timing of the start of data acquisition to coincide with the arrival of contrast agent in the vessels-of-interest is essential. It is crucial that the arterial enhancement coincide with the acquisition of central k-lines. Furthermore, for good arterial–venous differentiation, the central k-lines must be sampled before venous return. Three methods have been developed to ensure proper timing.

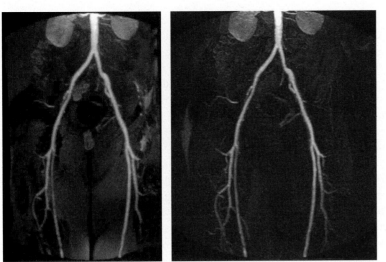

A,B

FIGURE 25.1. Nonsubtracted **(A)** and subtracted **(B)** contrast-enhanced MRA images of the aortoiliac region. The subtracted image shows higher a contrast-to-background ratio. More vessels can be seen on the subtracted image.

Test Bolus

Adequate timing can be achieved by measuring the circulation time after the intravenous injection of a small test bolus (1 to 2 mL) of contrast agent and the application of a rapid dynamic imaging sequence. With this dynamic series, the arrival of the test bolus after injection in the region-of-interest can be imaged, and the scan delay can then be calculated. To avoid pooling of the test bolus in veins, the tubing must be flushed with saline solution. Both the test bolus and the final infusion should be injected at the same rate. This timing method is fairly robust and easy to perform. A disadvantage is that it requires the administration of additional contrast agent. It lengthens the total procedure time by 2 to 3 minutes. Also, in patients with irregular heart action, the circulation time calculated from the test bolus may differ from that during injection of the final bolus.

Fluoroscopic Triggering

Fast imaging sequences can be used to visualize the influx of contrast into the region-of-interest. MRA data acquisition is then started automatically [SmartPrep; GE Medical Systems (11)] or manually [Bolus track; Philips Medical Systems (12)]. A disadvantage of this method is that a delay of 2 to 4 seconds occurs between visualization of the arrival of the contrast bolus and the actual start of acquisition. Also, the time for instructing the patient about breathing, if required, may be too short.

Time-Resolved Imaging

With ongoing improvements in hardware and gradient technology, the time required to image a large volume-of-interest with high resolution has been greatly reduced. At present, it is possible to image a coronal slab large enough to cover the entire anteroposterior diameter of the legs in 6 sec-

onds (13). Therefore, if a dynamic volumetric series is performed after the intravenous injection of the contrast agent, the arterial phase will always be included in one of the data sets, so that the need for bolus timing is obviated.

Imaging Strategies

Upper Limbs

For imaging the subclavian and brachial arteries, a moderately thick slab of 80 to 90 mm is required. Precontrast and postcontrast images are obtained during breath-holding. A bolus of 0.1 or 0.2 mmol of contrast agent per kilogram is injected at a rate of 2 to 3 mL/s. Venous overlap can be avoided by injecting contrast agent in the contralateral arm. Use of a body phased-array coil results in a higher signal-to-noise ratio.

Imaging the small vessels in the hand requires high-spatial-resolution scanning with the use of a head coil or preferably dedicated surface coils. The arteriovenous transit time in the hands is short (~12 seconds) and differs between the two hands in almost all cases (mean difference, 4.5 seconds) (14). Imaging the arteries in the hand requires accurate timing of the start of imaging with the use of elliptically reordered k-space sampling (14).

Lower Limbs

To image the leg vessels, a large anatomic region (~100 cm) must be covered. Because the longitudinal field of view of MR systems is limited to 45 to 50 cm, complete imaging of the lower extremity requires that several regions, or "stations," be imaged. This means that the patient must be repositioned to the isocenter of the magnet. Two methods for imaging the entire leg have been developed, so-called multistation imaging and the bolus chase method. In both techniques, one has to ensure sufficient overlap between the separate stations.

Multistation Imaging

In this technique, the three regions of the leg (aortoiliac, femoropopliteal, and infrapopliteal vessels) are imaged sequentially with two or three separate bolus injections of contrast medium (15). Imaging each station involves the acquisition of a mask data set, which is subtracted from the subsequent images obtained after contrast injection. Contrast agent can be injected at moderately high rates of 1 to 1.5 mL/s to ensure high signal intensity in the vessels. The advantage of this technique is that it can be applied on any clinical scanner without the use of special hardware, and imaging parameters can be tailored to every single station. The multistation technique, however, is not very time-efficient (30 to 45 minutes per patient), a total dose of contrast agent of 0.2 to 0.3 mmol/kg is required, and the contrast-to-noise ratio of the subtracted images becomes less at the second and third station because of circulating gadolinium (16) (Fig. 25.2). Using larger doses in the subsequent stages can partly circumvent this decrease in signal intensity. Surface coils can be used to image the different stations.

Bolus Chase or Stepping-Table Technique

In this technique, mask images of all three stations of the leg are made first (12,17–19). Then, during a slow, constant infusion of contrast agent, the flow of contrast through the leg is chased with a floating table. The technique requires the application of special hardware to move the table to predefined positions. Homemade table-stopping devices or special MR table hardware can be used. The advantage of the moving-table technique is that it is very rapid, covering the entire leg in less than 4 minutes, and requires a relatively low dose of contrast agent (approximately 30 mL).

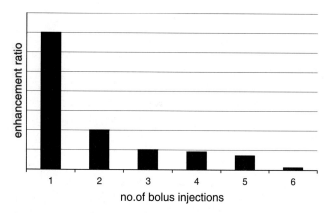

FIGURE 25.2. Enhancement ratios of subtracted images after repeated injection of Gd-DTPA (gadolinium diethylenetriamine pentaacetic acid) in a flowing phantom model. Repeated injections substantially reduce contrast-to-noise ratios. However, extravasation of contrast agent occurs *in vivo*. The effect of the intravascular accumulation of contrast is therefore lower *in vivo*. (From Watanabe Y, Dohke M, Okumura A, et al. Dynamic subtraction contrast-enhanced MR angiography: technique, clinical applications, and pitfalls. *Radiographics* 2000;20:135–152, with permission.)

Formerly, a disadvantage of the stepping-table technique was that the three stations were imaged sequentially although the scan preparation had been optimized for only a single station. Recently, the method has become more flexible (12), and even dedicated surface coils can be used (20).

Up to now no studies have compared the two methods.

Image Presentation

To encourage acceptance of the technique by referring clinicians, one has to provide them with images to which they are accustomed and that appear similar to conventional angiograms. The number of images should be limited as a practical concern for vascular surgeons. The images should be large so that they can be viewed from a distance; a four-on-one to six-on-one printing format should be used. Also, bony landmarks should be provided for better orientation, as on conventional angiograms (Fig. 25.3).

Pitfalls

Although signal loss caused by turbulence and in-plane saturation is usually not a problem in contrast-enhanced MRA, the length of a stenosis can still be overestimated, especially if velocities are high at the stenotic area and the concentration of contrast material is low (21).

Other artifacts can be encountered in contrast-enhanced MRA. In the subclavian region, for instance, susceptibility artifacts in the subclavian vein may cause signal void and artificial stenosis of the adjacent artery (22).

If the contrast agent arrives in the vessel-of-interest *after* sampling of the central k-lines as a consequence of improper timing, a central dark line may be seen in the vessel, a so-called pseudodissection (23).

Care must be taken to include all vessels-of-interest in the imaging volume. Inappropriate image coverage may create the appearance of occlusion of tortuous arteries, such as the external iliac arteries (24). It is therefore recommended that sagittal or transverse views also be obtained to demonstrate the entire imaging volume (Fig. 25.4).

Sometimes, a ghost or phase artifact can be seen parallel to vessels with very high signal intensity (23) (Fig. 25.5). Also, subtraction misregistration artifact may occur. Clips and metallic stents may cause signal voids resulting from susceptibility artifacts (Fig. 26.6).

CLINICAL APPLICATIONS OF PERIPHERAL MRA

Upper Limbs

Subclavian Steal Syndrome

Obstruction of the subclavian artery may give rise to the so-called subclavian steal syndrome. Blood supply to the arm is

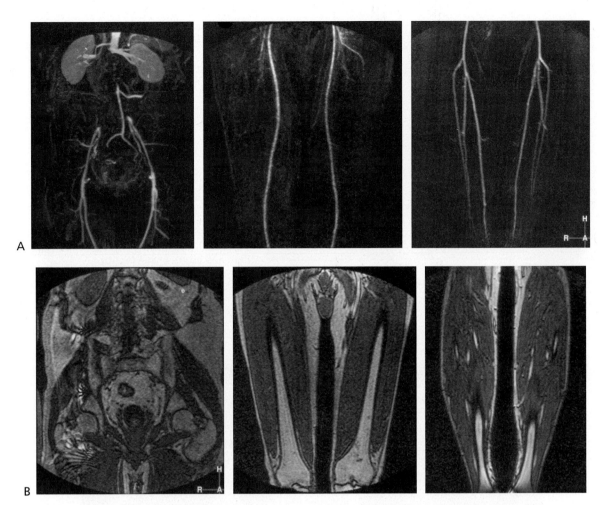

FIGURE 25.3. Peripheral MRA of the lower limbs in a patient with occlusion of the distal aorta and proximal common iliac arteries **(A)**. The nonsubtracted source images provide bony landmarks, especially of the joints **(B)**.

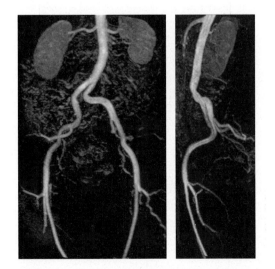

FIGURE 25.4. Coronal *(left)* and sagittal *(right)* contrast-enhanced MRA maximum intensity projection images of the aortoiliac region. The sagittal view especially shows the elongated external iliac arteries in this patient.

maintained by retrograde flow in the ipsilateral vertebral artery to the subclavian artery distal to the obstruction. Therefore, vertebrobasilar hypoperfusion may develop in patients with proximal subclavian artery stenosis when the ipsilateral arm is exercised. Contrast-enhanced MRA can demonstrate stenosis/occlusion in the proximal subclavian artery (Fig. 25.7), and retrograde flow in the vertebral arteries can be demonstrated in the same session with velocity mapping (25).

Takayasu Arteritis

Takayasu disease is a primary arteritis of unknown cause. It affects the aorta and its major branches in addition to the pulmonary artery. Stenosis is the most common angiographic finding in the aorta and its branches (Figs. 25.7 and 25.8), but occlusion, aneurysm, and dilatation may also be found (26) (Fig. 25.9). Conventional angiography in these patients is not without risk; the increased frequency of is-

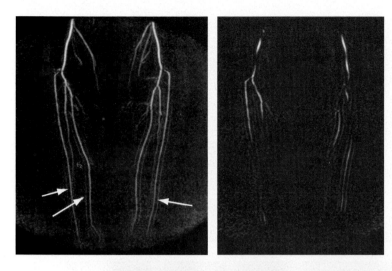

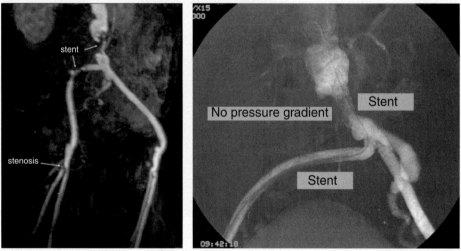

FIGURE 25.5. Example of ghost artifacts in images of the lower limbs *(arrows)*. Maximum intensity projection *(left)* and source image *(right)*.

FIGURE 25.6. Patient with aortoiliac bifurcation prosthesis and implanted stents in the distal aorta and right iliac leg of the prosthesis. At MRA *(left)*, susceptibility artifacts falsely suggest significant stenoses in the stents, but no pressure gradient was found on angiography *(right)*.

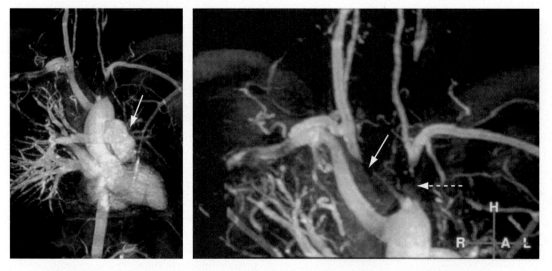

FIGURE 25.7. Stenosis at the origin of the left subclavian artery *(dashed arrow, right image)*. Distal filling of the subclavian artery by retrograde flow in the left vertebral artery (subclavian steal). This patient with Takayasu disease also has a common origin of the left and right carotid arteries with occlusion on the left and severe stenosis on the right *(arrow, right image)*. Occlusion of the left pulmonary artery *(arrow, left image)* is pathognomonic for Takayasu disease.

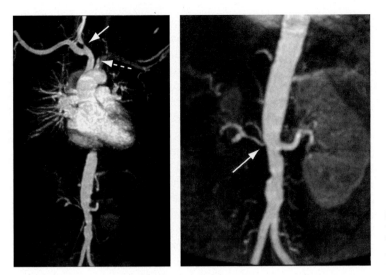

FIGURE 25.8. Patient with Takayasu disease. Stenosis in the right carotid artery *(arrow, left image)* and occlusion of the left carotid artery and left subclavian artery *(dashed arrow)*. In addition, a stenosis can be seen in the right renal artery *(arrow, right image).*

chemic complications is probably related to increased coagulative activity of their blood (26). In a study of 20 patients with Takayasu disease, all 80 lesions in the aorta and its branch vessels were detected with contrast-enhanced MRA (27). However, seven (9%) stenotic lesions in the branch vessels were overestimated as occlusions. This may have been related to a limitation in resolution. The advantage of contrast-enhanced MRA is that it can also demonstrate lesions in the pulmonary artery (Fig. 25.7). Pulmonary artery disease is specific to Takayasu arteritis and is not seen in atherosclerosis or other diseases in which systemic arterial lesions are present (28). Early inflammation of the aortic wall can be demonstrated by transverse spin-echo images after contrast injection (29).

Thoracic Outlet Syndrome

In thoracic outlet syndrome, neurovascular signs and symptoms result from compression of the subclavian vessels or brachial plexus in the costoclavicular area, caused by anatomically variable osseous structures in the region or by broad insertion of the scalenus muscle anteriorly on the clavicle. These patients may experience pain in the arm during elevation and a loss of sensation in the arm during exercise; a palpable thrill over the subclavian artery, diminished radial pulses, and a lowered brachial blood pressure may be present. Although in this syndrome neural compression is much more common than vascular compression, stenosis in the subclavian artery can be demonstrated by contrast-enhanced MRA.

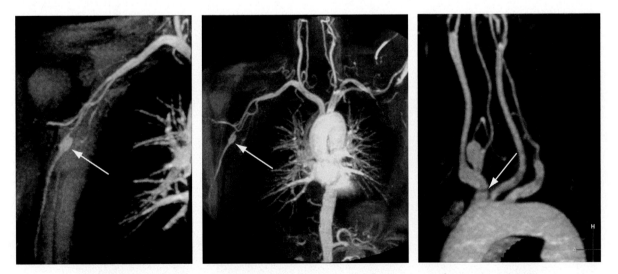

FIGURE 25.9. MRA of patient with Takayasu disease. Septal stenosis in the right brachiocephalic artery *(arrow, right image)* and aneurysm of the right brachial artery *(arrow, left and middle images).*

Dymarkowsky et al. (30) found arterial compression in three of five patients suspected of having a thoracic outlet syndrome. They performed time-resolved contrast-enhanced MRA of the subclavian arteries during adduction and hyperabduction of the arms. The cause of compression may be visible on T1-weighted spin-echo images.

Pathology of Hand Vessels

Atherosclerosis in the hand vessels is rare. Possible reasons to image the hand vessels are suspected presence of emboli from cardiac disease or atherosclerotic lesions in the subclavian artery, Raynaud syndrome, scleroderma, rheumatoid arthritis, vasculitis, and trauma. MRA of the hand vessels is still a challenge because of the limited arterial–venous time window and the need for high-resolution imaging.

Lower Limbs

Atherosclerosis

Atherosclerosis is a systemic process that may cause stenosis, occlusion, or aneurysmal dilatation of the affected arteries.

Steno-occlusive Disease

In patients with acute limb-threatening ischemia, angiographic imaging is performed as soon as possible, followed by thrombolytic therapy in the same session. MRA has no role in the management of this condition.

In patients with chronic ischemia, however, MRA has emerged as a valuable pretreatment alternative to catheter angiography. In analyzing MR angiograms of the lower limbs of patients with intermittent claudication, one must first understand what the treating physician wants to know. In other words, one has to "think like a vascular radiologist" and be familiar with the clinical issues and potential treatment options (31). It is important to analyze the proximal

inflow to a lesion, the distal outflow from the lesion, and the lesion itself. If the inflow is impaired, a distal arterial reconstruction may be endangered. On the other hand, if the outflow is limited, a proximal reconstruction may be compromised. A general rule in vascular surgery is to treat the most proximal lesions first because they usually have the greatest impact on flow to the limbs.

Regarding the lesion itself, it is important to report the localization, severity, and length of the stenosis. In general, hemodynamically significant stenoses, usually defined as luminal narrowings of more than 50%, require treatment. In cases of borderline stenosis (40% to 60%), it may be difficult to determine the hemodynamic significance of a lesion. However, the same holds true with conventional angiography, and in such cases, the intravascular pressure is measured to assess the hemodynamic implications of a lesion (32). In almost all studies evaluating the value of MRA, conventional digital subtraction angiography (DSA) is taken as the standard of reference. This standard, however, may not be as "gold" as one is inclined to believe. Eccentric plaques in the large proximal vessels may not be detected by DSA because the number of projections is limited (Fig. 25.10). In the renal arteries, we found a sensitivity of only 70% for DSA in the detection of hemodynamically significant stenoses in comparison with intravascular pressure measurement (33). In the iliac arteries, Wikström et al. (34) found sensitivities/specificities of 86%/88% for DSA, 81%/75% for MRA, and 72%/88% for duplex Doppler ultrasonography in the detection of significant stenoses when they used an aortofemoral pressure gradient of 20 mm Hg to indicate hemodynamic significance. Conventional angiography is probably also not an adequate standard of reference in analyzing runoff vessels; contrast-enhanced MRA demonstrated more patent vessels than did conventional angiography (35,36) (Fig. 25.11).

Duplex Doppler ultrasonography is an accurate method to detect stenoses in the carotid arteries, and it has also been shown to be a reliable noninvasive diagnostic modality in

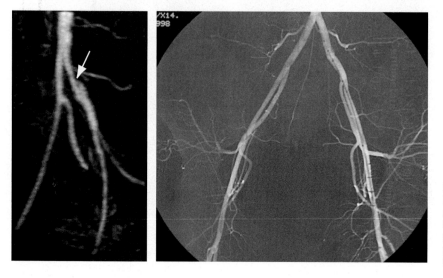

FIGURE 25.10. Patient with atherosclerotic lesion in the left common iliac artery as visualized on MRA *(left).* The stenosis is located on the dorsal wall of the vessel and not appreciated at angiography *(right),* although a pressure gradient of 25 mm Hg was measured.

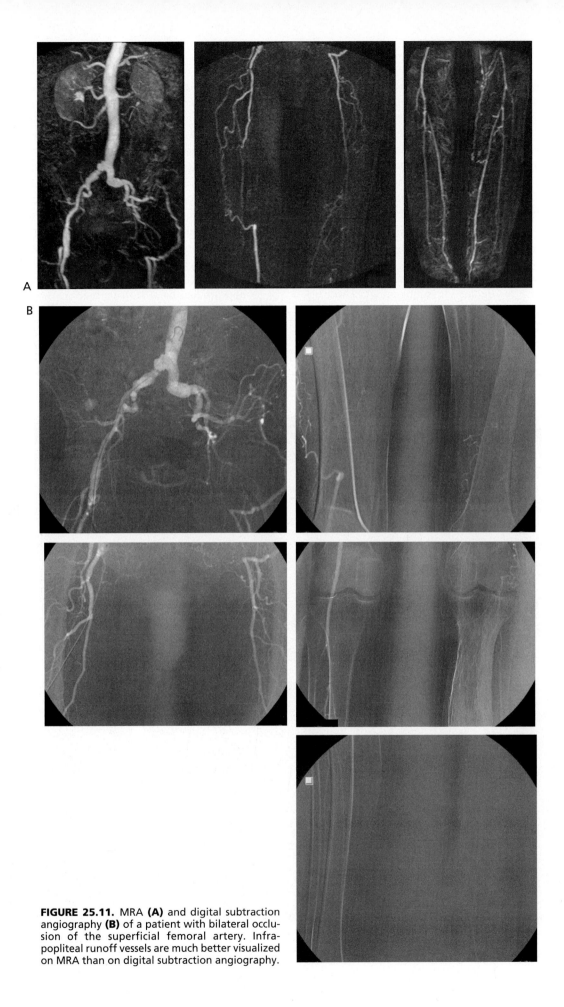

FIGURE 25.11. MRA **(A)** and digital subtraction angiography **(B)** of a patient with bilateral occlusion of the superficial femoral artery. Infrapopliteal runoff vessels are much better visualized on MRA than on digital subtraction angiography.

the lower limbs (37,38). Duplex ultrasonography, however, is operator-dependent and laborious, and it does not provide a complete road map for treatment planning.

Recently, a metaanalysis of nine studies of contrast-enhanced MRA (216 patients) and 18 studies of color-guided duplex ultrasonography (1,059 patients) was performed (39). In all these studies, conventional angiography was used as the gold standard. The pooled sensitivities of contrast-enhanced MRA for assessing arterial disease (i.e., >50% luminal reduction) in these studies was 97% (95% confidence interval, 95.7% to 99.3%), and that of duplex ultrasonography was 87.6% (95% CI, 84.4% to 90.8%). The pooled specificities were similar (96.2% for contrast-enhanced MRA and 94.7% for duplex ultrasonography). These figures for contrast-enhanced MRA correspond to those reported in the metaanalysis, previously mentioned, comparing 2D TOF with contrast-enhanced MRA (8).

Results for the different stations were reported in almost all the duplex ultrasonographic studies but in only five of the nine contrast-enhanced MRA studies. Stratification per anatomic site was therefore not possible. In general, the interval between contrast-enhanced MRA and conventional angiography was shorter (mean, 5 days) than that between duplex ultrasonography and angiography (mean, 17 days). One might expect that as the interval between the studied examination and the reference examination increased, the discriminatory power of the studied examination would decrease. This was indeed found for duplex ultrasonography. The lower sensitivity of duplex ultrasonography in the reported studies may therefore be partly attributed to the longer interval between duplex ultrasonography and angiography.

It appears that because of its high sensitivity and specificity, contrast-enhanced MRA may replace conventional angiography in the workup of patients with intermittent claudication (Fig. 25.12). Color-guided duplex ultrasonography will then be reserved to determine the hemodynamic significance of stenoses found on contrast-enhanced MRA.

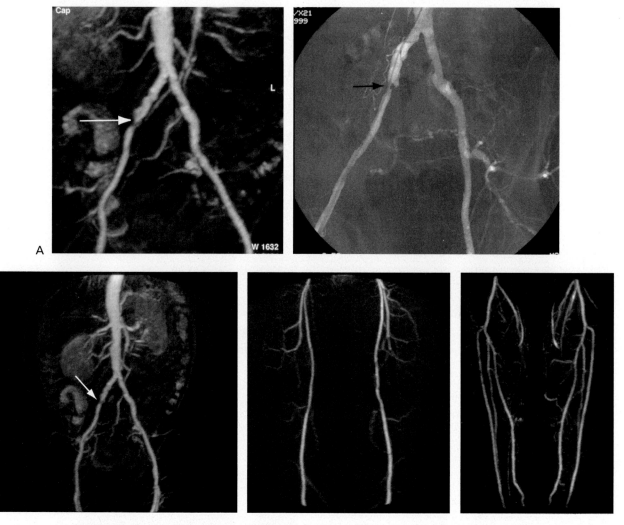

FIGURE 25.12. Comparison between MRA and digital subtraction angiography in a patient with stenosis of the right iliac artery **(A)**. The more distal vessels show no stenosis **(B)**.

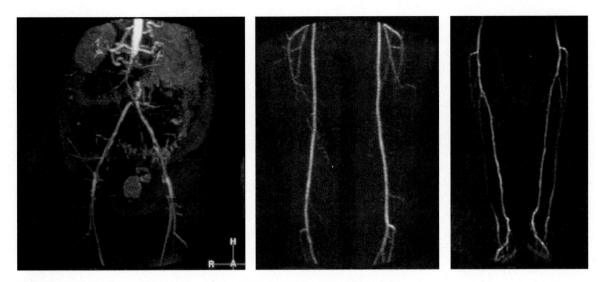

FIGURE 25.13. Patient with occlusion of the distal aorta (Leriche syndrome).

Intermittent claudication is commonly caused by stenosis or occlusion of the vessels in the legs. Sometimes, however, the symptoms may be caused by severe stenosis or occlusion of the aorta (Leriche syndrome). This entity can also be visualized with contrast-enhanced MRA (40) (Figs. 25.3 and 25.13).

Aneurysms

Contrast-enhanced MRA has been found adequate in demonstrating the extent of aortoiliac aneurysmal disease (41). Aneurysms may occur in the femoral and popliteal arteries. Popliteal aneurysm is an important entity because up to one-third of patients have either distal embolization or severe, acute limb ischemia caused by an unrecognized and nonpalpable popliteal aneurysm (42). Femoral aneurysms are less important and can be followed conservatively (43,44). In a study of 313 patients with abdominal aortic aneurysm, all of whom underwent ultrasonographic examination of the femoropopliteal region, Diwan et al. (45) encountered femoral and popliteal aneurysms in 12% (36 patients with 51 peripheral aneurysms, of which 31 were popliteal aneurysms). The peripheral aneurysms occurred only in the men with abdominal aortic aneurysm (incidence, 14%); no aneurysms were found in the 62 women with abdominal aortic aneurysm. The reason for this sex difference is not known. Peripheral occlusive disease was present in 14 (39%) of the 36 men with peripheral aneurysms, versus 20 (9%) of the 215 men without peripheral aneurysms.

Surprisingly, because it is a not infrequent and an important entity, popliteal aneurysms have not been reported in the studies of contrast-enhanced MRA of the peripheral arteries.

Diabetes

Diabetes-related angiopathy is an important cause of non-traumatic amputation of lower extremities in the industrial-ized world. Diabetic patients often have long segments of arterial occlusion, especially in the infrapopliteal vessels (Fig. 25.14). Surgical reconstitution of blood flow remains the most important therapeutic option for limb salvage in these patients. Improvements in bypass graft technology have made it possible to use the pedal arteries as target sites. To plan distal revascularizations, information on the distal vessels in the foot (including the pedal arch) is necessary. Some studies have indicated that even 2D TOF MRA can demonstrate patent distal vessels not visible on conventional angiography (34,46). Using the head coil for signal reception, Kreitner et al. (47) evaluated the value of contrast-enhanced MRA in 24 diabetic patients. All the patients underwent angiography for comparison within 5 days. Seven vascular segments were evaluated in each extremity: distal anterior tibial artery, distal posterior tibial artery, distal peroneal artery, dorsal pedal artery, lateral plantar artery, medial plantar artery, and plantar arch. Of a possible 168 segments, 74 were seen to be patent on DSA and 104 on contrast-enhanced MRA. Thirty vessel segments that were suitable for distal grafting in nine (38%) patients were seen exclusively on MRA. For seven of the nine patients, treatment plans were changed as a result. Therefore, this study shows that for diabetic patients with severe peripheral occlusive disease, contrast-enhanced MRA should be used in pedal bypass planning instead of DSA.

Surveillance of Peripheral Bypass Grafts

Contrast-enhanced MRA may be used in the postoperative follow-up of arterial bypass grafts. Peripheral bypass grafts may consist of autologous saphenous vein, expanded poly-tetrafluoroethylene (PTFE), or Dacron. Autologous venous grafts have a better patency rate than do the other grafts, but the incidence of bypass graft stenosis in the first postopera-

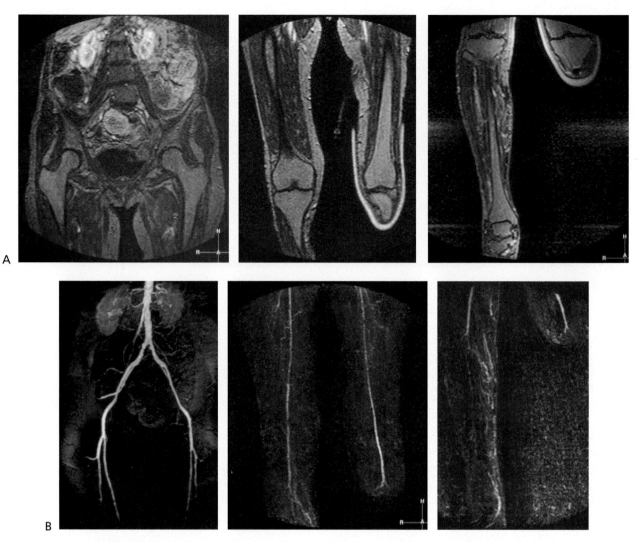

FIGURE 25.14. Patient with diabetes after amputation of the left lower leg **(A)**. Persistent ulceration and ischemia of the right lower leg are caused by occlusion of the infrapopliteal arteries **(B)**.

tive year is still 12%. Eighty percent of the cases of stenosis occur during the first postoperative year, and almost all occur in the first 18 months (48). In 60% of the cases of stenosis, no initial clinical symptoms are noted (48). Therefore, the bypass grafts are carefully monitored to detect stenosis in time to enable reconstitution of flow (secondary patency). Surveillance criteria such as the ankle–brachial index have been successfully tested. Duplex ultrasonography is also routinely performed for surveillance. The ratio of the midgraft peak systolic velocities proximal and distal to the stenosis can be calculated, or the entire graft can be visualized. Conventional angiography is performed when an abnormality is found at duplex ultrasonography or when a vascular intervention is needed.

Duplex ultrasonography can assess graft patency and detect stenoses adequately. However, duplex ultrasonography is limited in detecting collateral flow, and proximal lesions that may eventually endanger graft patency can be missed at duplex ultrasonography.

Two studies evaluated the use of contrast-enhanced MRA in the surveillance of lower limb grafts. Bertschinger et al. (49) evaluated 30 patients with 31 grafts who underwent both DSA and contrast-enhanced MRA. At contrast-enhanced MRA, 93 segments could be evaluated, and six graft segments could not be assessed because of artifacts caused by clips or stents. All abnormalities (10 stenoses, 9 occlusions, and 8 aneurysms or ectases) could be visualized by contrast-enhanced MRA (sensitivity 100%). Because six segments could not be evaluated, the specificity was 90.3%. Bendib et al. (50) selected 23 patients with 40 vascular grafts who had either clinical symptoms or abnormal findings on duplex ultrasonography. All patients also underwent x-ray angiography. MRA depicted 38 grafts (95%) with 28 abnormalities. Two stenoses were overestimated. Some grafts had more than one abnormality. The sensitivity of contrast-enhanced MRA for the detection of stenoses and occlusions was 91%, and the specificity was 95%. In five cases, contrast-enhanced MRA showed extra complications: four non-

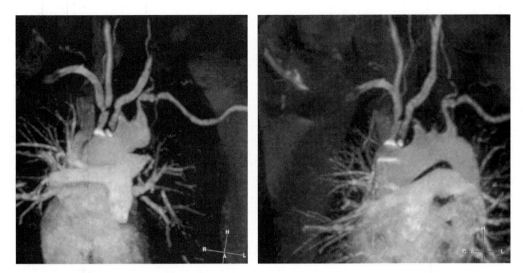

FIGURE 25.15. MRA of patient with atherosclerotic occlusions and reconstruction of the brachiocephalic artery and left carotid artery.

thrombotic ectases not seen on ultrasonography and one thrombotic ectasis overlooked at conventional angiography. Further study is required to assess whether contrast-enhanced MRA can be used as the only road map for additional reconstruction.

Contrast-enhanced MRA also appears useful in the surveillance of extra-anatomic bypass grafts. These grafts are made of PTFE or Dacron; veins cannot be used. Examples in the upper limbs are carotid–subclavian bypass, reconstruction of the innominate and subclavian arteries (Fig. 25.15), and axilloaxillary bypass. Possible reconstructions in the lower limbs are axillofemoral grafts (Fig. 16), femoro-femoral crossover bypasses, and thoracic aortofemoral artery bypass grafts (51).

Popliteal Entrapment

Intermittent claudication in younger patients without signs of atherosclerotic disease may be caused by the so-called popliteal entrapment syndrome. The incidence of the syndrome in the general population is 0.16% to 3.5% (52). It is associated with an anomalous relationship between the gastrocnemius muscle and the popliteal artery (53). The popliteal artery can have an anomalous course that is medial to the medial head of the gastrocnemius muscle. An abnormal insertion of the medial head of the gastrocnemius muscle may also result in compression of the popliteal artery during exercise. Finally, in "functional entrapment," the popliteal artery is compressed by a hypertrophic gastrocnemius muscle, even though the anatomic relationship between the two structures is normal (54). Potential treatment options are transection of the anomalous medial gastrocnemius head or stent implantation in the popliteal artery. Thus far, conventional angiography in rest and during active plantar flexion against resistance is the method of choice

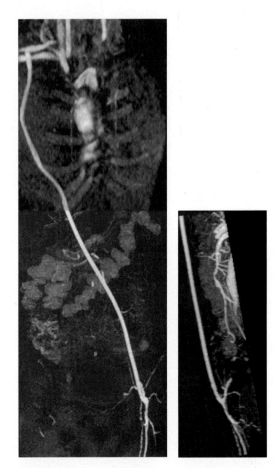

FIGURE 25.16. Coronal *(left)* and sagittal *(right)* maximum intensity projection reconstructions of an axillofemoral bypass from the right subclavian artery to the left common femoral artery.

to demonstrate popliteal artery compression during stress. DSA, however, does not show the cause of the entrapment syndrome.

Cross-sectional imaging may show the cause of entrapment. Di Cesare et al. (55) used 2D TOF MRA performed at rest and during active plantar flexion of the foot against resistance to examine six patients suspected of having popliteal entrapment. The compressed popliteal artery and anomalous anatomic relationships could be visualized in the transverse images obtained during stress.

The diagnosis of popliteal entrapment can also be made with contrast-enhanced MRA performed at rest and during stress. With reconstructions of the nonsubtracted 3D data set, the anomalous anatomy can be visualized. Figure 25.17 shows compression of the popliteal artery by the gastrocnemius muscle during stress as visualized by contrast-enhanced MRA.

NEW DEVELOPMENTS

MRI Techniques

Ongoing improvements in hardware and gradients have shortened scan times and enabled time-resolved imaging with a high degree of resolution. Time-resolved imaging will continue to improve with still better resolution, real-time reconstruction, and better viewing capabilities. Besides obviating the need for timing the contrast bolus, time-resolved imaging adds an extra dimension to images of the peripheral arteries. Because of the dynamic nature of the series, it is possible to visualize differences in influx of contrast agent in the two limbs, as in conventional angiography.

Dedicated coils for peripheral vascular imaging will probably be used more frequently. Such coils will provide images with a higher degree of resolution and improved signal-to-noise ratios and, in the case of phased-array coils, may re-

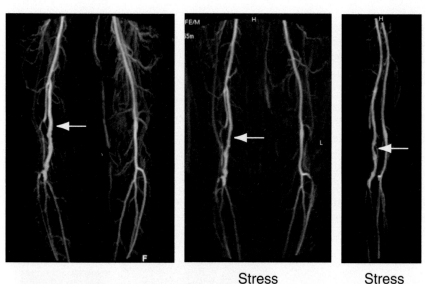

A

Stress   Stress

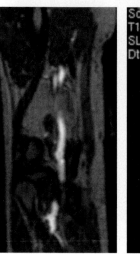

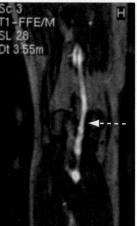

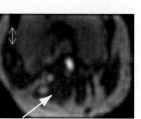

Stress

B   Stress

FIGURE 25.17. Images of a 27-year old male long-distance runner with recurrence of claudication. He previously underwent femoro-popliteal bypass grafting for severe stenosis of the right popliteal artery. At rest *(left)*, no stenosis is present. During plantar flexion of the foot with extension of the knee joint, compression of the bypass by the gastrocnemius muscle can be seen on MRA **(A)**: coronal *(middle)* and sagittal *(right)* maximum intensity projections. Coronal unsubtracted source image and transverse reconstructed image of the MRA study **(B)** show compression of the bypass between the medial and lateral heads of the gastrocnemius muscle and the medial femoral condyle.

duce imaging times by allowing the acquisition of data in parallel. With the so-called SMASH (simultaneous acquisition of spatial harmonics) (56) and SENSE (sensitivity encoding) (57) techniques, combinations of coils can be used to compensate for omitted gradient steps. The increase in imaging speed can be used to reduce acquisition times or increase the resolution of the scan.

Contrast Agents

In MR arteriography of the lower limbs, when extracellular contrast agents such as Gd-DTPA are administered at a slow infusion rate, venous enhancement occurs relatively late because contrast diffuses into the interstitium. A disadvantage of using slow infusion rates is the dilution of contrast agent in the bloodstream, so that enhancement is relatively moderate. Faster infusion rates result in a higher local concentration of contrast agent in the vessels-of-interest, but at the cost of faster venous return and a shorter arterial–venous time window for imaging. A possible solution to this problem may be the use of higher-concentration formulations, such as 1.0-M Gadovist (Schering, Berlin, Germany). However, the extravasation of extracellular contrast agents into the interstitium reduces contrast-to-background ratios.

Therefore, new contrast agents, the so-called blood pool agents, have been developed that remain within the blood compartment; little or no interstitial diffusion takes place. The term *blood pool agent* does not necessarily imply prolonged residence in the body. In fact, for safety reasons, it is desirable that blood pool agents be excreted rapidly, at almost "extracellular" speed or even faster. The first generation of blood pool agents exhibited little interstitial diffusion, but residence times in the blood were long, and the agents never reached clinical testing. They consisted of paramagnetic chelates covalently bound to macromolecules such as polylysine, albumin, polysaccharides, and lipids. The newer paramagnetic (gadolinium-based) blood pool agents have much faster clearing rates with little or no interstitial diffusion. These characteristics have been developed by producing agents that bind reversibly to macromolecules such as albumin (e.g., MS-325; Epix Medical, Cambridge, Massachusetts).

A separate paramagnetic contrast agent, MultiHance (Bracco Diagnostics, Princeton, New Jersey), which binds weakly to albumin, is being tested in clinical trials. Because of the weak protein binding, interstitial diffusion is diminished, but not absent. MultiHance is therefore not a blood pool agent *in sensu strictu*.

The blood pool agents of another class consist of superparamagnetic particles that contain iron oxide, such as PEG-Ferron (Nycomed Amersham, Buckinghamshire, United Kingdom), AngioMark (Epix Medical), and Combidex (Advanced Magnetics, Cambridge, Massachusetts).

The major advantage of both the paramagnetic and superparamagnetic intravascular agents, and also of Multi-Hance, is their greater relaxivity in comparison with that of the extracellular agents. This property can be used to obtain more intense signal in the vessels or to lower the required dose and injection volume.

The major disadvantage of the blood pool agents is early venous enhancement, which leaves a small time window for arterial imaging. Early venous enhancement is not a problem when the larger vessels are imaged, such as the iliac and femoral arteries, because selective projection reconstructions are possible. In the lower legs, however, venous overlap seriously degrades images of the arteries.

Considering the good results that have been obtained with extracellular agents, the problem of venous overlap must be solved before the blood pool agents can be successfully applied in peripheral MRA. A potential solution to this problem is the development of special postprocessing techniques, such as venous subtraction algorithms (58). Alternatively, algorithms may be developed that incorporate phase information into the image and provide it as an overlay indicating the direction of flow, so that arterial–venous differentiation will be possible, as in color Doppler ultrasonography (59).

SUMMARY

Because of major improvements in general MR technology and the application of contrast enhancement, MRA has become a serious alternative to conventional angiography. In fact, numerous studies have shown that contrast-enhanced MRA can replace DSA in diagnostic imaging of the peripheral arteries in both the arms and the legs. Although the resolution of DSA at present is still higher than that of MRA, in clinical practice, all relevant information regarding the patency of peripheral arteries can be obtained with contrast-enhanced MRA, which is a noninvasive means of providing multiplanar views of vessels that causes few side effects and can be performed on an outpatient basis.

The method can even be used safely in patients with impaired renal function, unlike DSA. Further improvements in MR technology will result in further reductions in scan times and higher degrees of spatial and contrast resolution. Whether blood pool agents will ever be used in peripheral MRA depends on the future development of software capable of removing excessive venous enhancement.

REFERENCES

1. Martin EC. Transcatheter therapies in peripheral and nonvascular disease. *Circulation* 1991;83:1–5.
2. Waugh JR, Sacharias N. Arteriographic complications in the DSA era. *Radiology* 1992;138:237–281.
3. Goldman K, Salvesen S, Hegedus V. Acute renal failure after contrast medium injection. *Invest Radiol* 1984;S19:S125.
4. Niendorf HP, Haustein J, Louton T, et al. Safety and tolerance

after intravenous administration of 0.3 mmol/kg Gd-DTPA: results of a randomized, controlled clinical trial. *Invest Radiol* 1991;26 (Suppl 1):221S–225S.

5. Ho KY, de Haan MW, Oei TK, et al. MR angiography of the iliac and upper femoral arteries using four different inflow techniques. *AJR Am J Roentgenol* 1997;169:45–53.

6. Ho KY, de Haan MW, Kessels AG, et al. Peripheral vascular tree stenosis: detection with subtracted and nonsubtracted MR angiography. *Radiology* 1998;206:673–681.

7. Poon E, Yucel EK, Pagan-Marin H, et al. Iliac artery stenosis measurements: comparison of two-dimensional time-of-flight and three-dimensional dynamic gadolinium-enhanced MR angiography. *AJR Am J Roentgenol* 1997;169:1139–1144.

8. Nelemans PJ, Leiner T, de Vet HCW, et al. Peripheral arterial disease: meta-analysis of the diagnostic performance of MR angiography. *Radiology* 2000;217:105–114.

9. Prince MR, Yucel EK, Kaufman JA, et al. Dynamic gadolinium-enhanced three-dimensional abdominal MR arteriography. *J Magn Reson Imaging* 1993;3:877–881.

10. Kopka L, Vosshenrich R, Rodenwaldt J, et al. Differences in injecting rates on contrast-enhanced breath-hold three-dimensional MR angiography. *AJR Am J Roentgenol* 1998;170:345–348.

11. Foo TKF, Saranathan M, Prince MR, et al. Automated detection of bolus arrival and initiation of data acquisition in fast, three-dimensional MR angiography image quality. *Radiology* 1997;203:275–280.

12. Leiner T, Ho KY, Nelemans PJ, et al. Three-dimensional contrast-enhanced moving-bed infusion-tracking (MoBi-track) peripheral MR angiography with flexible choice of imaging parameters for each field of view. *J Magn Reson Imaging* 2000;11:368–377.

13. Frayne R, Grist TM, Swan JS, et al. 3D MR DSA: effects of injection protocol and image masking. *J Magn Reson Imaging* 2000;12:476-487.

14. Winterer JT, Scheffler K, Paul G, et al. Optimization of contrast-enhanced MR angiography of the hands with a timing bolus and elliptically reordered 3D pulse sequence. *J Comput Assist Tomogr* 2000;24:903–908.

15. Watanabe Y, Dohke M, Okumura A, et al. Dynamic subtraction contrast-enhanced MR angiography: technique, clinical applications, and pitfalls. *Radiographics* 2000;20:135–152.

16. Westenberg JJM, Wasser MNJM, van der Geest RJ, et al. Scan optimization of gadolinium-enhanced three-dimensional MRA of peripheral arteries with multiple bolus injections and *in vitro* validation of stenosis quantification. *Magn Reson Imaging* 1999;17:47–57.

17. Ho KYJAM, Leiner T, De Haan MW, et al. Peripheral vascular tree stenoses: evaluation with moving-bed infusion-tracking MR angiography. *Radiology* 1998;206:683–692.

18. Wang Y, Lee HM, Khilnani NM, et al. Bolus-chase MR digital subtraction angiography in the lower extremity. *Radiology* 1998;207:263–269.

19. Meaney JFM, Ridgway JP, Chakraverty S, et al. Stepping-table gadolinium-enhanced digital subtraction MR angiography of the aorta and lower extremity arteries: preliminary experience. *Radiology* 1999;211:59–67.

20. Alley MT, Grist TM, Swan JS. Development of a phased-array coil for the lower extremities. *Magn Reson Med* 1995;34:260–267.

21. Mitsuzaki K, Yamashita Y, Onomichi M, et al. Delineation of simulated vascular stenosis with Gd-DTPA-enhanced 3D gradient echo MR angiography: an experimental study. *J Comput Assist Tomogr* 2000;24:77–82.

22. Neimatallah MA, Chenevert TL, Carlos RC, et al. Subclavian MR arteriography: reduction of susceptibility artifact with short echo time and dilute gadopentetate dimeglumine. *Radiology* 2000;217:581–586.

23. Maki JH, Prince MR, Londy FJ, et al. The effects of time-varying intravascular signal intensity and k-space acquisition order on three-dimensional MR angiography image quality. *J Magn Reson Imaging* 1996;6:642–651.

24. Korosec FR, Mistretta CA. MR angiography: basic principles and theory. *Magn Reson Imaging Clin N Am* 1998;6:223–256.

25. Van Grimberge F, Dymarkowski S, Budts W, et al. Role of magnetic resonance in the diagnosis of subclavian steal syndrome. *J Magn Reson Imaging* 2000;12:339–342.

26. Yamato M, Lecky JW, Hiramatsu K, et al. Takayasu arteritis: radiographic and angiographic findings in 59 patients. *Radiology* 1986;161:329–334.

27. Yamada I, Nakagawa T, Himeno Y, et al. Takayasu arteritis: diagnosis with breath-hold contrast-enhanced three-dimensional MR angiography. *J Magn Reson Imaging* 2000;11:481–487.

28. Yamada I, Numano F, Suzuki S. Takayasu arteritis: evaluation with MR imaging. *Radiology* 1993;188:89–94 .

29. Choe YH, Han BK, Koh EM, et al. Takayasu's arteritis: assessment of disease activity with contrast-enhanced MR imaging. *AJR Am J Roentgenol* 2000;175:505–511.

30. Dymarkowski S, Bosmans H, Marchal G, et al. Three-dimensional MR angiography in the evaluation of thoracic outlet syndrome. *AJR Am J Roentgenol* 1999;173:1005–1008.

31. Rofsky NM, Adelman MA. MR angiography in the evaluation of atherosclerotic peripheral vascular disease: what the clinician wants to know. *Radiology* 2000;214:325–338.

32. Kinney TB, Rose SC. Intraarterial pressure measurements during angiographic evaluation of peripheral vascular disease: techniques, interpretation, applications, and limitations. *AJR Am J Roentgenol* 1996;116:277–284.

33. Wasser MN, Westenberg J, van der Hulst VP, et al. Hemodynamic significance of renal artery stenosis: digital subtraction angiography versus systolically gated three-dimensional phase-contrast MR angiography. *Radiology* 1997;202:333–338.

34. Wikström J, Holmberg A, Johansson L, et al. Gadolinium-enhanced magnetic resonance angiography, digital subtraction angiography and duplex of the iliac arteries compared with intra-arterial pressure gradient measurements. *Eur J Vasc Endovasc Surg* 2000;19:516–523.

35. Owen RS, Carpenter JP, Baum RA, et al. Magnetic resonance imaging of angiographically occult runoff vessels in peripheral arterial occlusive disease. *N Engl J Med* 1992;326:1577–1581.

36. Carpenter JP, Owen RS, Baum RA, et al. Magnetic resonance angiography of peripheral vessels. *J Vasc Surg* 1992;16:807–813.

37. Koelemay MJW, Den Hartog D, Prins MH, et al. Diagnosis of arterial disease of the lower extremities with duplex ultrasonography. *Br J Surg* 1996;83:404–409.

38. Legemate DA, Teeuwen C, Hoeneveld H, et al. Value of duplex scanning compared with angiography and pressure measurement in the assessment of aortoiliac arterial lesions. *Br J Surg* 1991;78:1003–1008.

39. Visser K, Hunink MGM. Peripheral arterial disease: gadolinium-enhanced MR angiography versus color-guided duplex US—a meta-analysis. *Radiology* 2000;216:67–77.

40. Ruehm SG, Weishaupt D, Debatin JF. Contrast-enhanced MR angiography in patients with aortic occlusion (Leriche syndrome). *J Magn Reson Imaging* 2000;11:401–410.

41. Prince M, Narasimham D, Stanley J, et al. Gadolinium-enhanced magnetic resonance angiography of abdominal aortic aneurysms. *J Vasc Surg* 1995;21:656–669.

42. Whitehouse WM, Wakefield TW, Graham LM, et al. Limb-threatening potential of arteriosclerotic popliteal aneurysms. *Surgery* 1983;93:694–699.

43. Adiseshiah M, Bailey DA. Aneurysms of the femoral artery. *Br J Surg* 1977;64:174–176.

44. Graham LM, Zelenock GB, Whitehouse WM, et al. Clinical sig-

nificance of arteriosclerotic femoral artery aneurysms. *Arch Surg* 1980;115:502–507.

45. Diwan A, Sarkar R, Stanley JC, et al. Incidence of femoral and popliteal artery aneurysms in patients with abdominal aneurysms. *J Vasc Surg* 2000;31:863–869.

46. Baum RA, Rutter CM, Sunshine JH, et al. Multicenter trial to evaluate vascular magnetic resonance angiography of the lower extremity. *JAMA* 1995;274:875–880.

47. Kreitner KF, Kalden P, Neufang A, et al. Diabetes and peripheral arterial occlusive disease. Prospective comparison of contrast-enhanced three-dimensional MR angiography with conventional digital subtraction. *AJR Am J Roentgenol* 2000;174:171–179.

48. Berkowitz HD, Hobbs CL, Roberts B, et al. Value of routine vascular laboratory studies to identify vein graft stenosis. *Surgery* 1981;90:971–979.

49. Bertschinger K, Cassina PC, Debatin J, et al. Surveillance of peripheral arterial bypass grafts with three-dimensional MR angiography: comparison with digital subtraction angiography. *AJR Am J Roentgenol* 2001;176:215–220.

50. Bendib K, Berthezène Y, Croisille P, et al. Assessment of complicated arterial bypass grafts: value of contrast-enhanced subtraction magnetic resonance angiography. *J Vasc Surg* 1997;26: 1036–1042.

51. Krinsky G, Jacobowitz G, Rofsky N. Gadolinium-enhanced MR angiography of extraanatomic arterial bypass grafts. *AJR Am J Roentgenol* 1998;170:735–741.

52. Hamming JJ. Intermittent claudication at an early age due to anomalous course of the popliteal artery. *Angiology* 1959;10: 369–370.

53. Insua JA, Young JR, Humphries AV. Popliteal entrapment syndrome. *Arch Surg* 1970;101:771–775.

54. Mailis A, Lossing A, Ashby P, et al. Intermittent claudication of tibial vessels as a result of calf muscle hypertrophy: case report. *J Vasc Surg* 1992;16:116–120.

55. Di Cesare E, Marsili L, Marino G, et al. Stress MR imaging for evaluation of popliteal artery entrapment. *J Magn Reson Imaging* 1994;4:617–622.

56. Sodickson DK, McKenzie CA, Li W, et al. Contrast-enhanced 3D MR angiography with simultaneous acquisition of spatial harmonics: a pilot study. *Radiology* 2000;217:284–289.

57. Weiger M, Pruessmann KP, Kassner A, et al. Contrast-enhanced 3D MRA using SENSE. *J Magn Reson Imaging* 2000;12:671– 677.

58. Grist T, Korosec F, Peters D, et al. Steady-state and dynamic MR angiographic imaging with MS-325: initial experience in humans. *Radiology* 1998;207:539–544.

59. Nayak KS, Pauly JM, Kerr AB, et al. Real-time color flow MRI. *Magn Reson Med* 2000;43:251–258.

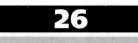

26

MRA OF CAROTID ARTERIES

CHARLES M. ANDERSON

It is now widely recognized that carotid artery stenosis may lead to stroke, that the risk for stroke increases with the severity of the lesion, and that correction of a stenotic lesion by surgical endarterectomy reduces the risk for stroke. The correction of carotid stenosis is of considerable medical significance. Stroke is the third leading cause of death in the United States and the major cause of disability among the elderly (1). Approximately 160 persons per 100,000 present with a first stroke each year. Four percent of middle-aged and elderly adults have carotid stenosis (2), a figure that increases with age (3). Nearly one-fourth of patients with coronary artery disease and one-third of patients with peripheral vascular disease also have carotid artery stenosis (4). These stenoses are often unsuspected before a debilitating stroke occurs. Many strokes could be avoided by the early detection of carotid artery plaque and subsequent endarterectomy.

The last decade has seen a rise in the use of noninvasive methods for imaging the carotid artery. The attitude, so prevalent 10 years ago, that all patients should undergo conventional catheter angiography before carotid surgery has given way to an understanding that noninvasive imaging techniques are both safer and cheaper and offer comparable clinical outcomes. This shift in practice favors the more widespread use of both Doppler ultrasonography and MRA. The carotid arteries are especially amenable to MRA. Unlike the heart, the neck is stationary during the cardiac and respiratory cycles. High-sensitivity coils for imaging the neck depict the carotid anatomy in great detail. Optimized carotid imaging sequences are widely available. Most importantly, the relationship between the degree of stenosis and clinical outcome is now understood, so that specific radiologic criteria are available to guide the selection of surgical candidates.

C. M. Anderson: Department of Radiology, University of California San Francisco, San Francisco, California.

TECHNIQUES

Acquisition Methods

The two sequences commonly used for carotid MRA are time-of-flight (TOF) and contrast-enhanced sequences. TOF MRA images the entry of blood into the imaging volume, whereas contrast-enhanced MRA images the distribution of contrast material (5–7), not blood motion per se. TOF MRA may be further categorized as two-dimensional (2D) (8) or three-dimensional (3D) (9), depending on whether the angiogram is constructed from multiple thin sections or from a single thick slab. A hybrid of the 2D and 3D techniques employs multiple overlapping thin-slab acquisition (MOTSA) (10). Each of these sequences has been successfully used to measure carotid stenosis. Each has its own strengths and weaknesses.

Two-Dimensional Time-of-Flight MRA

In 2D TOF MRA, one obtains a sequential series of slices that are transaxial to the neck and extend from the base of skull to the thoracic inlet. Tissues that remain stationary in a slice are pulsed by radio waves and become dark, whereas blood entering into the slice between the radiofrequency (RF) pulses has not been pulsed before and is bright. Each slice is fully acquired before the adjacent slice, so that blood does not have to pass through more than one slice. For adequate resolution, the slices should be 2 mm or less in thickness. If slices this thin cannot be achieved, then they can be overlapped to provide greater apparent resolution. A "walking" or "traveling" saturation band is placed just superior to each slice to remove any signal from the jugular veins. Because the sections in 2D TOF MRA are very thin, they are replaced with in-flowing blood, even when the vessel velocity is reduced. Therefore, the technique provides strong blood-to-background signal contrast in conditions of slow flow.

Three-Dimensional Time-of-Flight MRA

In 3D TOF MRA, the bifurcation is acquired by a thick slab that is transaxial to the neck. The slab is divided into very thin partitions by using a second, phase-encoding gradient. The partitions available in 3D TOF MRA are typically 1 mm or less—finer than the resolution available with 2D TOF MRA. The 3D method is effective only for relatively fast flow because blood may be pulsed several times and lose its signal before it traverses the width of the slab. As in 2D TOF MRA, a saturation band is placed superior and parallel to the acquisition slab to eliminate jugular venous signal.

Multiple Overlapping Thin-Slab Acquisition

In MOTSA, the angiogram is built up from many thin slabs. The slabs are acquired sequentially, as in 2D TOF MRA. Each slab is divided into thin partitions, as in 3D TOF. Because the slabs are relatively thin, on the order of 1 cm, blood can transverse the volume and the signal can be refreshed between RF pulses. Each slab partially overlaps the volume acquired by the prior slab. Only the central partitions of each slab are kept, to improve uniformity of signal. The need to overlap volumes results in a relatively inefficient acquisition time of 12 minutes or more.

Contrast-Enhanced MRA

Contrast-enhanced MRA has proved to be very effective for carotid angiography, combining speed of acquisition with an ability to visualize vessels in which flow is slow. Contrast is injected as a rapid bolus in a peripheral arm vein. When the bolus arrives in the carotid arteries, a fast 3D gradient-echo sequence is acquired. Because the contrast agent remains bright even when pulsed many times by radio waves, inflow does not have to be optimized. The acquisition slab may be oriented in the coronal plane to cover the entire length of the neck to the circle of Willis. The acquisition is completed before the jugular vein enhances, in 20 seconds or less.

Contrast-enhanced MRA is best performed on a modern machine with strong gradients of 20 mT/m or greater. With strong gradients, the acquisition time should be less than 20 seconds. The shorter the acquisition, the smaller the amount of contrast material that must be injected to sustain enhancement. Typically, 20 to 30 mL of gadolinium is required. Signal intensity, and hence the signal-to-noise ratio, improves with faster injection rates. Stronger gradients permit echo times (TEs) of less than 2 ms, which minimize flow and susceptibility artifacts.

The challenge in contrast-enhanced MRA is to initiate the brief acquisition at the time of arrival of contrast. The sequence can be initiated by one of several techniques:

1. A 2-mL test bolus can be administered, followed by a flush with 10 mL of saline solution. The vessel-of-interest is repeatedly acquired every second to determine the contrast transit time. The transit time is then used to calculate an imaging delay time for the subsequent full-dose injection. Although this technique is time-consuming, the incidence of failure is low.

2. As in helical computed tomography, some manufacturers have automated the process by programming the machine to initiate a sequence when it senses a signal change in the vessel (11). In this way, a separate test injection is avoided. This method of timing is often used with centric reordering of the phase-encoding steps. Centric reordering ensures that the large echoes are acquired early in the sequence, during peak enhancement; smaller, less important echoes are acquired later in the bolus. Elliptic centric reordering is a further refinement of the technique, in which the smallest echoes are not acquired at all.

3. Following the peripheral injection of intravenous contrast, the aortic arch can be imaged in real time with MR fluoroscopy. The fluoroscopy is terminated, and the angiography begun, when contrast is seen entering the aorta (12). As in automated detection, a centrically reordered acquisition is used (13).

4. If the acquisition time is very short, one can simply acquire several angiograms in succession. The angiogram corresponding to peak arterial enhancement is then retained. A more sophisticated implementation of this technique is to acquire only the large, central echoes several times during the passage of contrast and acquire the smaller echoes just once (14,15). Angiograms so acquired combine strong vessel signal with a high degree of resolution.

On contrast-enhanced MRA, noise may become visible as the pixel size is reduced. This problem is best compensated for by using a phase-array neck coil and by increasing the injected volume of contrast material. Another common solution is to acquire lower-resolution data, then calculate a higher-resolution image from those data by interpolation, a practice called *zero filling*. Zero filling improves apparent resolution but does not provide the same detail as true high-resolution acquisition.

It is advisable to obtain two acquisitions in rapid succession following the injection. The first, which is timed to peak arterial contrast, best demonstrates anatomy. The second acquisition shows late-filling vessels in conditions of exceptionally slow flow.

Methods Compared

Resolution

Three-dimensional TOF and contrast-enhanced MRA provide resolution superior to that of 2D TOF MRA in the direction of slice selection. This lack of resolution may impair the ability of 2D TOF MRA to detect ulcers, small plaques, or fibromuscular dysplasia.

Voxels should be 1 mm^3 or less to permit adequate measurements of luminal diameter. The diameter of the internal carotid artery (ICA) may be 5 or 6 mm. A pixel width of 1 mm appears to permit no better than 20% precision in the measurement of luminal width. In fact, the partial voluming of signal intensities results in greater precision when angiograms are interpolated and viewed at higher resolution. However, when the width of a lumen is measured under magnification, the limitations of interpolation become apparent. The use of a 512-image matrix improves accuracy. The margin of a vessel is more sharply defined on contrast-enhanced MRA than on 3D TOF MRA because slow flow at the vessel wall is as bright as faster flow in the center of the vessel, so that the perceived resolution of the gadolinium-enhanced technique is superior (Figs. 26.1 and 26.2).

Near-Occlusion

Three-dimensional TOF MRA is not suitable for this indication. Two-dimensional TOF MRA is better able to visualize vessels beyond a high-grade stenosis. Note that the ICA may be atretic when a flow-limiting lesion has been present for a long time and so be mistaken for a branch of the external carotid artery. Inspection of the carotid canals may help to differentiate an ascending pharyngeal artery from a small ICA. A congenitally small ICA can be differentiated

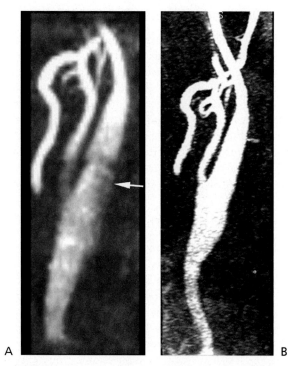

FIGURE 26.2. Greater uniformity of blood signal on contrast-enhanced MRA. **A:** Following endarterectomy, the distal common carotid artery and proximal internal carotid artery are patulous, so that blood flow is slower and signal weak *(arrow)*. **B:** On contrast-enhanced MRA, the signal intensity is uniform as a result of insensitivity to blood velocity.

from an atretic ICA by the small diameter of the bony canal. Contrast-enhanced MRA in the late arterial phase is thought to be the most sensitive sequence for detecting nearly occluded or reconstituted vessels (Fig. 26.3).

Reversal of Flow

A blood vessel in which the direction of flow is reversed (e.g., the vertebral artery in subclavian steal phenomenon) is invisible on TOF MRA because its signal is eliminated by a superior saturation band. If a vessel is not visible on TOF images, the acquisition can be repeated without a saturation band or with saturation inferior to the acquired volume. The fact that flow is reversed in a vessel may not be recognized on contrast-enhanced MRA because the vessel is already bright on the arterial phase image (Fig. 26.4).

Vessel Tortuosity

Horizontal segments of the carotid artery, such as one often encounters in the bulb, or down-going segments, such as may occur in redundant cervical loops, do not provide inflowing blood to a transaxial 2D TOF MRA section. As a result, horizontal and down-going segments are dark on 2D TOF angiograms. Collateral structures are often incompletely visualized when this sequence is used. Furthermore,

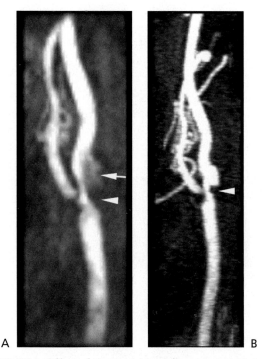

FIGURE 26.1. Effect of stagnant blood flow on signal intensity in multiple overlapping thin-slab acquisition (MOTSA) angiography. A moderately stenotic internal carotid artery origin is equally apparent by the MOTSA technique **(A)** and the contrast-enhanced MRA **(B)** technique *(arrowheads)*, but the vessel intensity is more uniform on contrast-enhanced MRA. In particular, blood flowing past the carotid bulb results in a relatively stagnant pool within the posterior bulb and weak signal intensity on MOTSA *(arrow)*.

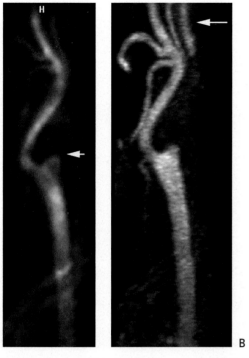

FIGURE 26.3. Internal carotid artery (ICA) reconstitution detected by contrast-enhanced MRA. **A:** An apparent occlusion of the ICA *(arrow)* on multiple overlapping thin-slab acquisition (MOTSA). **B:** With contrast-enhanced MRA, reconstitution of the ICA is noted in the midregion of the neck *(arrow)*. ICA reconstitution is rare but may occur, often resulting from vasa vasorum collaterals.

the signal intensity of a blood vessel may depend on the angle at which it enters the acquired slice. In contrast-enhanced MRA, which is not strongly dependent on the velocity of blood entry, signal is uniformly bright in a cervical loop. Furthermore, blood does not lose its signal on contrast-enhanced MRA as it dwells in the imaging volume.

Phase Dispersion and Overestimation of Stenosis

The intensity of the blood signal is diminished within the stenotic portion of an arterial lumen, and the degree of stenosis may be overestimated as a result. The reason for reduced signal intensity is twofold. First, the lumen may be smaller than the pixel diameter, in which case partial voluming of the signal takes place. Second, phase dispersion may occur within the lumen as the result of a high degree of variability of blood flow velocity and trajectory (16). This mechanism of cancellation of signal is loosely termed *turbulence,* although it may not fit the definition of truly turbulent flow. The amount of phase dispersion depends, among other things, on gradient strength and voxel size. In 2D TOF MRA, the slice-selection gradients are especially strong and the voxel especially large; as a result, signal cancellation is more pronounced. Phase dispersion is less pronounced in 3D TOF and contrast-enhanced MRA, so that signal is not lost until the luminal diameter is much smaller (Fig. 26.5).

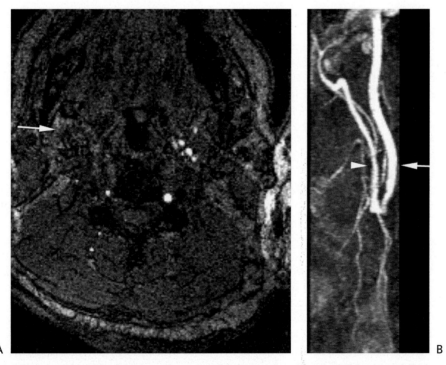

FIGURE 26.4. Arterial blood demonstrated without regard to direction of flow on contrast-enhanced MRA. **A:** No flow is visible in the right internal or external carotid artery on a two-dimensional (2D) time-of-flight (TOF) section *(arrow)*. **B:** On contrast-enhanced MRA, the common carotid artery is seen to be occluded, but the internal carotid artery *(arrow)* is reconstituted from reversal of a large external carotid artery branch *(arrowhead)*. Blood signal in this branch was eliminated by the superior saturation band used to suppress the jugular vein on 2D TOF MRA.

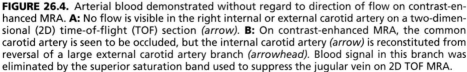

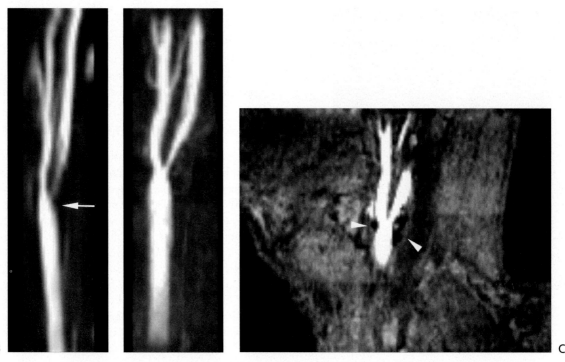

A,B   C

FIGURE 26.5. Overestimation of stenosis in two-dimensional (2D) time-of-flight (TOF) MRA. **A:** On 2D TOF MRA, the signal intensity is greatly diminished at the internal carotid artery origin *(arrow).* **B:** Intensity is much greater on 3D TOF MRA. **C:** On a parasagittal re-formation of the 3D TOF data, calculated through the plane of the bifurcation, dark structures are calcific plaque *(arrowheads).* The vessel width appears thicker and is more accurately portrayed on native sections or re-formations than it is on projections.

In general, fewer flow- and motion-related artifacts are encountered in contrast-enhanced MRA than in TOF MRA, for the following reasons: its relative insensitivity to blood velocity; the very short TE, during which the blood undergoes minimal displacement; and the brief total acquisition time, during which the patient is unlikely to move (Figs. 26.6 and 26.7). Whether overestimation of stenosis is less with 3D TOF or with contrast-enhanced MRA has not been established. A cause of weak signal within a narrowed lumen on contrast-enhanced MR angiograms appears to be a low signal-to-noise ratio (Fig. 26.8).

Plaque Visualization

Carotid plaque is visible on 3D TOF acquisitions, albeit at somewhat low levels of resolution. The signal of plaque is intermediate between that of bright blood and that of the dark, muscular arterial wall. Calcifications are devoid of signal, whereas hemorrhage is bright. The 3D volumetric data can be reformatted longitudinally in the plane of the bifurcation for a better demonstration of the location of plaque within the carotid bulb (Fig. 26.5). Another commonly used technique for plaque imaging is a dark blood sequence—usually a cardiac-gated, thin-slice, spin-echo series acquired perpendicular to blood flow (Fig. 26.9).

Protocols

The choice of acquisition parameters depends on both field strength and manufacturer. Each manufacturer provides imaging parameters that are optimized for their equipment.

Carotid Protocol

In a typical protocol, the patient is placed in a head and neck coil. Basic brain images might include diffusion (17) and fluid-attenuated inversion recovery (FLAIR) (18) to determine whether the patient has had a recent or remote stroke. Carotid imaging generally begins with a limited 2D TOF set to locate the bifurcations and identify vessels with occlusion or reversed flow. If a vertebral artery or other vessel is absent on the 2D images, the sequence should be repeated without presaturation bands to rule out reversal of flow. From the 2D TOF MRA, a MOTSA or contrast-enhanced MRA will be specified. The repetition time (TR) should be minimized on contrast-enhanced MRA. The TE should also be minimized, but not at the expense of resolution. Obtaining both MOTSA and contrast-enhanced MR angiograms for every patient provides a high degree of security during study interpretation and combines the strengths of each sequence (19).

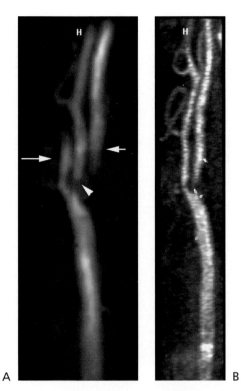

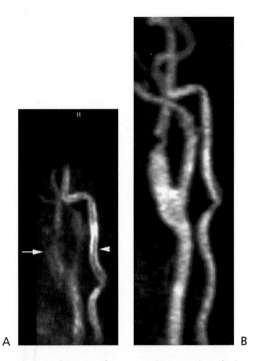

FIGURE 26.6. Reduction of gross patient motion on contrast-enhanced MRA. **A:** An apparent trifurcation of the carotid artery is seen on multiple overlapping thin-slab acquisition (MOTSA), with a stenosis at the origin of the external carotid artery *(arrowhead)* and two flanking vessels *(arrows)*. **B:** A simple bifurcation is noted on contrast-enhanced MRA. The artifact arose from gross motion of the head between two overlapping slabs of the MOTSA series.

FIGURE 26.7. Reduction of gross patient motion during rapid contrast-enhanced MRA acquisition. **A:** On a 12-minute multiple overlapping thin-slab acquisition (MOTSA), the vertebral artery is bright and distinct *(arrowhead),* whereas the carotid artery is faint *(arrow).* **B:** On a 20-second contrast-enhanced MRA acquisition, both vessels are clearly seen. The loss of carotid signal on MOTSA was caused by snoring.

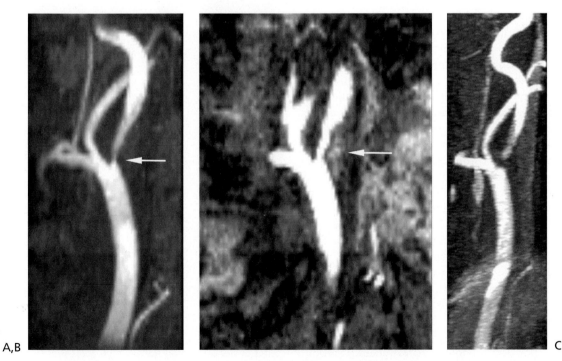

FIGURE 26.8. Overestimation of stenosis on contrast enhanced MRA. **A:** A stenotic internal carotid artery origin *(arrow)* on multiple overlapping thin-slab acquisition (MOTSA). **B:** The lumen is better seen on a parasagittal re-formation, which clearly depicts the plaque *(arrowhead).* **C:** In this example, the stenosis appears more severe on contrast-enhanced MRA.

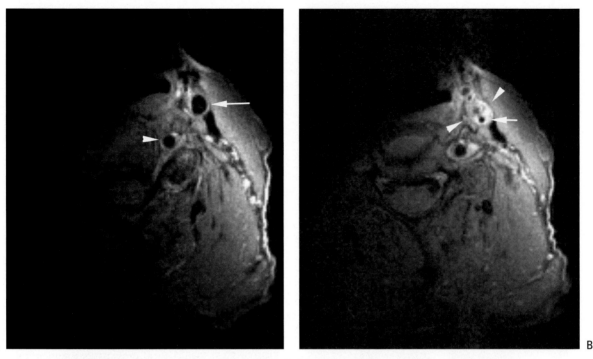

A   B

FIGURE 26.9. Carotid plaque imaging with a dark blood technique. **A:** Cardiac-gated spin-echo images of the neck, with use of a surface coil for signal reception, eliminates signal in the patent internal carotid artery *(arrow)* and vertebral artery *(arrowhead).* **B:** At the level of the carotid bifurcation, the lumen is greatly diminished *(arrow)* and surrounded by bright plaque *(arrowheads).*

Aortic Arch Protocol

TOF MRA has not proved successful for imaging the aortic arch and carotid origins. Reasons are artifacts caused by breathing motion, the diverse directions of blood flow encountered at the arch and therefore the inability to select a slice orientation that maximizes inflow for all arterial segments, and the presence of reciprocating flow within the aorta and proximal carotid arteries. For imaging the aortic arch and origins of the cervical vessels, contrast-enhanced MRA is the only effective option (20–22). Usually, the 3D slab is oriented in the coronal plane to show the entire length of the carotid and vertebral arteries in addition to the proximal subclavian vessels (Figs. 26.10 and 26.11). However, if the primary disease lies in the aortic arch, such as an aortic dissection that extends into the carotid arteries, then a parasagittal acquisition in the plane of the aortic arch ("candy cane" view) may be the best choice.

If both the arch and carotid arteries must be studied in one imaging session, two separate gadolinium angiograms can be obtained, the first optimized for the arch and the second for the carotid bifurcations. Venous enhancement will be present on the second study. Subtracting a preinjection from postinjection acquisition eliminates venous signal on the second angiogram. Alternatively, the arch and carotid arteries can be acquired in one slab with a large field of view. In that case, a 512-image matrix is recommended.

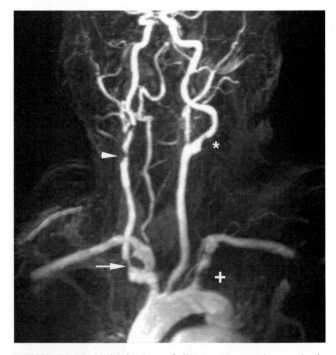

FIGURE 26.10. Multiple sites of disease portrayed on a single contrast-enhanced MR angiogram with a large field of view. A left anterior oblique projection has been calculated to show the sites of stenosis better. Narrowing is present at the origin of the right internal carotid artery (ICA) *(arrow)*, at the ICA bifurcation *(arrowhead)*, at the left carotid bulb *(*)*, and throughout the proximal left subclavian artery *(+)*. The left vertebral artery is occluded.

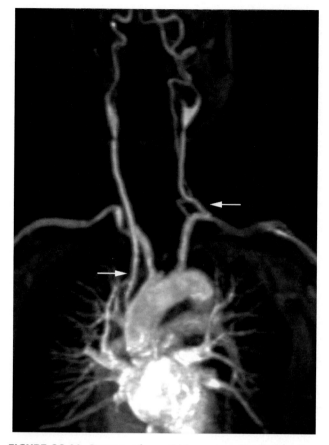

FIGURE 26.11. Patency of carotid bypass grafts displayed on contrast-enhanced MRA. An angiogram of the upper chest and neck demonstrates a left extrathoracic and a right aortic graft *(arrows)*, which were placed because of near-occlusion of the common carotid arteries.

Intracranial Vessels

Although beyond the scope of this chapter, it may be noted that the carotid siphons and cerebral arteries are best imaged with MOTSA. The intracranial vertebrobasilar arteries are also imaged with MOTSA. The extracranial vertebral arteries are best visualized by contrast-enhanced MRA.

Image Interpretation

When carotid MRA is interpreted, special care should be taken not to overestimate the degree of stenosis in an area of turbulent flow. This phenomenon is encountered within the decelerating jet beyond a critical lesion. The tendency to overestimate is greatly reduced if one interprets the study from source images or re-formations rather than from calculated projections (23,24). Maximum intensity projections (MIPs) aggravate signal loss and cause vessels to appear thinner because the algorithm selects not only the brightest intensities within the vessel but also the brightest intensities in the background (25). As a result, the average background intensity is elevated to exceed the signal at the edges of the vessel. MIP overestimation is a significant problem in 3D TOF MRA. It is less of a problem in contrast-enhanced MRA, in which background intensities are greatly suppressed; however, inspecting native partitions of contrast-enhanced MRA is still of value (Fig. 26.12).

An alternative to MIP is to calculate re-formations of 3D TOF sections in the plane of the bifurcation (Figs. 26.2 and 26.8). This method is very effective for displaying the location of plaque and allows one to trace a faint residual lumen that may not be recognizable on the native transaxial partitions.

Shaded surface displays (Fig. 26.13) are visually appealing but eliminate a great deal of useful signal information. In calculating these displays, one picks an intensity threshold that defines the margin of the vessel. Because the intensity is reduced within a stenotic lumen, the threshold inevitably exaggerates the degree of stenosis. If the intensity within the residual lumen is less than the threshold, continuity will be lost between the common carotid artery and the ICA.

Another common artifact is encountered at sharp turns in vessels. Blood velocity is greatest around outer curves, whereas blood flows more slowly along inner curves. On 3D TOF sequences, the inner portion of a curve may become saturated, and a false appearance of narrowing results. This artifact is often encountered where the carotid enters the

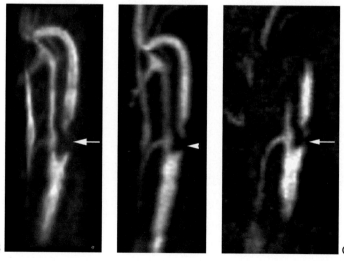

A,B   C

FIGURE 26.12. Demonstration of the need to view both native and projected images in the interpretation of MRA. **A:** A gap in the proximal internal carotid artery signal is present on a multiple overlapping thin-slab acquisition (MOTSA) *(arrow)*. **B:** In this example, the gap is slightly smaller on the contrast-enhanced MRA study *(arrowhead)*, possibly because some of the signal loss may have resulted from slow flow in the area beyond the plaque. **C:** The residual lumen is visible on a native partition through the stenosis *(arrow)*. Trace residual signal in the lumen was overwhelmed by background signal on maximum intensity projection.

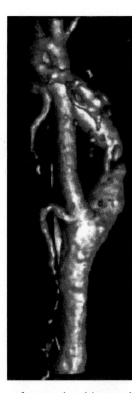

FIGURE 26.13. A surface-rendered image derived from a sub-millimeter-resolution, contrast-enhanced MR angiogram. Although this form of display eliminates background signal, all nuances of blood flow signal are lost. Variations in signal may be a valuable sign in the interpretation of MRA.

petrous bone and turns sharply (26). The problem is overcome by contrast-enhanced MRA.

In a very tight curve, especially within the carotid siphons, the direction of flow may differ substantially between the phase-encoding gradient and the frequency-encoding gradient. Mismapping and distortion of the vessel shape and the potential for a false stenosis are the result.

Metal susceptibility artifact in the neck may be caused by surgical clips or dental appliances. This artifact is recognized as a dark, circular signal void centered outside the vessel on cross-sectional localizing sequences. As in any type of MRI, the artifact is minimized by using a shorter TE and smaller voxels. Contrast-enhanced MRA, with its very short TE, is the preferred sequence when metal artifact is a concern (Fig. 26.14).

One should resist the temptation to interpret a study that is compromised by patient motion. Motion may mask a severe stenosis and generate a false stenosis.

Finally, the interpretation is most useful if one reports a stenosis as a percentage value rather than as a category or qualitative assessment. A computer workstation and measurement tools or film and a calibrated jeweler's loupe can be used for this purpose.

APPLICATIONS

The Carotid Artery and Stroke

Most plaques develop within the bulb of the carotid bifurcation. Atherosclerosis tends to occur at this site because of

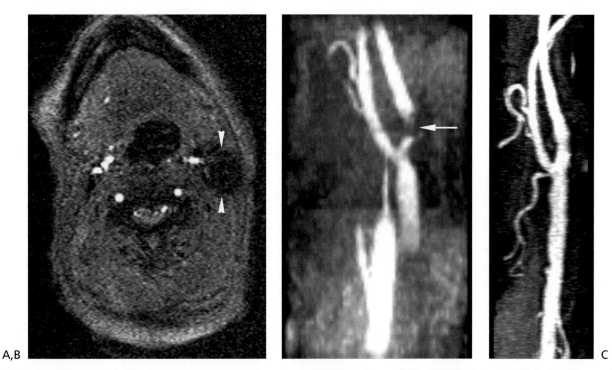

A,B   C

FIGURE 26.14. Metal clip artifact is minimized on contrast-enhanced MRA. **A:** A two-dimensional (2D) time-of-flight (TOF) image (echo time = 10 milliseconds) shows the prominent dark circle of a metal clip artifact *(arrowheads)*. **B:** The clip generated a false stenosis on 3D TOF MRA (echo time = 6 milliseconds) *(arrow)*. Note gross rotation of the neck during the study, so that the slabs are out of alignment. **C:** On contrast-enhanced MRA (echo time = 2 milliseconds), the clip artifact is greatly diminished. Metal susceptibility artifact is reduced by short echo times and small voxels.

"flow separation," a blood flow pattern that results in very low velocities along the posterior wall (27,28) (Figs. 26.15 and 26.16). Less common sites of carotid atherosclerosis include the common carotid origin and the internal carotid siphon. Carotid atherosclerosis is a known cause of stroke, but not the only one. Others are carotid wall dissection (29,30), fibromuscular dysplasia, kinking of a redundant carotid artery, cerebral artery thrombosis (31), and emboli arising from the heart (32) or aortic ulcerations (33).

Carotid atherosclerosis gives rise to stroke by two principal mechanisms: In thrombotic stroke, a vessel suddenly becomes occluded at the site of a stenosis, and in embolic stroke, material originating at the stenosis occludes intracranial branches. Emboli may be generated when plaque becomes necrotic and discharges its contents into the vessel lumen (34), when platelets and thrombin collect within an ulceration and then break free (35–37), or when thrombin forms within the flow eddies just beyond a stenosis (38). The idea that emboli can form without necrosis of plaque is supported by studies performed with transcranial Doppler ultrasonography, in which silent emboli are observed with great frequency (39). However, it is difficult to prove that emboli are the cause of stroke in a specific patient because the emboli are short-lived and may have resolved by the time angiography is performed (40). Furthermore, partially resolved emboli may mimic the appearance of an atheroma in an intracranial vessel.

Significance of Carotid Stenosis

Investigators have sought to define which morphologic features of atherosclerosis give rise to thrombosis or emboli, so

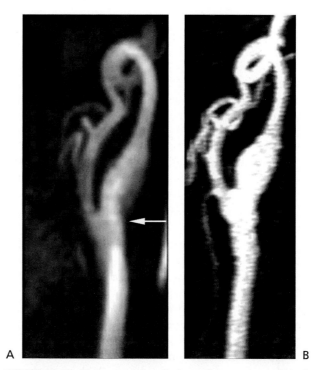

FIGURE 26.16. Flow separation. **A:** A nearly normal carotid bulb is brighter anteriorly than posteriorly. At the entrance to the bulb, a dark line extends from the posterior wall *(arrow)* at the site of flow separation. This is where carotid plaque most often forms. **B:** Flow separation is not apparent on contrast-enhanced MRA, which is less sensitive to blood velocity.

that intervention can be undertaken before a stroke occurs. Alterations in plaque composition and the development of a necrotic "core" could potentially be visualized by MRA (41–43), but as yet, only preliminary studies have related this information to the subsequent development of stroke (44,45). The only features of plaque that have been unequivocally linked to stroke are a high degree of luminal narrowing and the presence of a large ulcer. As stenosis becomes more severe, the risk for stroke increases. Following endarterectomy, the risk for stroke is diminished. This relationship has been confirmed by several well-publicized clinical trials.

The North American Symptomatic Carotid Endarterectomy Trial (NASCET) (46) examined 3,000 patients with recent transient ischemic attacks and bifurcation stenosis. Of those with stenosis greater than 70% of the vessel diameter, 24% went on to have a stroke within 18 months. Further, the risk for stroke in patients with 90% to 99% stenosis was greater than the risk for patients with 80% to 89% stenosis, which was in turn greater than the risk for patients with 70% to 79% stenosis. When endarterectomy was performed, the rate of stroke fell to 7% in 18 months. Surgery reduced the rate of stroke by 71% and the death rate by 58%.

The European Carotid Surgery Trial (ECST) (47) examined 2,518 symptomatic patients and concluded that

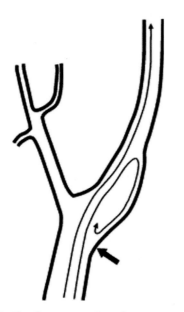

FIGURE 26.15. The flow separation phenomenon. The bloodstream separates from the proximal posterior bulb wall *(arrow)*, flowing cephalad in the anterior bulb, then recirculating to flow caudad in the posterior bulb. The point of flow separation is a common site of plaque formation.

endarterectomy in patients with stenosis greater than 70% reduced the risk for stroke within 3 years from 21.9% to 12.3%.

The Asymptomatic Carotid Atherosclerosis Study (ACAS) (48) examined 4,465 asymptomatic patients and found an advantage for endarterectomy even among this population, albeit a small one. The risk for stroke within 5 years in those with stenosis greater than 60% decreased from 11% to 5.1%

The advantages of endarterectomy are long-lived. The Veterans Affairs Cooperative Study Group (49) found that during a period of 8 years, 12% of surgical patients had cerebral events, versus 25% of those given medical treatment alone.

The surgical consequence of these studies has been that symptomatic patients with stenosis at least 70% of the vessel diameter are routinely referred for endarterectomy. In 1998, the NASCET investigators announced that after retrospective restratification of the data, they could recommend endarterectomy for patients with stenosis greater than 50% (50). This practice has not yet been generally adopted. The appropriate indication for endarterectomy in asymptomatic patients is a matter of debate. With a criterion of 60% stenosis, the value used for stratification in the ACAS, nearly 17 procedures would be performed to prevent one stroke in 5 years, or 85 procedures to prevent one stroke per year. In practice, many surgeon use a threshold of 80% to 85% to select symptomatic candidates for endarterectomy (51).

In the NASCET and the ACAS, stenoses were graded according to the narrowest diameter of the ICA at the lesion expressed as a percentage of the diameter of the normal ICA beyond the bulb (52,53) (Fig. 26.17). The decision to use diameter as a measure of stenosis, rather than residual cross-

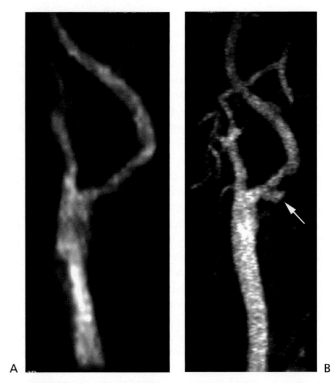

FIGURE 26.18. Ulcer detection on contrast-enhanced MRA. **A:** On multiple overlapping thin-slab acquisition (MOTSA), mild narrowing of a long segment of the proximal internal carotid artery is noted. **B:** On contrast-enhanced MRA, an ulcer is visible *(arrow)*. The ulcer was not visible on the time-of-flight image because of poor inflow into the ulcer cavity.

sectional area, was dictated by the choice of conventional catheter angiography, which portrays projectional anatomy.

Validation Studies

Investigations of imaging have focused on determining the relative accuracy rates of various modalities, among them Doppler ultrasonography, MRA, and catheter angiography, in detecting stenosis greater than 70% of the vessel diameter. The majority of studies have compared 3D TOF or MOTSA with catheter angiography (24,54–64). The median sensitivity for a high-grade lesion in these publications was 93%, and the median specificity was 88%. Studies comparing contrast-enhanced MRA with catheter angiography have shown very similar levels of accuracy (6,65–67). In addition, they have demonstrated better ulcer detection (Fig. 26.18) and better depiction of the length of stenosis and slow flow beyond a critical lesion (11). However, the signal-to-noise ratio of contrast-enhanced MRA was found to be inferior to that of MOTSA MRA. This was especially true if peak arterial enhancement was missed because of incorrect timing of the acquisition. The use of MOTSA and contrast-enhanced MRA together resulted in exceptionally high rates of accuracy in comparison with catheter angiography (19).

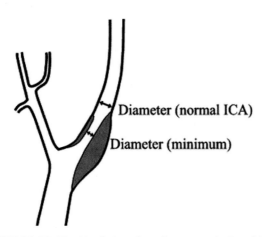

FIGURE 26.17. The North American Symptomatic Carotid Endarterectomy Trialists measured carotid artery stenosis by comparing the smallest residual luminal diameter in the bulb with the normal luminal diameter in the internal carotid artery beyond the bulb according to the following formula:
$[1 - (diameter_{minimum}/diameter_{normal\ ICA})] \times 100.$

Validation studies assume catheter angiography to be the gold standard. The problem with this assumption is that any errors in measurement by catheter angiography are counted as errors in MRA. Because the reproducibility of catheter angiography itself is no better than 94% (68–70), one can conclude that the actual sensitivities and specificities are better than those reported. In fact, preliminary data suggest that noninvasive imaging may be more sensitive than catheter angiography in some instances (56). In a comparison of catheter angiography, MRA, and Doppler ultrasonography in which surgical specimens rather than catheter angiography were used as the gold standard (71), Doppler ultrasonography and MRA each correlated better with the endarterectomy specimen than did catheter angiography. This discrepancy can be attributed to the fact that catheter angiography often does not appreciate the smallest diameter when the stenosis is elliptical or complex in shape. In fact, rotational angiography, a recently available technique for conventional angiography in which images are acquired from many orientations following a single catheter injection, has shown that catheter angiography may often underestimate the severity of a lesion by not viewing it from the most stenotic direction (72). That is to say, when MRA is compared with a gold standard of catheter angiography, one finds that MRA often overestimates, but when MRA is compared with a gold standard of rotational catheter angiography, no tendency to overestimate is found. The fact that the stenotic lumen is usually noncircular is particularly important in comparisons of catheter angiography and Doppler ultrasonography because Doppler velocities are determined by cross-sectional area rather than by diameter (73).

Information about the shape of plaque, known by MRA but not by catheter angiography, is ignored in the validation studies. The rationale for this approach has been that catheter angiography is the only modality known to reduce the incidence of stoke, by virtue of its use in clinical trials. Clinical trials on the scale of NASCET, with the use of MRA rather than catheter angiography to quantify stenosis, have never been undertaken. Therefore, MRA and Doppler ultrasonography are assumed to be effective only to the degree that they agree with measurements of diameter made by catheter angiography.

Cost-effectiveness

One would expect MRA to be more cost-effective than catheter angiography because of its lower cost and associated morbidity. The cost of MRA is on average one-third that of catheter angiography and three times that of Doppler ultrasonography. Typical costs of these modalities might be $300.00 (Doppler ultrasonography), $900.00 (MRA), and $2,700.00 (catheter angiography); however, these costs vary considerably among medical centers. In a capitated health care program, the target expense for carotid stenosis, including diagnosis, endarterectomy, and follow-up clinic visits, is approximately $15,000. This budget leaves little room for a catheter angiogram.

The frequency of stroke as a complication of catheter angiography is between 0.5% and 1.0% (74–76), and the perioperative surgical risk for stroke is 2% to 3% (46,48), so adding catheter angiography to the treatment plan substantially increases the overall complication rate. This fact was clearly demonstrated in the ACAS, in which the risks for stroke associated with catheter angiography and those associated with endarterectomy were found to be equal (77).

It is not surprising, therefore, that cost-effectiveness calculations have favored noninvasive imaging. These studies have used risk statistics from the NASCET and the ACAS, together with imaging accuracy statistics from the literature or from local practice, to predict the outcome of a hypothetical or actual cohort of patients, often as a function of the assumed prevalence of disease (60,78–83).

Kent et al. (60) examined the cost-effectiveness of various imaging strategies for a population of symptomatic patients. The use of Doppler ultrasonography alone resulted in a quality-adjusted life expectancy (QALE) of 9.619 years. Catheter angiography alone resulted in a QALE of 9.632 years, with an excessive incremental cost-effectiveness ratio of $99,200 per quality-adjusted life year (QALY). The combination of Doppler ultrasonography and MRA, followed by catheter angiography in the event of disparate results, maximized clinical outcome to 9.639 years at an incremental cost-effectiveness ratio of just $22,400.00 and was considered the optimal strategy. MRA alone was nearly identical to catheter angiography in outcome (QALE of 9.631 years) but was eliminated by dominance, and its marginal cost was not reported.

It is apparent from this example that the least and most expensive workup algorithms show little difference in outcome. The inclusion of catheter angiography may improve diagnostic accuracy, but it also introduces more complications.

Obuchowski et al. (83) assumed a 20% prevalence of surgical stenosis in patients who presented with a neck bruit. Three imaging strategies were examined: Doppler ultrasonography followed in selected cases by MRA, Doppler ultrasonography followed in selected cases by catheter angiography, and MRA alone. The QALE values of the three strategies were virtually identical, whereas the incremental costs per QALY were $2,922, $7,470, and $7,700, respectively. Doppler ultrasonography alone was not examined. This study again argues for a combined noninvasive approach (84).

When asymptomatic patients are screened, the advantages of noninvasive imaging are even stronger. Kuntz et al. (82) concluded that use of catheter angiography in this population actually resulted in a greater incidence of stroke (7.12% in 5 years) than did Doppler ultrasonography alone (6.35%), MRA alone (6.17%), or a combination of Doppler ultrasonography and MRA followed by catheter angiography if necessary (6.34%).

Limitations of Outcome Studies

The cost-effectiveness calculations assume that catheter angiography is completely accurate, whereas Doppler ultrasonography and MRA incorrectly categorize about 10% of surgical lesions. If one adopts the more likely assumption that catheter angiography, Doppler ultrasonography, and MRA are all capable of error, then the cost advantage of noninvasive imaging is even more dramatic.

Furthermore, the models assume that the 70% threshold, when NASCET risk statistics are used, and the 60% threshold, when ACAS risk statistics are used, represent hard boundaries between individuals with different expected surgical benefits. If the stroke prevalence statistics could be measured as a continuous variable of degree of stenosis, then minor differences in the measurement of stenosis would be much less important in determining outcome. However, gathering this data would necessitate an impractically large clinical trial.

In one respect, the models may underestimate the effect of imaging accuracy. The models assume proficiency in both Doppler ultrasonography and MRA, whereas in practice, the accuracy of noninvasive imaging is highly variable among medical centers. Howard et al. (85) pointed out this problem when they evaluated the Doppler ultrasonography data from various centers in the ACAS. The NASCET collected Doppler ultrasonography data and showed poor correlation with stroke risk, but uniformity or quality control among the contributors was minimal (86,87). The catheter angiography data, by comparison, were rigorously specified and read by a single well-trained interpreter (53). One should be cautioned, therefore, that the favorable outcomes predicted by the cost-effectiveness studies accrue only to those centers that perform imaging (and surgery) with a high level of experience (88).

Recommendations for Imaging

The workup of suspected carotid artery stenosis should begin with Doppler ultrasonography performed by an experienced, and preferably accredited, laboratory. If this study is technically adequate and reveals a lesion greater than 70%, and if the presence of a tandem lesion is not suggested based on the waveform, then the most cost-effective approach is to proceed directly to surgery. Typical technical limitations that might necessitate further imaging include the presence of a shadowing plaque, a deep course of the ICA, discordant gray scale and Doppler measurements, and contralateral disease. Tandem lesions are suggested by the presence of a dampened and delayed waveform (89) or unusually low diastolic velocities.

If patients require further imaging, they should be referred to an experienced MRA service with an active quality assurance program. In most cases, MRA will answer the question. Additional imaging is of marginal benefit for precisely determining the degree of stenosis—for example, for defining whether a stenotic lesion is just greater or just smaller than 70% in an otherwise adequate Doppler ultrasonogram (90). Rather, additional imaging should be used to clarify major uncertainties. If both MRA and Doppler ultrasonography are performed and the results agree, then the chance that these results will agree with those of conventional angiography is exceptionally high. In a study of patients who underwent Doppler ultrasonography, MRA, and catheter angiography for the detection of a 70% stenosis, Serfaty et al. (19) found that contrast-enhanced MRA had a sensitivity of 94% and a specificity of 85% in comparison with the gold standard of catheter angiography, but when contrast-enhanced MRA and Doppler ultrasonography were in agreement, the sensitivity and specificity were both 100%.

The use of catheter angiography should be minimized. However, patients' lesions are occasionally so atypical that they can be understood only with the high level of resolution and certain vascular contrast obtained in a catheter study. It may be argued that performing catheter angiography before each surgical procedure provides an additional margin of safety. In fact, the routine use of catheter angiography may worsen the average patient outcome. Furthermore, the quest for a highly precise measurement of diameter is meaningless for several reasons. First, luminal shape is highly complex, so that a single value for the diameter does not accurately express any hemodynamic phenomenon. Second, the association between stenosis and stroke is not perfect. Only about one-third of strokes result from a surgically accessible stenosis (91), and just 25% of patients with bifurcation stenosis greater than 70% have a stroke within 18 months (46). Among asymptomatic patients, only 21% with a high-grade lesion have a stroke within 3 years (48). These figures indicate that imaging cannot establish the benefit of endarterectomy for a specific patient. Rather, benefit accrues to the surgical population in aggregate. Third, catheter angiography subsequent to Doppler ultrasonography may occasionally find additional lesions but rarely changes therapy (92–97). Disease of the carotid origin occurs in only about 2% of patients with significant bifurcation stenosis (98), and embolization from this source is unusual (99). Fourth, the 70% surgical threshold is a result of the NASCET design and does not represent the absolute diameter below which no benefit can be obtained.

In practice, a majority of surgeons use primarily noninvasive imaging for presurgical assessment, and the use of catheter angiography has declined substantially.

Carotid Dissection

Carotid artery dissection (Fig. 26.19) is most frequently the result of trauma. Patients present with headache, neck pain, and sympathetic nerve paresis. The dissection, which may progress to thrombosis or give rise to an embolus, consists of

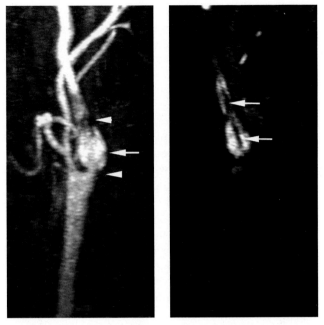

FIGURE 26.19. Dissection flap seen on native partitions. **A:** A contrast-enhanced MR angiogram of the carotid artery shows an aneurysm of the bulb *(arrow)* and focal stenoses *(arrowheads).* **B:** A dissection flap is noted on a native coronal partition *(arrows).* Intimal flaps are often hidden on maximum intensity projections.

a hemorrhage in the media that extends in some cases to the adventitia. An intimal flap may or may not be apparent. The flap often occurs within or just beyond the bulb and extends up the ICA for a variable distance. On angiography, a narrowing is seen that may be smooth or irregular (29,100). Because not all dissections are stenotic, spin-echo T1-weighted transverse images, preferably with fat saturation, help identify the false lumen (30).

The patient is usually treated conservatively with warfarin for several months as prophylaxis for stoke.

Fibromuscular Dysplasia

Fibromuscular dysplasia is a rare idiopathic disease of smooth muscle in which the vessel wall takes on a beaded appearance. It occurs most often in middle-aged women. The disease may progress to higher grades of stenosis, transient ischemic attacks, or even stroke. The administration of antiplatelet agents and dilation are common therapies. MRA is not as sensitive as catheter angiography for detecting mild cases of fibromuscular dysplasia. Two-dimensional TOF MRA may often miss fibromuscular dysplasia because of inadequate resolution. Moderate to advanced cases may be detected on contrast-enhanced MRA.

Vertebrobasilar Insufficiency

The term *vertebrobasilar insufficiency* refers to transient ischemic events of the posterior cerebral circulation. These may include loss of consciousness. Hypotension, arrhythmias, anemia, brain tumors, and subclavian steal phenomenon may all be mistaken for vertebral artery stenosis.

Stenosis typically occurs at the proximal vertebral origin, at the intracranial junction of the vertebral arteries, or within the basilar artery. MOTSA is typically used to image the intracranial posterior circulation but is a laborious technique in the cervical vertebral artery. The vertebral arteries are within the field of view of carotid contrast-enhanced MRA and are automatically acquired as part of the carotid study. The direction of flow is often not discernible on contrast-enhanced MRA. Subclavian steal must be diagnosed by 2D TOF MRA, acquired with an inferior and then with a superior saturation band to confirm reversal of vertebral blood flow.

Vertebral Dissection

Vertebral dissections usually occur between the C1 and C2 vertebral posterior elements as a result of twisting the neck. Patients present with a sudden onset of headache and neck pain and ischemic symptoms of the brainstem and cerebellum. The diagnosis is made on the basis of intramural hematoma, pseudoaneurysm, or vessel narrowing on MRI and MRA. Subarachnoid hemorrhage is a sign of intracranial dissection.

Aortic Arch and Carotid Origins

Transcutaneous Doppler ultrasonography cannot visualize the aortic arch and carotid origins directly, but proximal disease is implied by a dampened waveform or flow that is reversed in direction. Likewise, MRA of the carotid bifurcation may suggest the presence of a more proximal lesion when flow is reversed, or when the rate of inflow, and hence the degree of signal saturation on a 3D TOF acquisition, differs between the right and left vessels. In that event, a contrast-enhanced MRA acquisition of the arch provides a noninvasive alternative to catheter angiography.

The presence of thick aortic plaques or aortic ulcerations is a risk factor for stroke (101). These features are visible on contrast-enhanced MRA. However, mobile, free-floating plaques may be invisible as a result of time-averaged acquisition.

FUTURE APPLICATIONS

The trend toward MRI machines with ever-increasing gradient strength has substantially reduced the duration of sequence acquisition and permitted shorter and more concentrated injections of gadolinium. The MRI machines of the future will permit contrast-enhanced MRA acquisitions at even greater speed with better resolution and vascular signal intensity. Additionally, the TE will be still further reduced on these machines, so that both intrinsic and flow-related sources of signal cancellation will be eliminated. As a result, the tendency toward overestimation of the degree of stenosis may be alleviated.

As TEs become shorter and flow artifacts are reduced, contrast agents and blood inflow may no longer be necessary. Angiography may simply become a water-weighted sequence. In that case, the difference between MRI and MRA will disappear. Any number of vessel segments will be acquired in one procedure. Because carotid, coronary, and peripheral arterial diseases are strongly associated, a comprehensive screening study may include all three territories. Ironically, this innovation will bring us full circle to the earliest days of MRA, when blood imaging was attempted with cardiac-gated, T2-weighted spin-echo sequences.

Another potential approach for vascular imaging of the whole body is the use of experimental intravascular contrast agents. These agents persist in the blood pool for several hours, so that prolonged, high-resolution imaging sequences can be acquired. Contrast material may be administered before the patient enters the magnet, without the need for a timed injection. Preliminary reports have demonstrated strong image contrast and excellent correspondence with catheter angiography (102).

A potential innovation may result from a greater understanding of how the structure of plaque causes stroke. The NASCET considered only the diameter of a stenosis as a predictor of risk for stroke. It did not consider the plaque directly—its instability, morphology, and effect of blood flow patterns and wall shear. Currently, surgeons must perform five or more procedures before they can change the outcome of a single symptomatic patient. If plaque composition and shape, determined by high-resolution MRI, could provide a more specific index of patients at risk for stroke, unnecessary surgery would be greatly reduced.

Percutaneous carotid angioplasty with stent placement is a procedure that offers relief of a stenotic lesion with little or no need for hospitalization. However, considerable concern remains regarding whether angioplasty is as safe as surgical endarterectomy. Recent reviews indicate a complication rate exceeding that in the NASCET; however, many of the patients typically treated by angioplasty would not have qualified for inclusion in the NASCET because of the presence of comorbid conditions (103). If carotid intervention becomes universally accepted, then the utility of MRA may be greatly reduced. That is to say, patients will go directly from Doppler ultrasonography to the angiography suite for a procedure that will both confirm the findings of Doppler and correct the lesion. Indeed, the placement of a stent may preclude the subsequent performance of MRA because of an RF shielding effect.

Another unknown variable is the evolution of computed tomographic (CT) angiography (104,105). Recently introduced multiple-detector arrays permit rapid thin-slice acquisition throughout the length of the neck during the arterial phase of enhancement. CT angiography may eliminate the blood flow artifacts encountered in MRA and further improve the accuracy of noninvasive imaging.

SUMMARY

MRA of the carotid artery is a common imaging procedure that can be used to detect plaque and plaque ulceration, measure narrowing of the luminal diameter, confirm patency, identify reversal of flow, and visualize dissection flaps and hematomas. The two predominant sequences for carotid angiography are MOTSA and contrast-enhanced MRA. MOTSA does not require the injection of contrast material and so is cheaper and more convenient to use than contrast-enhanced MRA; however, contrast-enhanced MRA is gradually displacing MOTSA as the preferred sequence because it is relatively free from certain artifacts caused by blood flow and motion. The newer generation of MRI machines, with their strong gradients, have improved the quality of MR angiograms. The reliable interpretation of carotid MR angiograms requires an understanding of blood flow patterns in the carotid bulb and the recognition of common signal artifacts, especially the effects of turbulent flow and patient motion. The interpretation of MRA findings is improved by a program of quality control consisting of routine comparisons with other imaging modalities and surgical observations.

Noninvasive imaging of the carotid artery reduces cost, inconvenience, and risk. MRA competes with the other noninvasive modalities, Doppler ultrasonography and CT angiography, for the role of screening examination. As the least expensive study, Doppler ultrasonography may be recommended as the preferred screening modality. MRA is unique in its ability to study the brain and heart as an adjunct to angiography and can be recommended as a confirmatory or definitive examination.

REFERENCES

1. Kuller LH, Crook LP, Friedman GP. Survey of stroke epidemiology studies. Stroke 1972;3:579.
2. Colgan MP, Strode GR, Sommer JD, et al. Prevalence of asymptomatic carotid disease: results of duplex scanning in 348 unselected volunteers. *J Vasc Surg* 1998;8:674–679.
3. Fine-Edelstein JS, Wolf PA, O'Leary DH, et al. Precursors of extracranial carotid atherosclerosis in the Framingham study. *Neurology* 1994;44:1046–1050.
4. Schartz LB, Bridgman AH, Kieffer RW, et al. Asymptomatic carotid artery stenosis and stroke in patients undergoing cardiopulmonary bypass. *J Vasc Surg* 1995;21:146–153.
5. Cloft HJ, Murphy KJ, Prince MR, et al. 3D gadolinium-enhanced MR angiography of the carotid arteries. *Magn Reson Imaging* 1996;14:593–600.
6. Levy R, Prince M. Arterial-phase three-dimensional contrast-enhanced MR angiography of the carotid arteries. *AJR Am J Roentgenol* 1996;67:211–215.

7. Prince M, Chenevert T, Foo T, et al. Contrast-enhanced abdominal MR angiography: optimization of imaging time by automating the detection of contrast arrival time in the aorta. *Radiology* 1997;203:109–114.

8. Keller PJ, Drayer BP, Fram EK, et al. MR angiography with two-dimensional acquisition and three-dimensional display. *Radiology* 1989;173:527–532.

9. Masaryk TJ, Modic MT, Ruggiere PM, et al. Three-dimensional (volume) gradient echo imaging of the carotid bifurcation: preliminary clinical experience. *Radiology* 1989;171:801–806.

10. Parker DL, Yuan C, Blatter DD. MR angiography by multiple thin slab 3D acquisition. *Magn Reson Med* 1991;17:434–451.

11. DeMarco JK, Schonfeld S, Keller I, et al. Contrast-enhanced carotid MR angiography with commercially available triggering mechanism and elliptic centric phase encoding. *AJR Am J Roentgenol* 2001;176:221–227.

12. Riederer SJ, Bernstein MA, Breen JF, et al. Three-dimensional contrast-enhanced MR angiography with real-time fluoroscopic triggering: design specifications and technical reliability in 330 patient studies. *Radiology* 2000;215:584–593.

13. Huston J, Fain SB, Riederer SJ, et al. Carotid arteries: maximizing arterial to venous contrast in fluoroscopically triggered contrast-enhanced MR angiography with elliptic centric view ordering. *Radiology* 1999;211:265–273.

14. Korosec F, Grist T, Frayne R, et al. Time-resolved contrast-enhanced 3D MR angiography. *Magn Reson Med* 1996;36:345–351.

15. Mistretta CA, Grist TM, Korosec FR, et al. 3D time-resolved contrast-enhanced MR DSA: advantages and tradeoffs. *Magn Reson Med* 1998;40:571–581.

16. Urchuk S, Plewes D. Mechanism of flow-induced signal loss in MR angiography. *J Magn Reson Imaging* 1992;2:453–462.

17. Le Bihan, ed. *Diffusion and perfusion magnetic resonance imaging.* Philadelphia: Lippincott–Raven Publishers, 1995.

18. Brandt-Zawadski M, Atkinson D, Detrick M, et al. Fluid-attenuated inversion recovery (FLAIR) for assessment of cerebral infarction: clinical experience in 50 patients. *Stroke* 1996;27:1187–1191.

19. Serfaty JM, Chirossel P, Chevallier JM, et al. Accuracy of three-dimensional gadolinium-enhanced MR angiography in the assessment of extracranial carotid artery disease. *AJR Am J Roentgenol* 2000;175:455–463.

20. Prince MR. Body MR angiography with gadolinium contrast agents. *Magn Reson Imaging Clin N Am* 1996;4:11–24.

21. Krinsky G, Maya M, Rofsky N, et al. Gadolinium-enhanced 3D MRA of the aortic arch vessels in the detection of atherosclerotic cerebrovascular disease. *J Comput Assist Tomogr* 1998;22:167–178.

22. Carpenter JP, Holland GA, Golden MA, et al. Magnetic resonance angiography of the aortic arch. *J Vasc Surg* 1997;25:125–151.

23. DeMarco JK, Nesbit GM, Wesbey GE, et al. Prospective evaluation of extracranial carotid stenosis: MR angiography with maximum intensity projections and multiplanar reformation compared with conventional angiography. *AJR Am J Roentgenol* 1994;163:1205–1212.

24. Anderson CM, Lee RL, Levin DL, et al. Measurement of internal carotid artery stenosis from source MR angiograms. *Radiology* 1994;193:219–226.

25. Rossnick S, Laub G, Braeckle R. Three-dimensional display of blood vessels in MRI. In: *Proceedings of the IEEE Computers in Cardiology.* New York: Institute of Electrical and Electronic Engineers, 1986:193–195.

26. van Tyen R, Saloner D, Jou LD, et al. MR imaging of flow through tortuous vessels: a numerical simulation. *Magn Reson Med* 1994;31:184–195.

27. Zarins C, Giddens D, Balasubramanian L, et al. Carotid plaques localized in regions of low flow velocity and shear stress. *Circulation* 1981;64:44.

28. Shaaban AM, Duerinckx AJ. Wall shear and early atherosclerosis: a review. *AJR Am J Roentgenol* 2000;174:1657–1665.

29. Levy C, Laissy JP, Raveau V, et al. Carotid and vertebral artery dissections: three-dimensional time-of-flight MR angiography and MR imaging versus conventional angiography. *Radiology* 1994;190:97–103.

30. Provenzale JM. Dissection of the internal carotid and vertebral arteries: imaging features. *AJR Am J Roentgenol* 1995;165:1099–1104.

31. Marzewski DJ, Furlan AJ, St. Louis P, et al. Intracranial internal carotid artery stenosis: long-term prognosis. *Stroke* 1981;13:821–824.

32. Castaigne P, Lhermitte F, Gautier J, et al. Internal carotid artery occlusion: a study of 61 instances in 50 patients with postmortem data. *Brain* 1970;93:321.

33. Amarenco P, Duyckaerts C, Tzourio C, et al. The prevalence of ulcerated plaques in the aortic arch in patients with stroke. *N Engl J Med* 1992;326:221–225.

34. Mohr J, Gautier J, Pessin M. Internal carotid artery disease. In: Barnett H, Mohr J, Stein B, et al., eds. *Stroke.* New York: Churchill Livingstone, 1992:285–335.

35. Winberger J, A R. Neurologic symptoms associated with nonobstructive plaque at carotid bifurcation: analysis by real-time B-mode ultrasonography. *Arch Neurol* 1983;40:489–492.

36. Dixon S, Pais S, Raviola C, et al. Natural history of nonstenotic asymptomatic ulcerative lesions of the carotid artery: a further analysis. *Arch Surg* 1982;117:1493.

37. Eliasziw M, Streifler JY, Fox AJ, et al. Significance of plaque ulceration in symptomatic patients with high-grade carotid stenosis. North American Carotid Endarterectomy Trial. *Stroke* 1994;25:304–308.

38. Beal M, Williams R, Richardson E, et al. Cerebral embolism as a cause of transient ischemic attacks and cerebral infarction. *Neurology* 1981;31:860.

39. Akiyama Y, Sakaguchi M, Yoshimoto H, et al. Detection of microemboli in patients with extracranial carotid artery stenosis by transcranial Doppler sonography. *No Shinkei Geka* 1997;25:41–45.

40. Bozzao L, Fantozzi L, Bastianello S, et al. Ischemic supratentorial stroke: angiographic findings in patients examined in the very early phase. *J Neurol* 1989;236:340.

41. Wildy KS, Yuan C, Ferguson MS, et al. Atherosclerosis of the carotid artery: evaluation by magnetic resonance angiography. *J Magn Reson Imaging* 1996;6:726–732.

42. Davies MJ, Richardson PD, Woolf N, et al. Risk of thrombosis in human atherosclerotic plaques: role of extracellular lipid, macrophage, and smooth muscle cell content. *Br Heart J* 1993;69:377–381.

43. Martin AJ, Ryan LK, Gottlieb AL, et al. Arterial imaging: comparison of high resolution US and MR imaging with histologic correlation. *Radiographics* 1997;17:189–202.

44. el-Barghouti N, Nicolaides AN, Tegos T, et al. The relative effect of carotid plaque heterogeneity and echogenicity on ipsilateral cerebral infarction and symptoms of cerebrovascular disease. *Int Angiol* 1996;15:300–306.

45. Kardoulas DG, Katsamouris AN, Gallis PT, et al. Ultrasonographic and histologic characteristics of symptom-free and symptomatic carotid plaque. *Cardiovasc Surg* 1996;4:580–590.

46. Barnett HJM. North American Symptomatic Carotid Trial Collaborators. Beneficial effect of carotid endarterectomy in symptomatic patients with high-grade carotid stenosis. *N Engl J Med* 1991;325:445–453.

47. European Carotid Surgery Trialists' Collaborative Group. MRC European carotid surgery trial: interim results for symptomatic patients with severe (70–99%) or with mild (0–29%) carotid stenosis. *Lancet* 1991;337:1235–1243.

48. Executive Committee for the Asymptomatic Carotid Atherosclerosis Study. Endarterectomy for asymptomatic carotid artery stenosis. *JAMA* 1995;273:1421–1428.

49. Hobson RW, Strandness DE. Editorial: Carotid artery stenosis: what's in the measurement? *J Vasc Surg* 1993;18:1069–1070.

50. Barnett HJ, Taylor DW, Eliasziw M, et al. Benefit of carotid endarterectomy in patients with symptomatic moderate or severe stenosis. *N Engl J Med* 1998;339:1415–1425.

51. Barnett HJM, Meldrum HE, Eliasziw M. Atherosclerotic disease of the carotid arteries: a medical perspective. In: Barnett HJM, Mohr JP, Stein MB, et al., eds. *Stroke.* New York: Churchill Livingston, 1998:1189–1198.

52. Barnett HJM, Warlow CP. Editorial: Carotid endarterectomy and the measurement of stenosis. *Stroke* 1993;24:1281–1284.

53. Fox J. How to measure carotid stenosis. *Radiology* 1993;186:316–318.

54. Korogi Y, Takahashi M, Mabuchi N, et al. Intracranial vascular stenosis and occlusion: diagnostic accuracy of three-dimensional, Fourier transform, time-of-flight MR angiography. *Radiology* 1994;193:187–193.

55. Levi CR, Mitchell A, Fitt G, et al. The accuracy of magnetic resonance angiography in the assessment of extracranial carotid artery occlusive disease: a comparison with digital subtraction angiography using NASCET criteria for stenosis measurement. *Cerebrovasc Dis* 1996;6:231–236.

56. Liberopoulos K, Kaponis A, Kokkinis K, et al. Comparison study of magnetic resonance angiography, digital subtraction angiography, duplex ultrasound examination with surgical and histological findings of atherosclerotic carotid bifurcation disease. *Int Angiol* 1996;15:131–137.

57. Link J, Brinkmann G, Steffens JC, et al. MR angiography of the carotid arteries in 3D TOF technique with sagittal double-slab acquisition using a new head-neck coil. *Rofo Fortschr Geb Rontgenstr Neuen Bildgeb Verfahr* 1996;165:544–550.

58. Vanninen RL, Manninen HI, Partanen PL, et al. Carotid artery stenosis: clinical efficacy of MR phase-contrast flow quantification as an adjunct to MR angiography. *Radiology* 1995;194:459–467.

59. Vogl TJ, Heinzinger K, Juergens M, et al. Multiple slab MR angiography of the internal carotid artery: a preoperative comparative study. *Rofo Fortschr Geb Rontgenstr Neuen Bildgeb Verfahr* 1995;162:404–411.

60. Kent KC, Kuntz KM, Mahesh RP, et al. Perioperative imaging strategies for carotid endarterectomy: analysis of morbidity and cost-effectiveness in symptomatic patients. *JAMA* 1995;274:888–893.

61. Nicholas GG, Osborne MA, Jaffe JW, et al. Carotid artery stenosis: preoperative noninvasive evaluation in a community hospital. *J Vasc Surg* 1995;22:9–16.

62. Patel MR, Kuntz KM, Roman AK, et al. Preoperative assessment of the carotid bifurcation: can magnetic resonance angiography and duplex ultrasonography replace contrast arteriography? *Stroke* 1995;26:1753–1758.

63. Mittl RL, Broderick M, Carpenter JP, et al. Blinded reader comparison of magnetic resonance angiography and duplex ultrasonography for carotid artery bifurcation stenosis. *Stroke* 1994;25:4–10.

64. Young GR, Humphrey PR, Shaw MD, et al. Comparison of magnetic resonance angiography, duplex ultrasound, and digital subtraction angiography in assessment of extracranial internal carotid artery stenosis. *J Neurol Neurosurg Psychiatry* 1994;57:1466–1478.

65. Willig DS, Turski PA, Frayne R, et al. Contrast-enhanced 3D MR DSA of the carotid artery bifurcation: preliminary study of comparison with unenhanced 2D and 3D time-of-flight MR angiography. *Radiology* 1998;208:447–451.

66. Slosman F, Stolpen AH, Lexa FJ, et al. Extracranial atherosclerotic carotid artery disease: evaluation of non–breath-hold three-dimensional gadolinium-enhanced MR angiography. *AJR Am J Roentgenol* 1998;170:489–495.

67. Enochs WS, Ackerman RH, Kaufman JA, et al. Gadolinium-enhanced MR angiography of the carotid arteries. *J Neuroimaging* 1998;8:185–190.

68. Gagne PJ, Matchett J, MacFarland D, et al. Can the NASCET technique for measuring carotid stenosis be reliably applied outside the trial? *J Vasc Surg* 1996;24:449–455.

69. Young GR, Sandercock PA, Slattery J, et al. Observer variation in the interpretation of intra-arterial angiograms and the risk of inappropriate decisions about carotid endarterectomy. *J Neurol Neurosurg Psychiatry* 1996;60:152–157.

70. Eliasziw M, Fox AJ, Sharpe BL, et al. Carotid artery stenosis: external validity of the North American Symptomatic Carotid Endarterectomy Trial measurement method. *Radiology* 1997;204:229–233.

71. Pan XM, Saloner D, Reilly LM, et al. Assessment of carotid artery stenosis by ultrasonography, conventional angiography, and magnetic resonance angiography: correlation with *ex vivo* measurement of plaque stenosis. *J Vasc Surg* 1995;21:82–88.

72. Elgersma OE, Wust AFJ, Buijs PC, et al. Multidirectional depiction of internal carotid artery stenosis: three-dimensional time-of-flight MR angiography versus rotational and conventional digital subtraction angiography. *Radiology* 2000;216:511–516.

73. Prestigiacomo CJ, Connolly ES, Quest DO. Use of carotid ultrasound as a preoperative assessment of extracranial carotid artery blood flow and vascular anatomy. *Neurosurg Clin N Am* 1996;7:577–587.

74. Hankey GJ, Warlow CP, Sellar RJ. Cerebral angiographic risk in mild cerebrovascular disease. *Stroke* 1990;21:209–222.

75. Grzyska U, Freitag J, Zeumer H. Selective arterial intracerebral DSA: complication rate and control of risk factors. *Neuroradiology* 1990;32:296–299.

76. Polak JF. Noninvasive carotid evaluation: carpe diem. *Radiology* 1993;186:329–331.

77. Young B, Moore WS, Robertson JT, et al. An analysis of perioperative surgical mortality and morbidity in the asymptomatic carotid atherosclerosis study. Asymptomatic Carotid Arteriosclerosis Study Investigators. *Stroke* 1996;27:2216–2224.

78. Cronenwett JL, Birkmeyer JD, Nackman GB, et al. Cost-effectiveness of carotid endarterectomy in asymptomatic patients. *J Vasc Surg* 1997;25:298–309.

79. Derdeyn CP, Powers WJ. Cost-effectiveness of screening for asymptomatic carotid atherosclerotic disease. *Stroke* 1996;27:1944–1950.

80. Lee TT, Solomon NA, Heidenreich PA, et al. Cost-effectiveness of screening for carotid stenosis in asymptomatic persons. *Ann Intern Med* 1997;126:337–346.

81. Vanninen R, Manninen H, Soimakallio S. Imaging of carotid artery stenosis: clinical efficacy and cost-effectiveness. *AJNR Am J Neuroradiol* 1995;16:1875–1883.

82. Kuntz KM, Skillman JJ, Whittemore AD, et al. Carotid endarterectomy in asymptomatic patients—is contrast angiography necessary? A morbidity analysis. *J Vasc Surg* 1995;22:706–714.

83. Obuchowski NA, Modic MT, Magdinec M, et al. Assessment of the efficacy of noninvasive screening for patients with asymptomatic neck bruits. *Stroke* 1997;28:1330–1339.

84. Carriero A, Ucchino S, Magarelli N, et al. Carotid bifurcation stenosis: a comparative study between MR angiography and duplex scanning with respect to digital subtraction angiography. *J Neuroradiol* 1995;22:103–111.

85. Howard G, Baker WH, Chambless LE, et al. An approach for the use of Doppler ultrasound as a screening tool for hemodynamically significant stenosis (despite heterogeneity of Doppler performance). A multicenter experience. Asymptomatic Carotid Atherosclerosis Study Investigators. *Stroke* 1996;27:1951–1957.

86. Hobson RW 2d, Weiss DG, Fields WS, et al. VA Cooperative Trial: Efficacy of Carotid Endarterectomy for Asymptomatic Carotid Stenosis. The Veterans Affairs Cooperative Study Group. *N Engl J Med* 1993;328:221–227.

87. Eliasziw M, Rankin RN, Fox AJ, et al. Accuracy and prognostic consequences of ultrasonography in identifying severe carotid artery stenosis. North American Symptomatic Carotid Endarterectomy Trial (NASCET) Group. *Stroke* 1995;26:1747–1752.

88. Horrow MM, Stassi J, Shurman A, et al. The limitations of carotid sonography: interpretative and technology-related errors. *AJR Am J Roentgenol* 2000;174:189–194.

89. Kotval PS. Doppler waveforms parvus and tardus: a sign of proximal flow obstruction. *J Ultrasound Med* 1988;8:435–440.

90. Kallmes DF, Omary RA, Dix JE, et al. Specificity of MR angiography as a confirmatory test of carotid artery stenosis. *AJNR Am J Neuroradiol* 1996;17:1501–1506.

91. Mohr JP, Caplan LR, Melski JW, et al. The Harvard Cooperative Stroke Registry: a prospective registry. *Neurology* 1978;28:754.

92. Khaw KT. Does carotid duplex imaging render angiography redundant before carotid endarterectomy? *Br J Radiol* 1997;70:235–238.

93. Golledge J, Wright R, Pugh N, et al. Colour-coded duplex assessment alone before carotid endarterectomy. *Br J Surg* 1996;83:1234–1237.

94. Ballard JL, Deiparine MK, Bergan JJ, et al. Cost-effective evaluation and treatment for carotid disease. *Arch Surg* 1997;132:268–271.

95. Hansen F, Bergqvist D, Lindblad B, et al. Accuracy of duplex sonography before carotid endarterectomy—a comparison with angiography. *Eur J Vasc Endovasc Surg* 1996;12:331–336.

96. Jackson MR, Chang AS, Robles HA, et al. Determination of 60% or greater carotid stenosis: a prospective comparison of magnetic resonance angiography and duplex ultrasound with conventional angiography. *Ann Vasc Surg* 1998;12:236–243.

97. Saouaf R, Grassi CJ, Hartnell GG, et al. Complete MR angiography and Doppler ultrasound as the sole imaging modalities prior to carotid endarterectomy. *Clin Radiol* 1998;53:759–786.

98. Akers D, Markowitz I, Kerstein M, et al. The evaluation of the aortic arch in the evaluation of cerebrovascular insufficiency. *Am J Surg* 1987;154:230.

99. Provan JL. Arteriosclerotic occlusive arterial disease of brachiocephalic and arch vessels. In: Rutherford RB, ed. *Vascular Surgery*. Philadelphia: WB Saunders, 1989:822.

100. Djouhri H, Guillon B, Brunereau L, et al. MR angiography for the long-term follow-up of dissection aneurysms of the extracranial internal carotid artery. *AJR Am J Roentgenol* 2000;174:1137–1140.

101. The French Study of Aortic Plaques in Stroke Group. Atherosclerotic disease of the aortic arch as a risk factor for recurrent ischemic stroke. *N Engl J Med* 196;334:1216–1221.

102. Bluemke AB, Stillman AE, Bis KG, et al. Carotid MR angiography: phase II study of safety and efficacy for MS-325. *AJR Am J Roentgenol* 2001;219:114–122.

103. Phatouros CC, Higashida RT, Malek AM, et al. Carotid artery stent placement for atherosclerotic disease: rationale, technique and current status. *Radiology* 2000;217:26–41.

104. Leclerc X, Godefroy O, Lucas C, et al. Internal carotid arterial stenosis: CT angiography with volume rendering. *Radiology* 1999;210:673–682.

105. Link J, Brossman J, Grabner M, et al. Spiral CT angiography and selective digital subtraction angiography of internal carotid artery stenosis. *AJNR Am J Neuroradiol* 1996;17:89–94.

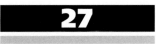

ATHEROSCLEROTIC PLAQUE IMAGING

ZAHI A. FAYAD

ATHEROSCLEROTIC PLAQUES

Atherosclerosis, a systemic disease of the vessel wall that occurs in the aorta and the carotid, coronary, and peripheral arteries, is the primary cause of heart disease and stroke (1). It is responsible for 50% of all deaths in Western societies. The main components of atherosclerotic plaque are the following: (a) fibrous elements such as connective tissue extracellular matrix, including collagen, proteoglycans, and fibronectin elastic fibers; (b) lipids such as crystalline cholesterol, cholesteryl esters, and phospholipids; and (c) inflammatory cells such as monocyte-derived macrophages, T lymphocytes, and smooth-muscle cells (2). The occurrence of these components in varying proportions in different plaques gives rise to a spectrum of lesions (1,3,4). Furthermore, the characteristics of "high-risk" or "vulnerable" plaque vary depending on the arterial region (i.e., coronaries, carotids, or aorta) in which it is located.

Coronary Artery Vulnerable Plaques

Rupture-prone plaques in the coronary arteries, so-called vulnerable plaques, tend to have a thin (~65 to 150 μm) fibrous cap and a large lipid core. An acute coronary syndrome often results from the rupture of a modestly stenotic vulnerable plaque (3,4) that is often not visible by x-ray angiography (3).

In brief, according to the criteria of the American Heart Association Committee on Vascular Lesions, the different lesion types depend in part on stage or phase of progression (1,4). The coronary "vulnerable" types IV and Va lesions (phase 2) and the "complicated" type VI lesion (phase 4) are the most relevant to acute coronary syndrome. Types IV and Va lesions, although not necessarily stenotic at angiography, are prone to disruption, with the macrophage-dependent release of proteolytic enzymes such as metalloproteases (2,5). Type IV lesions consist of extracellular lipid intermixed with fibrous tissue covered by a fibrous cap, whereas type Va lesions possess a predominantly extracellular lipid core covered by a thin fibrous cap. Disruption of a type IV or Va lesion leads to the formation of a thrombus or "complicated" type VI lesion. The lipid core is made highly thrombogenic by the presence of tissue factor (1,6). The type VI lesion that results in acute coronary syndrome, rather than being characterized by a small mural thrombus, consists of an occlusive thrombus.

Small types IV and Va coronary lesions by angiography may eventually account for as many as two-thirds of patients in whom unstable angina or other acute coronary syndromes develop (3). These relatively nonstenotic plaques with large lipid cores are vulnerable and at high risk for rupture and thrombosis; the caps are often thinnest at the shoulder regions, where macrophages (7) and mast cells (8) accumulate and disruption is a frequent occurrence (5). In contrast, the most severely stenotic plaques at angiography, which have a high content of smooth-muscle cells and collagen and little lipid, are less susceptible to rupture.

Carotid Artery High-Risk Plaques

In contrast to vulnerable plaques in the coronary arteries, which are characterized by a high lipid content and thin fibrous cap, high-risk plaques in the carotid arteries are severely stenotic. We use the term *high-risk* rather than the classic term *vulnerable* because *vulnerable* implies the presence of a lipid-rich core. Indeed, high-risk carotid plaques are not necessarily lipid-rich but rather heterogeneous, and they are very rich in fibrous tissue. When they rupture, an

Z. A. Fayad: Departments of Radiology and Medicine, Mount Sinai School of Medicine, and Cardiovascular Imaging Department, Mount Sinai Medical Center, New York, New York.

intramural hematoma or dissection often develops that is probably related to the impact of blood during systole against a resistant area of stenosis (9). Because the carotid arteries are superficial and not subject to significant motion, they are much easier to image than the coronary arteries (10). This is also true of the peripheral vessels (i.e., in the lower extremities), in which the pathobiology of vascular atherosclerotic disease is similar to that in the carotid arteries. However, more information is available about the imaging of carotid plaque than of peripheral vascular lesions.

Aortic Vulnerable Plaques

Studies performed at autopsy (11) and with transesophageal echocardiography (TEE) (12) have shown that atherosclerosis in the thoracic aortic is a significant marker for coronary disease. In fact, parameters such as aortic wall thickness, luminal irregularities, and plaque composition are strong predictors of future vascular events (13,14). Thus, with the use of TEE, the French Aortic Plaque Study (FAPS) investigators found a significantly increased risk for all vascular events (stroke, myocardial infarction, peripheral embolism, and cardiovascular death) in patients who had noncalcified aortic plaques with a thickness of more than 4 mm (13,14). It is thought that these noncalcified plaques, relatively easy to assess and characterize by imaging methods, are frequently lipid-laden plaques (American Heart Association types IV and Va) (14), which in the coronary arteries are considered to be "vulnerable" plaques, prone to rupture and thrombosis.

TECHNIQUES

The direct visualization of atherosclerotic plaques should enhance our understanding of the natural history of this disease. Several invasive imaging techniques, such as x-ray angiography, intravascular ultrasonography, angioscopy, and optical coherence tomography, in addition to noninvasive imaging techniques, such as surface B-mode ultrasonography and ultrafast computed tomography, can be used to assess atherosclerotic vessels. Most of the standard techniques identify the luminal diameter or stenosis, wall thickness, and plaque volume.

However, none of these imaging methods can completely characterize the composition of the atherosclerotic plaque and therefore are incapable of identifying vulnerable or high-risk plaques (15).

High-resolution MR has emerged as the potential leading noninvasive imaging modality for characterizing atherosclerotic plaque *in vivo*. MR differentiates plaque components on the basis of biophysical and biochemical parameters, such as chemical composition and concentration, water content, physical state, molecular motion, and diffusion (16). MR provides a method of imaging without the need for ionizing radiation that can be repeated sequentially over time.

APPLICATIONS

MR *Ex Vivo* Studies of Plaque

The early work on the application of MR techniques to characterize plaque focused on lipid assessment with nuclear MR spectroscopy and chemical shift imaging (17–24). Unfortunately, the concentration of lipid in plaque is very low in comparison with that of water, and these techniques suffer from poor signal-to-noise ratio (SNR) (18,21,25). Therefore, it has been difficult to apply them *in vivo*. Current studies are focused on MRI of water protons.

MR Multicontrast Plaque Imaging

Following an *ex vivo* MRI study of iliac artery specimens by Kaufman et al. (26), Herfkens et al. (27) performed the first *in vivo* imaging study of aortic atherosclerosis in a patient. Only the anatomic or morphologic features of the atherosclerotic lesions, such as wall thickening and luminal narrowing, were assessed.

Following improvements in MR techniques (e.g., faster imaging and detection coils), high-resolution and contrast imaging became possible, and studies were undertaken of the different components of plaque with multicontrast MR generated by T1, T2, and proton density weighting (15). The characterization of atherosclerotic plaque by MR is based on the signal intensities (Table 27.1) and morphologic appearance of plaque on T1-weighted, proton density-

TABLE 27.1. PLAQUE CHARACTERIZATION WITH MAGNETIC RESONANCE

	Relative MR signal intensity[a]		
	T1W	PDW	T2W
Calcium	Hypointense	Hypointense	Hypointense
Lipid	Hyperintense	Hyperintense	Hypointense
Fibrous tissue	Isointense	Hyperintense	Isointense to hyperintense
Thrombus[b,c]	Variable	Variable	Variable

[a] Relative to that of background (muscle).
[b] Surface irregularities.
[c] Variable signal intensity may be a consequence of organizational changes in the thrombus.
T1W, T1-weighted; PDW, proton density-weighted; T2W, T2-weighted.

weighted, and T2-weighted images, as previously validated (10,25,28–33).

The fibrous tissues of plaque, consisting of extracellular matrix elaborated by smooth-muscle cells, are associated with a short T1. This T1 shortening (increased signal intensity on T1-weighted images) is the consequence of specific interactions between protein and water (34).

Plaque lipids consist primarily of unesterified cholesterol and cholesteryl esters and are associated with a short T2 (25). The short T2 (decreased signal intensity on T2-weighted images) of the lipid components is in part a consequence of the micellar structure of lipoproteins, their de-

naturation by oxidation, or an exchange between cholesteryl esters and water molecules (both from the fatty chain or the cholesterol ring), with a further interchange between free and bound water (25,35,36). Perivascular fat, mainly composed of triglycerides, differs in appearance on MR images from atherosclerotic plaque lipids (37). The signal intensities of the calcified regions of plaque, which consist primarily of calcium hydroxyapatite, are low on MR images because of their low proton density and diffusion-mediated susceptibility effects (26,38).

The MR appearance and evolution of thrombus or hemorrhage in the central nervous system (39), pelvis (40), and

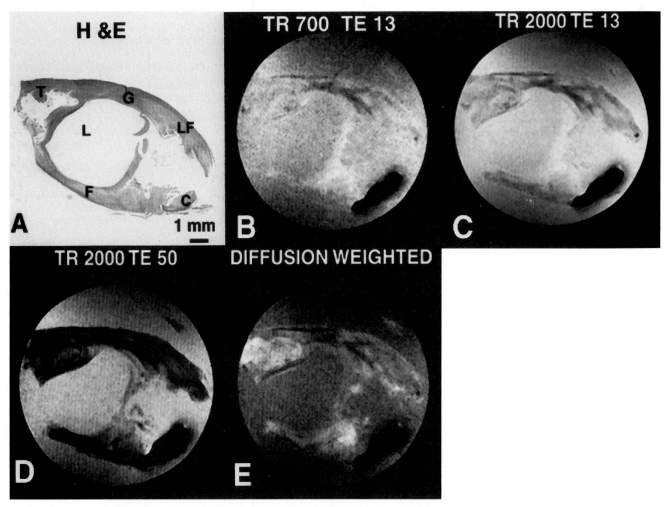

FIGURE 27.1. High-resolution *ex vivo* MR images of a human carotid endarterectomy specimen. All MRI images are 256 × 256, with a field of view of 12.4 mm, a slice thickness of 500 μm, and an in-plane resolution of 48 μm. **A** Low-magnification photomicrograph of the matched hematoxylin and eosin-stained section. The T1-weighted **(B)**, proton density-weighted **(C)**, T2-weighted **(D)**, and diffusion-weighted (b = 636 s/mm^2) **(E)** images were used to characterize the plaque. For orientation, the lumen *(L)*, regions of calcification *(C)*, fibrocellular tissue *(F)*, fibrocellular regions containing extracellular lipid *(LF)*, thrombus *(T)*, and the necrotic lipid-rich core (sometimes called *gruel*) *(G)* are labeled. Calcified tissue appears dark on all MRI images, whereas the lipid core appears dark on the T2-weighted image (D) but light on the T1-weighted (B) and proton density-weighted (C) images. Note that thrombus appears bright on the diffusion-weighted image (E). (From Shinnar M, Fallon JT, Wehrli S, et al. The diagnostic accuracy of *ex vivo* magnetic resonance imaging for human atherosclerotic plaque characterization. *Arterioscler Thromb Vasc Biol* 1999;19:2756–2761, with permission.)

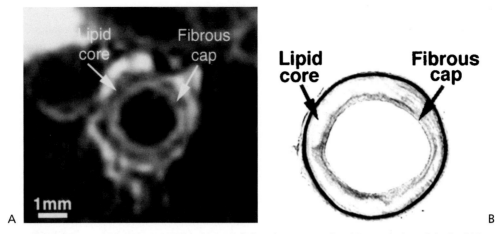

FIGURE 27.2. *In vivo* MR T2-weighted image **(A)** and corresponding histopathology **(B)** of rabbit atherosclerotic aorta. The lipid core is hypointense, and the fibrous cap is hyperintense. (From Helft G, Worthley SG, Fuster V, et al. Atherosclerotic aortic component quantification by noninvasive magnetic resonance: an *in vivo* study in rabbits. *J Am Coll Cardiol* 2001;37:1149–1154, with permission.)

aorta (41,42) have been previously studied. The appearance of hemorrhage depends on the structure of hemoglobin and its oxidation state. At various stages, blood clots contain different products (i.e., oxyhemoglobin, deoxyhemoglobin, methemoglobin, hemosiderin/ferritin). Each of these has a set of specific MR relaxation properties (T1 and T2) that produce different signal intensities (43–47). Blood shortens the T1 and T2 of water. T1 shortening is presumed to be caused by the formation of methemoglobin (which is paramagnetic) from hemoglobin. T2 shortening is caused by magnetic susceptibility. In this regard, ferritin- or hemosiderin-rich mature thrombus is associated with marked signal loss on T2-weighted images.

We analyzed 22 human carotid endarterectomy specimens with *ex vivo* MR and histopathologic examination (48). Sixty-six cross sections were matched on multicontrast MR images and histopathology. The overall sensitivity and specificity for each component were very high. Calcification, fibrous tissue, lipid core, and thrombus were readily identified. Diffusion imaging, which probes the motion of water molecules, was found to be useful for thrombus detection, as has been demonstrated previously (49) (Fig. 27.1).

In Vivo MRI Experimental Studies

MR has been used to study plaques in several animal models, including mice (50), rats (51), rabbits (52), pigs (53), and nonhuman primates (54). In atherosclerotic rabbits, we validated the ability of MRI to quantify lipid-rich and fibrous components of lesions. The plaques were induced in the thoracic and abdominal aorta by a combination of atherogenic diet and double-balloon denudation (55) (Fig. 27.2). Fast spin-echo sequences were obtained with an in-plane resolution of 0.35 mm and a slice thickness of 3 mm.

Proton density- and T2- weighted images were obtained. A significant correlation between MRI and histology was observed in the analysis of lipid-rich and fibrous areas.

In two separate serial studies (56,57), MRI demonstrated significant regression of aortic plaque *in vivo* in atherosclerotic rabbits who underwent cholesterol lowering. In these studies, after aortic balloon injury and feeding of a high cholesterol diet, one group of rabbits was continued on the atherogenic diet (atherosclerosis progression), and another group was placed on a normal-chow, low-cholesterol diet (atherosclerosis regression). A significant reduction in both vessel wall area and mean wall thickness was observed in the dietary regression group, and an increase was seen in the dietary progression group. A significant reduction in the lipid-rich component of plaques was also observed in the dietary regression group, and an increase in the dietary progression group. A small, nonsignificant increase in the fibrous plaque components was noted in the dietary regression group, but a significant decrease in the fibrous composition of lesions in the progression group. A significant correlation was found between MR and histopathology for atherosclerotic burden and plaque composition (57).

Another serial MRI study (58), on the effect of lipid-lowering therapy with hepatic hydroxymethylglutaryl coenzyme A (HMG CoA) reductase inhibitors (statins) and a novel class of agents, the acylcholesterol acyltransferase (ACAT) inhibitors, showed beneficial effects in a Watanabe rabbit. The combination of statins and ACAT inhibitors induced a significant regression of previously established atherosclerotic lesions.

We have also shown in the rabbit model of aortic atherosclerosis that MRI can be used to document arterial remodeling (59). With conventional MR systems (i.e., 1.5 T), an in-plane spatial resolution of 300 μm or more can be achieved with sufficient SNR and contrast-to-noise ratio for *in vivo* imaging of the vessel wall. To study small structures, such as the abdominal aorta of mice (<1 mm in luminal diameter), it is necessary to increase the SNR by using high-magnetic-field scanners equipped with small radiofrequency (RF) coils and strong magnetic field gradients (60). Using a 9.4-T (89-mm) bore system, we studied atherosclerosis in live animals (60). The achievable in-plane spatial resolution with MR microscopy was approximately 50 to 97 μm, and the slice thickness was 500 μm. Using transgenic apolipoprotein E knockout mice, we showed an excellent agreement between MR microscopy and histologic findings for aortic plaque size, shape, and characteristics. We have recently extended this study to follow the rapid progression of atherosclerosis in animals with lesions of varying severity (61) (Fig. 27.3). High-resolution MRI and MR microscopy may allow the convenient and noninvasive quantitative assessment of serial changes in atherosclerosis in different animal models of disease progression and regression (62).

In Vivo MRI Studies of Human Carotid Artery Plaque

MR has been used to study atherosclerotic plaque in human carotid (10,63), aortic (64), peripheral (65), and coronary (66) arterial disease. *In vivo* images of advanced lesions in carotid arteries have been obtained from patients referred for endarterectomy (10). The carotid arteries, with a superficial location and relative absence of motion, present less of a technical challenge for imaging than do vessels such as the aorta and coronary arteries. Short-T2 components were quantified *in vivo* before surgery, and the values were correlated with values obtained *in vitro* after surgery (10). Some

of the MR studies of carotid arterial plaques include imaging and characterization of normal and pathologic arterial walls (10), quantification of plaque size (63), and detection of fibrous cap "integrity" (67).

As mentioned previously, most *in vivo* studies of MRI imaging and characterization of plaque have been performed in a multicontrast approach (i.e., T1, proton density, and T2 weighting) with high-resolution black blood spin-echo and fast spin-echo MR sequences. As the name implies, the signal from flowing blood is rendered black by the use of preparatory pulses (e.g., RF spatial saturation or inversion recovery pulses) for better visualization of the adjacent vessel wall. Hatsukami et al. (67) introduced the use of bright blood imaging (i.e., three-dimensional fast time-of-flight imaging) to visualize fibrous cap thickness and morphologic integrity. That sequence provides enhancement of the signal from flowing blood and a mixture of T1 and proton density contrast weighting, which highlights the fibrous cap.

MRA and high-resolution black blood imaging of the vessel wall can be combined (Fig. 27.4). MRA demonstrates the severity of stenotic lesions and their spatial distribution, whereas the high-resolution black blood wall characterization technique may show the composition of plaques and facilitate risk stratification and the selection of treatment modality. Spatial resolution has recently been improved (≤250 μm) with the design of new phased-array coils (68,69) tailored for carotid imaging (70) and new imaging sequences, such as long-echo-train fast spin-echo imaging with "velocity-selective" flow suppression and double inversion recovery preparatory pulses (black blood imaging) (64,66).

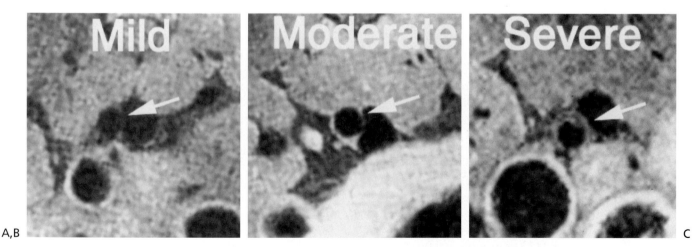

A,B   C

FIGURE 27.3. MR microscopy images (proton density-weighted) of the abdominal aorta *(arrows)* in three ApoE⁻/⁻ (apolipoprotein E knockout) mice showing varying degrees of severity of atherosclerotic lesions. **A:** The mild lesion is from an ApoE⁻/⁻ mouse on a Western diet for 8 weeks. **B:** The moderate lesion is from an ApoE⁻/⁻ mouse on a Western diet for 20 weeks. **C:** The severe lesion is taken from a transplant study; the donor mouse was on a Western diet for 27 weeks, and the recipient was on a Western diet for 20 weeks. All MR images have a pixel size of 109 × 109 × 500 μm and were acquired with a 9.4-T Bruker system. (From ref. 61, with permission.)

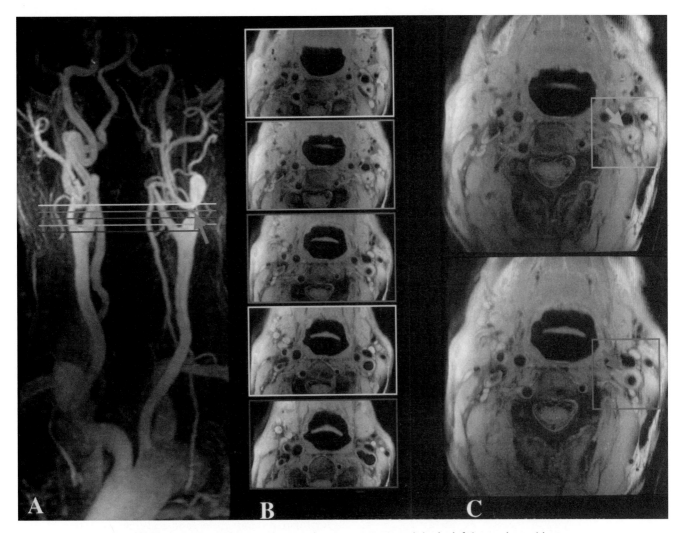

FIGURE 27.4. A: Carotid MR angiogram shows a severe stenosis in the left internal carotid artery *(arrow)*. The MR angiogram was obtained with a contrast-enhanced (gadolinium diethylenetriamine pentaacetic acid, or Gd-DTPA) three-dimensional fast gradient-echo sequence and a carotid aortic arch phased-array coil. **B:** Cross-sectional high-resolution MR black blood images of the carotid arteries are shown. A display of the MR slice positions appears in the left panel *(top line corresponds to the top image, the second line refers to the second image from the top, and so on)*. **C:** Magnified views of some of the carotid plaques *(second and third from the top in panel B)* are also shown. The *arrows* indicate the carotid plaques. (From ref. 15, with permission.)

In Vivo MRI Studies of Human Aortic Plaque

In vivo black blood MR characterization of atherosclerotic plaque in the human aorta has been reported (64,71). The principal challenges associated with MRI of the thoracic aorta are obtaining sufficient sensitivity for submillimeter imaging and excluding artifacts caused by respiratory motion and blood flow. Summers et al. (71) used MRI to show that the wall thickness of the ascending aorta is increased in patients with homozygous familial hypercholesterolemia. Only conventional T1-weighted spin-echo images were obtained, and therefore plaque composition was not analyzed. Fayad et al. (64) assessed the composition of plaque in the thoracic aorta with T1-, proton density-, and T2-weighted images.

Rapid high-resolution imaging was performed with a fast spin-echo sequence in conjunction with "velocity-selective" flow suppression preparatory pulses. The results of matched cross-sectional aortic imaging with MR and TEE correlated strongly for plaque composition and mean maximal plaque thickness. A patient with plaques in the descending aorta rich in both lipid and fibrous tissue is shown in Fig. 27.5.

In asymptomatic subjects from the Framingham Heart Study (FHS), MR showed that the prevalence and burden (i.e., plaque volume/aortic volume) of aortic atherosclerosis increase significantly with age and are higher in the abdominal than in the thoracic aorta (72). It was also found that long-term measures of risk factors and the FHS coronary risk score are strongly associated with asymptomatic aortic atherosclerosis as detected by MR (73).

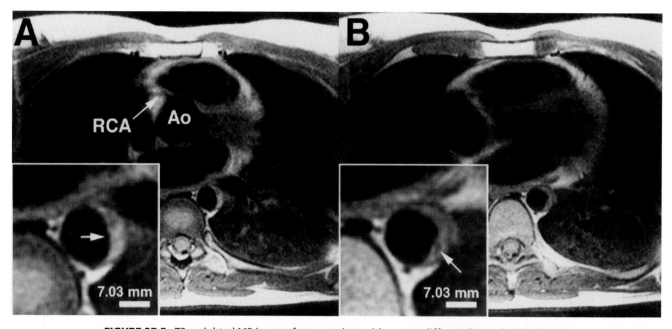

FIGURE 27.5. T2-weighted MR images from a patient with severe, diffuse atherosclerotic disease in the descending thoracic aorta. The plaques differ in appearance and characteristics from one location to another. Plaque characterization was based on the information obtained from T1-, proton density-, and T2- weighted MR images. The inserts in each panel represent magnified views of the descending thoracic aorta. **A:** A "stable" plaque rich in fibrous tissue *(arrow of inset)* is shown. **B:** An "unstable" lipid-rich plaque *(arrow of inset) is shown.* The MR images are 5 mm thick, were acquired with no interslice gap, and are displayed in a cephalic (A) to caudal (B) direction. The origin of the right coronary artery *(RCA, arrow in A)* is clearly seen originating from the aortic root *(Ao).* (From ref. 64, with permission.)

In Vivo MRI Studies of Coronary Artery Plaque

The ultimate goal is noninvasive imaging of plaque in the coronary arteries. Preliminary studies in a pig model showed that the difficulties encountered in imaging the coronary wall are caused by a combination of cardiac and respiratory motion artifacts and the tortuous course, small size, and location of the coronary arteries (33,74). We applied the black blood MR methods used in the human carotid artery and aorta to image the coronary arterial lumen and wall (66). The imaging method was validated in coronary lesions induced in Yorkshire albino swine with balloon angioplasty (74). The intraobserver and interobserver assessment of variability by intraclass correlation for both MRI and histopathology showed good reproducibility, with the intraclass correlation coefficients ranging from .96 to .99. MRI was also able to visualize intralesional hematoma (sensitivity of 82% and specificity of 84%).

After the animal experiments, high-resolution black blood MRI of both normal and atherosclerotic human coronary arteries was performed. The difference in maximal wall thickness between normal subjects and patients ($\geq$40% stenosis) was statistically significant. Figure 27.6 shows an *in vivo* MR image of plaque in the left anterior descending coronary artery of a patient. The study of Fayad et al. (66) of MRI of coronary plaque was performed during breath-holding to minimize respiratory motion. To alleviate the need for breath-holding, Botnar et al. (75) combined the black blood fast-spin echo method with a real-time navigator for respiratory gating and real-time correction of slice position.

Human *In Vivo* Monitoring of Therapy with MRI

As has been shown in experimental studies, MR is a powerful tool for investigating serially and noninvasively the progression and regression of atherosclerotic lesions *in vivo*. We have demonstrated in a recent study that MR can be used *in vivo* to measure the effect of lipid-lowering therapy (statins) in asymptomatic untreated patients with hypercholesterolemia and carotid and aortic atherosclerosis (76). Atherosclerotic plaques were visualized and measured with MR at different times after the initiation of lipid-lowering therapy. Significant regression of atherosclerotic lesions was observed. Importantly, despite the early and expected hypolipidemic effect of the statins, a minimum of 12 months was needed to observe changes in the vessel wall. In fact, no changes were detected at 6 months. A decrease in the vessel wall area but no change in the luminal area was noted at 12 months. These findings are in agreement with those of previous experimental studies (56,58).

High-resolution MR of the popliteal artery and the response to balloon angioplasty have been reported by Coulden et al. (65). In all patients, the extent of atherosclerotic plaque could be defined, such that even in segments of vessel that were angiographically "normal," atherosclerotic lesions with cross-sectional areas ranging from 49% to 76% of the potential luminal area were identified. Following angioplasty, plaque fissuring and local dissection were easily identified, and serial changes in luminal diameter, blood flow, and lesion size were documented. This study showed that high-resolution MR can define the extent of atherosclerotic plaque in the peripheral vasculature and demonstrate the changes of remodeling and restenosis following angioplasty.

FUTURE APPLICATIONS

Improvements in MR Techniques for Imaging Plaque

The spatial resolution of current MR techniques for imaging plaque is limited mainly by the available SNR. One way to increase the SNR directly is to improve the receiver coils.

New External Coils

We have designed and tested a new cardiac coil for high-resolution (≤0.5 mm in-plane resolution) MRI of human coronary plaques (69). Our new coil consists of an array (four-el-

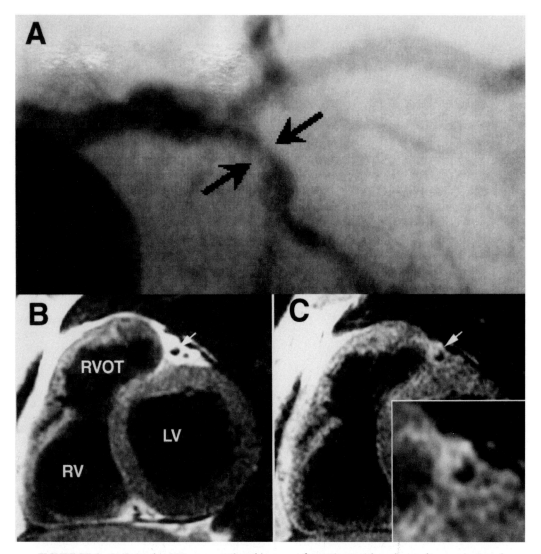

FIGURE 27.6. A–C: *In vivo* MR cross-sectional images of a patient with a plaque *(arrows in A and B)* in the left anterior descending artery (LAD). The *inset in C* shows a magnified view of the plaque in the LAD. A selective coronary x-ray angiogram (A) shows LAD stenosis *(arrows).* The MR images are 4 mm thick with an in-plane spatial resolution of 750 μm and were acquired during a suspended respiration (<16 seconds) with long-echo-train fast spin-echo imaging and "velocity-selective" flow suppression. *RV,* right ventricle; *LV,* left ventricle; *RVOT,* right ventricular outflow tract. (From Fayad ZA, Fuster V, Fallon JT, et al. Noninvasive *in vivo* human coronary artery lumen and wall imaging using black-blood magnetic resonance imaging. *Circulation* 2000;102:506–510, with permission.)

ement phased-array coil: two square coils, each 7.3 × 7.3 cm, and two rectangular coils, each 6.4 × 9.7 cm) in which all the coils are placed on the surface of the chest. MRI was performed on a 1.5-T imager. We compared the SNRs in various regions of the heart with the new four-element anterior coil and with a general whole heart coil (two anterior and two posterior elements, each 20 × 12 cm). High-resolution imaging of the coronary wall and plaque was performed with two-dimensional spiral and black blood fast spin-echo sequences in 15 normal subjects and patients with proximal coronary disease. Figure 27.7 shows the SNR plot as a function of depth for the two coil arrays. It is evident from the curves that the anterior array has an SNR advantage for depths to about 12 cm. High-resolution imaging of coronary plaque (≤0.5 mm in-plane resolution and 3- to 4-mm slice thickness) was achieved with our four-element anterior phased-array coil in all subjects. Proximally, our new coil produced images superior to those obtained with a general whole heart coil. We believe this new approach can play an important role in applications such as high-resolution MR characterization of the wall in atherosclerotic proximal coronary arteries.

Internal Coils

Another way to improve SNR and spatial resolution is with internal coils; these include perivascular coils, which are implanted around a vessel-of-interest (77–79); intravascular coils, which are inserted directly inside a vessel (30,80–96); and transesophageal coils, which are placed in the esophagus (97). However, with these approaches, the characterization of MR plaque becomes an invasive procedure.

The advantages of perivascular implantation of an MR coil are that the same area-of-interest is imaged without positioning the coil and that a high signal is obtained only from within the tissue-of-interest. With the use of an inductively coupled coil, no external wires are needed. Summers et al.

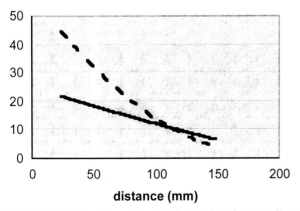

FIGURE 27.7. Signal-to-noise ratio (vertical axis) versus distance from the surface for the standard whole heart phased-array coil *(solid line)* and the newly designed four-element anterior phased-array coil *(broken line)*.

(79), utilizing an implanted coil at 7 T, demonstrated wall changes after angioplasty in a rat carotid artery. In that study, a primary injury model was used to demonstrate the response of a normal vessel to angioplasty. Their results showed a good correlation between values for arterial wall thickness measured with MR and those obtained with histology. With an external surface coil, maximal SNR is achieved at the skin; the SNR becomes progressively lower at deeper levels. The implanted design has the added advantage that the maximal SNR is at the level of the artery, with little noise contributed by surrounding tissues. The implanted coil technique is a useful tool for experimental research in animal models of plaque progression and treatment. In a New Zealand rabbit model of hypercholesterolemia, Ford et al. (77) implanted a coil around a balloon-injured aorta to demonstrate spatial resolution and SNR sufficient for following morphologic changes over time. Quantitative MR morphometry corresponded well with morphologic measurements based on angiography and histology. In a research model, *in vivo* MRI with an implanted coil eliminates the need to perform multiple invasive procedures to follow the induction of atherosclerosis and restenosis. The technique is an improvement over conventional histologic techniques, which require the sacrifice of multiple animals to assess chronologic change, and it improves statistical power by providing high-resolution images of the arterial wall sequentially within the same animal. This technique remains a research tool for investigating plaque morphology and development in animal models.

Perivascular imaging combines adequate spatial resolution with sufficient signal strength and homogeneity to provide high-resolution imaging of plaque, but it is limited to animal work because of the need for permanent surgical implantation. Intravascular MRI, although similarly invasive, provides direct contact between the imaging coil and the vessel wall to create maximal spatial resolution. The coil can be placed intravascularly by percutaneous methods and can be removed after imaging. When the coil is positioned next to the vascular wall, the plaque is within the area of maximal coil sensitivity. Although, unlike perivascular coil implantation, the technique does not facilitate the temporal evaluation of wall plaque, it provides better spatial detail in comparison with surface external coils. Problems associated with intravascular MR techniques are artifacts caused by blood flow and vessel wall pulsation, rapid radial falloff in signal intensity, and poor flexibility (98). Improvements to alleviate the first two of these problems were reported by Zimmerman-Paul et al. (88,89), who designed a coil consisting of a loop of wire enclosed by an inflatable balloon to be immobile against the vessel wall. One problem with intravascular MR with this balloon technique is the need to occlude the vessel during imaging for several minutes. The technique may be acceptable in evaluating the peripheral arteries, but it prevents analysis of the carotid or coronary arteries. Possible solutions include shorter imaging times or new catheter designs that allow flow through the imaging area (86,95,99).

Two recent and promising coil designs are by Ocali and Atalar (99) and Shinnar et al. (95). The device by Ocali and Atalar is formed by short-circuiting one end of a coaxial cable and exposing a critical length of the inner conductor. The advantages of this design over previous ones include its small diameter, a high degree of flexibility, and a high signal intensity that allows most of the associated electronics to be placed remote from the catheter. The device by Shinnar et al. has similar features. This catheter coil is 1.3 mm in diameter and is positioned over a guidewire. The probe is not mounted on a balloon and thus does not obstruct blood flow during image acquisition. The coil was tested *in vivo* in a rabbit model of atherosclerosis. The SNR allowed the acquisition of high-resolution images with a 78-µm in-plane resolution and a 1- to 2-mm slice thickness with no significant motion artifacts. Plaque components (e.g., lipid core, fibrous cap) were easily identified. A comparison between *in vivo* imaging with an external surface coil and the intravascular coil is shown in Figure 27.8. The new nonobstructive design of the intravascular coil holds great promise for further high-resolution MRI characterizations of atherosclerotic plaque *in vivo*. The ability to position the probe with a guidewire makes it possible to place it under fluoroscopic or MRI guidance (84), and its size is compatible with human coronary arteries. Future work will concentrate on coronary imaging in animals and the possible use of MR for interventional purposes (83,98,100).

MRI provides the necessary spatial resolution and tissue characterization to aid in the evaluation of high-risk plaques. Newer coil designs that acquire signal from the surface of a vessel, around it, and from within it will make possible the evaluation and diagnosis of plaques at risk. As these techniques become more clinically useful, percutaneous therapy will be applied in the hope of improving outcomes and decreasing acute ischemic syndromes. In addition, these techniques will enable us to understand better the pathology of the vessel wall that leads to the formation of high-risk plaque.

Further Possible Improvements in MR Techniques for Imaging Plaque

Thinner slices, such as those obtained with three-dimensional acquisition techniques, may further improve artery wall imaging (101). Coils with specially tailored designs, such as smaller anterior four-element phased-array coils, may improve spatial resolution and allow the identification of substructures within coronary atherosclerotic lesions (69). Additional MR techniques, such as water diffusion weighting (48,49), magnetization transfer weighting (102), and contrast enhancement (53,103), may provide complementary structural information and allow a more detailed characterization of plaque. Slowly flowing blood near vessel walls is another phenomenon that may potentially influence the accuracy of vessel wall imaging with black blood techniques. Our preliminary results of using a black blood MR sequence in the coronary arteries and brain (66,74) suggest that this effect is minimal. However, new and more robust methods of blood suppression are needed for accurate plaque imaging, especially at the carotid arterial bifurcation (104).

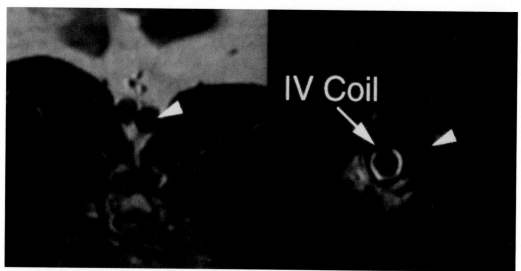

FIGURE 27.8. *In vivo* imaging of aortic plaque *(arrowhead)* in a rabbit model of atherosclerosis. External imaging with a surface coil and intravascular MR imaging are compared. **A:** The image was acquired with an in-plane resolution of 350 µm and a slice thickness of 3 mm. **B:** The image was acquired with the intravascular MR coil *(IV coil)* and an in-plane resolution of 78 µm and a 2-mm slice thickness.

SUMMARY

Techniques for imaging atherosclerotic plaque are essential to identify vulnerable plaques. Several invasive and noninvasive imaging techniques are available to assess atherosclerotic vessels. Most of the standard techniques determine luminal diameter or stenosis, wall thickness, and plaque volume. These imaging techniques are ineffective for identifying plaques that are unstable or are at high risk for and vulnerable to thrombosis. *In vivo* high-resolution, multicontrast MRI holds the greatest promise for the noninvasive imaging of high-risk plaques. MR allows the serial assessment of the progression and regression of atherosclerosis. The application of MRI opens up entirely new areas for the diagnosis, prevention, and treatment (e.g., lipid-lowering drug regimens) of atherosclerosis in all arterial locations.

ACKNOWLEDGMENTS

This work was supported in part by grants from the Radiological Society of North America, New York; Community Trust; the National Institutes of Health (NHLBI-NIH P50-HL-54469, R01-HL-61801, R01-HL-61814); Merck; Magna Laboratories; and GE Medical Systems; and by funds from the Zena and Michael A. Wiener Cardiovascular Institute and the Department of Radiology of the Mount Sinai School of Medicine. The authors acknowledge the assistance of Drs. Gilbert Aguinaldo, Juan J. Badimon, Robin P Choudhury, Roberto Corti, Burton Drayer, John T. Fallon, Valentin Fuster, Edward A. Fisher, Gerard Helft, Meir Shinnar, Ernane Reis, Jean Francois Toussaint, Steve G. Worthley. We are also grateful for the assistance of Drs. Thomas Foo, Herman Flick, and Chris Hardy; Mrs. Bronwyn Medley, and Mr. Manoj Saranathan of GE Medical Systems and GE Corporate Research and Development; Dr. Michele Mercuri of Merck; and Dr. Lawrence Minkoff of Magna Laboratories. Karen Metroka, Stella Palencia, and Mary Ann Whelan-Gales assisted in patient selection and recruitment. Finally, we thank Frank Macaluso, Paul Wisdom, and John Abela for their help in MRI scanning.

REFERENCES

1. Fuster V, Fayad ZA, Badimon JJ. Acute coronary syndromes: biology. *Lancet* 1999;353(Suppl 2):SII5–SII9.
2. Libby P. Molecular bases of the acute coronary syndromes. *Circulation* 1995;91:2844–2850.
3. Falk E, Shah PK, Fuster V. Coronary plaque disruption. *Circulation* 1995;92:657–671.
4. Fuster V. Lewis A. Conner Memorial Lecture. Mechanisms leading to myocardial infarction: insights from studies of vascular biology. *Circulation* 1994;90:2126–2146.
5. Richardson PD, Davies MJ, Born GV. Influence of plaque configuration and stress distribution on fissuring of coronary atherosclerotic plaques. *Lancet* 1989;2:941–944.
6. Toschi V, Gallo R, Lettino M, et al. Tissue factor modulates the thrombogenicity of human atherosclerotic plaques. *Circulation* 1997;95:594–599.
7. Moreno PR, Falk E, Palacios IF, et al. Macrophage infiltration in acute coronary syndromes. Implications for plaque rupture. *Circulation* 1994;90:775–778.
8. Kaartinen M, Penttila A, Kovanen PT. Accumulation of activated mast cells in the shoulder region of human coronary atheroma, the predilection site of atheromatous rupture. *Circulation* 1994;90:1669–1678.
9. Glagov S, Zarins C, Giddens DP, et al. Hemodynamics and atherosclerosis. Insights and perspectives gained from studies of human arteries. *Arch Pathol Lab Med* 1988;112:1018–1031.
10. Toussaint JF, LaMuraglia GM, Southern JF, et al. Magnetic resonance images lipid, fibrous, calcified, hemorrhagic, and thrombotic components of human atherosclerosis *in vivo*. *Circulation* 1996;94:932–938.
11. Solberg LA, Strong JP. Risk factors and atherosclerotic lesions. A review of autopsy studies. *Arteriosclerosis* 1983;3:187–198.
12. Fazio GP, Redberg RF, Winslow T, et al. Transesophageal echocardiographically detected atherosclerotic aortic plaque is a marker for coronary artery disease. *J Am Coll Cardiol* 1993;21:144–150.
13. The French Study of Aortic Plaques in Stroke Group. Atherosclerotic disease of the aortic arch as a risk factor for recurrent ischemic stroke. *N Engl J Med* 1996;334:1216–1221.
14. Cohen A, Tzourio C, Bertrand B, et al. Aortic plaque morphology and vascular events: a follow-up study in patients with ischemic stroke. FAPS Investigators. French Study of Aortic Plaques in Stroke. *Circulation* 1997;96:3838–3841.
15. Fayad ZA, Fuster V. Clinical imaging of the high-risk or vulnerable atherosclerotic plaque. *Circ Res* 2001;89:305–316.
16. Wood ML, Wehrli FW. Principles of magnetic resonance imaging. In: Stark DD, Bradley WG, eds. *Magnetic resonance imaging*, vol 1. St. Louis: Mosby, 1999:1–14.
17. Soila K, Nummi P, Ekfors T, et al. Proton relaxation times in arterial wall and atheromatous lesions in man. *Invest Radiol* 1986;21:411–415.
18. Maynor CH, Charles HC, Herfkens RJ, et al. Chemical shift imaging of atherosclerosis at 7.0 tesla. *Invest Radiol* 1989;24:52–60.
19. Pearlman JD, Zajicek J, Merickel MB, et al. High-resolution ^{1}H NMR spectral signature from human atheroma. *Magn Reson Med* 1988;7:262–279.
20. Mohiaddin RH, Firmin DN, Underwood SR, et al. Chemical shift magnetic resonance imaging of human atheroma. *Br Heart J* 1989;62:81–89.
21. Vinitski S, Consigny PM, Shapiro MJ, et al. Magnetic resonance chemical shift imaging and spectroscopy of atherosclerotic plaque. *Invest Radiol* 1991;26:703–714.
22. Gold GE, Pauly JM, Glover GH, et al. Characterization of atherosclerosis with a 1.5-T imaging system. *J Magn Reson Imaging* 1993;3:399–407.
23. Altbach MI, Mattingly MA, Brown MF, et al. Magnetic resonance imaging of lipid deposits in human atheroma via a stimulated-echo diffusion-weighted technique. *Magn Reson Med* 1991;20:319–326.
24. Toussaint JF, Southern JF, Fuster V, et al. ^{13}C-NMR spectroscopy of human atherosclerotic lesions. Relation between fatty acid saturation, cholesteryl ester content, and luminal obstruction. *Arterioscler Thromb* 1994;14:1951–1957.
25. Toussaint JF, Southern JF, Fuster V, et al. T2-weighted contrast for NMR characterization of human atherosclerosis. *Arterioscler Thromb Vasc Biol* 1995;15:1533–1542.

26. Kaufman L, Crooks LE, Sheldon PE, et al. Evaluation of NMR imaging for detection and quantification of obstructions in vessels. *Invest Radiol* 1982;17:554–560.

27. Herfkens RJ, Higgins CB, Hricak H, et al. Nuclear magnetic resonance imaging of atherosclerotic disease. *Radiology* 1983; 148:161–166.

28. Merickel MB, Carman CS, Brookeman JR, et al. Identification and 3-D quantification of atherosclerosis using magnetic resonance imaging. *Comput Biol Med* 1988;18:89–102.

29. Yuan C, Tsuruda JS, Beach KN, et al. Techniques for high-resolution MR imaging of atherosclerotic plaque. *J Magn Reson Imaging* 1994;4:43–49.

30. Martin AJ, Gotlieb AI, Henkelman RM. High-resolution MR imaging of human arteries. *J Magn Reson Imaging* 1995;5:93–100.

31. Yuan C, Murakami JW, Hayes CE, et al. Phased-array magnetic resonance imaging of the carotid artery bifurcation: preliminary results in healthy volunteers and a patient with atherosclerotic disease. *J Magn Reson Imaging* 1995;5:561–565.

32. von Ingersleben G, Schmiedl UP, Hatsukami TS, et al. Characterization of atherosclerotic plaques at the carotid bifurcation: correlation of high-resolution MR imaging with histologic analysis—preliminary study. *Radiographics* 1997; 17:1417–1423.

33. Worthley SG, Helft G, Fuster V, et al. High resolution *ex vivo* magnetic resonance imaging of in situ coronary and aortic atherosclerotic plaque in a porcine model. *Atherosclerosis* 2000; 150:321–329.

34. Edzes HT, Samulski ET. Cross relaxation and spin diffusion in the proton NMR or hydrated collagen. *Nature* 1977;265:521–523.

35. Fisel CR, Ackerman JL, Buxton RB, et al. MR contrast due to microscopically heterogeneous magnetic susceptibility: numerical simulations and applications to cerebral physiology. *Magn Reson Med* 1991;17:336–347.

36. Witztum JL, Steinberg D. Role of oxidized low density lipoprotein in atherogenesis. *J Clin Invest* 1991;88:1785–1792.

37. Rapp JH, Connor WE, Lin DS, et al. Lipids of human atherosclerotic plaques and xanthomas: clues to the mechanism of plaque progression. *J Lipid Res* 1983;24:1329–1335.

38. Kucharczyk W, Henkelman RM. Visibility of calcium on MR and CT: can MR show calcium that CT cannot? *AJNR Am J Neuroradiol* 1994;15:1145–1148.

39. Bradley WG Jr. MR appearance of hemorrhage in the brain [see Comments]. *Radiology* 1993;189:15–26.

40. Yamashita Y, Hatanaka Y, Torashima M, et al. Magnetic resonance characteristics of intrapelvic haematomas. *Br J Radiol* 1995;68:979–985.

41. Murray JG, Manisali M, Flamm SD, et al. Intramural hematoma of the thoracic aorta: MR image findings and their prognostic implications [see Comments]. *Radiology* 1997;204: 349–355.

42. Bluemke DA. Definitive diagnosis of intramural hematoma of the thoracic aorta with MR imaging [Editorial; Comment]. *Radiology* 1997;204:319–321.

43. Rapoport S, Sostman HD, Pope C, et al. Venous clots: evaluation with MR imaging. *Radiology* 1987;162:527–530.

44. Bryant RG, Marill K, Blackmore C, et al. Magnetic relaxation in blood and blood clots. *Magn Reson Med* 1990;13:133–144.

45. Bass JC, Hedlund LW, Sostman HD. MR imaging of experimental and clinical thrombi at 1.5 T. *Magn Reson Imaging* 1990;8:631–635.

46. Erdman WA, Jayson HT, Redman HC, et al. Deep venous thrombosis of extremities: role of MR imaging in the diagnosis. *Radiology* 1990;174:425–431.

47. Totterman S, Francis CW, Foster TH, et al. Diagnosis of femoropopliteal venous thrombosis with MR imaging: a com-

parison of four MR pulse sequences. *AJR Am J Roentgenol* 1990;154:175–178.

48. Shinnar M, Fallon JT, Wehrli S, et al. The diagnostic accuracy of *ex vivo* magnetic resonance imaging for human atherosclerotic plaque characterization. *Arterioscler Thromb Vasc Biol* 1999;19:2756–2761.

49. Toussaint JF, Southern JF, Fuster V, et al. Water diffusion properties of human atherosclerosis and thrombosis measured by pulse field gradient nuclear magnetic resonance. *Arterioscler Thromb Vasc Biol* 1997;17:542–546.

50. Fayad ZA, Fallon JT, Shinnar M, et al. Noninvasive *in vivo* high-resolution magnetic resonance imaging of atherosclerotic lesions in genetically engineered mice. *Circulation* 1998;98: 1541–1547.

51. Chandra S, Clark LV, Coatney RW, et al. Application of serial *in vivo* magnetic resonance imaging to evaluate the efficacy of endothelin receptor antagonist SB 217242 in the rat carotid artery model of neointima formation. *Circulation* 1998;97: 2252–2258.

52. Skinner MP, Yuan C, Mitsumori L, et al. Serial magnetic resonance imaging of experimental atherosclerosis detects lesion fine structure, progression and complications *in vivo*. *Nat Med* 1995;1:69–73.

53. Lin W, Abendschein DR, Haacke EM. Contrast-enhanced magnetic resonance angiography of carotid arterial wall in pigs. *J Magn Reson Imaging* 1997;7:183–190.

54. Kaneko E, Yuan C, Skinner MP, et al. Serial magnetic resonance imaging of experimental atherosclerosis allows visualization of lesion characteristics and lesion progression *in vivo*. *Ann N Y Acad Sci* 1997;811:245–252; discussion 252–254.

55. Helft G, Worthley SG, Fuster V, et al. Atherosclerotic aortic component quantification by noninvasive magnetic resonance: an *in vivo* study in rabbits. *J Am Coll Cardiol* 2001;37:1149–1154.

56. McConnell MV, Aikawa M, Maier SE, et al. MRI of rabbit atherosclerosis in response to dietary cholesterol lowering. *Arterioscler Thromb Vasc Biol* 1999;19:1956–1959.

57. Helft G, Worthley SG, Fuster V, et al. Progression and regression of atherosclerotic lesions: monitoring with serial noninvasive magnetic resonance imaging. *Circulation* 2002; 105:993–998.

58. Worthley SG, Helft G, Osende JI, et al. Serial evaluation of atherosclerosis with *in vivo* MRI: study of atorvastatin and avasimibe in WHHL rabbits. *Circulation* 2000;102:II-809.

59. Worthley SG, Helft G, Fuster V, et al. Serial *in vivo* MRI documents arterial remodeling in experimental atherosclerosis. *Circulation* 2000;101:586–589.

60. Fayad ZA, Fallon JT, Shinnar M, et al. Noninvasive *in vivo* high-resolution magnetic resonance imaging of atherosclerotic lesions in genetically engineered mice. *Circulation* 1998;98:1541–1547.

61. Choudhury RP, Aguinaldo JG, Rong JX, et al. Atherosclerotic lesions in genetically modified mice quantified *in vivo* by noninvasive high-resolution magnetic resonance microscopy. *Atherosclerosis* 2002;162:315–321.

62. Pohost GM, Fuisz AR. From the microscope to the clinic: MR assessment of atherosclerotic plaque. *Circulation* 1998;98: 1477–1478.

63. Yuan C, Beach KW, Smith LH Jr, et al. Measurement of atherosclerotic carotid plaque size *in vivo* using high resolution magnetic resonance imaging. *Circulation* 1998;98:2666–2671.

64. Fayad ZA, Nahar T, Fallon JT, et al. *In vivo* MR evaluation of atherosclerotic plaques in the human thoracic aorta: a comparison with TEE. *Circulation* 2000;101:2503–2509.

65. Coulden RA, Moss H, Graves MJ, et al. High resolution magnetic resonance imaging of atherosclerosis and the response to balloon angioplasty. *Heart* 2000;83:188–191.

66. Fayad ZA, Fuster V, Fallon JT, et al. Noninvasive *in vivo* human coronary artery lumen and wall imaging using black-blood magnetic resonance imaging. *Circulation* 2000; 102:506–510.

67. Hatsukami TS, Ross R, Polissar NL, et al. Visualization of fibrous cap thickness and rupture in human atherosclerotic carotid plaque *in vivo* with high-resolution magnetic resonance imaging. *Circulation* 2000;102:959–964.

68. Fayad ZA, Connick TJ, Axel L. An improved quadrature or phased-array coil for MR cardiac imaging. *Magn Reson Med* 1995;34:186–193.

69. Fayad ZA, Hardy CJ, Giaquinto R, et al. Improved high resolution MRI of human coronary lumen and plaque with a new cardiac coil. *Circulation* 2000;102:II-399.

70. Hayes CE, Mathis CM, Yuan C. Surface coil phased arrays for high-resolution imaging of the carotid arteries. *J Magn Reson Imaging* 1996;6:109–112.

71. Summers RM, Andrasko-Bourgeois J, Feuerstein IM, et al. Evaluation of the aortic root by MRI: insights from patients with homozygous familial hypercholesterolemia. *Circulation* 1998;98:509–518.

72. Jaffer FA, O'Donnell CJ, Kissinger KV, et al. MRI assessment of aortic atherosclerosis in an asymptomatic population: the Framingham Heart Study. *Circulation* 2000;102:II-458.

73. O'Donnell CJ, Larson MG, Jaffer FA, et al. Aortic atherosclerosis detected by MRI is associated with contemporaneous and longitudinal risk factors: the Framingham Heart Study (FHS). *Circulation* 2000;102:II-836.

74. Worthley SG, Helft G, Fuster V, et al. Noninvasive *in vivo* magnetic resonance imaging of experimental coronary artery lesions in a porcine model. *Circulation* 2000;101:2956–2961.

75. Botnar RM, Stuber M, Kissinger KV, et al. Noninvasive coronary vessel wall and plaque imaging with magnetic resonance imaging. *Circulation* 2000;102:2582–2587.

76. Corti R, Fayad ZA, Fuster V, et al. Effects of lipid-lowering by simvastatin on human atherosclerotic lesions: a longitudinal study by high-resolution, noninvasive magnetic resonance imaging. *Circulation* 2001;104:249–252.

77. Ford JC, Shlansky-Goldberg RD, Golden M. MR microscopy of the arterial wall in an experimental model of atherosclerosis: preliminary results. *J Vasc Interv Radiol* 1997;8:93–99.

78. Carpenter TA, Hodgson RJ, Herrod NJ, et al. Magnetic resonance imaging in a model of atherosclerosis: use of a collar around the rabbit carotid artery. *Magn Reson Imaging* 1991;9: 365–371.

79. Summers RM, Hedlund LW, Cofer GP, et al. MR microscopy of the rat carotid artery after balloon injury by using an implanted imaging coil. *Magn Reson Med* 1995;33:785–789.

80. Yeung CJ, Atalar E. RF transmit power limit for the barewire loopless catheter antenna [In Process Citation]. *J Magn Reson Imaging* 2000;12:86–91.

81. Yang X, Bolster BD Jr, Kraitchman DL, et al. Intravascular MR-monitored balloon angioplasty: an *in vivo* feasibility study. *J Vasc Interv Radiol* 1998;9:953–959.

82. Correia LC, Atalar E, Kelemen MD, et al. Intravascular magnetic resonance imaging of aortic atherosclerotic plaque composition. *Arterioscler Thromb Vasc Biol* 1997; 17:3626–3632.

83. Ladd ME, Debatin JF. Interventional and intravascular MR angiography. *Herz* 2000;25:440–451.

84. Quick HH, Ladd ME, Nanz D, et al. Vascular stents as RF antennas for intravascular MR guidance and imaging. *Magn Reson Med* 1999;42:738–745.

85. Quick HH, Ladd ME, Zimmermann-Paul GG, et al. Single-loop coil concepts for intravascular magnetic resonance imaging. *Magn Reson Med* 1999;41:751–758.

86. Quick HH, Ladd ME, Hilfiker PR, et al. Autoperfused balloon catheter for intravascular MR imaging. *J Magn Reson Imaging* 1999;9:428–434.

87. Ladd ME, Quick HH. Reduction of resonant RF heating in intravascular catheters using coaxial chokes. *Magn Reson Med* 2000;43:615–619.

88. Zimmermann GG, Erhart P, Schneider J, et al. Intravascular MR imaging of atherosclerotic plaque: *ex vivo* analysis of human femoral arteries with histologic correlation. *Radiology* 1997;204: 769–774.

89. Zimmermann-Paul GG, Quick HH, Vogt P, et al. High-resolution intravascular magnetic resonance imaging: monitoring of plaque formation in heritable hyperlipidemic rabbits. *Circulation* 1999;99:1054–1061.

90. Martin AJ, McLoughlin RF, Chu KC, et al. An expandable intravenous RF coil for arterial wall imaging. *J Magn Reson Imaging* 1998;8:226–234.

91. Martin AJ, Henkelman RM. Intravascular MR imaging in a porcine animal model. *Magn Reson Med* 1994;32:224–229.

92. Martin AJ, Ryan LK, Gotlieb AI, et al. Arterial imaging: comparison of high-resolution US and MR imaging with histologic correlation. *Radiographics* 1997;17:189–202.

93. Kandarpa K, Jakab P, Patz S, et al. Prototype miniature endoluminal MR imaging catheter. *J Vasc Interv Radiol* 1993;4: 419–427.

94. Hurst GC, Hua J, Duerk JL, et al. Intravascular (catheter) NMR receiver probe: preliminary design analysis and application to canine iliofemoral imaging. *Magn Reson Med* 1992;24:343–357.

95. Shinnar M, Worthley SG, Helft G, et al. A new non-obstructive intravascular MRI probe for high resolution *in vivo* imaging of atherosclerotic plaques. *J Am Coll Cardiol* 2000;35:479A.

96. Rogers WJ, Prichard JW, Hu YL, et al. Characterization of signal properties in atherosclerotic plaque components by intravascular MRI. *Arterioscler Thromb Vasc Biol* 2000;20:1824–1830.

97. Shunk KA, Lima JA, Heldman AW, et al. Transesophageal magnetic resonance imaging. *Magn Reson Med* 1999;41:722–726.

98. Lardo AC. Real-time magnetic resonance imaging: diagnostic and interventional applications. *Pediatr Cardiol* 2000;21:80–98.

99. Ocali O, Atalar E. Intravascular magnetic resonance imaging using a loopless catheter antenna. *Magn Reson Med* 1997;37: 112–118.

100. Tello R, Mitchell PJ, Melhem ER, et al. Interventional catheter magnetic resonance angiography with a conventional 1.5-T magnet: work in progress. *Australas Radiol* 1999;43:435–439.

101. Luk-Pat GT, Gold GE, Olcott EW, et al. High-resolution three-dimensional *in vivo* imaging of atherosclerotic plaque. *Magn Reson Med* 1999;42:762–771.

102. Pachot-Clouard M, Vaufrey F, Darasse L, et al. Magnetization transfer characteristics in atherosclerotic plaque components assessed by adapted binomial preparation pulses. *MAGMA* 1998;7:9–15.

103. Yu X, Song SK, Chen J, et al. High-resolution MRI characterization of human thrombus using a novel fibrin-targeted paramagnetic nanoparticle contrast agent. *Magn Reson Med* 2000; 44:867–872.

104. Steinman DA, Rutt BK. On the nature and reduction of plaque-mimicking flow artifacts in black blood MRI of the carotid bifurcation. *Magn Reson Med* 1998;39:635–641.

WHOLE BODY THREE-DIMENSIONAL MRA

MATHIAS GOYEN
STEFAN G. RUEHM
JÖRG F. DEBATIN

Peripheral vascular disease is a major health problem, accounting for more than 100,000 surgical procedures annually in the United States alone (1). The disease interferes with activities of daily living, resulting in loss of independence and economic productivity. Peripheral vascular disease is caused by the systemic process of atherosclerosis and is frequently associated with coronary, renal, and carotid arterial disease. The management of a patient with peripheral vascular disease has to be planned in the context of the epidemiology of the disease and, in particular, the apparent risk factors or markers predicting spontaneous deterioration (2). It is obvious that the proper management of arterial disease requires a comprehensive assessment of the underlying vascular morphology. Localizing and gauging the severity of arterial lesions is crucial for therapeutic decision making. For this purpose, several imaging modalities, including conventional catheter angiography, duplex ultrasonography, computed tomographic angiography, and MRA, are in clinical use.

To date, the peripheral arterial system has been displayed with catheter-based x-ray angiography. However, the high cost, invasiveness, and associated risks (3–5) of this procedure have motivated the development and evaluation of noninvasive peripheral vascular imaging techniques, including ultrasonography, computed tomographic (CT) angiography, and MRA. The advantages of MRA relative to CT angiography include a large field-of-view, the use of contrast material that is not nephrotoxic, and a lack of ionizing radi-

ation. In comparison with ultrasonography, MRA is less operator-dependent and overcomes difficulties related to limited acoustic windows. The lack of ionizing radiation and the safety of the contrast agents (6), in conjunction with a high rate of diagnostic accuracy, have driven the rapid implementation of MRA as the modality of choice for assessing arterial disease in many centers throughout the world (7–10).

CONCEPT OF WHOLE BODY MRA

Because atherosclerotic disease effects the entire arterial system, extended coverage allowing the simultaneous assessment of the arterial system from the supraaortic arteries to the distal runoff vessels appears desirable. Originally, subsequent parenchymal enhancement and limitations of the contrast dose curtailed contrast-enhanced three-dimensional (3D) MRA to a display of the arterial territory contained within a single field-of-view extending over 40 to 48 cm. The implementation of "bolus chase" techniques extended coverage to encompass the entire runoff vasculature, including the pelvic, femoral, popliteal and trifurcation arteries (11–14). The implementation of faster gradient systems has laid the foundation for a further extension of the bolus chase technique; coverage of the whole body with 3D MRA, from the carotid arteries to the runoff vessels, has become possible in a mere 72 seconds (15).

The concept of whole body MRA is based on the acquisition of five slightly overlapping 3D data sets in immediate

M. Goyen, S. G. Ruehm, and J. F. Debatin: Department of Diagnostic and Interventional Radiology, University Hospital Essen, Essen, Germany.

succession. The first data set covers the aortic arch, supraaortic branch arteries, and thoracic aorta, and the second data set covers the abdominal aorta with its major branches, including the renal arteries. The third data set displays the pelvic arteries, and the last two data sets cover the arteries of the thighs and calves, respectively.

TECHNIQUE

After the 3D acquisitions have been planned with a "moving vessel scout" and the arrival time of the contrast determined with the test bolus technique, a commercially available fast gradient-echo 3D sequence is employed (Magnetom Sonata; Siemens, Erlangen, Germany: repetition time/echo time, 2.1/0.7 milliseconds; flip angle, 25 degrees; 40 partitions interpolated by zero filling to 64; slab thickness, 120 mm; slice thickness, 3.0 mm interpolated to 1.9 mm; field-of-view, 390 × 390 mm; matrix, 256 × 225 interpolated by zero filling to 512 × 512; readout bandwidth, 863 Hz per pixel; acquisition time, 12 seconds). To avoid any gaps, the 3D data sets are overlapped by 3 cm to obtain a craniocaudal coverage of 176 cm. Each 3D data set is collected over 12 seconds (16).

A weight-adjusted dose of 0.2 mmol of a gadolinium chelate per kilogram of body weight is diluted with 0.9% normal saline solution to a total volume of 60 mL (17). The contrast medium (MR Spectris; Medrad, Pittsburgh, Pennsylvania) is automatically injected according to a biphasic protocol; the first half is injected at a rate of 1.3 mL/s, and the second half at a rate of 0.7 mL/s. The contrast is flushed with 30 mL of saline solution injected at a rate of 1.3 mL/s.

DIAGNOSTIC ACCURACY

Correlation with a limited number of regional diagnostic subtraction angiography examinations revealed the diagnostic performance of whole body MRA to be sufficient to warrant use as a noninvasive alternative to digital subtraction angiography (15). In comparison with conventional catheter angiography, according to the findings of two independent and masked readers, whole body MRA had overall sensitivities of 91% (95% confidence interval, 0.76 to 0.98) and 94% (95% CI, 0.8 to 0.99) and specificities of 93% (95% CI, 0.85 to 0.97) and 90% (95% CI, 0.82 to 0.96) for the detection of substantial vascular disease (luminal narrowing >50%). Interobserver agreement for the assessment of whole body magnetic angiograms was very good (κ = 0.94; 95% CI, 0.9 to 0.98).

ANGIOSURF IN WHOLE BODY MRA

The performance of whole body 3D MRA is further improved by using an angiographic system for unlimited

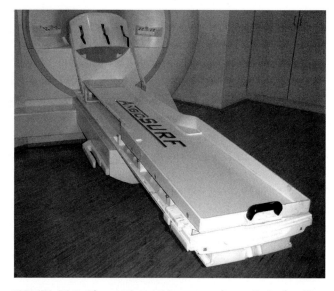

FIGURE 28.1. The angiographic system for unlimited rolling fields of view (AngioSURF) is a manually driven table platform for acquiring high-resolution contrast-enhanced whole body three-dimensional (3D) MRA. The AngioSURF, which can be installed on top of the original table of a Siemens MR scanner, allows the patient to be moved manually between the circular polarized spine and the circular polarized body array surface coils. The technique makes it possible to perform whole body 3D data acquisition through stepwise movement of the volunteer/patient relative to the surface coils. With this approach, the achievable signal-to-noise ratio is significantly enhanced in comparison with that of data acquired with the body coil of the scanner. A high-resolution whole body MR angiogram, for example, can be acquired in 72 seconds with the administration of a single bolus of contrast.

rolling fields of view (AngioSURF; MR-Innovation, Essen, Germany) (Fig. 28.1), which integrates the torso surface coil for signal reception to improve spatial resolution. Use of the surface coil resulted in high values of the signal-to-noise ratio and contrast-to-noise ratio, which translated into a sensitivity of 95.3% and a specificity of 95.2% for the detection of significant stenoses (luminal narrowing >50%) in peripheral vascular disease of the lower extremities (18).

For the AngioSURF examination, all patients are placed feet first within the bore of the magnet and examined in the supine position on the fully MR-compatible AngioSURF platform, which is placed on a table (Fig. 28.1). The AngioSURF platform fits on most standard MR systems manufactured by Siemens. The platform, 240 cm in length, is placed on seven pairs of roller bearings, which are anchored to the table used for the examination. Up to six 400-mm 3D data sets can be acquired in immediate succession. Markers permit adjustment of the desired field-of-view. Signal reception is accomplished by using posteriorly located spine coils and an anteriorly located torso phased-array coil, which remains stationary within the bore. The two utilized elements of the spine coil are integrated in the table used for the examination, and the standard torso phased-array coil is

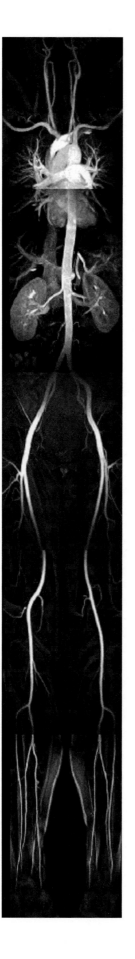

anchored to a height-adjustable holder, which remains fixed to the stationary table. Thus, data for all five stations are collected with the same stationary set of coils positioned at the isocenter of the magnet.

Despite the recognition that atherosclerotic disease is a systemic disease affecting the entire arterial system, the diagnostic approach to atherosclerosis has remained segmental, largely because of the limitations inherent to the imaging modalities currently employed, including radiation exposure, limitations of the contrast dose, invasiveness, and economic factors. MRI can provide images of the vascular system by virtue of the fact that moving blood looks bright in comparison with tissues that are not moving when certain special acquisition modes are used. Many of the limitations of nonenhanced MRA studies have been overcome by administering gadolinium-based MR contrast media. If dynamically infused during data acquisition, gadolinium-based contrast agents shorten the T1 relaxation time of flowing blood, and a selective display of the arterial system is obtained (19,20).

The time needed to acquire a complete 3D data set can be significantly reduced by using the latest high-performance scanner and gradients. If the repetition time is shortened to 2.1 milliseconds, a 3D data set can be collected in just 12 seconds. Thus, up to five 3D data sets can be collected within the short intraarterial contrast phase of slightly more than 60 seconds (Fig. 28.2). Improved signal within the arterial system obtained by using a phased-array torso surface coil directly translates into an increase in achievable spatial resolution, which amounts to 0.8 × 0.8 × 2 mm (post-interpolation pixel size) in the applied protocol. This enables a better delineation of the smaller vessels, especially the tibial vessels.

In patients with peripheral vascular disease, it is desirable to localize and gauge the severity of occlusive arterial lesions to assist in planning an intervention (Fig. 28.3). The TransAtlantic Inter-Society Consensus (TASC) on the management of peripheral arterial disease recommends that depending on local availability, experience, and cost, duplex

FIGURE 28.2. Three-dimensional whole body MR angiogram obtained with AngioSURF consisting of five three-dimensional (3D) data sets collected over 72 seconds. The acquisition time for each 3D data set was 12 seconds. During a 3-second break in the acquisition, the table was manually repositioned to the center of the subsequent image volume. With five successive acquisitions, craniocaudal coverage thus extended over 180 cm, and the total data acquisition time amounted to 72 seconds. MultiHance (Bracco Diagnostics, Princeton, New Jersey) was administered at a dose of 0.2 mmol/kg of body weight and at a rate of 1.3 mL/s for the first half and 0.7 mL/s for the second half of the contrast volume, followed by a 30-mL flush of saline solution administered with an automated injector (MR Spectris). The scan delay was determined with a 2-mL test bolus at the level of the descending aorta. The quality of the whole body MR angiogram is sufficient to assess the arterial system from the supraaortic arteries to the runoff vessels.

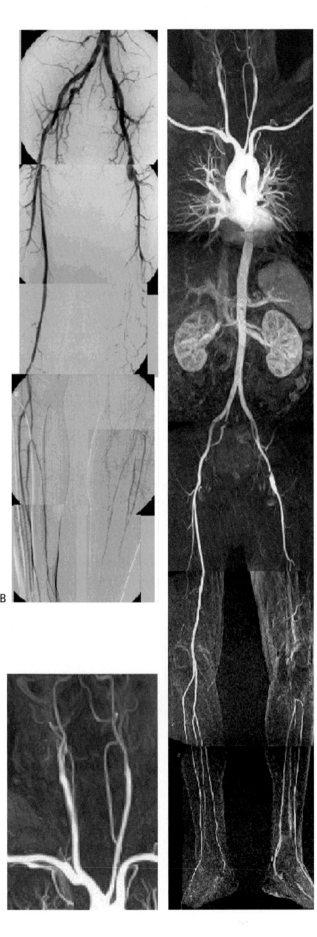

A,B

C

scanning or MRA be used as a preliminary noninvasive examination before angiography (21).

APPLICATIONS IN PERIPHERAL VASCULAR DISEASE

In a series of 100 consecutive patients with peripheral vascular disease who were initially referred for an assessment of the peripheral vasculature with MRA, the AngioSURF examination revealed additional clinically relevant disease in 25 patients (33 segments), including renal artery narrowing (15 cases), carotid arterial stenosis (12 cases), subclavian artery stenosis (2 cases), and abdominal aortic aneurysm (4 cases). The high degree of concomitant arterial disease in patients with peripheral vascular disease is not surprising and underscores the systemic nature of atherosclerosis. Patients with intermittent claudication are at particularly high risk for atherosclerotic disease in other parts of the circulation. Because peripheral vascular disease is caused by atherosclerosis, it is rarely an isolated disease process.

The extent of coexisting cardiovascular disease must be appreciated to ensure that the clinician will treat peripheral vascular disease in the proper context. Studies on the prevalence of coronary artery disease in patients with peripheral vascular disease show that the history, clinical examination, and electrocardiography typically indicate the presence of coronary artery disease in 40% to 60% of such patients, although it may often be asymptomatic and masked because they are capable of only limited exercise (22,23). The link between peripheral vascular disease and cerebrovascular disease seems to be weaker than that between peripheral vascular and coronary artery disease. Duplex ultrasonography has revealed carotid disease in 26% to 50% of patients with peripheral vascular disease (24,25). Most of these patients have a history of cerebral events or a carotid bruit and seem to be at increased risk for further events (26).

The fact that 12 unsuspected carotid lesions were identified in 10 patients in our series highlights the fact that the history is often too focused on symptoms. Because all the patients we studied presented with symptoms suggestive of peripheral vascular disease, our history taking focused on

---

FIGURE 28.3. Invasive catheter angiogram **(A)** and whole body MR angiogram **(B)** in a 54-year-old man with peripheral vascular disease and a history of a bypass graft in the left leg. The catheter angiogram shows a high-grade stenosis of the proximal anastomosis of the bypass graft and an occlusion of the superficial femoral artery/popliteal artery on the left. The whole body MR angiogram reveals these pathologic findings equally well. **C:** In addition, because of the extended coverage of the anatomy, a high-grade stenosis of the right internal carotid artery was detected that was not suspected clinically.

that region. Only very direct questioning revealed additional symptomatology suggestive of carotid disease in three patients.

Approximately one-fourth of patients with peripheral vascular disease have hypertension, and the possibility of narrowing of the renal arteries should be considered in these cases. Thirteen patients (13%) had renal artery disease with luminal narrowing greater than 50%.

Arguments are ongoing about the value of screening all patients with peripheral vascular disease, symptomatic or not, for carotid disease and aortic aneurysms (25,27). Patients with claudication are undoubtedly more likely to have significant asymptomatic disease in these areas than the general population, but the treatment of asymptomatic carotid disease remains controversial, and the issue of the yield versus the cost of such screening tests is significant.

It must be mentioned that our examination, although referred to as *whole body MRA,* does not include the intracranial or coronary arteries, for which a dedicated approach to diagnostic assessment is still required. However, the noninvasiveness, 3D features, extended coverage, and high level of contrast of whole body MRA combine to allow a quick, risk-free, and comprehensive evaluation of the arterial system in patients with atherosclerosis.

NEW MRA CONTRAST AGENTS

Currently, only extracellular, nonbinding gadolinium chelates have received regulatory approval as MRA agents for use in humans (28). Modified paramagnetic gadolinium-based agents with varying degrees of protein and superparamagnetic compounds are currently undergoing clinical evaluation (29). Some new agents, such as MultiHance (Bracco Diagnostics, Princeton, New Jersey), have a higher relaxivity and different routes of excretion but still distribute into the extracellular spaces. Higher-concentration formulations of contrast compounds, such as 1.0-*M* Gadovist (Schering, Berlin, Germany), may be advantageous for arterial enhancement (30) in comparison with 0.5-*M* extracellular contrast agents. Blood pool or intravascular contrast agents are large enough or bind to sufficiently large molecules when injected that they do not leak out of the capillaries; rather, they remain within the intravascular compartment. In view of the rapid progress of MRA techniques based on the use of extracellular agents, the future of intravascular contrast agents for the morphologic imaging of the arterial vascular tree outside the coronary arteries remains questionable.

REFERENCES

1. Rutkow IM, Ernst CB. An analysis of vascular surgical manpower requirements and vascular surgical rates in the United States. *J Vasc Surg* 1986;3:74–83.

2. TransAtlantic Inter-Society Consensus (TASC). Management of peripheral arterial disease (PAD). *J Vasc Surg* 2000;31(Suppl Part 2):S5.

3. Hessel SJ, Adams DF, Abrams HL. Complications of angiography. *Radiology* 1981;138:273–281.

4. AbuRahma AF, Robinson PA, Boland JP, et al. Complications of arteriography in a recent series of 707 cases: factors affecting outcome. *Ann Vasc Surg* 1993;7:122–129.

5. Shehadi WH. Contrast media adverse reactions: occurrence, recurrence, and distribution patterns. *Radiology* 1982;143:11–17.

6. Shellock FG, Kanal E. Safety of magnetic resonance imaging contrast agents. *J Magn Reson Imaging* 1999;10:477–484.

7. Prince MR. Gadolinium-enhanced MR aortography. *Radiology* 1994;191:155–164.

8. Prince MR, Narasimham DL, Stanley JC, et al. Breath-hold gadolinium-enhanced MR angiography of the abdominal aorta and its major branches. *Radiology* 1995;197:785–792.

9. Meaney JF, Weg JG, Chenevert TL, et al. Diagnosis of pulmonary embolism with magnetic resonance angiography. *N Engl J Med* 1997;336:1422–1427.

10. Goyen M, Debatin JF, Ruehm SG. Peripheral MR-angiography. *Top Magn Res Imaging* 2001;12:327–335.

11. Meaney JF, Ridgway JP, Chakraverty S, et al. Stepping-table gadolinium-enhanced digital subtraction MR angiography of the aorta and lower extremity arteries: preliminary experience. *Radiology* 1999;211:59–67.

12. Ho KY, Leiner T, de Haan MW, et al. Peripheral vascular tree stenoses: evaluation with moving-bed infusion-tracking MR angiography. *Radiology* 1998;206:683–692.

13. Ruehm SG, Hany TF, Pfammatter T, et al. Pelvic and lower extremity arterial imaging: diagnostic performance of three-dimensional contrast-enhanced MR angiography. *AJR Am J Roentgenol* 2000;174:1127–1135.

14. Goyen M, Ruehm SG, Barkhausen J, et al. Improved multistation peripheral MR angiography with a dedicated vascular coil. *J Magn Reson Imaging* 2001;13:475–480.

15. Ruehm SG, Goyen M, Barkhausen J, et al. Rapid magnetic resonance angiography for detection of atherosclerosis. *Lancet* 2001;357:1086–1091.

16. Ruehm SG, Goyen M, Quick HH, et al. Whole-body MRA on a rolling table platform (AngioSURF). *Rofo Fortschr Geb Rontgenstr Neuen Bildgeb Verfahr* 2000;172:670–674.

17. Goyen M, Herborn CU, Lauenstein TC, et al. Optimization of contrast dosage for gadobenate dimeglumine-enhanced high-resolution whole-body 3D magnetic resonance angiography. *Invest Radiol* 2002;37:263–268.

18. Goyen M, Quick HH, Debatin JF, et al. Whole-body 3D MR angiography using AngioSURF: initial clinical experience. *Radiology (in press).*

19. Prince MR, Chenevert TL, Foo TK, et al. Contrast-enhanced abdominal MR angiography: optimization of imaging delay time by automating the detection of contrast material arrival in the aorta. *Radiology* 1997; 203:109–114.

20. Cavagna FM, Maggioni F, Castelli PM, et al. Gadolinium chelates with weak binding to serum proteins. A new class of high-efficiency, general purpose contrast agents for magnetic resonance imaging. *Invest Radiol* 1997;32:780–796.

21. TransAtlantic Inter-Society Consensus (TASC). Management of peripheral arterial disease (PAD). *J Vasc Surg* 2000;31(Suppl Part 2):S69.

22. Von Kemp K, van den Brande P, Peterson T, et al. Screening for concomitant diseases in peripheral vascular patients. Results of a systematic approach. *Int Angiol* 1997;16:114–122.

23. Hertzer NR, Beven EG, Young JR, et al. Coronary artery disease in peripheral vascular patients. A classification of 1000 coronary

angiograms and results of surgical management. *Ann Surg* 1984; 199:223–233.

24. Klop RB, Eikelboom BC, Taks AC, et al. Screening of the internal carotid arteries in patients with peripheral vascular disease by colour-flow duplex scanning. *Eur J Vasc Surg* 1991;5: 41–45.

25. Alexandrova NA, Gibson WC, Norris JW, et al. Carotid artery stenosis in peripheral vascular disease. *J Vasc Surg* 1996; 23:645–649.

26. McDaniel MD, Cronenwett JL. Basic data related to the natural history of intermittent claudication. *Ann Vasc Surg* 1989;3:273–277.

27. Marek J, Mills JL, Harvich J, et al. Utility of routine carotid duplex screening in patients who have claudication. *J Vasc Surg* 1996;24:572–577; discussion 577–579.

28. Goyen M, Ruehm SG, Debatin JF. MR-angiography: the role of contrast agents. *Eur J Radiol* 2000;34:247–256.

29. Knopp MV, von Tengg-Kobligk H, Floemer F, et al. Contrast agents for MRA: future directions. *J Magn Reson Imaging* 1999; 10:314–316.

30. Goyen M, Lauenstein TC, Herborn CU, et al. 0.5 *M* Gd-chelate (Magnevist) vs. 1.0 *M* Gd-chelate (Gadovist): dose-independent effect on image quality of pelvic 3D MRA. *J Magn Reson Imaging* 2001;14:602–607.

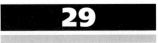

ENDOVASCULAR INTERVENTIONAL MRI

ARNO BÜCKER

MRA is on the verge of supplanting x-ray angiography as a diagnostic technique. This change has come about because of technical progress in sequence development and improvements in hardware. Although the study of coronary arteries using MRA is still a challenge, the advent of fast gradients with short repetition times (TR) and echo times (TE), which enable the acquisition of three-dimensional (3D) contrast-enhanced angiograms during breath-holding, represents a breakthrough in the clinical application of MRA in the region of the aorta, its branches, and even runoff vessels. In an ideal MR sequence to control vascular interventions, a 3D data set would be acquired with real-time upgrades of the background anatomy and interventional device. Of course, the vascular anatomy and interventional device would both have to be depicted with a high degree of spatial resolution. The application of contrast media should not be necessary, as it is when the technique of diagnostic breath-hold 3D MRA is applied directly, because toxic concentrations of commercially available contrast agents must be avoided in cases that require multiple injections. Although the application of blood pool agents can circumvent this problem, the resulting overlap of arterial and venous anatomy is undesirable.

So far, we are struggling even to approach the ideal situation of real-time 3D imaging to control vascular MR interventions. The acquisition of 3D data sets is still too slow for this purpose. However, first attempts at vascular interventions have been successfully performed by using road maps of 3D data sets in conjunction with real-time projection of a catheter tip onto previously reconstructed maximum intensity projections (MIP) (1). In addition to a high level of temporal resolution, excellent spatial resolution is needed to visualize small vessels and interventional instruments. These instruments must be made of nonferromagnetic material if large artifacts are to be avoided. Furthermore, because safety aspects have to be considered, metallic devices such as guidewires, which can act as antennae, cannot be used (2).

Many of the above mentioned "challenges" have now been met at least partially, although the ideal solution is yet to be found. As this book is written, active research is ongoing that will further modify currently applied techniques so that they can be integrated into routine clinical practice. At present, almost all the applications reported thus far have been performed only in animal studies. Nonetheless, I am convinced that with further technical developments, real-time imaging to control endovascular interventional MRI will eventually be applied clinically and therefore will have a tremendous impact on clinical practice.

TECHNIQUES

The various requirements for endovascular interventional MRI outlined above must be fulfilled simultaneously. A real-time imaging sequence will not provide acceptable control of interventions if it displays the vascular anatomy without depicting the interventional devices at the same time. For didactic reasons, the different technical aspects are discussed separately. However, it must be kept in mind that because of the need for coordinated functionality and simultaneous fulfillment of all the major prerequisites, the MRI control of vascular interventions is a demanding and challenging field of research.

A. Bücker: Department of Diagnostic Radiology, University Clinic Aachen, Aachen, Germany.

Real-Time MRI

As early as 1984, real-time MRI was described in the literature applying echo-planar imaging (3). However, the spatial resolution of these images is quite low; the basic physics of MRI cause a tradeoff between spatial and temporal resolution in the now routinely used cartesian acquisition of MR images. Because each imaging point must be measured individually, the spatial resolution of an MR image is directly proportional to the acquisition time. Therefore, standard MR techniques yield either images with high spatial and low temporal resolution, or vice versa. New imaging strategies, such as radial and spiral scanning, have become essential for vascular MR-guided interventions and are discussed here because an understanding of the technical details is necessary to perform interventions; furthermore, the new techniques are expected to become important in real-time diagnostic imaging, especially of the heart.

Hardware Considerations

The requirement for speed favors systems with a high field strength in interventional MRI. On the other hand, such systems offer less access to the patient than do open MR scanners with an intermediate or low field strength (4). A further disadvantage of systems with a high field strength is an increase in susceptibility artifacts, which can be a problem when metallic devices are used (5). When the need for high-quality diagnostic MR angiograms and the prerequisites for real-time imaging capabilities are taken into account, it can be concluded that scanners with a high field strength are preferable for guiding vascular interventions, although systems with an intermediate field strength have been successfully applied (1). Up-to-date high gradients are also mandatory for state-of-the-art imaging. These provide the short TR and TE needed not only for speed but also for the high-quality imaging of so-called true FISP (fast imaging with steady-state precession) sequences, which already play a major role in diagnostic imaging of the heart and are eventually expected to do so in interventions. Despite the fact that many articles have been written about the possible applications of magnets with a low field strength in interventional MR in general, as in biopsies and thermoablation (6,7), no reports have been published about vascular interventions performed with low-field-strength systems that provide reasonable imaging speed and quality.

If vascular interventions are to be performed under MR guidance, additional modifications of the hardware are required. An in-room monitor must be kept beside the magnet for direct control of the intervention. It should be possible to change the slice position and at least some of the scan parameters on the fly to have sufficient flexibility to optimize image quality by changing the TR, TE, and flip angle. At least at present, an angiographic backup system is needed for control of MR-guided vascular interventions and as preparation for possible complications and emergencies. In addition, dedicated real-time MR sequences require special hardware for the real-time reconstruction of raw data. Different interventional setups fulfill these requirements at least partially and are described in the literature (8–10).

Sequence Design

MR images are created by collecting raw data in so-called k-space. The standard acquisition scheme at present is cartesian imaging to fill k-space with lines; each line represents one phase-encoding step (Fig. 29.1). With standard gradient-echo or spin-echo sequences, the acquisition of one k-space line requires one TR. Consequently, an MR gradient-echo image with a 256 matrix (256 phase-encoding steps) and a TR of 4 milliseconds requires a total acquisition time of 1 second. The application of fast spin-echo or gradient-echo techniques or echo-planar imaging makes it possible to sample more than one phase-encoding step during one TR period, so that the speed of image acquisition is increased. Although imaging in subseconds is possible with either technique, we have found neither the image contrast nor the acquisition speed sufficient for guiding vascular interventions, at least in comparison with other k-space strategies, de-

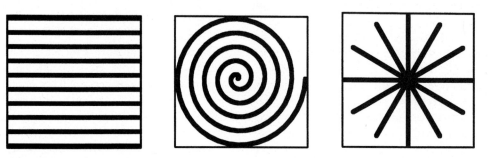

FIGURE 29.1. The filling of k-space can be accomplished by different strategies. Cartesian *(left),* spiral *(middle),* and radial scanning are schematically demonstrated. To reconstruct an MR modulus image, both the central and outer parts of k-space must be covered. The central parts are mainly responsible for contrast and signal. In spiral or radial scanning, the number of spirals or radials is not directly related to spatial resolution.

scribed below. However, Bakker et al. (11) used cartesian imaging to guide interventions with MR. They showed that background subtraction on the fly greatly increases the visibility of interventional instruments. Special hardware modifications were required to calculate and display the images fast enough (12). The frame rate achieved was about one image every 2 seconds, representing an image acquisition time of 0.5 to 1 second and additional latency for image calculation and display. Despite the relatively slow imaging speed, these investigators were able to perform balloon dilations *in vitro* and *in vivo* under MR control (13).

In terms of fast k-space coverage, spiral scanning is one of the most efficient ways to sample data. As the name implies, one or more spirals are acquired to fill k-space (Fig. 29.1). In theory, one spiral is sufficient to reconstruct an MR image. Usually, more than one spiral is acquired, and the different spirals are interleaved. The effects of this and more refined techniques, such as partial k-space coverage, are beyond the scope of this text, and the interested reader is referred to the literature (14,15). Depending on the exact form of the spiral and its length, the acquisition time for one spiral will vary. Spiral scanning does allow acquisition times for one image in the range of 100 milliseconds, so that, for example, real-time visualization of the beating heart is possible. Therefore, this technique is interesting for diagnostic imaging (Fig. 29.2). Because no cardiac triggering is required, no problems are caused by an irregular heart rhythm. The speed of spiral scanning is combined with a flow sensitivity that yields good contrast of the cardiac chambers and vessels, so that this technique can be applied

for vascular interventions. One drawback of spiral scanning is the need for a homogeneous magnetic field to avoid major artifacts. This requirement can cause problems when metallic devices are used, which usually interfere with the necessary homogeneity.

Another technique for sampling k-space is radial scanning (16). As in cartesian scanning, multiple lines are acquired, but these lines fill k-space in a radial manner (Fig. 29.1). In comparison with spiral scanning, this technique is much less time-efficient because a relatively high number of radials must be collected to avoid streaking artifacts caused by severe undersampling and to achieve a sufficient signal-to-noise ratio. Because the acquisition time for each radial line is comparable with that in cartesian scanning, relatively long imaging times result. Nonetheless, radial scanning is fast enough to guide vascular interventions successfully (17). Either of two techniques is used. Some degree of undersampling can be accepted for radial scanning because the spatial resolution is not directly related to the number of radial lines. Therefore, the spatial resolution is not essentially reduced by undersampling (18), and only a few radials are needed to depict a structure with a high level of contrast (Fig. 29.3). In addition, radial scanning can be ideally combined with the sliding window reconstruction technique, also called *view sharing* (19). This reconstruction technique uses partially new data in conjunction with old data to calculate new MR images with a frame rate higher than the acquisition speed required for a single complete MR image (Fig. 29.4). As a result, an MR movie is produced in which fast movements are partially frozen by averaging. Although this feature makes the technique at least theoretically less well suited for the diagnostic imaging of heart function, it visualizes a moving interventional device on a basically unchanging background anatomy extremely well. One further advantage of this technique is its lack of susceptibility to motion artifacts (20), so that, for example, it can be applied to detect pulmonary embolism without the need for breath-holding (21). Many of the images in this chapter were acquired by radial scanning in combination with the sliding window reconstruction technique, which yielded a frame rate of 20 images per second. Because in the past the time needed to acquire one complete MR image was in the range of seconds, a minor latency occurred between the movement of the interventional instrument on the real-time images and the actual movement.

All real-time imaging sequences currently used for the MR guidance of vascular interventions acquire only a single slice. Three-dimensional imaging is still too slow to be even close to real-time imaging, not to mention the difficulties of maintaining good contrast between vessels and background anatomy. Because of the need for contrast, the principle of projection imaging cannot be applied in interventional MRI. In comparison with x-ray angiography, the tomographic nature of MR is clearly a disadvantage in this regard. To cover the vascular anatomy of interest, including tortu-

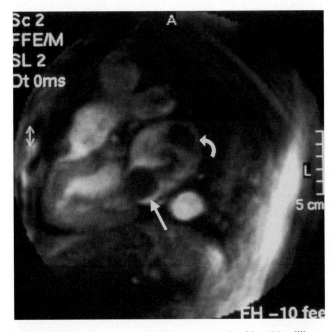

FIGURE 29.2. A real-time spiral image acquired in 120 milliseconds demonstrates a left atrial myxoma *(arrow)* on this long-axis view. The dark areas in the left atrium, caused by turbulent flow, were easily distinguished from a mass on real-time imaging.

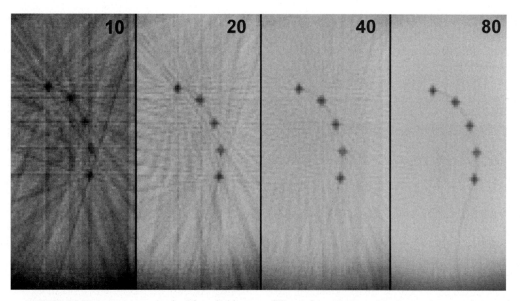

FIGURE 29.3. Images acquired with radial k-space filling of a catheter with dysprosium markers (see also Fig. 29.7) in a water bath. The numbers in the images, which indicate the number of radials acquired to calculate the MR image, demonstrate how few radials are needed to depict the structure of the catheter markers. Additionally, increasing the number of radials can be seen to yield a higher signal-to-noise ratio and diminish streaking artifacts, which are caused by undersampling.

ous vessels, the acquired single slice must be as thick as possible, yet good contrast must be maintained between the vascular anatomy and the background. At the same time, of course, the depiction of interventional devices has to be considered. The application of blood pool agents has been shown to be advantageous (22); however, the slice thickness that can be used is limited. Figure 29.5 shows radial images of a ureter. The signal intensity is high because of the earlier application of Gd-DTPA (gadolinium diethylenetriamine pentaacetic acid), so that the ureter simulates a vessel filled with a blood pool agent. The growing loss of contrast be-

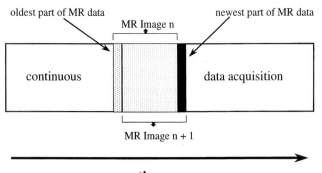

FIGURE 29.4. The sliding window reconstruction technique calculates images with a speed higher than the acquisition speed for a single image. This is achieved by using old and new data to calculate the next image. Although this technique can in principle be applied to all k-space–filling strategies, it is especially useful for radial scanning because a single radial line acquires inner and outer parts of k-space and adds fresh low- and high-frequency components to the newly calculated image.

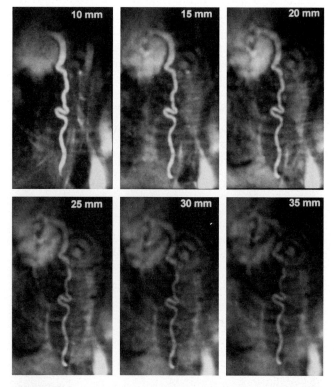

FIGURE 29.5. Images of increasing slice thickness acquired with radial k-space filling. The gadolinium-filled ureter simulates a vessel, which is filled with a blood pool agent that constantly reduces the intraluminal longitudinal relaxation time T1. Despite use of the contrast agent, thicker slices yield a progressively diminishing contrast of the ureter against the background. The ringlike artifacts are caused by the radial filling of k-space.

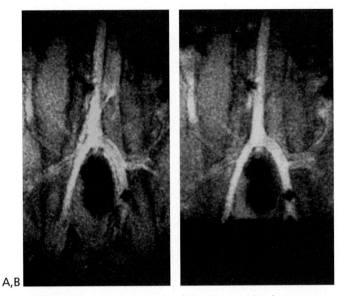

FIGURE 29.6. Radial scanning of the iliac arteries demonstrates the intrinsic contrast of this gradient-echo technique. **A:** For the first image, arteries and veins are superimposed. **B:** The second image was acquired after placement of a saturation band distal to the imaged area, which resulted in a complete suppression of the venous signal to allow a clear depiction of the iliac arteries.

tween structures containing contrast agent and the background as slice thickness increases is a principle that holds true for all MR sequences; therefore, the maximal slice thickness is limited. Furthermore, the use of blood pool agents causes an overlap of venous and arterial anatomy, which can significantly degrade the image quality. This is illustrated in Figure 29.6, which shows the intrinsic contrast of radial images. One image displays veins in addition to arteries. The other image was acquired with a saturation band, which saturates the venous flow and thereby allows a much clearer depiction of the arterial anatomy.

INSTRUMENT VISUALIZATION

Despite the progress that has been made in real-time imaging, the quality of the images acquired with the various techniques is still poor in comparison with the quality of those acquired with x-ray fluoroscopy, as becomes especially apparent when a small catheter is visualized on an MR image acquired in real time. Plastic catheters usually appear black on MR images because they lack protons. Interventional devices are small and so can be seen only if the spatial resolution of an MR image is high enough. In addition, the background must be sufficiently bright to provide a reasonable contrast with the low signal intensity of the instruments. So far, the spatial resolution and contrast characteristics of real-time imaging sequences are not good enough to depict an interventional instrument reliably. Therefore, special means have been introduced to visualize devices. These are divided

into passive and active techniques. *Passive visualization* is defined as direct visualization of the instrument in the acquired MR image. No changes are made in the MR sequence or scanner hardware for passive visualization. *Active visualization,* on the other hand, requires special hardware and usually modifications of the MR imaging sequence to exploit the abilities of MR to localize a dedicated coil in 3D space. This information is used to project the position of the coil *actively* onto the MR image.

Passive Visualization with Susceptibility Markers

In 1990, Rubin et al. (23) noted that standard conventional radiographic catheters on MR images were characterized by a small signal void, so that they could not be reliably detected on MR images. Therefore, they applied an even coating of ferromagnetic material to the polyethylene catheters. Depending on the concentration of the ferromagnetic material, a susceptibility artifact resulted that exceeded the actual catheter size, and the catheter became easily visible on MR images. However, the artifact behavior of the ferromagnetic catheters largely depended on their orientation to the main magnetic field (B_0). Because this parameter cannot be controlled during angiography but is determined by the vascular anatomy, such catheters are not well suited for MR interventions. The problem of the dependence of susceptibility artifacts on the orientation to B_0 was solved by Bakker et al. (24), who placed ringlike markers of dysprosium oxide around catheters (Fig. 29.7). Dysprosium belongs to the

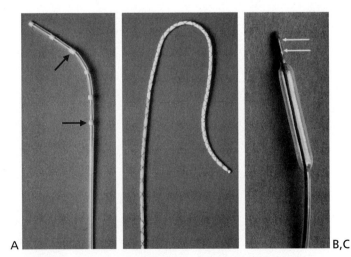

FIGURE 29.7. Passive visualization can be achieved with **(A)** susceptibility markers *(arrows)* or with the field inhomogeneity principle **(B),** in which a copper wire forms a loop along the catheter shaft. If the wire is wound like double helix, as in this example, a small current sent through the insulated copper wire causes a signal drop around the whole length of the catheter shaft. **C:** For active visualization, a microcoil is needed at the catheter tip to localize its position *(arrows).*

group of lanthanides (rare earth metals), as does the well-known element gadolinium. High concentrations of lanthanides cause signal voids because of differences between their ability to become magnetized, called *susceptibility,* and that of the surrounding human tissue. (Signal voids are therefore termed *susceptibility artifacts.*) The ability to visualize catheters reliably was proved *in vitro* and in a human volunteer (25). Although the dependence of susceptibility markers on the orientation to B_0 was solved, the size of the marker on the MR image still depended on the sequence parameters, the TE being the most important one. Because real-time MRI is difficult to perform, it is not desirable to have to adapt imaging parameters to visualize interventional instruments optimally. Furthermore, the tomographic nature of MRI means that a large signal void is advantageous so long as the instrument is located in a large vessel like the aorta. This ensures that the device can be localized even if it is not positioned in the middle of the imaged slice. On the other hand, with smaller vessels, large susceptibility artifacts obscure the vascular anatomy. Many dedicated interventional scanners allow sequence parameters to be adapted on the fly and so can at least partly influence the size of susceptibility markers, but if one considers the TEs that are reasonable for real-time scanning, the effect is relatively small (Fig. 29.8).

Passive Visualization with the Field Inhomogeneity Concept

So that the size of an instrument could be changed on an MR image independently of the sequence parameters, the field inhomogeneity concept was developed (26). A loop of insulated copper wire is wound around the instrument from the hub to the tip and back (Fig. 29.7). A small energy source is connected to the copper wire loop to allow a small amount of direct current to flow through the wire. According to the rule of thumb, the flowing current creates a local magnetic field, which causes a local field inhomogeneity and thereby a signal loss. Depending on the strength of the current, the artifact size can be varied (Fig. 29.9). The signal void can be shaped by different wire configurations; therefore, only local markers can be created at the beginning and end of a balloon, or the whole length of a catheter can be marked. As in the passive method first proposed by Bakker and colleagues (24), the wire can be wound to cause signal voids independently of the catheter orientation to B_0 (27). The small currents of up to 150 mA needed to produce sufficiently large areas of signal void during *in vivo* experiments are too small to be a safety problem (28), especially when the insulated copper wires are positioned inside the catheter walls, as is done with standard braiding. Nonetheless, the wires can act as antennae, and in case of resonance, they can heat up significantly (2). This safety aspect is discussed in further detail in a later section.

The field inhomogeneity concept has been evaluated in animal experiments showing its advantage for visualizing interventional devices in vessels of different sizes (29) (Fig. 29.10). By applying a larger current of about 150 mA, it was possible to visualize the full length of a catheter constantly in the aorta of a pig. As soon as the catheter was steered into the renal artery, the signal void obscured the vascular anatomy. This problem could be simply solved by switching the current off while the MRI sequence parameters were kept constant (30).

Although the catheter could be visualized in the proximal part of the renal artery, it was very difficult to find the correct imaging plane to depict the full course of the renal artery. As described above, the tomographic nature of MR is a disadvantage in finding smaller vessels or depicting a tortuous vascular anatomy. Active visualization can help to solve these problems.

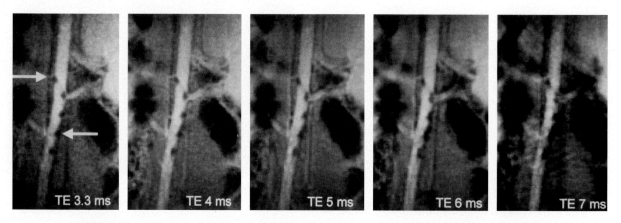

FIGURE 29.8. The size of passive susceptibility markers can be changed by modifying the echo time (TE). Longer TEs yield bigger signal voids around the markers, as can be seen on the radial gradient-echo images acquired with increasing TEs. Because the increase in TE lengthens image acquisition and degrades image quality, the possibility of changing the effect of susceptibility markers is limited.

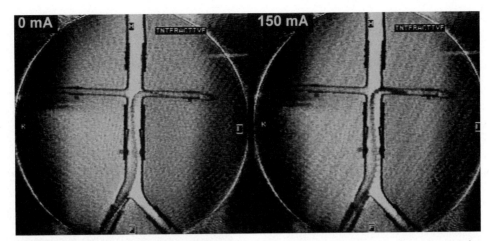

FIGURE 29.9. With the field inhomogeneity principle, a catheter is imaged in a flow phantom by radial scanning. The artifact around the catheter can be increased by sending a current, in this example 150 mA, through the copper wire running along the catheter shaft.

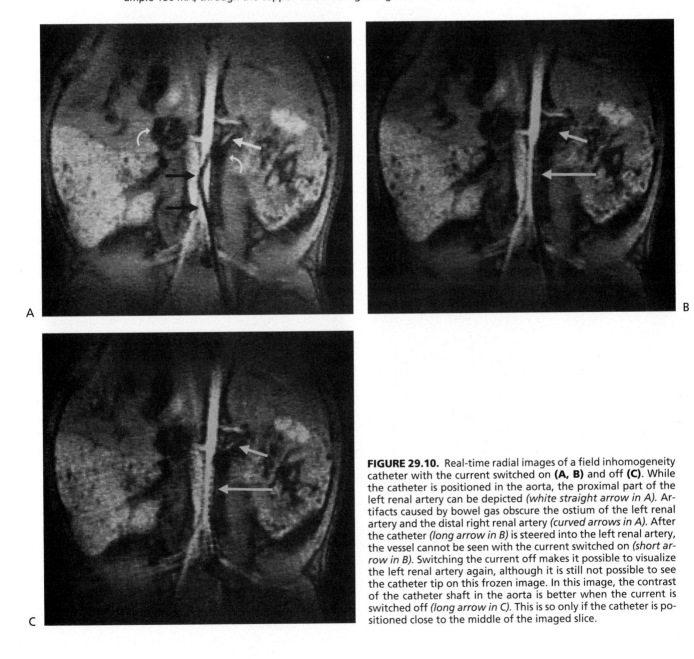

FIGURE 29.10. Real-time radial images of a field inhomogeneity catheter with the current switched on **(A, B)** and off **(C)**. While the catheter is positioned in the aorta, the proximal part of the left renal artery can be depicted *(white straight arrow in A)*. Artifacts caused by bowel gas obscure the ostium of the left renal artery and the distal right renal artery *(curved arrows in A)*. After the catheter *(long arrow in B)* is steered into the left renal artery, the vessel cannot be seen with the current switched on *(short arrow in B)*. Switching the current off makes it possible to visualize the left renal artery again, although it is still not possible to see the catheter tip on this frozen image. In this image, the contrast of the catheter shaft in the aorta is better when the current is switched off *(long arrow in C)*. This is so only if the catheter is positioned close to the middle of the imaged slice.

Active Visualization

In active visualization, a small microcoil is mounted on an instrument (Fig. 29.7). The sensitivity of an MR coil is related to its size. Therefore, a small microcoil used for receiving MR signal yields a signal only in close proximity to the microcoil. If an adequate MR sequence is applied, the frequency of the signal can be used to localize the position of the microcoil in 2D (Fig. 29.11) or even 3D space (31). If the microcoil is placed on the tip of a catheter, the position of the catheter tip can be calculated and projected onto an MR image (1,32) (Fig. 29.12). Additionally, knowledge of the position of the microcoil in 3D space can be used to position the MRI plane in real time to contain the microcoil, so-called slice tracking (33). It has been shown that the number of microcoils can be increased, albeit at the cost of reducing the speed with which the coil position can be updated (34). Furthermore, the shape of the microcoil can be changed to cover the length of an instrument—for example, to visualize a longer segment of a guidewire. This technique, called *MR profiling* (35), can also be used in combination with other microcoils.

Initially, the technique of MR tracking was used to superimpose the position of a microcoil onto a previously acquired MIP image (1). The 3D data set was acquired in a breath-hold after the application of a bolus of contrast material. Therefore, a real-time update of the background anatomy was not possible, and any movement of the patient or even bending of a vessel during catheter manipulation

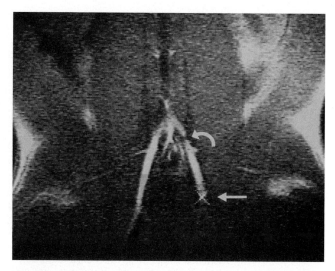

FIGURE 29.12. The position of an active tip-tracking catheter is projected onto this real-time radial image, indicated by a blinking cross *(straight arrow)*. The plain gradient-echo image demonstrates a stenosis in the proximal iliac artery *(curved arrow)*, which could be successfully dilated by real-time tip tracking of the active balloon catheter.

could lead to the false impression that the microcoil was positioned outside the vascular tree. Nonetheless, balloon occlusion, embolization, and puncture of the portal venous system were successfully performed with this technique (1). An *in vitro* comparison of active MR catheter tracking and x-ray guidance of catheter steering showed that the same amount of time was needed for both techniques (36). It has not yet been shown whether this holds true for the more complex anatomy of *in vivo* conditions. To avoid movement artifacts with the active tip-tracking technique, real-time imaging of the vascular anatomy in addition to real-time tip tracking is desirable. Simultaneous real-time depiction of the anatomy and the catheter tip is accomplished by applying a 2D radial scanning technique *in vitro* (33) and *in vivo* (37). Multiple MR receiver channels are necessary to collect data from the microcoil and the standard MR coil simultaneously. For the 2D imaging technique, it is necessary to position the vessel-of-interest in the imaged slice. This can be accomplished with the slice-tracking technique, which uses knowledge of the position of the microcoil to change the position of the imaged slice. The general slice orientation must be known to ensure that a longer part of the vessel-of-interest is included in the scan plane. In an even more sophisticated technique, three microcoils are mounted on the catheter tip (38). The microcoils are needed to calculate two points near the catheter tip and thereby provide information about the orientation of the interventional instrument. In addition, software is programmed to define a point-of-interest—for example, a stenosis. The three points can be used to define automatically the optimal imaging plane for an intervention, containing the instrument tip and the target region. The additional hardware and software modifications and the

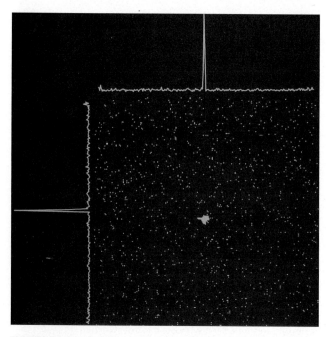

FIGURE 29.11. A microcoil receives signal only from the immediately surrounding area, which creates an image that consists of a small, high-intensity region. Analysis of this signal makes it possible to calculate the position of the microcoil, which can be projected onto a "standard" MR image.

implementation on a 0.2-T scanner do not allow for real-time imaging. Nonetheless, if this sophisticated approach can be fully automated and combined with a real-time imaging sequence, the whole procedure could be applied clinically despite its complexity.

Other Techniques

The difficulty and complexity of visualizing interventional instruments by fast MRI techniques is demonstrated by the number of different approaches. Besides those already described, other techniques are used that vary greatly in regard to potential imaging speed, available spatial resolution, and other general advantages and disadvantages. Small tuned antennae at the tips of catheters have been described as fiducial markers (39), and electron spin resonance (40) and the Overhauser effect (41) have also been exploited for instrument visualization. Catheters filled with contrast material are used in various imaging strategies (42–44). Intravascular MRI has been applied to guide aortic dilation in rabbits (45). This list is far from complete, and the interested reader is referred to the respective literature.

Safety Aspects

Provided that the general contraindications are respected, MR is a safe examination technique. Of course, no ferromagnetic materials can be used close to an MR scanner. However, even with nonferromagnetic metals, safety problems can be caused by heating (46) or the induction of electric currents (47). A danger of interventional instruments is that they can act as antennae as soon as a critical length of the instrument is reached. Heating is caused by resonance of the instrument, which leads to a constant feeding of radiofrequency energy into the device and subsequent heating. Like a radio antenna, which is tuned to a radio station, the interventional device can be tuned (resonant) to the radiofrequency transmitted by the body coil of the MR scanner. The conditions at which resonance occurs are very difficult to predict under clinical conditions. It is impossible to simulate a worst-case scenario and measure the maximal heating for one sequence. Besides the position of the instrument inside the magnet bore, its orientation and the shape of the patient being examined play a major role. The amount of radiofrequency energy applied by an MR sequence is also important, but in the case of resonance, even a sequence with a low specific absorption rate can in theory cause significant and potentially harmful heating. An *in vitro* experiment performed with an active tip-tracking catheter found no significant heating at 0.5 T, but a temperature increase of up to 20° at 1.5 T (48). Another *in vitro* study examined guidewires and found a temperature increase of only 15° at 1.5 T and no significant heating at 0.2 T (49). Experiments performed with guidewires at 1.5 T observed heating of almost 50° in 30 seconds that reached a maximum of 74°C (2). Touching a stan-

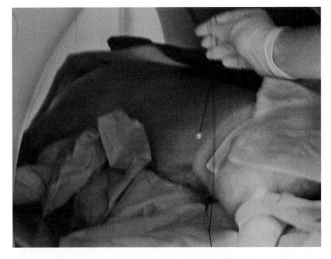

FIGURE 29.13. A 40-kg pig is placed as far off center in the magnet bore as possible. The tip of the nitinol guidewire is positioned in the aorta, and the distal end is bent backward in the magnet to touch the dead animal. Sparks, which caused skin burns, can be seen at the distal end of the guidewire.

dard nitinol guidewire resulted in skin burns in one case in this study. During *in vivo* animal experiments, we measured a temperature increase of 35°C at the tip of a standard nitinol guidewire placed in the aorta of a living pig. The pig itself was placed as far off center in the magnet bore as possible (Fig. 29.13). Furthermore, we could repeatedly produce sparks at the distal end of the standard nitinol guidewire simply by bending the tip to touch the animal (Fig. 29.13). Thus far, we do not know whether a similar effect can be created at the end of the guidewire that is inserted into the animal.

First steps to solve the safety problems of metallic wires and other metallic instruments have been undertaken. The insertion of chokes along wires has been proposed, and the feasibility of this technique to prevent heating has been shown (50). In another method, photoresistors and photo-optic methods are applied to eliminate the need for an electric connection between the MR scanner and a microcoil, so that heating caused by resonance is impossible (51). Another approach is to use a laser fiber to deliver energy to a small coil at the catheter tip; this causes intravoxel dephasing, as described by the field inhomogeneity concept, without the need for a conducting wire (52). So far, no safe MR-compatible guidewires are available commercially, which is one of the main reasons why so few MR-guided vascular interventions have been performed clinically.

ENDOVASCULAR APPLICATIONS OF INTERVENTIONAL MRI

Because of the unresolved safety problems of standard metallic instruments, almost all the MR-guided interventions performed thus far have been carried out *in vitro* or in animals. The steadily growing number of applications will surely stimulate further research and the commercial production of instruments that can be used safely with currently available techniques.

MR-Guided Percutaneous Dilation

Percutaneous transluminal angioplasty (PTA) was one of the first interventions to be performed under MR guidance. Initially, active tip tracking was used to project the catheter tip onto an MIP of a previously acquired contrast-enhanced 3D data set (1). Despite the fact that this method lacks real-time updates of the vascular anatomy, it was successfully applied in a patient in an open 0.5-T scanner for PTA of an iliac artery. Simultaneous real-time active tip tracking and real-time visualization of the vascular anatomy were performed to dilate iliac artery stenoses in a pig model (37). Passive visualization was applied in dilations of the aorta, iliac arteries, and dialysis shunts (11,13,53). In two studies, clinical trials were performed in humans. One relied on the visualization of standard nitinol guidewires, stents, and gadolinium-filled balloons for PTA of the iliac arteries (54). No side effects were caused by the use of metallic guidewires in this study; nonetheless, the risk for heating of nitinol guidewires, especially in systems with high field strengths, should not be neglected. Potential radiofrequency heating of guidewires *in vitro* has been described by several groups (2,49,55,56) (Fig. 29.13). Another clinical study involved

patients with stenotic hemodialysis shunts (57). Passive visualization with dysprosium markers was successfully applied in conjunction with a subtraction technique. Renal artery dilation under MR guidance has also been performed in an animal model (58).

MR-Guided Stent Placement

One drawback of contrast-enhanced 3D MRA is poor visualization of stent lumina and therefore the inability to quantify in-stent restenosis (59). Nonetheless, some stents cause only minor artifacts on MR images, so that they can be placed under MR guidance (60). The feasibility of real-time control of MR-guided stent placement with radial scanning and passive visualization was first demonstrated in animal experiments (61). Passive visualization was also used for the first MR-guided stent placement in humans (54). In this study, no real-time MR control was used to perform the intervention. The artifact behavior of stents depends on both the type of stent and the imaging sequences applied. When real-time radial images of ZA stents (Cook Europe, Bjaeverskov, Denmark) (62) were compared with the slower standard gradient-echo images of Memotherm stents (BARD, Salt Lake City, Utah, USA) used in the only clinical study performed thus far (54), the quality of the real-time images was better. *In vitro* comparisons of the artifact behaviors of these two types of stents indicated that they were similar.

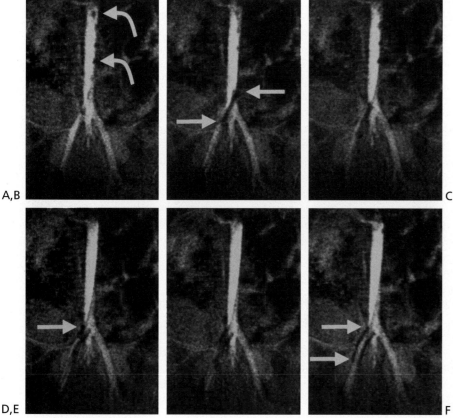

FIGURE 29.14. Real-time radial images acquired during the MR-guided placement of a ZA stent. **A:** A guidewire with dysprosium markers *(arrows)* is shown in the aorta of a living pig. **B:** The stent is introduced into the aorta *(arrows)*. After the stent is withdrawn **(C)**, it is partially **(D,E)** and then completely deployed **(F)**. (From Bücker A, Neuerburg JM, Adam G, et al. Real-time MR fluoroscopy for MR-guided iliac artery stent placement. *J Magn Reson Imaging* 2000;12:616–622, with permission.)

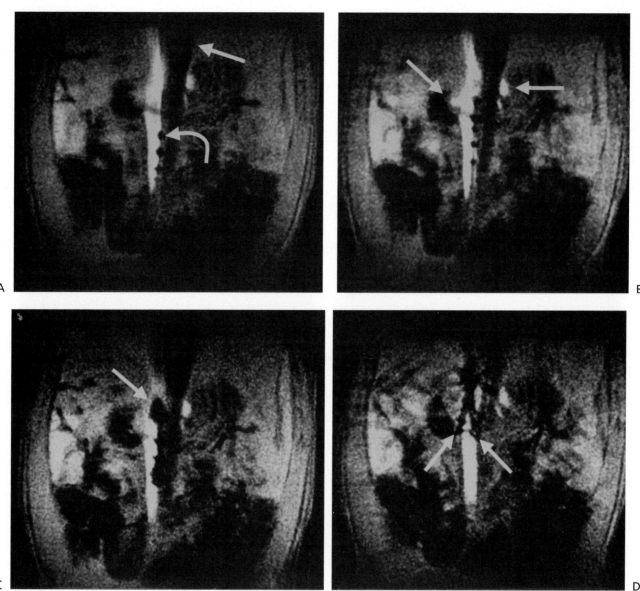

FIGURE 29.15. Real-time radial images with a cranially positioned saturation slab yield a black aorta *(straight arrow in A)*. The introducer sheath of an MR-eye Günther tulip inferior vena cava filter (Cook Europe, Bjaeverskov, Denmark) is advanced *(curved arrow in A)* up to the renal veins *(arrows in B)*. The filter head *(arrow in C)* is positioned at the ostium of the left renal vein. After deployment, the filter legs *(arrows in D)* can be seen, in addition to the position of the filter head.

Thus, progress has been made in improving real-time image quality (Fig. 29.14), although the hardware and software demands are quite high (63). In another study, active visualization was used for stent placement, with the stent functioning as a receiver antenna (64).

MR-Guided Placement of Vena Cava Filters

The placement of a vena cava filter is a relatively simple intervention, which therefore can be performed under MR guidance with relatively slow MRI techniques (65–67). All studies have been performed with passive visualization of the instruments, including the various vena cava filters. Like the artifact behavior of stents, that of vena cava filters varies with the filter type and the imaging sequence used. Real-time radial imaging can be also used to place vena cava filters; it depicts the renal veins and inferior vena cava, so that fast and precise positioning of the filter is possible (68) (Fig. 29.15).

MR-Guided Transjugular Portosystemic Shunt Procedures

In 1994, MR was used to facilitate the planning of a transjugular intrahepatic portosystemic shunt (TIPS) before the procedure itself was performed under x-ray guidance (69). Reports of MR-guided TIPS procedures have been published (1,70). In my experience, MR guidance is helpful only for puncture of the portal vein. Stent placement is particularly difficult and time-consuming under MR guidance because the slice must be oriented along the plane of the TIPS tract (71). The tomographic nature of MR is a disadvantage in visualizing the TIPS tract, portal vein, and inferior vena cava in one imaging plane. Special planscan tools, active tip tracking, and slice tracking are needed to localize the ideal MRI plane for controlling the TIPS procedure in a reasonable time.

MR-Guided Radiofrequency Ablation of the Heart

The heart is an especially difficult challenge for MR-guided interventions because of its constant movement and complex anatomy. Because a catheter was successfully steered through the aorta, one article claims that MR-guided catheterization of the coronary arteries is possible (72). Radiofrequency ablation of the heart has been performed under MR guidance by means of passive catheter visualization (73). Besides controlling the intervention, MRI made it possible to visualize the success of the transmural ablation directly. The difficulty of defining the correct scan plane, which contains the catheter, was apparent during this study, and the authors suggest that active tip tracking be introduced to solve this problem (73).

MR-Guided Coil Embolization

In addition to MR-guided dilation of the renal arteries, coil embolization has been performed in pigs (74). The tortuous anatomy of the renal arteries makes it difficult to depict their entire length with the real-time radial scanning technique.

The application of blood pool contrast agents might make it possible to acquire thicker slices yet maintain the vessel-to-background contrast, but they were not used in this study. The passive visualization of platinum and nitinol coils made it possible to place them correctly, and the flow-sensitive technique of radial scanning made it possible to judge the success of the embolization directly. However, the artifacts of the coils and the relatively low level of spatial resolution in comparison with that of x-ray angiography made it impossible to visualize the coil shape exactly by real-time MRI.

The successful closure of surgically created carotid artery aneurysms in dogs has been reported. In this study, a gadolinium-filled catheter was superimposed onto an MIP of a previously acquired MR angiogram (75). Nearly real-time visualization (about three images per second) was achieved by incorporating time-resolved imaging contrast kinetics elements (TRICKS, an apt acronym) and a projection dephaser (44). The technique did not allow direct visualization of the Guglielmi detachable coils; this was achieved by repeatedly acquiring new MR angiograms and so could not be controlled in real time.

FUTURE PERSPECTIVES

The most obvious advantage of MRI is that radiation is not involved, and consequently it can rival x-ray angiography as a method to guide interventions. In addition to the lack of radiation, MRI offers several other potential benefits: the ability to visualize vascular anatomy without the administration of contrast material, depict vessel walls and differentiate between lipid-rich and calcified plaques, and measure blood flow, to name only a few. Of course, these advantages are offset by difficulties associated with the tomographic nature of MRI, problems involved in the use and visualization of standard interventional instruments, the complexity of

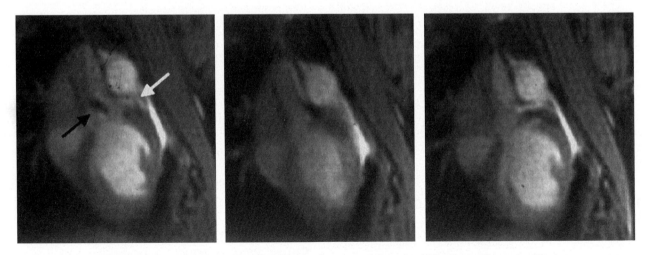

FIGURE 29.16. Real-time MR radial images show a stainless steel Flex Force Coronary Stent (Aachen Resonance, Aachen, Germany) *(black arrow)* that was placed in the left anterior descending artery *(white arrow)* under MR guidance.

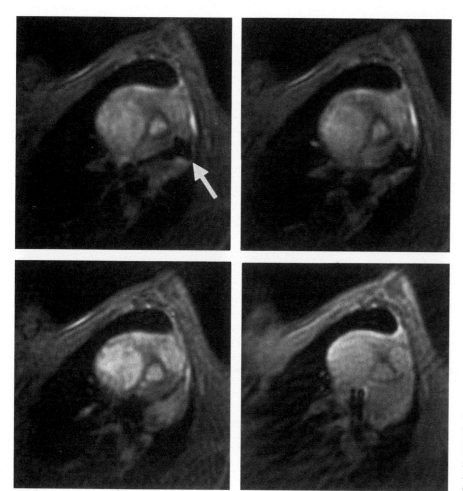

FIGURE 29.17. MR-compatible occluder placement under real-time MR imaging. After deployment of the first half of the septal occluder in the left atrium *(arrow),* the occluder is withdrawn against the septum, and its second half is deployed in the right atrium.

the MR technique, and the longer time required for the acquisition of image data in comparison with high-resolution real-time x-ray imaging. However, all these problems have been solved completely or partially during the past few years. We are now about to explore a new area for the application of interventional MRI: the heart (73,76,77) (Figs. 29.16 and 29.17). As a result, both investigators and manufacturers will be motivated to undertake further research. For example, the possibility of confirming transmural ablation or sparing pediatric patients with heart disease the administration of radiation during electrophysiologic examinations would be a definite advantage in the field of cardiology. In light of the progress that has been made thus far, endovascular interventional MRI will undoubtedly eventually become part of the clinical routine and make it possible to offer better patient care.

SUMMARY

If MR-guided vascular interventions are to be successful, two main challenges must be overcome. The first is high-quality real-time imaging, which has been developed very effectively during the past few years. The second is the interventional instrumentarium. Interventionalists have become very spoiled by the successful development of sophisticated guidewires and catheters for selective catheterizations. These high-quality instruments have evolved during many years, and time will be needed to adapt them to the MR environment. The large number of approaches attempted mirrors the complexity of the task. On the other hand, the manifold applications of MR guidance, used successfully in animal experiments and even clinically, clearly demonstrate its potential. As soon as the interventional instruments become available and the safety problems have been solved, clinical applications in specialized centers will be undertaken to compare MR with x-ray guidance and monitoring. Only after this comparison has been completed will the role of MR in vascular interventions, currently restricted to pure research, be defined in the clinical routine.

REFERENCES

1. Wildermuth S, Debatin JF, Leung DA, et al. MR imaging-guided intravascular procedures: initial demonstration in a pig model. *Radiology* 1997;202:578–583.

2. Konings MK, Bartels LW, Smits HF, et al. Heating around intravascular guidewires by resonating RF waves. *J Magn Reson Imaging* 2000;12:79–85.

3. Mansfield P. Real-time echo-planar imaging by NMR. *Br Med Bull* 1984;40:187–190.

4. Adam G, Bucker A, Glowinski A, et al. Interventional MR tomography: equipment concepts [in German]. *Radiologe* 1998;38:168–172.

5. Lewin JS, Duerk JL, Jain VR, et al. Needle localization in MR-guided biopsy and aspiration: effect of field strength, sequence design, and magnetic field orientation. *AJR Am J Roentgenol* 1996;166:1337–1345.

6. Duerk JL, Lewin JS, Wendt M, et al. Remember true FISP? A high SNR, near 1-second imaging method for T2-like contrast in interventional MRI at .2 T. *J Magn Reson Imaging* 1998;8:203–208.

7. Busch M, Bornstedt A, Wendt M, et al. Fast "real time" imaging with different k-space update strategies for interventional procedures. *J Magn Reson Imaging* 1998;8:944–954.

8. Adam G, Neuerburg J, Bucker A, et al. Interventional magnetic resonance. Initial clinical experience with a 1.5-tesla magnetic resonance system combined with c-arm fluoroscopy. *Invest Radiol* 1997;32:191–197.

9. Silverman SG, Jolesz FA, Newman RW, et al. Design and implementation of an interventional MR imaging suite. *AJR Am J Roentgenol* 1997;168:1465–1471.

10. Paley M, Mayhew JE, Martindale AJ, et al. Design and initial evaluation of a low-cost 3-tesla research system for combined optical and functional MR imaging with interventional capability. *J Magn Reson Imaging* 2001;13:87–92.

11. Bakker CJ, Smits HF, Bos C, et al. MR-guided balloon angioplasty: *in vitro* demonstration of the potential of MRI for guiding, monitoring, and evaluating endovascular interventions. *J Magn Reson Imaging* 1998;8:245–250.

12. van der Weide R, Zuiderveld KJ, Bakker CJ, et al. Image guidance of endovascular interventions on a clinical MR scanner. *IEEE Trans Med Imaging* 1998;17:779–785.

13. Smits HF, Bos C, van der Weide R, et al. Endovascular interventional MR balloon angioplasty in a hemodialysis access flow phantom [corrected] [published erratum appears in *J Vasc Interv Radiol* 1998 Nov-Dec;9(6):1024]. *J Vasc Interv Radiol* 1998;9:840–845.

14. Spielman DM, Pauly JM, Meyer CH. Magnetic resonance fluoroscopy using spirals with variable sampling densities. *Magn Reson Med* 1995;34:388–394.

15. Pipe JG, Ahunbay E, Menon P. Effects of interleaf order for spiral MRI of dynamic processes. *Magn Reson Med* 1999;41:417–422.

16. Rasche V, de Boer RW, Holz D, et al. Continuous radial data acquisition for dynamic MRI. *Magn Reson Med* 1995;34:754–761.

17. Bücker A, Adam G, Neuerburg JM, et al. Real-time MRI with radial k-radial scanning technique for control of angiographic interventions [in German]. *Rofo Fortschr Geb Rontgenstr Neuen Bildgeb Verfahr* 1998;169:542–546.

18. Peters DC, Korosec FR, Grist TM, et al. Undersampled projection reconstruction applied to MR angiography. *Magn Reson Med* 2000;43:91–101.

19. Riederer SJ, Tasciyan T, Farzaneh F, et al. MR fluoroscopy: technical feasibility. *Magn Reson Med* 1988;8:1–15.

20. Glover GH, Pauly JM. Projection reconstruction techniques for reduction of motion effects in MRI. *Magn Reson Med* 1992;28:275–289.

21. Haage P, Bucker A, Kruger S, et al. Radial k-scanning for real-time MR imaging of central and peripheral pulmonary vasculature [in German]. *Rofo Fortschr Geb Rontgenstr Neuen Bildgeb Verfahr* 2000;172:203–206.

22. Bakker CJ, Bos C, Weinmann HJ. Passive tracking of catheters and guidewires by contrast-enhanced MR fluoroscopy. *Magn Reson Med* 2001;45:17–23.

23. Rubin DL, Ratner AV, Young SW. Magnetic susceptibility effects and their application in the development of new ferromagnetic catheters for magnetic resonance imaging. *Invest Radiol* 1990;25:1325–1332.

24. Bakker CJ, Hoogeveen RM, Weber J, et al. Visualization of dedicated catheters using fast scanning techniques with potential for MR-guided vascular interventions. *Magn Reson Med* 1996;36:816–820.

25. Bakker CJ, Hoogeveen RM, Hurtak WF, et al. MR-guided endovascular interventions: susceptibility-based catheter and near-real-time imaging technique. *Radiology* 1997;202:273–276.

26. Glowinski A, Adam G, Bucker A, et al. Catheter visualization using locally induced, actively controlled field inhomogeneities. *Magn Reson Med* 1997;38:253–258.

27. Glowinski A, Kursch J, Adam G, et al. Device visualization for interventional MRI using local magnetic fields: basic theory and its application to catheter visualization. *IEEE Trans Med Imaging* 1998;17:786–793.

28. Adam G, Glowinski A, Neuerburg J, et al. Catheter visualization in MR-tomography: initial experimental results with field-inhomogeneity catheters [in German]. *Rofo Fortschr Geb Rontgenstr Neuen Bildgeb Verfahr* 1997;166:324–328.

29. Adam G, Glowinski A, Neuerburg J, et al. Visualization of MR-compatible catheters by electrically induced local field inhomogeneities: evaluation *in vivo*. *J Magn Reson Imaging* 1998;8:209–213.

30. Bücker A, Adam G, Neuerburg JM, et al. Real-time MRI with radial k-space scanning technique for control of angiographic interventions [in German]. *Rofo Fortschr Geb Rontgenstr Neuen Bildgeb Verfahr* 1998;169:542–546.

31. Ackerman JL, Offutt MC, Buxton RB, et al. Rapid 3-D tracking of small RF coils. In: *Proceedings of the International Society of Magnetic Resonance in Medicine* 1986:1131.

32. Dumoulin CL, Souza SP, Darrow RD. Real time position monitoring of invasive devices using magnetic resonance imaging. *Magn Reson Med* 1993;29:411–415.

33. Rasche V, Holz D, Kohler J, et al. Catheter tracking using continuous radial MRI. *Magn Reson Med* 1997;37:963–968.

34. Ladd ME, Zimmermann GG, McKinnon GC, et al. Visualization of vascular guidewires using MR tracking. *J Magn Reson Imaging* 1998;8:251–253.

35. Ladd ME, Erhart P, Debatin JF, et al. Guidewire antennas for MR fluoroscopy. *Magn Reson Med* 1997;37:891–897.

36. Zimmermann-Paul GG, Ladd ME, Pfammatter T, et al. MR versus fluoroscopic guidance of a catheter/guidewire system: *in vitro* comparison of steerability. *J Magn Reson Imaging* 1998;8:1177–1181.

37. Bücker A, Adam G, Neuerburg J, et al. MR-guided PTA applying radial k-space filling and active tip tracking: simultaneous real-time visualization of the catheter tip and the anatomy. In: *Proceedings of the International Society of Magnetic Resonance in Medicine* 1999:575.

38. Zhang Q, Wendt M, Aschoff AJ, et al. Active MR guidance of interventional devices with target-navigation. *Magn Reson Med* 2000;44:56–65.

39. Coutts GA, Gilderdale DJ, Chui M, et al. Integrated and interactive position tracking and imaging of interventional tools and internal devices using small fiducial receiver coils. *Magn Reson Med* 1998;40:908–913.

40. Ehnholm GJ, Vahala ET, Kinnunen J, et al. Electron spin resonance (ESR) probe for interventional MRI instrument localization. *J Magn Reson Imaging* 1999;10:216–219.

41. Joensuu RP, Sepponen RE, Lamminen AE, et al. A shielded Overhauser marker for MR tracking of interventional devices. *Magn Reson Med* 2000;43:139–145.

42. Nanz D, Weishaupt D, Quick HH, et al. TE-switched double-contrast enhanced visualization of vascular system and instruments for MR-guided interventions. *Magn Reson Med* 2000;43:645–648.

43. Omary RA, Unal O, Koscielski DS, et al. Real-time MR imaging-guided passive catheter tracking with use of gadolinium-filled catheters. *J Vasc Interv Radiol* 2000;11:1079–1085.

44. Unal O, Korosec FR, Frayne R, et al. A rapid 2D time-resolved variable-rate k-space sampling MR technique for passive catheter tracking during endovascular procedures. *Magn Reson Med* 1998;40:356–362.

45. Yang X, Atalar E. Intravascular MR imaging-guided balloon angioplasty with an MR imaging guide wire: feasibility study in rabbits. *Radiology* 2000;217:501–506.

46. Buchli R, Boesiger P, Meier D. Heating effects of metallic implants by MRI examinations. *Magn Reson Med* 1988;7:255–261.

47. Peden CJ, Collins AG, Butson PC, et al. Induction of microcurrents in critically ill patients in magnetic resonance systems. *Crit Care Med* 1993;21:1923–1928.

48. Wildermuth S, Erhart P, Leung DA, et al. Active instrumental guidance in interventional MR tomography: introduction to a new concept [in German]. *Rofo Fortschr Geb Rontgenstr Neuen Bildgeb Verfahr* 1998;169:77–84.

49. Liu CY, Farahani K, Lu DS, et al. Safety of MRI-guided endovascular guidewire applications. *J Magn Reson Imaging* 2000;12:75–78.

50. Ladd ME, Quick HH. Reduction of resonant RF heating in intravascular catheters using coaxial chokes. *Magn Reson Med* 2000;43:615–619.

51. Wong ME, Zhang Q, Duerk J, et al. An optical system for wireless detuning of parallel resonant circuits. *J Magn Reson Imaging* 2000;12:632–638.

52. Konings MK, Bartels LW, van Swol CF, et al. Development of an MR-safe tracking catheter with a laser-driven tip coil. *J Magn Reson Imaging* 2001;13:131–135.

53. Godart F, Beregi JP, Nicol L, et al. MR-guided balloon angioplasty of stenosed aorta: *in vivo* evaluation using near-standard instruments and a passive tracking technique. *J Magn Reson Imaging* 2000;12:639–644.

54. Manke C, Nitz WR, Lenhart M, et al. Stent angioplasty of pelvic artery stenosis with MRI control: initial clinical results [in German]. *Rofo Fortschr Geb Rontgenstr Neuen Bildgeb Verfahr* 2000;172:92–97.

55. Nitz WR, Oppelt A, Renz W, et al. On the heating of linear conductive structures as guide wires and catheters in interventional MRI. *J Magn Reson Imaging* 2001;13:105–114.

56. Wildermuth S, Dumoulin CL, Pfammatter T, et al. MR-guided percutaneous angioplasty: assessment of tracking safety, catheter handling and functionality. *Cardiovasc Intervent Radiol* 1998;21:404–410.

57. Smits HF, Bos C, van der Weide R, et al. Interventional MR: vascular applications. *Eur Radiol* 1999;9:1488–1495.

58. Omary RA, Frayne R, Unal O, et al. MR-guided angioplasty of renal artery stenosis in a pig model: a feasibility study. *J Vasc Interv Radiol* 2000;11:373–381.

59. Meyer JM, Buecker A, Schuermann K, et al. MR evaluation of stent patency: *in vitro* tests of 22 metallic stents and the possibility of determining their patency by MR angiography. *Invest Radiol* 2000;35:739–746.

60. Manke C, Nitz WR, Lenhart M, et al. Magnetic resonance monitoring of stent deployment: *in vitro* evaluation of different stent designs and stent delivery systems. *Invest Radiol* 2000;35:343–351.

61. Bücker A, Neuerburg JM, Adam G, et al. Stentplazierung unter Echtzeit-MR-Kontrolle: erste tierexperimentelle Erfahrungen. *Fortschr Röntgenstr* 1998;169:655–657.

62. Bücker A, Neuerburg JM, Adam GB, et al. Real-time MR fluoroscopy for MR-guided iliac artery stent placement. *J Magn Reson Imaging* 2000;12:616–622.

63. Bücker A, Adam G, Neuerburg JM, et al. Interventional magnetic resonance imaging—non-invasive imaging for interventions [in German]. *Rofo Fortschr Geb Rontgenstr Neuen Bildgeb Verfahr* 2000;172:105–114.

64. Quick HH, Ladd ME, Nanz D, et al. Vascular stents as RF antennas for intravascular MR guidance and imaging. *Magn Reson Med* 1999;42:738–745.

65. Neuerburg J, Bücker A, Adam G, et al. Kavafilterimplantation unter MRT-Kontrolle: Experimentelle In vitro- und In vivo-Untersuchungen. *Fortschr Röntgenstr* 1997;167:418–424.

66. Bartels LW, Bos C, van Der Weide R, et al. Placement of an inferior vena cava filter in a pig guided by high-resolution MR fluoroscopy at 1.5 T. *J Magn Reson Imaging* 2000;12:599–605.

67. Frahm C, Gehl HB, Lorch H, et al. MR-guided placement of a temporary vena cava filter: technique and feasibility. *J Magn Reson Imaging* 1998;8:105–109.

68. Bücker A, Neuerburg JM, Adam G, et al. Real-time MR guidance for inferior vena cava filter placement. *J Vasc Interv Radiol* 2001;12:753–756.

69. Muller MF, Siewert B, Stokes KR, et al. MR angiographic guidance for transjugular intrahepatic portosystemic shunt procedures. *J Magn Reson Imaging* 1994;4:145–150.

70. Kee ST, Rhee JS, Butts K, et al. MR-guided transjugular portosystemic shunt placement in a swine model. *J Vasc Interv Radiol* 1999;10:529–535.

71. Bücker A, Neuerburg JM, Adam GB, et al. MR-guidance of TIPS procedures performed at 1.5 T. *Eur Radiol* 2000;10(Suppl 1):171.

72. Serfaty JM, Yang X, Aksit P, et al. Toward MRI-guided coronary catheterization: visualization of guiding catheters, guidewires, and anatomy in real time. *J Magn Reson Imaging* 2000;12:590–594.

73. Lardo AC, McVeigh ER, Jumrussirikul P, et al. Visualization and temporal/spatial characterization of cardiac radiofrequency ablation lesions using magnetic resonance imaging. *Circulation* 2000;102:698–705.

74. Bücker A, Adam G, Neuerburg J, et al. Coil embolisation of renal arteries under real-time MR control exploiting radial k-space filling: *in vivo* animal experiments. In: *Proceedings of the International Society of Magnetic Resonance in Medicine* 2000:1316.

75. Strother CM, Unal O, Frayne R, et al. Endovascular treatment of experimental canine aneurysms: feasibility with MR imaging guidance. *Radiology* 2000;215:516–519.

76. Bücker A, Grabitz R, Spuentrup E, et al. MR-guided placement of an atrial septal closure device in an animal model. *Circulation* 2000 *(in press)*.

77. Spuentrup E, Ruebben A, Schaeffter T, et al. MR-guided coronary stent placement in a pig model. *Circulation* 2002;105:874–879.

SUBJECT INDEX

Page numbers followed by 'f' indicate figures. Page numbers followed by 't' indicate tables.